PRINCIPLES AND PRACTICE
OF SEX THERAPY

Principles and Practice of Sex Therapy

FIFTH EDITION

Yitzchak M. Binik
Kathryn S. K. Hall
Editors

THE GUILFORD PRESS
New York   London

© 2014 The Guilford Press
A Division of Guilford Publications, Inc.
370 Seventh Avenue, Suite 1200, New York, NY 10001
www.guilford.com

Printed in the United States of America

This book is printed on acid-free paper.

Last digit is print number: 9 8 7 6 5 4

The authors have checked with sources believed to be reliable in their efforts to provide information that is complete and generally in accord with the standards of practice that are accepted at the time of publication. However, in view of the possibility of
human error or changes in behavioral, mental health, or medical sciences, neither the
authors, nor the editors and publisher, nor any other party who has been involved in
the preparation or publication of this work warrants that the information contained
herein is in every respect accurate or complete, and they are not responsible for any
errors or omissions or the results obtained from the use of such information. Readers
are encouraged to confirm the information contained in this book with other sources.

Library of Congress Cataloging-in-Publication Data

Principles and practice of sex therapy. — Fifth edition / edited
by Yitzchak M. Binik, Kathryn S. K. Hall.
    pages cm
  Includes bibliographical references and index.
  ISBN 978-1-4625-1367-3 (hardback : acid-free paper)
  I. Binik, Yitzchak M., editor of compilation.   II. Hall, Kathryn S. K.,
editor of compilation.
  RC557.P75 2014
  616.85′8306—dc23
                                                        2014006124

This book is dedicated to the memory of our friend and colleague Dr. Sandra R. Leiblum. Sandy, as she was affectionately known, was an unabashed advocate for sex therapy, and her enthusiasm for the discipline is reflected in her vision and editorship of four editions of *Principles and Practice of Sex Therapy*. This book embodies the scientist-practitioner model that Sandy herself exemplified. She was a talented sex therapist and a skilled sex researcher. Her writings (both empirical and clinical) remain seminal contributions to the field. In both her professional and personal life Sandy was engaging, entertaining, energetic, and effervescent. Her quick wit, her high energy, her crackling intelligence, and her ebullient smile made her a captivating speaker and teacher.

Sandy thought her greatest talent was finding, encouraging, and promoting the talents of others. She employed this skill in her numerous collaborations, as well as in her teaching, mentoring, and supervising of sex therapists and researchers. *Principles and Practice of Sex Therapy* was Sandy's way of creating a community in which knowledge could be shared and ideas could inspire. We are honored to continue the tradition that Sandy started, and we proudly dedicate this fifth edition of *Principles and Practice of Sex Therapy* to her memory. We miss her greatly.

About the Editors

Yitzchak (Irv) M. Binik, PhD, is Professor in the Department of Psychology at McGill University and Director of the Sex and Couple Therapy Service at McGill University Health Center in Montreal. Dr. Binik is a Fellow of the Canadian Psychological Association and a Diplomate of the American Board of Sexology. He was a member of the DSM-5 work group on sexual and gender disorders. Dr. Binik is a recipient of the Distinguished Contribution to Professional Psychology Award from the Canadian Psychological Association and the Masters and Johnson Award for Lifetime Achievement from the Society for Sex Therapy and Research (SSTAR). He has published more than 100 refereed articles in the areas of health psychology/psychosomatics and sexuality. His main research interest is sexual dysfunction, with a particular interest in genito-pelvic pain/penetration disorder.

Kathryn S. K. Hall, PhD, is a clinical psychologist in private practice in Princeton, New Jersey. She began her career in sex therapy working with Drs. Sandra R. Leiblum and Raymond C. Rosen at the Sexual Counseling Service at the University of Medicine and Dentistry of New Jersey (now Rutgers Biomedical and Health Sciences). She has conducted research on a variety of sex-related topics and has presented at national and international conferences. Her current research interests include desire in arranged marriages and cultural variations in the experience and treatment of sexual problems. Dr. Hall is coeditor of *The Cultural Context of Sexual Pleasure and Problems: Psychotherapy with Diverse Clients*; author of *Reclaiming Your Sexual Self: How You Can Bring Desire Back into Your Life*, winner of the SSTAR Consumer Book Award; and book review editor for the *Journal of Sex and Marital Therapy*.

Contributors

Marc E. Agronin, MD, Medical Director for Mental Health and Clinical Research, Miami Jewish Health Systems, and Affiliate Associate Professor of Psychiatry and Neurology, University of Miami Miller School of Medicine, Miami, Florida

Stanley E. Althof, PhD, Executive Director, Center for Marital and Sexual Health of South Florida, West Palm Beach, Florida, and Professor Emeritus, Case Western Reserve University School of Medicine, Cleveland, Ohio

Sophie Bergeron, PhD, Associate Professor of Psychology, University of Montreal, Montreal, Quebec, Canada

Yitzchak (Irv) M. Binik, PhD, Professor of Psychology, McGill University, and Director, Sex and Couple Therapy Service, McGill University Health Center, Montreal, Quebec, Canada

Erin Breckon, BA, master's student in Counselling Psychology, University of British Columbia, Vancouver, British Columbia, Canada

Lori Brotto, PhD, Head of the Division of Gynaecologic Specialties and Associate Professor of Gynaecology and Psychiatry, University of British Columbia, Vancouver, British Columbia, Canada

Nicola Brown, PhD, staff psychologist, Gender Identity Clinic for adults, Centre for Addiction and Mental Health, Toronto, Ontario, Canada

Rebecca P. Cameron, PhD, Professor of Psychology, California State University, Sacramento, California

James M. Cantor, PhD, Associate Professor of Psychiatry, University of Toronto Faculty of Medicine, and Senior Scientist, Campbell Family Mental Health Research Institute, Centre for Addiction and Mental Health, Toronto, Ontario, Canada

Judith C. Daniluk, PhD, Professor, Counselling Psychology, University of British Columbia, Vancouver, British Columbia, Canada

Paul Enzlin, PhD, Associate Professor of Sexology and Program Director, Institute for Family and Sexuality Studies, Department of Development and Regeneration, KU Leuven, and Head of the Sex Therapy Team, Context: Center for Couple, Family and Sex Therapy, UPC KU Leuven, Leuven, Belgium

Thomas M. Facelle, MD, resident in urology, University of Medicine and Dentistry of New Jersey, University Hospital, Newark, New Jersey

William A. Fisher, PhD, Distinguished Professor, Department of Psychology and Department of Obstetrics and Gynaecology, University of Western Ontario, Waterloo, Ontario, Canada

David Goldmeier MD, FRCP, Clinical Lead, Jane Wadsworth Sexual Function Clinic, St Mary's Hospital, London, United Kingdom

Cynthia A. Graham, PhD, Senior Lecturer, Department of Psychology, University of Southampton, Southampton, United Kingdom; Research Fellow, Kinsey Institute for Research in Sex, Gender, and Reproduction, Indiana University; and visiting Research Fellow, Rural Center for AIDS/STD Prevention, Indiana University, Bloomington, Indiana

Kathryn S. K. Hall, PhD, clinical psychologist, Princeton, New Jersey

Stephen Holzapfel, MD, Director, Sexual Medicine Counselling Unit, Family Practice Health Centre, Women's College Hospital, and Associate Professor, Department of Family and Community Medicine and Department of Obstetrics and Gynaecology, University of Toronto, Toronto, Ontario, Canada

Martin P. Kafka, MD, Clinical Associate Professor of Psychiatry, Harvard Medical School, Boston, Massachusetts, and Senior Clinical Associate, McLean Hospital, Belmont, Massachusetts

Peggy J. Kleinplatz, PhD, Professor of Medicine and Clinical Professor of Psychology, University of Ottawa, Ottawa, Ontario, Canada

Emily Koert, MA, PhD candidate in Counselling Psychology, University of British Columbia, Vancouver, British Columbia, Canada

Stephen B. Levine, MD, Clinical Professor of Psychiatry and Co-director, Center for Marital and Sexual Health, Case Western Reserve University School of Medicine, Cleveland, Ohio

Mijal Luria, MD, Director, Center for Sexual Health, Hadassah Mt. Scopus Medical Center, Jerusalem, Israel

Marta Meana, PhD, Professor of Psychology and Dean of the Honors College, University of Nevada, Las Vegas, Las Vegas, Nevada

Martin M. Miner, MD, Director, Men's Health Center of The Miriam Hospital, and Clinical Associate Professor of Family Medicine and Urology and Co-Director of the Men's Health Center, Warren Alpert Medical School, Brown University, Providence, Rhode Island

Linda R. Mona, PhD, Director of Psychology Postdoctoral Training, VA Long Beach Healthcare System, Long Beach, California

Margaret Nichols, PhD, Founder and Executive Director, Institute for Personal Growth, New Jersey Psychotherapy Center, Highland Park, New Jersey

Lucia F. O'Sullivan, PhD, Professor, Department of Psychology, University of New Brunswick, Fredericton, New Brunswick, Canada

Vickie Pasterski, PhD, Research Psychologist, Department of Paediatrics, Addenbrooke's Hospital, University of Cambridge, Cambridge, United Kingdom

Michael A. Perelman, PhD, Clinical Professor of Psychiatry, Reproductive Medicine, and Urology, Weill Medical College, Cornell University, and Co-Director, Human Sexuality Program, Payne Whitney Clinic of the New York Presbyterian Hospital, New York, New York

Caroline F. Pukall, PhD, Associate Professor, Department of Psychology, and Director, Sex Therapy Service, Psychology Clinic, Queen's University, Kingston, Ontario, Canada

Elke D. Reissing, PhD, Professor, School of Psychology; Director, Human Sexuality Research Laboratory; and Supervisor of sex therapy training, Centre for Psychological Services and Research, University of Ottawa, Ottawa, Ontario, Canada

Alessandra H. Rellini, PhD, Associate Professor, Department of Psychology, University of Vermont, Burlington, Vermont

Natalie O. Rosen, PhD, Assistant Professor, Department of Psychology and Neuroscience, Dalhousie University, and cross-appointed, Department of Obstetrics and Gynaecology, IWK Health Centre, Halifax, Nova Scotia, Canada

Raymond C. Rosen, PhD, Chief Scientist, New England Research Institutes, Watertown, Massachusetts; and former Co-Director, Sex and Marital Therapy Center, and former Chief Psychologist and Director of the Human Sexuality Program, Robert Wood Johnson Medical School, Rutgers, The State University of New Jersey, Piscataway, New Jersey

Hossein Sadeghi-Nejad, MD, Professor of Surgery/Urology, New Jersey Medical School, Rutgers, The State University of New Jersey, Piscataway, New Jersey; Chief of Urology, VA New Jersey Health Care System, East Orange, New Jersey; and Director, Center for Male Reproductive Medicine (private practice) at the Hackensack University Medical Center, Hackensack, New Jersey

Sabina Sarin, MS, MPhil, PhD candidate in Clinical Psychology, McGill University, Montreal, Quebec, Canada

Eric T. Steiner, PhD, Department of Psychology, National University, San Diego, California

Maggie L. Syme, PhD, MPH, Research Assistant Professor, San Diego State University, San Diego, California

Moniek M. ter Kuile, PhD, Associate Professor, Department of Gynaecology, Leiden University Medical Center, Leiden, The Netherlands

Michael W. Wiederman, PhD, Professor of Psychology, Columbia College, Columbia, South Carolina

John P. Wincze, PhD, Associate Director, Men's Health Center, The Miriam Hospital, and Clinical Professor, Department of Psychiatry and Human Behavior and the Department of Psychology, Brown University, Providence, Rhode Island

Kenneth J. Zucker, PhD, Psychologist-in-Chief and Head of the Gender Identity Service for children and adolescents in the Child, Youth, and Family Program, Centre for Addiction and Mental Health; and Professor, Department of Psychiatry, University of Toronto, Toronto, Ontario, Canada

Preface

Sexual problems are ubiquitous. We know that thanks to large-scale national and multinational epidemiological surveys. Furthermore, community and clinical samples verify that sexual dysfunction and dissatisfaction are widespread. And yet, clinical training programs in psychology, psychiatry, family therapy, and related fields give at best passing attention to this area. Moreover, to adequately address sexual problems, clinicians now need to be cognizant of advances in sexual medicine as well. It is not surprising that many of us in the field feel a need for more education and training on how to conceptualize and treat sexual problems. This book offers just that—a means for all of us, seasoned, novice, and student practitioners alike, to deepen our knowledge and enhance our skills so that we can provide effective treatment for the sexual problems of our clients.

Since the first edition was published in 1980, *Principles and Practice of Sex Therapy* has been the major text in its field. It has succeeded because of its adherence to a basic guiding principle: the integration of current research with clinical practice. This fifth edition continues and expands upon this principle and tradition. All chapters are authored by internationally recognized experts who synthesize the often separate worlds of sex research and clinical practice. As a result of these syntheses, each chapter presents empirically validated clinical interventions for the sexual disorder under consideration. This volume will be an invaluable aid for aspiring students as well as seasoned clinicians and clinical researchers wishing to keep current with innovations in the field.

What you will find in this fifth edition is a multidisciplinary perspective designed to provide evidence-based treatment approaches to the common, challenging, and/or complex sexual issues facing individuals and couples today. Because reconciling the differing views in practice can be challenging, most chapters include an assessment and treatment algorithm, a GPS as it were for the current clinical terrain.

The timing of this new edition is not arbitrary. In the 7 years since the publication of the previous edition, sex therapy has undergone unprecedented growth and change. This has been prompted by an explosion of sex research fueled, in part, by the pharmaceutical industry's quest to find the next Viagra, and by new technologies that can more precisely measure physiological sexual responses. Unpredictably, sex therapy and sexual medicine are rather companionable bedfellows. Often sexual medicine interventions aid function (provide blood flow for an erection, hormones for desire), while sex therapy provides the opportunity and context to be sexual. Removing the psychological barriers to sexual pleasure, dealing with relational issues, and providing cognitive-behavioral interventions for sexual dysfunction continue to be the mainstays of sex therapy. In addition, sex therapy has always addressed the important connection between mind and body, and continues to incorporate new techniques, most recently mindfulness meditation.

The timing of the publication of this fifth edition of *Principles and Practice of Sex Therapy* also coincides with the newly released DSM-5. Whereas DSM-IV had one chapter on sexual disorders, there are now three separate DSM-5 chapters, one on sexual dysfunction, one on gender dysphoria, and one on paraphilia. This suggests a major theoretical shift in recognizing that there exist three distinct categories of pathology. For sexual dysfunction diagnoses, there are notable changes that reflect long-standing concerns about the adequacy of Masters and Johnson's triphasic model and its underlying assumption of parallelism in sexual response between men and women. These changes and the implications for clinical practice and research are critically reviewed in this volume.

The structure of this edition reflects the changes that have transpired in the practice of sex therapy. The first section, a third of the book, is devoted to updating and incorporating new research and treatment for sexual dysfunctions, while the second section deals with the expanded scope of sex therapy in providing treatment for other sexual concerns, including hypersexuality (often referred to as sexual addiction), nonviolent paraphilic sexual interests, pedophilia, persistent genital arousal in women, and gender dysphoria. The final section of the book deals with new challenges for sex therapy in terms of its expanding clientele. Adolescents, aging adults, ethnic and sexual minorities, disabled individuals, and those dealing with sexual trauma, chronic illness, and sexually transmitted infection are presenting for sex therapy with increasing frequency. We are fortunate to have expert authors who have written sensitively on the ways that sex therapy can be adapted to be more inclusive.

This volume reflects the basic idea that sex therapy should no longer be the sole domain of a small, highly specialized group of clinicians. While *Principles and Practice of Sex Therapy* is the definitive text for expert clinicians and researchers, we hope this book will encourage others to enter the field.

We are extraordinarily grateful that many of the leaders in sex research and therapy contributed chapters to this book. We were aided in our editing duties by several very able assistants, including Caroline Maykut, Jackie Huberman, Marie Faaborg-Andersen, and Tanya D'Amours. Dr. Sandra Leiblum first brought the idea of *Principles and Practice of Sex Therapy* to The Guilford Press in 1978. She edited and coedited this book through its first four editions, setting the standard for excellence. Those of you who knew Sandy and her work will recognize her imprint and influence in almost every chapter. We thank Guilford for continuing to believe in this volume, and we especially thank Senior Editor Jim Nageotte for his wisdom, his advice, and his guidance in moving this book forward to publication.

Contents

Medical Problems

Lifespan Changes

INTRODUCTION

The Future of Sex Therapy

Yitzchak (Irv) M. Binik and Kathryn S. K. Hall

Once characterized by a clearly defined set of procedures designed to treat a narrow list of sexual dysfunctions, the scope of sex therapy has significantly broadened. This new edition of *Principles and Practice of Sex Therapy* reflects the tremendous growth that has taken place in the field and challenges previous perceptions of what sex therapy is and what a sex therapist does. The sexual dysfunction chapters take up only a third of the book and are located in the first section, "Sex Therapy for Sexual Dysfunction." Most of the current edition is organized into two new sections titled "Sex Therapy for Other Sexual Disorders" and "Therapeutic Challenges for Sex Therapy." These sections replace the section in the fourth edition called "Special Issues," which dealt with a variety of topics ranging from the paraphilias to childhood sexual abuse. In our view, these topics are no longer "special" but part of a sex therapist's everyday work.

Despite these significant changes from the previous edition, the organizing principle has not changed. Since its first edition (Leiblum & Rosen, 1980), *Principles and Practice of Sex Therapy* has been unique for its sophisticated synthesis of up-to-date research with clinical practice. Its goal has been and remains to critically review the available research with a view to informing and directing the clinician. In fact, the choice of editors for this edition reflects this goal. Although both editors would consider themselves clinician scientists, Kathryn S. K. Hall spends most of her time as a private practice clinician, whereas Yitzchak M. Binik is chiefly an academic researcher. We hope that both clinicians and researchers will benefit from our collaboration.

SEX THERAPY FOR SEXUAL DYSFUNCTION

The eight chapters in the first section reflect the "bread and butter" work of traditional sex therapy, that is, the assessment and treatment of sexual dysfunction. For better or worse, sexual dysfunction has been defined, at least in North America, as those dysfunctions listed in the fifth edition of the *Diagnostic and Statistical Manual of Mental Disorders* (DSM-5; American Psychiatric Association, 2013). Despite some name changes, most of these sexual dysfunctions date from the publication of DSM-III-R (American Psychiatric Association, 1987), and most sex therapists still treat premature (early) and delayed ejaculation, erectile dysfunction, low desire, vaginismus, and orgasmic dysfunction.

Despite this continuity, there are some notable changes in DSM-5 (American Psychiatric Association, 2013) and, as a result, in this edition. Sexual aversion disorder does not appear in DSM-5 nor as a chapter in this edition. The rationale for this omission is fairly simple. Based on available statistics, sexual aversion disorder was rarely diagnosed, and there was a minimal research literature on it (Brotto, 2010). During the DSM-5 development process, when the American Psychiatric Association asked for public and professional feedback about this potential deletion, no one who responded seemed to mind. In fact, it was hard to reconstruct why sexual aversion disorder had ever become a DSM sexual dysfunction. One theory is that it was due to the important influence of Helen Singer Kaplan (1987), who wrote a book on this topic, *Sexual Aversion, Sexual Phobias, and Panic Disorder.* Although few would deny that there are patients who are phobic or disgusted about various aspects of sexuality, it seemed unlikely to the DSM-5 committee that these reactions exist as a distinct and valid diagnostic category. In our view, the appearance and disappearance of this diagnosis reflects both poorly and well on the field. On the one hand, exciting new ideas are welcomed and integrated; on the other, such ideas should be carefully vetted before entering the canon. How to balance these opposing tendencies remains a challenge for the field.

Another notable change is the omission of female sexual arousal disorder (FSAD) as a separate diagnostic category. This problem has not disappeared, but its diagnosis has been combined with hypoactive sexual desire disorder (HSDD) in women into a new category called "sexual interest arousal disorder." The rationale for this change is discussed in detail by Brotto and Luria in Chapter 1. Although few mourned the passing of sexual aversion disorder, there has been a storm of controversy about the amalgamation of FSAD and HSDD (Clayton, Derogatis, Rosen, & Pyke, 2012). For the moment, there does not seem to be a lot of concern about the loss of female sexual arousal disorder as a separate category; what is motivating the controversy is the disappearance of HSDD as a distinct category in women. Historians and sociologists will ultimately sort out the meaning of this controversy, but it is tempting to speculate that the interest in preserving low desire in women as a distinct and separate category is motivated, in part, by the pharmaceutical lobby and the impending appearance of drugs for low desire. The good news is that controversy often breeds interest and new research leading to treatment innovation. This will be welcome, as we are currently stalled pharmacologically and psychologically concerning the treatment of difficulties of desire and arousal in women.

This kind of controversy is not reflected in the chapters concerning arousal or desire problems in men. However, Meana and Steiner, in Chapter 2, propose a very controversial hypothesis for many men diagnosed with HSDD. They suggest the tantalizing idea that many men diagnosed with low desire actually have desire, but not for their partners. Whether this reflects a true gender difference or our lack of knowledge about low desire in men remains to be seen. Not surprisingly, no one is currently suggesting amalgamating the diagnosis of low sexual desire in men with erectile dysfunction. In fact, in Chapter 3, Rosen and colleagues outline the enormous progress made in understanding the biological mechanisms of erectile disorder. Despite this progress, the authors make it clear that traditional and new sex therapy interventions are necessary for up-to-date treatment.

The final major change in DSM-5 (American Psychiatric Association, 2013) classification is the collapsing of the categories of vaginismus and dyspareunia into one new diagnosis called "genito-pelvic pain/penetration disorder." This descriptive mouthful of a name reflects the significant overlap in symptomatology between the disorders and the many conceptual difficulties in defining them (Binik, 2010a, 2010b). Despite our conceptual agreement with the change in DSM, we have opted to keep two separate chapters concerning these dysfunctions. The main reason is that recent and exciting clinical innovations concerning the treatment of vaginismus (defined as the woman's inability to have desired intercourse) suggest a strong divergence from the treatment of dyspareunia (defined as pain experienced during intercourse), even if the diagnoses merge. These treatment innovations are spelled out by ter Kuile and Reissing (Chapter 8) and are based on the "fear/avoidance" model of pain rather than on the traditional vaginal spasm model. Bergeron et al. (Chapter 7) summarize the continuing progress in research and clinical intervention for genital pain (dyspareunia) while emphasizing couple interactional aspects and their effect on this pain. We have asked each author in this section to critically evaluate the DSM-5 changes.

These DSM-5 changes reflect the diminishing importance of gender parallelism in our understanding and treatment of sexual dysfunction. As discussed earlier, the conceptualizations and interventions for desire and arousal in men and women have almost totally diverged. Dyspareunia was defined in DSM-IV (American Psychiatric Association, 1994) as a diagnosis for both women and men, despite the fact that it was rarely applied to men. In DSM-5 (American Psychiatric Association, 2013), male dyspareunia is not a formal diagnosis because of the lack of sufficient data and research. Paradoxically, there is a small but growing body of research on urological chronic pelvic pain syndrome (UCPPS) in men, which suggests that a diagnosis similar to male dyspareunia may have a future (Davis, Binik, & Carrier, 2009). Bergeron et al. review this work in Chapter 7. The ultimate fate of gender differences in diagnoses is not clear and will probably evolve with gender politics, theory, and clinical practice.

There has been little gender controversy, however, about premature (early) and delayed ejaculation. Although surveys suggest that "premature orgasm" may be a problem for some women, this issue seldom comes to clinical attention (Laumann, Gagnon, Michael, & Michaels, 1994). The diagnostic criteria for premature (early) ejaculation have undergone a major overhaul in DSM-5 by the inclusion of a specific time specification of approximately 1 minute or less. This change, however, does not greatly affect Althof's recommendation (Chapter 5) that clinicians carefully consider a "combination therapy" (psychotherapy and pharmacotherapy) approach. This combination approach does not simply target time as the solution to premature (early) ejaculation; it considers ejaculatory latency in the context of the couple's relationship and the male's feelings of masculinity. A similar approach is taken by Perelman in discussing delayed ejaculation (Chapter 6). Perelman expands his discussion to also include the whole range of ejaculatory/orgasmic problems for men (e.g., anejaculation; painful ejaculation; retrograde ejaculation; reductions in volume, force, sensation of ejaculation; postorgasmic illness syndrome).

The last "traditional sexual dysfunction" reviewed in Part I is female orgasmic disorder. Graham (Chapter 4) points out that "directed masturbation" continues to be the mainstay of treatment for this problem because it has shown to be highly effective. In fact, it is the only sex therapy technique that is acknowledged by current standards to be efficacious, at least for lifelong anorgasmia (Heiman, 2002). Although it is wonderful to have such an efficacious treatment, we cannot help wondering whether the success of this treatment has hindered further research concerning the nature and function of female orgasm. We still do not fully understand the tremendous variability in women's ability to experience orgasm.

Overall, the single most important influence on the practice of sex therapy for the traditional DSM sexual dysfunctions is the continuing development of sexual medicine. As a result, we requested that each author in this section review the relevant sexual medicine research and discuss how such work can be integrated into practice. Most authors recommended a multidisciplinary or interdisciplinary assessment and treatment model. As a result, we asked them to reify this model with an assessment and treatment algorithm. The net result is a far cry from the solo sex therapy practitioner model that was the standard 20 years ago.

Many will argue that such multidisciplinary models are a luxury affordable only in developed countries, and even there only in major centers. Although this may be true, it is important to differentiate between what is possible and what may be necessary or ideal. Even when resources are available, the question of how to integrate multiple disciplines effectively is a continuing health care management problem.

SEX THERAPY FOR OTHER SEXUAL DISORDERS

The relationship between sexual dysfunction and the other sexual disorders might be best characterized as a DSM-arranged marriage. Paraphilia and gender-dysphoria clinicians and researchers have usually not been sex therapists. Yet in the view of previous DSMs and most of the North American mental health community, all sexual and gender issues are alike. The net result is that the sexual dysfunctions, paraphilias, and gender identity disorders have all been thrown into a single DSM chapter. This is not true in the World Health Organization (WHO) *International Classification of Diseases* (ICD) classification..

Whether sexuality is an important defining characteristic for gender dysphoria is a matter of some controversy. Brown and Zucker (Chapter 11) point out that autogynephilia—that is, sexual arousal to the idea of oneself being a woman—may be a crucial mechanism in male-to-female gender dysphoria and that this "erotic location error" is considered by some as a sexual orientation. This theory has aroused bitter controversy, as evidenced by the recent brouhaha between J. Michael Bailey of Northwestern University and some militant gender activists (see special issue of *Archives of Sexual Behavior*, June 2008). Brown and Zucker also review the intervention literature and summarize the substantive changes in the DSM-5 diagnosis.

The difficulty in classifying problems as sexual or not is also exemplified by the discussion of persistent genital arousal disorder in Chapter 12. This problem was originally referred to as persistent sexual arousal disorder. This name change suggests an obvious change in conceptualization. Goldmeier and colleagues argue that the presence of persistent physical genital symptoms of arousal is not sufficient to define a problem as sexual. Nonetheless, sex therapists will often treat such problems because they interfere with sexual and relationship functioning; most other health professionals will avoid such conversations. This same controversy exists with respect to hypersexuality, or, as it is popularly known, sexual compulsivity/addiction. Kafka points out, in Chapter 13, that the jury is still out in deciding whether this problem is a sexual one or whether it is better characterized as an attachment or obsessional disorder. Despite the growth in clinical and popular interest in this problem, it is not classified as a sexual disorder in DSM-5. Whether this disorder will ultimately become part of the canon or go the way of sexual aversion disorder remains to be seen.

The conceptual and clinical issues involving the paraphilias are somewhat different. There is little doubt that unusual or alternative objects of sexual arousal/desire are the key defining features; there is, however, much doubt about whether such symptoms are indications of psychopathology, the result of unfortunate developmental outcomes, or the failure of societal tolerance. Whatever the origin, clinicians are often faced with problems in dealing with the legal system and public opinion, in addition to the welfare of their clients. Kleinplatz, in Chapter 9, and Cantor, in Chapter 10, suggest very different intervention strategies for dealing with paraphilic attractions and behaviors. Kleinplatz advocates an existential psychotherapy approach to effect deep personality change, whereas Cantor describes a community containment model that aims to control rather than change pedophilic attraction. These differences in approach not only reflect basic theoretical differences but may also reflect different therapeutic strategies for dealing with the potential societal and legal implications resulting from the coercive versus noncoercive paraphilias.

Although the somewhat unhappy arranged marriage among sexual dysfunction, gender dysphoria, and paraphilias has lasted for many years, it appears to be ending. DSM-5 appears to have arranged a "legal separation" (i.e., separate chapters) in an attempt to coordinate the metadiagnostic structures of the next WHO classification (ICD-11) and DSM-5. This will no doubt facilitate international collaboration, though it does not really solve the conceptual issues of whether these categories are really similar or not. Whether there will be a reconciliation or a full divorce in the future remains to be seen.

The modern sexual medicine movement has not been heavily involved in the treatment of paraphilias and gender dysphoria, but physicians always have. Endocrinologists and surgeons are often required for the management of gender dysphoria, and psychiatrists are often called upon to prescribe sex-drive-reducing medication for the "chemical castration" of convicted sex offenders. Whereas psychologists have often been heavily involved in the treatment of sex offenses and gender dysphoria, sex therapists have often shied away from these groups. We have, therefore, asked each of the authors in Part II to address the role of sex therapy directly. Clearly, the problem-solving skills and achievement of comfort involved in talking about sexual and relationship issues that are required for sex therapy will be very useful in dealing with the paraphilias and gender dysphoria.

THERAPEUTIC CHALLENGES FOR SEX THERAPY

The chapters in Part III address the clinical and research challenges facing sex therapy today. Some of the issues (e.g., culture, trauma, infidelity, illness, aging) affect all psychological problems and therapies. They are, however, so frequently encountered in sex therapy practice that it is, in our view, necessary to deal with them directly and specifically in any sex therapy text. This reflects our view that traditional sex therapy, as exemplified by Masters and Johnson's cognitive-behavioral type interventions, is no longer sufficient to characterize actual practice. Considering what we now know about the long-term efficacy of traditional sex therapy interventions, it is perhaps not surprising that this is the largest section of this edition.

We have organized these "therapeutic challenges" into three different subsections. The first is the most varied and deals with groups for which standard practice must often be adapted to the nature of the group. Obvious examples include sexual minorities—lesbians, gays, and bisexuals (LGBs)—as well as individuals from non-Western cultures. In fact, LGBs are characterized by Nichols in Chapter 14 as coming from a different sexual culture than the typical heterosexual sex therapy client. For many years, LGBs avoided heterosexual and institutionally based treatment environments because of their anti-gay biases. It is our strong impression that both the "institutional" and the LGB communities have changed. Although non-gay-friendly therapists still exist, their number is diminishing; in most public and many private health institutions, homophobia is also greatly reduced. It also appears to us that LGB treatment seekers are changing. Not so long ago, they felt compelled, often for good reason, to limit their therapist choices to members of their own community. Today, the frame of reference appears to be enlarged to "who will be the best therapist for me," independent of his or her sexual orientation. The LGB community has expanded and welcomed transgender, questioning, and queer individuals, so the moniker now frequently reads LGBTQ. Transgender clients have often felt misunderstood by mainstream therapists, physicians, and sex therapists. Nichols points out that the role of therapists is shifting from gatekeepers of medical/surgical intervention to advocates. Hall and Graham (Chapter 15) extend this theme of adapting standard practice into a multicultural and intercultural context. They point out that the cultural context of the client (couple) and the culturally unique meaning of the sexual problem are crucial to understand in order to implement effective intervention with respect to sexual issues.

Two "new" chapters for this volume concern infidelity and body image. These are not new issues for sex therapists, who often receive referrals for sexual dysfunctions such as lack of desire or arousal in which the underlying issues may be infidelity or body image. Most sex therapists will opt to deal with the underlying issues in conjunction with the sexual dysfunction. How to do therapy in this way is not immediately obvious, because the research literatures related to infidelity and body image are not well developed and often not linked to practical clinical intervention. Wiederman and Sarin (Chapter 16) connect the growing social psychological literature on body image to clinical reality by pointing out that it is body image specific to sexual situations, not global measures of body image, that are the best predictors of sexual functioning. Levine (Chapter 18) points out that a therapeutic understanding of the ongoing experience of partners who are living with infidelity is more crucial than adoption of a particular treatment model or set of techniques.

Chapter 17 addresses the long-standing issue of how to deal with sexual abuse. Rellini integrates the available research data and cautions the clinician about making unwarranted causal assumptions linking the abuse to sexual dysfunction. She also presents useful therapeutic insights into how to practically deal with a history of abuse that is, in fact, interfering with current sexuality.

The second subsection within Part III is titled "Medical Problems." Sex therapists are often called on to consult and treat individuals suffering from the sexual effects of an illness, accident, or medical situation. It is often hard to disentangle the effects of chronic illness from age, as these are highly correlated. It is also often tempting to attribute sexual difficulties to the direct effects of a particular illness. Enzlin (Chapter 20) provides us with a general model for explicating the interaction of chronic illness and sexuality. This model differentiates between the direct, indirect, and iatrogenic effects of chronic illness on sexuality. Enzlin also provides us with a "stepped-care" approach for dealing with the ensuing problems. Sexually transmitted infections (STIs) constitute an instance of illness that requires a special chapter (Chapter 22). This special case is important because of the enormous influence of HIV on society and because STIs, as opposed to most other illnesses affecting sexuality, disproportionately affect younger populations. Sex therapists should now be able to educate their clients about STI risks and to treat couples in which one member is affected. In their chapter, titled "Suppose They Gave an Epidemic and Sex Therapy Didn't Attend," Fisher and Holzapfel point out how sex therapy has failed to take up this task.

One of the legitimate criticisms of previous editions was that they failed to differentiate adequately between illness and disability. Disability is no longer conceptualized as a solely medical condition. Mona and colleagues (Chapter 21) point out that individuals suffering from disabilities constitute the largest minority group in the world and that disability must be seen as a "multicultural variable." This reconceptualization has dramatic implications for treatment models.

Chapter 19 deals with a specific medical/interpersonal issue: infertility. Although sociocultural changes and modern advances in contraception have decreased the interdependence of sexuality and reproduction, modern technological advances in infertility treatment have made sex therapists key members of infertility treatment teams. In Chapter 19, Daniluk and colleagues point out that couples, prior to a diagnosis of infertility, do not have higher rates of sexual dysfunction than the general population. However, the psychological and medical stresses following such a diagnosis take their toll. The authors present assessment and counseling strategies appropriate to each stage of the infertility treatment, including invaluable guidelines for the therapist working in this area.

The third subsection within Part III represents a new direction for *Principles and Practice of Sex Therapy*. It emphasizes a developmental/lifespan view of sexuality. In our sex therapy training years, we rarely saw clients younger than 25 or older than 50. In today's world, clients under 20 and over 70 are not uncommon. O'Sullivan and Pasterski (Chapter 23) point out that our conceptualizations of sexual problems and our treatment strategies are still based on 25- to 50-year-olds and that there are no systematic treatment studies of sexual dysfunction for individuals under 18. They nonetheless provide case examples to guide clinicians until more information is available. Agronin (Chapter 24) deals with a similar lack of information about aging populations. In addition to the "normal" changes in sexuality experienced with healthy aging, he discusses the interpersonal and ethical issues raised by individuals and couples attempting to continue their sexual lives when faced with memory loss and institutionalization. Finally, in the previously discussed Chapter 11, Brown and Zucker discuss children and adolescents with gender dysphoria, who are now raising many ethical and treatment questions about when it is appropriate to start hormonal and medical treatment. Although dealing with the sexual problems of 25- to 50-year-olds continues to be challenging, we believe that the field must expand to take into account the reality of sexual behavior throughout the lifespan.

THE FUTURE OF SEX THERAPY

The different editions of *Principles and Practice of Sex Therapy*, starting with the first in 1980, reflect the history of our field. We hope this new edition also will foreshadow future developments. The immediate future of sex therapy depends on new blood and new ideas. Fortunately, we have been able to recruit several relatively junior but highly accomplished clinicians and researchers (Beckon, Facelle, Koert, N. O. Rosen, Sadeghi-Nejad, Sarin, Steiner) who are forcing the field to confront the new realities of the 21st century. In addition, there are a relatively large number of established professionals who are first-time contributors to *Principles and Practice of Sex Therapy* (Agronin, Brotto, Brown, Cameron, Cantor, Daniluk, Enzlin, Fisher, Goldmeier, Graham, Holzapfel, Kleinplatz, ter Kuile, Levine, Luria, Meana, Miner, Mona, O'Sullivan, Pasterski, Pukall, Reissing, Rellini, Syme, Wiederman, Wincze, Zucker). Last but not least, we have induced some of our past stars (Althof, Bergeron, Kafka, Nichols, Perelman, R. C. Rosen) to either update their 4th-edition chapters or write new chapters. The net result is that the majority of the content of the book is new or written from a new perspective.

Our author list probably also reflects some of the ongoing professional trends. Five nonpsychiatric physicians (one gynecologist, one genitourinary sexual medicine specialist, one general practitioner, and two urologists) are now contributors. This reflects the continuing influence and importance of sexual medicine. Among the mental health professionals contributing to this volume, the vast majority are clinical psychologists, whereas only two are psychiatrists. Perhaps this reflects a lessening of interest in sex therapy among psychiatrists. For some topics, it proved very difficult to find a lead author who was both a seasoned clinician and a researcher. In such cases, we played matchmaker and linked a nonclinical researcher with a clinician. The results were excellent. We are worried, however, about the growing divergence between clinicians and researchers. Our goal in this volume was to integrate up-to-date research with clinical practice. This goal is achievable only if training programs and professionals insist on both.

One continuing trend is the internationalization of sex therapy. In this edition, there are authors from Belgium, Canada, England, the Netherlands,

Israel, and the United States. We expect this trend to continue and expect that future editions will include contributors from non-Western countries. It is interesting that the single largest group of authors is Canadian. It appears that Canada, a country with a population of approximately 35 million people, has become a major center for sex therapy and research.

In the concluding chapter, "Sex Therapy in Transition: Are We There Yet?," Meana, Binik, and Hall have brought into focus some of the basic issues that are raised in many of the individual chapters and that concern the field as a whole. Perhaps the central question is whether the concept of sexual dysfunction is still valid or useful. The authors of DSM-5 have punted on this issue by declining to define the concept of sexual dysfunction. Many classification gurus believe that the ultimate basis of classification is mechanism; unfortunately, we are nowhere close to understanding the mechanisms of most sexual dysfunctions. Other gurus believe that sexual dysfunctions are social constructions not easily classifiable by traditional methods. It seems likely to us that neither mechanism nor construction can currently deal with the phenomena of sexual dysfunction and that a combined classificatory approach is the next stage.

Meana and colleagues also raise important issues concerning the future relationship between sex therapy and sexual medicine, about the influence of the DSM diagnostic manuals, and about the pressing need for treatment outcome evaluation. In the final chapter, as in this introduction, we exhort readers, novices and seasoned practitioners alike, to continue questioning and challenging assumptions about the nature of sexual problems and, most important, to continue to develop and refine treatments. Sex therapy began as a challenge to psychotherapy, which had woefully neglected sexuality. We think the future of our field depends on the very attitude that ushered sex therapy into existence. We are pleased to offer this edition of *Principles and Practice of Sex Therapy* as a guidepost along the way of what has been, and what we hope will continue to be, an amazing journey.

REFERENCES

American Psychiatric Association. (1987). *Diagnostic and statistical manual of mental disorders* (3rd ed., rev.). Washington, DC: Author.

American Psychiatric Association. (1994). *Diagnostic and statistical manual of mental disorders* (4th ed.). Washington, DC: Author.

American Psychiatric Association. (2013). *Diagnostic and statistical manual of mental disorders* (5th ed.). Arlington, VA: Author.

Binik, Y. M. (2010a). The DSM diagnostic criteria for dyspareunia. *Archives of Sexual Behavior, 39*(2), 278–291.

Binik, Y. M. (2010b). The DSM diagnostic criteria for vaginismus. *Archives of Sexual Behavior, 39*(2), 292–303.

Binik, Y. M., & Meana, M. (2009). The future of sex therapy: Specialization or marginalization? *Archives of Sexual Behavior, 38*(6), 1016–1027.

Brotto, L. A. (2010). The DSM diagnostic criteria for sexual aversion disorder. *Archives of Sexual Behavior, 39*(2), 271–277.

Clayton, A. H., Derogatis, L. R., Rosen, R. C., & Pyke, R. (2012). Intended or unintended consequences? The likely implications of raising the bar for sexual dysfunction diagnosis in the proposed DSM-V revisions: I. For women with incomplete loss of desire or sexual receptivity. *Journal of Sexual Medicine, 9*(8), 2027–2039.

Davis, S. N., Binik, Y. M., & Carrier, S. (2009). Sexual dysfunction and pelvic pain in men: A male sexual pain disorder? *Journal of Sex and Marital Therapy, 35*(3), 182–205.

Heiman, J. R. (2002). Psychologic treatments for female sexual dysfunction: Are they effective and do we need them? *Archives of Sexual Behavior, 31*(5), 445–450.

Kaplan, H. S. (1987). *Sexual aversion, sexual phobias, and panic disorder.* New York: Brunner/Mazel.

Laumann, E. O., Gagnon, J. H., Michael, R. T., & Michaels, S. (1994). *The social organization of sexuality: Sexual practices in the United States.* Chicago: University of Chicago Press.

Leiblum, S. R., & Rosen, R. C. (Eds.). (1980). *Principles and practice of sex therapy* (1st ed.). New York: Guilford Press.

PART I

SEX THERAPY FOR SEXUAL DYSFUNCTION

Desire and Arousal

CHAPTER 1

Sexual Interest/Arousal Disorder in Women

Lori Brotto and Mijal Luria

Brotto and Luria say, "A lack of interest in sexual activity that creates personal distress and strains relationship satisfaction is the most common reason that women seek sex therapy." And yet as Brotto and Luria point out, this seemingly straightforward problem is actually complex and resistant to treatment. The search for the elusive "cure" ultimately led to a renewed interest in research regarding the nature of female sexual desire and has resulted in a major reformulation of the diagnosis. Sexual interest arousal disorder (SIAD) is a new DSM-5 sexual dysfunction that merges the DSM-IV dysfunctions of hypoactive sexual desire disorder (HSDD) and female sexual arousal disorder (FSAD). The DSM-5 committee (of which Brotto was a member) noted that women often present clinically with both low sexual desire and diminished capacity for sexual arousal. Citing long-standing concerns about the adequacy of Masters and Johnson's triphasic and gender-neutral model of sexual response, the DSM-5 committee turned instead to the empirically based incentive motivation model, in which biological, psychological, and contextual factors interact to elicit sexual interest, as well as sexual arousal. The fact that no such diagnostic change was proposed for male HSDD reflects the growing divergence in theoretical conceptualizations between male and female sexuality. An important therapeutic implication of the new diagnosis and underlying model is that effective treatment of SIAD will often involve medication, individual or conjoint sex, therapy or some combination thereof.

Lori Brotto, PhD, is Head of the Division of Gynaecologic Specialties at the University of British Columbia, Associate Professor of Gynaecology and Psychiatry, and a Registered Psychologist in the province of British Columbia. Her research focuses on developing and testing mindfulness-based interventions for women with sexual difficulties and genital pain. Dr. Brotto is Associate Editor for the *Archives of Sexual Behavior* and *Sexual and Relationship Therapy*. She was a member of the Sexual and Gender Identity Disorders work group for DSM-5.

Mijal Luria, MD, is the Director of the Center for Sexual Health at the Hadassah Mt. Scopus Medical Center in Jerusalem, Israel, where she is an attending obstetrician–gynecologist and sex therapist. She was a member of the committee on Women's Sexual Desire and Arousal Disorders during the Third International Consultation on Sexual Medicine held in Paris in 2009. She is a board member of the International Society for the Study of Women's Sexual Health.

A lack of interest in sexual activity that creates personal distress and strains relationship satisfaction is the most common reason that women seek sex therapy. Described frequently by patients as "I've lost my libido," or "It takes a long time for me to get sexually excited," or "I would be content if we never had sex again!" the presence of little or no desire for sex has received widespread attention from clinicians, researchers, and the lay public because of its complexity and relative resistance to treatment. A new disorder, sexual interest/arousal disorder (SIAD), has been included in the fifth edition of the *Diagnostic and Statistical Manual of Mental Disorders* (DSM-5; American Psychiatric Association, 2013) to replace hypoactive sexual desire disorder (HSDD) and female sexual arousal disorder (FSAD) from the DSM-IV-TR (American Psychiatric Association, 2000) due to long-standing dissatisfaction with HSDD and FSAD. In particular, criticisms have included the following: (1) HSDD and FSAD rely on Masters and Johnson's (1966) linear sexual response cycle, which may not fit the experiences of all women; (2) the frequency and intensity of desire for sex is only one aspect of how women describe their experience of sexual desire (or lack thereof); (3) reliance on sexual fantasies as an indicator of sexual desire is problematic because many women with satisfactory levels of desire report not having sexual fantasies; (4) "persistent and recurrent" are ambiguously interpreted in the DSM-IV-TR criteria; and (5) the use of the term "hypoactive" in HSDD is misleading, as it implies an underlying biological etiology to low sexual desire (Brotto, 2010; Graham, 2010) that is usually impossible to conclude in the clinical scenario. The following vignette illustrates a typical case of female SIAD.

Miranda presented for sex therapy with the primary complaint of "I don't feel any sexual excitement any longer." Upon being asked by her therapist, she revealed that she rarely thought about sex with her partner, although she continued to have sexual intercourse on a weekly basis. She did not initiate sexual activity, and she only reluctantly accepted her partner's sexual solicitations for fear of losing the relationship. Sexual touching elicited few, if any, positive sexual sensations, and she was minimally aware of vaginal lubrication. On most occasions of sexual activity, the encounter ended with her feeling physically and emotionally dissatisfied; however, on a few occasions she was able to become somewhat sexually aroused in her mind. These problems had existed for the past 5 years and had led Miranda to withdraw emotionally from her 15-year relationship.

The criteria for SIAD are polythetic and require that a woman experience a minimum of three symptoms for at least 6 months. Possible manifestations of SIAD include: lack of interest in sexual activity; reduced or absent erotic thoughts; lack of initiation and receptivity to sexual activity; reduced pleasure during sex; reduced or absent desire emerging during a sexual encounter; and a reduction in genital and nongenital sexual sensations. The criteria hinge upon a conceptualization of sexual interest/arousal that emphasizes its responsive nature. In other words, because some women may not experience desire for sex at the outset of sexual activity but are able to become sexually responsive *during* the sexual encounter (Carvalheira, Brotto, & Leal, 2010), a diagnosis of "dysfunction" is inappropriate for those women with the sole complaint of low or absent sexual desire before or at the start of a sexual encounter. The latter group may present for treatment on the basis of a dissatisfied partner who mourns her loss of innate sexual desire or because a woman herself believes that desire *should* be felt often and independent of potential inhibitory or excitatory forces. For example, Sarah (age 32, married) in the past experienced spontaneous sexual desire and a very robust sexual arousal response until the birth of her third child, when she experienced a marked decline in the frequency of sexual urges. She continued, however, to become sexually aroused and orgasmic during sexual activity, particularly if she was well rested, and this triggered responsive desire during the encounter. Sarah would not, in our view, meet criteria for SIAD.

The use of "persistent and recurrent" in previous editions of the DSM has also been criticized due to its lack of objectivity in defining a sexual dysfunction and for the potential to overpathologize normal variations in sexual experience or behavior. Not all individuals seeking sex therapy have a diagnosable sexual dysfunction, and some, perhaps even many, require education and information to challenge sex-related myths. Thus the criteria for SIAD require symptoms to be present for a minimum duration of 6 months. Some of the symptoms must have been present in all or almost all (approximately 75%) sexual encounters to rule out common normative variations in sexual interest (which may be adaptive to the particular context). As in the case of Miranda, it is the repeated experience of sexual interest/arousal concerns over a prolonged period of time that signal the likely presence of SIAD.

The introduction of polythetic criteria means that two women with different symptom expressions may both meet criteria for SIAD. For example, Mary may lack interest in sexual activity, have no erotic or sexual thoughts, and reject her partner's sexual invitations. Barbara, on the other hand, may have great difficulty becoming mentally sexually excited, have a reduced sexual desire response during sexual activity, and lack signs of physical sexual arousal. Because they experience three of six symptoms for 6 months or longer, both Mary and Barbara would meet SIAD criteria. The advantages of a polythetic system (with SIAD) over DSM-IV-TR's monothetic criteria (with HSDD) are that (1) it addresses the finding that sexual behavior alone is an unreliable referent for sexual desire; (2) it acknowledges that sexual response difficulties may be expressed differently across different women; (3) it expands the narrow focus on lubrication as a sole indicator of sexual arousal; and (4) it seeks to depathologize normal variations (and reductions) in sexual response by requiring that symptoms occur on most sexual encounters for a minimum duration of 6 months.

EPIDEMIOLOGY

Given that SIAD is a new disorder in DSM-5, its prevalence is unknown (for a review of prevalence studies, see Brotto, 2010, and Graham, 2010). Focusing on the symptom of "lack of interest in sex" for the preceding month, the second wave of the British National Survey of Sexual Attitudes and Lifestyles (NATSAL) found a prevalence of 40.6% among women ages 16–44 (Mercer, Fenton, Johnson, Wellings, Macdowall, et al. (2003). However, when a more stringent 6-month duration of symptoms was used, this figure dropped to 10.2%. This figure was also found in the more recent Prevalence of Female Sexual Problems Associated with Distress and Determinants of Treatment Seeking (PRESIDE) study (Shifren, Monz, Russo, Segreti, & Johannes, 2008). Because less than 28% of sexual difficulties with a 1-month duration persist for 6 months or more (Hayes, Bennett, Fairley, & Dennerstein, 2006), only persisting symptoms of low sexual interest should be considered to fulfill a diagnosis of SIAD. Multinational studies find higher rates of low sexual interest in Middle East and Southeast Asian countries (Laumann, Nicolosi, Glasser, Paik, Gingell, et al., 2005), emphasizing the importance of cultural sensitivity when assessing sexual interest and arousal.

A diagnosis of SIAD requires the presence of clinically significant distress and it is usually distress that brings women in for treatment. There is evidence from the Women's International Study of Health and Sexuality (WISHeS) that low desire is more distressing for younger as compared with older, menopausal women, challenging the view that low desire becomes more prevalent with age.

Even considering the drop in prevalence when low desire and distress together are experienced over several months, loss of sexual interest continues to be the most frequent complaint seen in sex therapy clinics, and the majority of women with any sexual difficulty (i.e., desire, arousal, orgasm, or pain-related) believe that their low sexual desire is the cause of their sexual difficulties (Hayes et al., 2006).

Women with SIAD may also experience a reduction in or absence of genital and/or nongenital sensations during sexual activity; however, the prevalence of this symptom is unknown, because past studies assessing FSAD have tended to focus on lack of lubrication, which ranges in prevalence from 2.6% to 31.2% (Graham, 2010). When a composite measure of arousal that included feeling aroused during sex, having pleasant tingling in genitals, and enjoying genitals being touched was assessed, the prevalence over the past month was 12.2%.

In the clinical scenario, women often report difficulties with both sexual interest and capacity for sexual arousal. For example, Brynne had a long history of dry vulvar tissue, some pain with penetration, and great difficulty reaching orgasm. Despite these concerns, she continued to have interest in sex and would masturbate once per week. However, as her health deteriorated over time and necessitated the use of a cocktail of medications, her sleep became disrupted, her mood dropped, and she and her partner began to have increasing relational discord. Brynne's motivation for sex precipitously declined, which further hampered her ability to become sexually aroused. Brynne's situation is not unique. In fact, several studies have found a high degree of comorbidity between HSDD and FSAD, and desire and arousal scores using validated instruments are usually highly correlated (see Brotto, Graham, Binik, Segraves, & Zucker, 2011, for a review). A central tenet of the incentive motivation model for sexual response is that sexual desire and sexual arousal emerge together, in response to effective sexual cues. Sexual desire and sexual arousal may even represent different sides of the same sexual coin.

ETIOLOGY AND MODELS

The incentive motivation model of sexual response, which arose from a large number of elegant Dutch studies, provides an integrative model in which biological, psychological, and contextual factors interact to elicit sexual interest and arousal (see Laan & Both, 2008, for a review). It posits that sexual desire results from an interplay between a sexual response system and effective stimuli that activate this system (Toates, 2009). Early views (Kaplan, 1977, 1979; Lief, 1977) likened sexual desire to other drive states, such as hunger and thirst, which were based on the premise that these appetitive reactions originated from within an individual and progressively increased with time and that, once satiated, an individual could continue on for a period of time before the desire started to build again. However, this conceptualization does not mirror what patients report clinically. They lament the loss of touch that once triggered an electrifying arousal response or the desire for sex that was cultivated during a close dance with an attractive partner. In comparison with former linear models of sexual response, the incentive motivation model fits the experiences of women with and without sexual concerns because it emphasizes the important role of real or imaginary stimuli that trigger motivation and response. Within such a framework, sexual desire and sexual arousal are seen as simultaneous responses to a sexually relevant stimulus (i.e., a stimulus that the individual perceives as being sufficiently sexual) and are, therefore, not distinct constructs. This model places a heavy emphasis on the role of stimuli. However, within incentive motivation theory, stimuli become effective only in the context of a system that allows for sexual responsiveness. Biological and psychological factors can influence the responsiveness of the sexual system, as well as the effectiveness of sexual stimuli to elicit sexual response; thus an evaluation of biological, psychological, and sociocultural influences must form a part of a thorough assessment of SIAD.

Basson (2002a, 2002b), took the empirical findings from incentive motivation theory and applied them clinically to formulate a circular model of sexual response that has gained widespread interest. The model notes that women begin sexual encounters for any variety of sexual or nonsexual reasons and that awareness of any innate feelings of desire may be absent for women (note that although Basson originally conceptualized her model as applying to both men and women, in recent years scholars have applied it mostly to understanding women). During a sexual encounter, if a woman experiences some sexual arousal and excitement, this then triggers "responsive sexual desire"—a desire for the sexual activity to continue for now more sexual reasons, in addition to whatever initial incentives were present. If the outcome is rewarding (emotionally and/or physically), she might have more motivation to initiate or respond to cues in the future. Women with and without sexual difficulties often relate to this experience of "responsive desire" more than any initial awareness of sexual desire (Carvalheira et al., 2010; Goldhammer & McCabe, 2011), and they sometimes report relief when a clinician normalizes their lessening sexual desire that comes about with age and relationship duration. Interestingly, even among women who reported high levels of sexual arousal, the majority (85%) reported that they at least occasionally began a sexual encounter with no desire but then experienced responsive desire as sex progressed (Carvalheira et al., 2010).

Hormones, Neurotransmitters, and Medical Factors Affecting Sexual Response

Hormones may affect the responsivity of the sexual system and therefore should be considered in the woman with SIAD, both at the time of assessment and as treatment unfolds. In the context of a mental health practice, it may be necessary for multidisciplinary medical colleagues (e.g., primary care physician, gynecologist, endocrinologist) to play a role. Steroid hormones activate mechanisms of sexual excitation by directing the synthesis of enzymes and receptors for several neurochemical systems (Kruger, Hartmann, & Schedlowski, 2005; Pfaus, 2009). Those include dopamine, norepinephrine, melanocortin, and oxytocin systems.

The most abundant and potent hormone before menopause is 17ß-estradiol (known as "estradiol"; E2), produced by the granulosa cells of the ovaries. After menopause, estrogen is produced in extragonadal intracellular sites in small amounts. In a number of studies using varying methodologies (assessment at diverse menopausal transition stages, different study designs and questionnaires), a weak correlation between lower levels of estradiol and decreased sexual desire has been found by some (Freeman et al., 2007; Guthrie, Dennerstein, Taffe, Lehert, & Burger, 2004) but not by others (Avis, Stellato, Crawford, Johannes, & Longcope, 2000; Tungphaisal, Chandeying, Sutthijumroon, Krisanapan, & Udomratn, 1991); thus measurement of serum estradiol is not helpful for diagnosing a woman with low sexual desire. Nevertheless, an adequate level of estradiol is important for maintaining vaginal lubrication and avoiding dyspareunia (Guthrie et al., 2004; Sarrel, 1990).

Androgen levels peak when women are in their 20s and drop gradually with age, so that women in their 40s have approximately half the level of circulating total testosterone as women in their 20s. Despite long-held popular beliefs, population-based studies have shown minimal or no correlation between testosterone levels and sexual desire in women (Davis, Davison, Donath, & Bell, 2005; Guthrie et al., 2004; Santoro et al., 2005). The lack of accuracy of current assays to measure testosterone is a well-known limitation because most clinically available assays are designed to measure testosterone in the male range or to identify hyperandrogenic states in women (Davis, Guay, Shifren, & Mazer, 2004). Because of the intracrinology of sex hormones, measuring androgen metabolites might identify cases of true androgen deficiency and differentiate women who will benefit from therapy from those who will not, but to date even these approaches have not been useful clinically for identifying women with a sexual desire disorder (Basson, Brotto, Petkau, & Labrie, 2010). Another confounding factor is the great variability in the responsiveness of women to androgens. For example, there are contradictory findings on the effects of the oral contraceptive pill, which increases the concentration of sex-hormone-binding globulin (SHBG), thereby lessening the bioavailable testosterone, on sexual interest (Burrows, Basha, & Goldstein, 2012). It is possible that polymorphic variations in the androgen receptor gene may also influence women's responses to androgens.

Dopamine is considered to be the major neurotransmitter involved in sexual arousal, due to its actions in mesolimbic and hypothalamic circuits. Some women given dopaminergic drugs such as bupropion or apomorphine have reported increased sexual desire and response (Caruso et al., 2004), though these agents are usually not used clinically to boost sexual motivation. There was much promise for flibanserin, a 5-hydroxytryptophan 1A (5-HT$_{1A}$) receptor agonist, 5-HT$_{2A}$ receptor antagonist, and dopamine D4 receptor partial agonist in the treatment of loss of sexual desire (Goldfischer et al., 2011); however, it was not approved by the Food and Drug Administration (FDA) and therefore remains unavailable clinically. Much is unknown about the role of neurosteroids (i.e., steroids synthesized de novo within the brain) in mediating sexual interest in women, but they are speculated to play a role in sexual motivation. Clinically, it is, at present, impossible to directly measure neurosteroid levels.

Although progesterone receptors are found in many of the same brain areas as estrogen receptors, including the hypothalamus and the limbic system, there are few data on its effects on human sexual behavior. There is some evidence in humans that synthetic progestins may have negative effects on sexual desire (Sherwin, 1999).

Medical conditions affecting the circulatory, endocrine, musculoskeletal, and central nervous systems are important to take into account in the presence of sexual interest and arousal complaints. However, their impact on sexual response may be indirect and illustrate the biopsychosocial complexity of SIAD. For example, whereas cancer treatment may stop ovarian function and contribute to vaginal stenosis, dryness, and pain, the impact of cancer on sexual self-esteem and body image may exert even greater negative effects on sexual motivation.

Taken together, it is important that the clinician be mindful of the myriad medical and organic contributors to SIAD, yet not become blindsided by their presence to the exclusion of other important relational and psychological factors.

Relational Aspects

The link between sexual function and relationship well-being has been repeatedly confirmed. Sexual problems might be both the cause and the result of unsatisfactory relationships. The woman who lacks motivation for sexual contact as a result of her low emotional intimacy, trust, or respect toward her partner is unfortunately a very common finding in the clinical scenario. A woman's feelings for her partner are a major determinant of her sexual desire, above and beyond any hormonal contributors (Dennerstein, Dudley, & Burger, 2001; Guthrie et al., 2004).

Formalization of the relationship can also influence sexual desire: feelings of love, security, partner support, commitment, and emotional closeness are less likely to lead to sexual desire by married women than by single women (McCall & Meston, 2006). In married women, feelings of institutionalization of the relationship, overfamiliarity, and desexualization of roles can dampen sexual desire (Sims & Meana, 2010). Relationship experts, such as Perel (2006), argue that in cultivating security, stability, love, and commitment, a couple is at risk of losing the very ingredients that fuel their eroticism (e.g., passion, danger, the unknown). In the clinical scenario, a therapist must therefore balance concerns about a woman's complaints of loss of motivation for once highly passionate and erotic sex in the context of her now 10-year relationship. Specific partner-related attributes can also affect her sexual desire, including a partner with a high sexual interest who asks for (or even demands) sex with minimal efforts to elicit her sexual response; a partner with poor sexual technique or particularly rigid sexual beliefs about sexual technique; a partner with sexual needs that the woman believes she cannot satisfy; and a partner to whom the woman is not attracted (Witting et al., 2008). His sexual dysfunction can also adversely affect her interest in sex, and improvement in his sexual function can simultaneously increase hers. Within an incentive motivation model, partner factors that influence the range and intensity of stimuli used and the woman's response to those cues become an important focus in the clinical scenario.

Mood

Along with relationship factors, mood is a major correlate of women's sexual health. Mood instability, low self-esteem, and having an introverted personality style have been associated with decreased sexual interest and may all influence the responsivity of the sexual system. Having depression significantly increases the odds of having low sexual interest by at least twofold among women ages 40–80 (Laumann et al., 2005), and loss of sexual desire is common in major depressive disorder (MDD), which is defined by a "loss of interest or pleasure." Sexual dysfunction secondary to antidepressant therapy is also well documented though such complaints tend to focus more on orgasmic functioning and not sexual desire. In the case of Leslie, a 24-year-old single female student who became severely depressed following the unexpected death of her mother, her lack of motivation to masturbate would not warrant a diagnosis of SIAD, even though this represents a marked reduction from her previous frequency of two to three times a week. If the low sexual interest/arousal is attributable to a nonsexual psychiatric disorder (such as MDD in Leslie's case), then the clinician would not apply a diagnosis of SIAD.

Sociocultural Influences

Sexuality has always been subject to the influence of social constructs. Negative messages about masturbation in girls and the view of women as passive recipients of men's sexual desires and actions may encourage a passive attitude to sexual activity and inhibit their sexual interest (Boul, Hallam-Jones, & Wylie, 2009). In the last 10 years a different theoretical framework, the "new view of women's sexual problems" (Tiefer, 2001; Tiefer, Hall, & Tavris, 2002), has emerged in response to the medicalization of sexual difficulties that may have been perpetuated by previous DSMs and by pharmaceutical interests. The new view stresses the importance of social factors as a cause of women's sexual avoidance or distress and deemphasizes the focus on hormonal and/or biological factors. Inadequate sex education, failure to meet cultural norms concerning sexual attractiveness or sexual response, fatigue due to family and work obligations, or conflict between the sexual norms of culture of origin and those of the dominant culture may be at the heart of many sexual problems (Tiefer et al., 2002) and therefore deserve attention clinically.

Another important sociocultural influence on women's sexual desire concerns ethnicity. Cross-cultural studies find markedly disparate rates of low desire depending on a woman's ethnic background (Cain et al., 2003; Laumann et al., 2005), and certain variables, such as sex guilt and religiosity, mediate the association between a woman's culture and her level of sexual desire (Woo, Brotto, & Gorzalka, 2011; Woo, Morshedian, Brotto, &

Gorzalka, 2012). In the absence of qualitative data on how women from various ethnocultural groups experience sexual motivation, however, one must be cautious in assuming that a lack of motivation for sex is a necessary sign of a sexual dysfunction among ethnic minority women. There is much we do not know about the triggers of desire and arousal across cultures and whether a loss of sexual response is experienced as distressing. If ethnocultural factors do have an impact on sexual response, their mechanism of influence may include a biological propensity of the sexual system, as well as responses to sexual cues that are influenced by nonbiological factors.

Assessment/Treatment Algorithm

We have devised an assessment/treatment algorithm useful in guiding the clinician (Figure 1.1). In evaluating the criteria for SIAD, the clinician must inquire about both frequency and intensity of sexual interest, fantasies/erotic thoughts, pleasure during sex, and physical sensations. The rationale stems from the finding that some women may identify more with how often they do (or do not) experience sexual interest/arousal, whereas other women may recognize changes in the intensity of their response. The range of sexual stimuli that might elicit a woman's sexual interest and arousal should also be explored, along with her current and past responses to such stimuli given that women with low desire have a more restricted range of effective stimuli that elicit their desire (McCall & Meston, 2006). The clinician should also assess typical patterns of initiation between the couple, given that a woman's lack of initiating sexual activity may not necessarily point to a problem with her sexual motivation as men, in general, are more likely to initiate sex (Baumeister, Catanese, & Vohs, 2001).

ASSESSMENT AND DIAGNOSTIC ISSUES

The assessment of women with sexual interest and arousal problems is based on three main elements: a structured interview, a physical examination, and, to a smaller extent, laboratory investigation. In keeping with incentive motivation theory and Basson's (2002a, 2002b) circular model of sexual response, the clinician must inquire about both frequency and intensity of sexual interest, fantasies/erotic thoughts, pleasure during sex, and physical (including genital and nongenital) sensations. As reviewed, hormonal factors may influence the responsiveness of the sexual system but may also have an impact on reasons to engage in sex. Similarly, psychological and sociocultural processes may affect one's sexual propensity, his or her reasons for engaging in sex, and responses to sexual cues. A complete assessment of SIAD requires that the clinician be attentive to the myriad psychosocial and biological contributors and how they may interact to influence a woman's motivation for sex and her subsequent response.

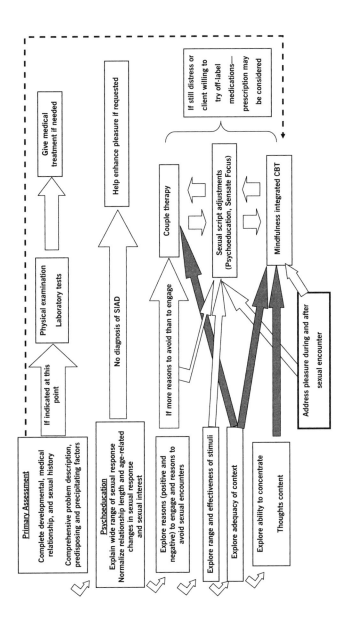

FIGURE 1.1. Assessment and treatment algorithm. After initial assessment, if medical problems are found, further medical examination and treatment are warranted. If psychological or couple issues are first detected, the client may benefit from treatment focusing on cognitive processing, mindfulness skills, and behavioral changes. In some cases, couple therapy is needed. Psychoeducation is imperative to overcome unfavorable beliefs and to define and adjust expectations. If there are few or no motivations to be sexual, sexual stimuli are not satisfactory, thought content is distracting or disturbing, mindfulness-integrated CBT is recommended. Address sexual scripts and develop alternatives as needed. Address pleasure. Off-label medications are indicated only if previous steps were unsuccessful, after the client received full explanation on the limitations and possible risks of medical treatment.

Structured Interview

A thorough biopsychosocial assessment should comprise a complete medical history (including hormonal status and mood), a demographic overview (along with sociocultural and family-of-origin issues that may have affected views on sexuality), and a physical and emotional developmental history (including past sexual experiences—wanted and unwanted). If the woman is currently in a relationship, assessment of nonsexual aspects of the relationship, level of commitment, partner's perspective on symptoms, and partner's sexual function should be assessed. An interview with the partner (together and alone) can be invaluable. Specific to evaluating the diagnostic criteria for SIAD, the clinician should assess the woman's motivations (or lack of motivation) for sexual activity, as well as disincentives to engage sexually. The range of stimuli and current and past response to such stimuli, her ability to stay focused and experience responsive desire, and the sexual outcome—whether the sexual experience is emotionally and/or physically satisfying or pleasurable—should also be assessed. Even if a woman describes only few effective cues that elicit her sexual desire/arousal, it is still crucial to evaluate her partner's sexual technique and other partner-related factors that may be explaining her symptoms (Laan & Both, 2011). In the case of Laura, a 50-year-old woman in a committed 3-year lesbian relationship, her self-definition was "I never was much of a sexual person," and she only minimally enjoyed sex throughout each of her long-term relationships. In the context of her structured interview, Laura revealed that foreplay was always minimal, that she was highly distractible during sexual activity and would worry about upsetting her partners, and that she experienced great discomfort in communicating to her partners about what was pleasurable to her. Moreover, Laura felt that each of her partners, except her current one, was more interested in her own orgasms than in learning how to please Laura sexually. In Laura's case, the role of partner-related factors and insufficient stimulation may be especially pertinent to assess and subsequently address in treatment.

There are a large number of self-report and clinician-administered scales and interviews that assess sexual desire in women (for a review, see Brotto, Bitzer, Laan, Leiblum, & Luria, 2010). Although these can be useful for screening sexual symptoms in a busy medical setting, they are of unknown reliability in making a diagnosis of SIAD. It is noteworthy that when a self-report validated measure of sexual functioning is used, the prevalence of low desire is considerably higher than when computerized or face-to-face interviews are employed (Witting et al., 2008)

Physical Examination

The physical examination, when a woman presents with symptoms of low sexual interest/arousal, is a good setting to explore her perceptions, beliefs, and attitudes in response to her own anatomy and to educate and encourage a positive approach to her genitals and body. In the case in which a mental health professional is providing care, a referral to a primary care physician or specialist may be warranted. A gynecological examination should include an evaluation of the level of voluntary control of the pelvic floor muscles, pelvic floor muscle tone, presence of vaginal atrophy, size of introitus, presence of discharge or evidence of infection, epithelial disorders, and/or pain, as well as an evaluation of the pelvic organs. Vulvovaginal hypotrophy or atrophy is common after menopause, in breastfeeding women, in women treated with low-estrogen or progesterone-only contraceptives, and in hypothalamic or pituitary disease. Ruling out these contributors to low desire/arousal is essential.

Laboratory Investigations

Laboratory evaluation is seldom of use in the identification of female sexual desire and arousal problems. Estrogen deficiency is best detected by history and a physical examination. If the menopausal status in a hysterectomized woman is unclear, measurements of estradiol and follicle-stimulating hormone (FSH) are indicated. If irregular menstrual patterns, unexplained amenorrhea, or fertility problems are present, prolactin and thyroid-stimulating hormone (TSH) levels should be tested as well. Androgen serum levels do not correlate with sexual function and are currently not recommended. Assessment of genital sexual response with vaginal photoplethysmography similarly is not used clinically, as it is found to correlate poorly with women's subjective experiences (Chivers, Seto, Lalumière, Laan, & Grimbos, 2010).

Specialized Examinations

A number of specialized tests, which are available to evaluate vascular and neurological parameters of women's sexual function, are usually available only in research settings. Their use in identifying women with SIAD is currently unknown, and they are not used clinically.

APPROACHES TO TREATMENT

Figure 1.1 outlines our treatment algorithm, which is based on the principles of incentive motivation (i.e., that sexual desire/arousal emerge in response to effective cues and that each individual has a predisposition to sexual responsiveness that is influenced by both biology and psychology) and on the circular model of sexual response that highlights the importance of incentives for sex, stimuli, and context. Each of these aspects is addressed in treatment, and identification of "breaks" in the cycle is used to guide treatment. For example, treatment of Jane, who states that her only motivation for sex is to avoid her husband's outbursts of anger and that she derives no personal benefit from sex, may include couple therapy focused on nonsexual dynamics, possibly including couple communication and emotional regulation skills for Jane's husband. On the other hand, Michelle reports having a variety of positive reasons to engage in sex but derives little to no pleasure from sexual touch and therefore limits foreplay with her boyfriend to just a few brief moments prior to intercourse. Michelle and her partner may benefit from couple exercises in sensate focus and exploration of stimuli through skills in sexual technique. This may include psychoeducation on the nature of the sexual response, including the role of age, relationship duration, and sexual myths. Next we review the brief literature exploring nonpharmacological and pharmacological treatments that may be useful for SIAD.

Nonpharmacological Treatments for SIAD

The literature on nonpharmacological treatments for low desire/arousal is sparse, and there is insufficient evidence for a single "evidence-based" treatment. However, there is considerable interest in evaluating psychological treatments, in particular, cognitive-behavioral therapy (CBT) and mindfulness-based interventions (MBIs). At present, we can conclude that there is promising evidence for these methods in improving women's low desire and arousal, but future research should focus on more carefully evaluating these methods in large samples of women with SIAD compared with a control group.

Cognitive-Behavioral Therapy

Early sex researchers identified anxiety surrounding sexual performance as one of the most important precipitants of sexual dysfunction (Masters & Johnson, 1970). Spectating was thought to lead one to evaluate and monitor his or her own performance instead of focusing on the pleasurable sensory aspects of the sexual encounter. The resulting preoccupation with performance and critical thoughts then disrupted the processes of sexual functioning and hindered sexual response. Such cognitive interference, which distracts the person from focusing on the erotic encounter, can also activate the autonomic nervous system, triggering negative affect that is not synonymous with sexual arousal or pleasure. This anxiety creates further cognitive interference, perhaps giving rise to thoughts such as "I'm a failure" or "I'll never be able to experience desire," which in turn hinder the sexual response. Behavioral avoidance is a natural consequence, which further exacerbates the anxiety about performance (Barlow, 1986). Such cognitive catastrophizing and behavioral avoidance are common among women seeking treatment for sexual response concerns.

   Although much of the early research focused on men, there is evidence that cognitive distraction during sexual activity negatively affects women's sexual esteem, sexual satisfaction, and sexual response. Compared with women without sexual difficulties, those with sexual dysfunction hold stronger negative beliefs about the influence of age and body image on sexuality, and this makes them more vulnerable to activation of negative self-schemas (specifically those of incompetence) when confronted with a negative sexual situation (Nobre & Pinto-Gouveia, 2006). These self-critical schemas then trigger negative automatic thoughts, which prevent the woman from focusing on sexual stimuli and elicit negative affect, which further impairs sexual response.

These findings provide a strong justification for the use of CBT skills such as challenging problematic thoughts and shifting attention allocation through performance-based exercises. Unfortunately, only few studies have evaluated CBT for women's low sexual desire or arousal (see Brotto et al., 2010, for a review).

There is evidence that 8 weeks of individual CBT (including sensate focus, directed masturbation, and the coital alignment technique) significantly increases sexual desire and leads to lasting improvements 6 months later. There is also evidence that CBT administered in group format over 12 weeks to women with HSDD significantly reduces HSDD severity, with sustained gains even a year after treatment. The finding that CBT for low desire, administered with minimal intervention and using a self-help manual, led to only marginal improvements suggests that this approach may be inadequate to address the complexity of loss of sexual interest within a relationship.

In two studies that evaluated CBT for women with complaints of lack of sexual arousal, treatment significantly improved self-reported subjective arousal to the level of that of women in the nonclinical group or in comparison with a placebo control condition. In one study, CBT also resulted in a trend toward increased concordance between self-reported and physiologically measured sexual arousal, suggesting that one mechanism by which CBT is effective is in assisting women to appreciate their genital arousal response, which, in turn, may influence their subjective experience.

Neither study found an effect of CBT on physiological sexual arousal measured with a vaginal photoplethysmograph. This concurs with evidence that women's genital arousal response is usually robust even if a woman is reporting a complete lack of subjective sexual arousal and suggests that treatments focused on strengthening the physiological sexual response may do nothing to alter a woman's reported sexual difficulties. It is perhaps not surprising, therefore, that all proposals to the FDA for pharmaceutical agents to treat women's sexual dysfunction have been rejected on the grounds of inadequate efficacy (as well as questionable long-term safety data).

Mindfulness-Based Interventions

Mindfulness is an ancient Eastern practice that embodies present-moment, nonjudgmental awareness. It made its debut into western healthcare in the 1970s through treatment of chronic pain and the work of Kabat-Zinn, who developed mindfulness-based stress reduction (Kabat-Zinn, 1990). Since then, it has been adapted for a variety of populations and uses, including the prevention of depressive relapse, and found to be effective for a large range of psychological and health-related conditions. Clinically, women with SIAD may describe their symptoms as "a disconnect between my mind and my body" and may declare an absence of pleasure despite the genital arousal response remaining robust. MBIs, which aim to cultivate active awareness of the body in an accepting, nonjudgmental, and compassionate manner, might be ideally suited to help with the complaints of low sexual desire (Brotto & Heiman, 2007). A three-session mindfulness-based CBT group treatment for women with low sexual desire has been found to significantly improve sexual desire, sex-related distress, and perceptions of genital tingling. The treatment included in-session mindfulness practices followed by daily at-home mindfulness practice, and exercises included an eating meditation, followed by body-scan, mindfulness-of-breath, and finally mindfulness-of-thoughts exercises. When women became more accustomed to practicing mindfulness in their day-to-day lives, exercises that bridged mindful awareness with sexual activity were then introduced. When applied to women with primarily sexual arousal complaints, this four-session mindfulness-based CBT treatment significantly improved women's perception of their genital arousal during an erotic film. Moreover, their self-reported sexual arousal during sexual activity, desire, orgasm, and sexual satisfaction all improved. Although the absence of a control group makes it difficult to delineate the precise mechanisms by which this MBI was effective, the finding that these effects were replicated in four studies to date suggests that skills in mindful awareness may be useful in the treatment of SIAD.

Pharmacological Treatments for SIAD

The search for a pharmacological means to cure women's low desire has been fierce. The main paths under investigation include hormonal treatment, dopaminergic agonists, melanocortin-stimulating hormones, α-adrenergic antagonists, nitric oxide delivery systems, and prostaglandins. Because most of these agents have been tested in women meeting criteria for HSDD or FSAD, their efficacy in treating SIAD is largely unknown.

Hormonal Treatment: Estrogen

Desire disorders emerging from vulvovaginal atrophy can benefit from estrogen treatment. Given the direct causal relationship between low estrogen levels and atrophy, estrogen therapy, unless contraindicated, is the current standard of care for treating this condition (Tan, Bradshaw, & Carr, 2012). Local delivery is the preferred method of treatment. Systemic estrogen is indicated in the presence of other climacteric symptoms, specifically hot flashes.

   Local estrogen therapy can be given as tablets, pessaries/vagitories, cream, or a vaginal ring. Therapy is available as conjugated equine estrogens, estradiol, estriol, or estrone. Concurrent progestogen therapy is not indicated, nor is annual endometrial surveillance, in asymptomatic women using vaginal estrogen. For women with a history of hormone-dependent cancer, management is decided in consultation with the oncologist balancing quality-of-life concerns and risk of recurrence.

Hormonal Treatment: Testosterone

The controversy surrounding the use of testosterone for the treatment of low sexual desire has a long history and continues to be hotly debated today. Despite the fact that testosterone therapy did not meet regulatory approval for the treatment of HSDD, estimates suggest that 4.1 million prescriptions for off-label testosterone are made annually in the United States alone (Davis & Braunstein, 2012). Studies in naturally and surgically menopausal estrogen-replete and nonreplete women who reported a decline in their desire for sex have found a benefit of a 300 µg/day testosterone patch. Concerns about the high rate of androgenic side effects (30% of the sample) and the finding of more new cases of breast cancer not found in the placebo group remain, however. Findings for a testosterone spray in premenopausal women with HSDD are significant, though the actual increase amounted to only one sexually satisfying event per month. Most recently, there was much excitement about a topical gel formulation of testosterone (Libigel) as providing "a clear path to FDA approval"; however, a lack of significant benefit over placebo in all study endpoints, and the finding that the placebo effect was more beneficial than drug on some endpoints (BioSante Pharmaceuticals, 2012), suggests that sex researchers would do well to capitalize on these findings and attempt to understand what the mechanisms are by which the placebo response is so effective (Bradford & Meston, 2009). In all of these trials, only women with a baseline frequency of two to three sexually satisfying episodes per month were enrolled, as opposed to what is commonly seen in clinical practice, in which women consistently report few or no sexually satisfying encounters.

Currently the use of transdermal testosterone for reduced sexual desire in surgically postmenopausal women has been approved by the European Medicines Agency (since 2010) but not by the FDA or Health Canada. The main concerns are the inconsistent evidence of the androgen effects on breast tissue proliferation and the unknown effects on insulin resistance, metabolic syndrome, and cardiovascular disease. The 2009 International Consultation on Sexual Medicine supported the investigational use of testosterone in postmenopausal estrogen-replete women in specific cases and with clear guidelines (see Basson, Wierman, van Lankveld, & Brotto, 2010, for more information).

Selective Tissue Estrogenic Activity Regulator: Tibolone

Available in 90 countries (but not in North America), tibolone is a 19-nor testosterone derivative and a selective tissue estrogenic activity regulator (STEAR) that is metabolized into metabolites with estrogenic, progestagenic, and androgenic properties. Tibolone therapy has shown increases in sexual desire, frequency of arousability, sexual fantasies, and vaginal lubrication versus placebo (Laan, van Lunsen, & Everaerd, 2001). In two studies without a placebo control group, women receiving either tibolone or two different estrogen–progesterone preparations (Nijland et al., 2008; Uygur, Yeşildaglar, & Erkaya, 2005) showed an overall improvement in sexual function. Tibolone has been found to increase the risk of recurrence of breast cancer (Kenemans et al., 2009) and the risk of stroke in older women (60–85 years; Cummings et al., 2008). Its efficacy and safety in women with SIAD is unknown.

Hormone Precursor Replacement Therapy: DHEA

A recent comprehensive review on the use of systemic dehydroepiandrosterone (DHEA) has found no convincing data to support its use to improve sexual function, with contradictory findings regarding its safety. However, vaginal application of DHEA for postmenopausal vaginal atrophy significantly improves sexual desire/interest, sexual arousal, orgasm, and pain (Labrie et al., 2009a, 2009b). This effect is attributed to the tissue local conversion of DHEA into androgens as well as estrogens, possibly exerting benefits on all the three layers of the vaginal wall, and does not significantly increase serum levels of these hormones. This may be especially beneficial for women in whom the use of estrogen is contraindicated. More information on the use of vaginal DHEA is warranted, particularly in women with SIAD.

Centrally Acting Investigational Medications for Low Desire/Arousal

Centrally acting medications to improve sexual desire remain strictly off-label, and their efficacy and safety in women with SIAD is unknown. However, there is limited evidence for the beneficial effects of buproprion (a norepinephrine and dopamine reuptake inhibitor); intranasal bremelanotide (an alpha-melanocyte-stimulating hormone analogue), though there have been concerns about cardiovascular side effects; apomorphine (a dopaminergic agent), though it had a high incidence of side effects; and flibanserin (a 5-HT_{1A} receptor agonist, 5-HT_{2A} receptor antagonist, and dopamine D4 receptor partial agonist).

Peripherally Acting Investigational Medications for Low Desire/Arousal

Pharmacological agents that target genital congestion may not be clinically relevant given that most women who present for treatment because of sexual interest or arousal concerns have normal genital congestion when measured in the laboratory. If difficulties with genital sexual sensations predominate the clinical picture and/or if the genital arousal response is related to spinal cord injury or diabetes, sildenafil may be considered (see Brotto et al., 2010, for review). Although a number of other peripherally acting agents have been tested in controlled trials, findings have not been conclusive, and, as such, they are not considered frontline treatments for sexual interest/arousal concerns.

Taken together, the literature reviewed suggests there is much work to be done in terms of evaluating treatments for women with SIAD. The algorithm in Figure 1.1 suggests that if medically indicated, pharmaceutical treatment may be useful, though the clinician must bear in mind that their use remains off-label. Although nonpharmacological treatments such as sensate focus, CBT, and mindfulness skills have a long history, evidence of their efficacy in the scientific literature is minimal. Nonetheless, we advocate a stepwise treatment plan that includes psychoeducation and clarification of myths early on, followed by more concentrated couple and/or individual therapy at subsequent stages. If lack of motivation/incentives for sex, difficulties with effective stimuli, or a problematic context are contributing to the SIAD symptoms, we advocate strongly for involvement of the partner in therapy.

Although a multidisciplinary treatment team may be warranted in some cases (particularly if there are biomedical contributors such as significant endocrine disorder, genital pain affecting desire/arousal, or medical disease affecting response, such as spinal cord disease or multiple sclerosis), our experience is that this is not necessary for the successful treatment of SIAD. We do, however, believe that sex therapy plays an important role in treatment, and this may be delivered by a skilled practitioner in any of the fields known to interact with women with sexual concerns (e.g., psychology, psychiatry, family medicine, gynecology, social work, nursing).

CASE DISCUSSION: MINDFULNESS-BASED COGNITIVE THERAPY IN THE TREATMENT OF SIAD

Patricia was a 48-year-old full-time teacher, married to Edward, a hospital administrator, and they had one child together. Patricia had been married previously and had one adult child from that relationship. They presented for treatment after struggling with discrepant desire in their relationship for the full duration of their 15-year marriage. She reported having had a very low interest in sexual activity for her entire life and rarely experienced any erotic thoughts. She did not initiate sexual activity with Edward but responded to his attempts to initiate approximately 50% of the time. In the past 5 years, however, Edward initiated sex less and less frequently, as he perceived Patricia's lack of receptivity as a personal rejection. She had difficulty identifying any triggers for her sexual desire or response, though she did describe sexual activity with him as enjoyable once she was able to relax and focus on the present moment, which occurred only very rarely. Sex was occasionally painful due to lack of lubrication, and she could not identify nongenital signs of arousal within her body. She struggled with a lifelong history of anxiety—particularly centered around a fear of negative evaluation—and she experienced physical symptoms of anxiety during stressful situations daily. She also had a more generalized difficulty in identifying positive emotions and struggled when trying to label her mood during positive events. Patricia was otherwise healthy, perimenopausal, and not taking any medications. During her individual interview Patricia noted that she occasionally masturbates, mostly as a method of stress reduction. However, Edward was unaware of this, as she worried that he might perceive her interest in masturbation as indicating that she specifically was not interested in sex with him. She and Edward were in a loving and mutually respectful relationship and were clearly very committed to one another. In his individual assessment, however, Edward declared that he could not envision himself remaining in this relationship if Patricia's sexual difficulties did not improve.

Because Patricia had reduced interest in sex and an absence of erotic thoughts/fantasies, rejected Edward's sexual invitations, and displayed a lack of sexual response to cues that would normally elicit desire and a lack of physical signs of excitement, she met diagnostic criteria for SIAD. A physical examination revealed signs of vulvar-vaginal atrophy, and Patricia was prescribed a topical estrogen, which, over a period of weeks, restored some positive genital sensation.

The entire first treatment session was spent providing psychoeducation and describing the circular model of sexual response, as well as principles of incentive motivation theory. Patricia acknowledged that she was not completely aware of what "turned her on," and she expressed discomfort about communicating to Edward the particular touches and stimuli that she found arousing. As a result, her motivations for sex stemmed primarily from a need to keep Edward happy, even though she derived no personal satisfaction out of sex. Early sessions focused on exploring possible positive incentives to engage in sex. Although Patricia would accept that sex was probably good for her relationship, she also maintained that because the rest of their nonsexual relationship was very rewarding, she was not as motivated as Edward to work on improving her desire. Moreover, because she had never experienced a pronounced sexual response or sexual pleasure in the past, Patricia felt as if she was in pursuit of something she had no personal experience with. Indeed, the lifelong nature of her symptoms posed a challenge to our treatment. Some cognitive challenging of fixed beliefs, such as "It is inappropriate to share with Edward my sexual wants" and "Every time Edward touches me, he is communicating to me that he only wants sex" was useful early in the therapy process.

Patricia was introduced to mindfulness skills, initially for up to 10 minutes in session and subsequently 30 minutes' daily practice of the body scan at home. She was encouraged to suspend any attachment toward needing to "be fixed" but, rather, to be with her moment-to-moment sensations. After a period of weeks, this allowed Patricia to begin to identify body sensations that were experienced as positive, and her practice also allowed her to explore her anxiety more fully in a compassionate and nonjudgmental manner. She learned that from her earliest interactions, sex had been quite stressful for her, due to having partners who blamed her for not reaching orgasm. Her more general restricted range of emotions stemmed from an emotionally invalidating environment as a child, combined with extreme pressure placed on her to excel in competitive swimming throughout her childhood and adolescence. Patricia was then introduced to mindfulness-of-thoughts skills, in which she was able to view her worries as "mental events," and she began to identify bodily sensations that accompanied these mental events. After a few months of daily mindfulness practice, Patricia began to explore the use of mindfulness during solo sexual activity. She would place her hand on different parts of her body and then fully attend to any resulting sensations without judgment. The exercises became gradually more sexual. She started to experience some pleasure during the exercises and could guide her mind fully to the present. Distractions could fade into the background landscape and were no longer seen as an impediment to being sexual. The exercises were then generalized to partnered sexual activity with Edward, during which Patricia learned to accept her state of sexual neutrality at the beginning of sexual interactions but then welcomed her responses as the encounter ensued. Edward responded positively to Patricia's newfound response and therefore began to initiate non-intercourse sexual encounters more often. The introduction of sensate-focus exercises then encouraged Patricia to verbalize what she experienced as pleasurable to Edward. By the end of 1 year of treatment, Patricia felt that she had gained some interest in sexual activity, was fully aware of the responsive nature of her sexual desire, and found their sexual interactions to be pleasurable. There was ongoing work to do in terms of her own generalized anxiety and fear of negative evaluation, though Patricia felt that the mindfulness skills learned in sex therapy had a positive effect on her mental well-being and self-esteem more generally. During the next stage of therapy, the couple and therapist focused on exploring varied forms of sexual stimuli that might effectively elicit Patricia's sexual interest and arousal. Patricia's more generalized anxiety was an obstacle at times to exploring new triggers, and this was addressed through a combination of mindful self-compassion, as well as gentle probing of her articulated thought biases.

CONCLUSIONS

Because SIAD is a new disorder in DSM-5, empirical research testing the reliability and validity of this condition has not yet been carried out. However, on the basis of long-standing concerns about the reliance on Masters and Johnson's sex response cycle to categorize and define sexual desire and arousal complaints, this new diagnosis offers an alternative conceptualization that is based on an incentive motivation model and the concept of responsive sexual desire. Insufficient evidence exists to suggest that SIAD applies as well to men as it does to women. Compared with research on men's sexual difficulties, there is still much that is unknown about effective treatments for women's sexual interest/arousal difficulties, and psychological treatment outcome studies are rare. As the race continues to identify an effective and safe pharmaceutical treatment for women's sexual difficulties, the diagnosis of SIAD offers researchers and clinicians an opportunity to evaluate broader domains of the sexual motivation construct, which takes into account the observation of wide individual differences in how desire is experienced and expressed.

REFERENCES

American Psychiatric Association. (2000). *Diagnostic and statistical manual of mental disorders* (4th ed., text rev.). Washington, DC: Author.

American Psychiatric Association. (2013). *Diagnostic and statistical manual of mental disorders* (5th ed.). Arlington, VA: Author.

Avis, M. E., Stellato, R., Crawford, S. L., Johannes, C. B., & Longcope, C. (2000). Is there an association between menopause status and sexual functioning? *Menopause, 7*(5), 297–309.

Barlow, D. H. (1986). Causes of sexual dysfunction: The role of anxiety and cognitive interference. *Journal of Consulting and Clinical Psychology, 54*(2), 140–148.

Basson, R. (2002a). A model of women's sexual arousal. *Journal of Sex and Marital Therapy, 28*(3), 1–10.

Basson, R. (2002b). Rethinking low sexual desire in women. *British Journal of Obstetrics and Gynecology, 109*(4), 357–363.

Basson, R., Brotto, L. A., Petkau, J. A., & Labrie, F. (2010). Role of androgens in women's sexual dysfunction. *Menopause, 17*(5), 962–971.

Basson, R., Wierman, M. E., van Lankveld, J., & Brotto, L. A. (2010). Summary of the recommendations on sexual dysfunctions in women. *Journal of Sexual Medicine, 7*(1), 314–326.

Baumeister, R. F., Catanese, K. R., & Vohs, K. D. (2001). Is there a gender difference in strength of sex drive?: Theoretical views, conceptual distinctions, and a review of relevant evidence. *Personality and Social Psychology Review, 5*(3), 242–273.

BioSante Pharmaceuticals. (2012). *LibiGel.* Retrieved May 1, 2012, from *www.biosantepharma.com/libigel.php.*

Boul, L., Hallam-Jones, R., & Wylie, K. R. (2009). Sexual pleasure and motivation. *Journal of Sex and Marital Therapy, 35*(1), 25–39.

Bradford, A., & Meston, C. M. (2009). Placebo response in the treatment of women's sexual dysfunctions: A review and commentary. *Journal of Sex and Marital Therapy, 35*(3), 164–181.

Brotto, L. A. (2010). The DSM diagnostic criteria for hypoactive sexual desire disorder in women. *Archives of Sexual Behavior, 39*(2), 221–239.

Brotto, L. A., Bitzer, J., Laan, E., Leiblum, S., & Luria, M. (2010). Women's sexual desire and arousal disorders. *Journal of Sexual Medicine, 7*, 586–614.

Brotto, L. A., Graham, C. A., Binik, Y. M., Segraves, R. T., & Zucker, K. J. (2011). Should sexual desire and arousal disorders in women be merged?: A response to DeRogatis, Clayton, Rosen, Sand, and Pyke (2010). *Archives of Sexual Behavior, 40*, 221–225.

Brotto, L. A., & Heiman, J. R. (2007). Mindfulness in sex therapy: Applications for women with sexual difficulties following gynecologic cancer. *Sexual and Relationship Therapy, 22*(1), 3–11.

Burrows, L. J., Basha, M., & Goldstein, A. T. (2012). The effects of hormonal contraceptives on female sexuality: A review. *Journal of Sexual Medicine, 9*, 2213–2223.

Cain, V. S., Johannes, C. B., Avis, N. E., Mohr, B., Schocken, M., Skurnick, J., et al. (2003). Sexual functioning and practices in a multi-ethnic study of midlife women: Baseline results from SWAN. *Journal of Sex Research, 40*(3), 266–276.

Caruso, S., Agnello, C., Intelisano, G., Farina, M., Di Mari, L., & Cianci, A. (2004). Placebo-controlled study on efficacy and safety of daily apomorphine sl intake in premenopausal women affected by hypoactive sexual desire disorder and sexual arousal disorder. *Urology, 63*(5), 955–959.

Carvalheira, A. A., Brotto, L. A., & Leal, I. (2010). Women's motivations for sex: Exploring the Diagnostic and Statistical Manual, Fourth Edition, Text Revision criteria for hypoactive sexual desire and female sexual arousal disorders. *Journal of Sexual Medicine, 7*(4), 1454–1463.

Chivers, M. L., Seto, M. C., Lalumière, M. L., Laan, E., & Grimbos, T. (2010). Agreement of self-reported and genital measures of sexual arousal in men and women: A meta-analysis. *Archives of Sexual Behavior, 39*(1), 5–56.

Cummings, S. R., Ettinger, B., Delmas, P. D., Kenemans, P., Stathopoulos, V., Verweij, P., et al. (2008). The effects of tibolone in older postmenopausal women. *New England Journal of Medicine, 359*(7), 697–708.

Davis, S. R., & Braunstein, G. D. (2012). Efficacy and safety of testosterone in the management of hypoactive sexual desire disorder in postmenopausal women. *Journal of Sexual Medicine, 9*, 1134–1148.

Davis, S. R., Guay, A. T., Shifren, J. L., & Mazer, N. A. (2004). Endocrine aspects of female sexual dysfunction. *Journal of Sexual Medicine, 1*(1), 82–86.

Dennerstein, L., Dudley, E., & Burger, H. (2001). Are changes in sexual functioning during midlife due to aging or menopause? *Fertility and Sterility, 76*(3), 456–460.

Freeman, E. W., Sammel, M. D., Lin, H., Gracia, C. R., Pien, G. W., Nelson, D. B., et al. (2007). Symptoms associated with menopausal transition and reproductive hormones in midlife women. *Obstetrics and Gynecology, 110*(2, Pt. 1), 230–240.

Goldfischer, E., Breaux, J., Katz, M., Kaufman, J., Smith, W. B., Kimura, T., et al. (2011). Continued efficacy and safety of flibanserin in premenopausal women with hypoactive sexual desire disorder (HSDD): Results from a randomized withdrawal study. *Journal of Sexual Medicine, 8*, 3160–3172.

Goldhammer, D. L., & McCabe, M. P. (2011). A qualitative exploration of the meaning and experience of sexual desire among partnered women. *Canadian Journal of Human Sexuality, 20*, 19–29.

Graham, C. A. (2010). The DSM diagnostic criteria for female sexual arousal disorder. *Archives of Sexual Behavior, 39*(2), 240–255.

Guthrie, J. R., Dennerstein, L., Taffe, J. R., Lehert, P., & Burger, H. G. (2004). The menopausal transition: A 9–year prospective population-based study. The Melbourne women's midlife health project. *Climacteric, 7*(4), 375–389.

Hayes, R. D., Bennett, C. M., Fairley, C. K., & Dennerstein, L. (2006). What can prevalence studies tell us about female sexual difficulty and dysfunction? *Journal of Sexual Medicine, 3*(4), 589–595.

Kabat-Zinn, J. (1990). *Full catastrophe living: Using the wisdom of your body and mind to face stress, pain, and illness*. New York: Delacorte.

Kaplan, H. S. (1977). Hypoactive sexual desire. *Journal of Sex and Marital Therapy, 3*, 3–9.

Kaplan, H. S. (1979). *Disorders of sexual desire*. New York: Brunner/Mazel.

Kenemans, P., Bundred, N. J., Foidart, J. M., Kubista, E., von Schoultz, B., Sismondi, P., et al. (2009). LIBERATE study group. safety and efficacy of tibolone in breast-cancer patients with vasomotor symptoms: A double-blind, randomised, non-inferiority trial. *Lancet Oncology, 10*(2), 135–146.

Kruger, T. H., Hartmann, U., & Schedlowski, M. (2005). Prolactinergic and dopaminergic mechanisms underlying sexual arousal and orgasm in humans. *World Journal of Urology 23*(2), 130–138.

Laan, E., & Both, S. (2008). What makes women experience desire? *Feminism and Psychology, 18*(4), 505–514.

Laan, E., & Both, S. (2011). Sexual desire and arousal disorders in women. *Advances in Psychosomatic Medicine, 31*, 16–34.

Laan, E., van Lunsen, R. H. W., & Everaerd, W. (2001). The effects of tibolone on vaginal blood flow, sexual desire and arousability in postmenopausal women. *Climacteric, 4*, 28–41.

Labrie, F., Archer, D., Bouchard, C., Fortier, M., Cusan, L., Gomez, J., et al. (2009a). Effect of intravaginal dehydroepiandrosterone (prasterone) on libido and sexual dysfunction in postmenopausal women. *Menopause, 16*(5), 923–931.

Labrie, F., Archer, D., Bouchard, C., Fortier, M., Cusan, L., Gomez, J., et al. (2009b). Serum steroid levels during 12-week intravaginal dehydroepiandrosterone administration. *Menopause, 16*(5), 897–906.

Laumann, E. O., Nicolosi, A., Glasser, D. B., Paik, A., Gingell, C., Moreira, E., et al. (2005). Sexual problems among women and men aged 40–80 years: Prevalence and correlates identified by the Global Study of Sexual Attitudes and Behaviors. *International Journal of Impotence Research, 17*(1), 39–57.

Lief, H. I. (1977). Inhibited sexual desire. *Medical Aspects of Human Sexuality, 7*, 94–95.

Masters, W. H., & Johnson, V. E. (1966). *Human sexual response*. Boston: Little, Brown.

Masters, W. H., & Johnson, V. E. (1970). *Human sexual inadequacy*. Boston: Little, Brown.

McCall, K., & Meston, C. (2006). Cues resulting in desire for sexual activity in women. *Journal of Sexual Medicine, 3*(5), 838–852.

Mercer, C. H., Fenton, K. A., Johnson, A. M., Wellings, K., Macdowall, W., McManus, S., et al. (2003). Sexual function problems and help seeking behavior in Britain: National probability sample survey. *British Medical Journal, 327*, 426–427.

Nijland, E. A., Schultz, W. C. M. W., Nathorst-Boös, J., Helmond, F. A., Van Lunsen, R. H. W., Palacios, S., et al. (2008). Tibolone and transdermal E_2/NETA for the treatment of female sexual dysfunction in naturally menopausal women: Results of a randomized active-controlled trial. *Journal of Sexual Medicine, 5*(3), 646–656.

Nobre, P., & Pinto-Gouveia, J. (2006). Dysfunctional sexual beliefs as vulnerability factors for sexual dysfunction. *Journal of Sex Research, 43*(1), 68–75.

Perel, E. (2006). *Mating in captivity: Reconciling the erotic and the domestic*. New York: HarperCollins.

Pfaus, J. G. (2009). Pathways of sexual desire. *Journal of Sexual Medicine, 6*(6), 1505–1533.

Santoro, N., Torrens, J., Crawford, S., Allsworth, J. E., Finkelstein, J. S., Gold, E. B., et al. (2005). Correlates of circulating androgens in mid-life women: The study of women's health across the nation. *Journal of Clinical Endocrinology and Metabolism, 90*(8), 4836–4845.

Sarrel, P. M. (1990). Sexuality and menopause. *Obstetrics and Gynecology, 75*(4, Suppl.), 26S–30S.

Sherwin, B. B. (1999). Progestogens used in menopause: Side effects, mood and quality of life. *Journal of Reproductive Medicine, 44*(2, Suppl.), 227–232.

Shifren, J. L., Monz, B. U., Russo, P. A., Segreti, A., & Johannes, C. B. (2008). Sexual problems and distress in United States women. *Obstetrics and Gynecology, 112,* 970–978.

Sims, K. A., & Meana, M. (2010). Why did passion wane?: A qualitative study of married women's attributions for declines in sexual desire. *Journal of Sex and Marital Therapy, 36*(4), 360–380.

Tan, O., Bradshaw, K., & Carr, B. R. (2012). Management of vulvovaginal atrophy-related sexual dysfunction in postmenopausal women: An up-to-date review. *Menopause, 19*(1), 109–117.

Tiefer, L. (2001). A new view of women's sexual problems: Why new? Why now? *Journal of Sex Research, 38*(2), 89–96.

Tiefer, L., Hall, M., & Tavris, C. (2002). Beyond dysfunction: A new view of women's sexual problems. *Journal of Sex and Marital Therapy, 28*(Suppl. 1), 225–232.

Toates, F. (2009). An integrative theoretical framework for understanding sexual motivation, arousal, and behavior. *Journal of Sex Research, 46*(2–3), 168–193.

Tungphaisal, S., Chandeying, V., Sutthijumroon, S., Krisanapan, O., & Udomratn, P. (1991). Postmenopausal sexuality in Thai women. *Asia–Oceania Journal of Obstetrics and Gynaecology, 17*(2), 143–146.

Uygur, D., Yeşildaglar, N., & Erkaya, S. (2005). Effect on sexual life: A comparison between tibolone and continuous combined conjugated equine estrogens and medroxyprogesterone acetate. *Gynecological Endocrinology, 20*(4), 209–212.

Witting, K., Santtila, P., Varjonen, M., Jern, P., Johansson, A., von der Pahlen, B., et al. (2008). Female sexual dysfunction, sexual distress, and compatibility with partner. *Journal of Sexual Medicine, 5*(11), 2587–2599.

Woo, J. S. T., Brotto, L. A., & Gorzalka, B. B. (2011). The role of sex guilt in the relationship between culture and women's sexual desire. *Archives of Sexual Behavior, 40*(2), 385–394.

Woo, J. S. T., Morshedian, N., Brotto, L. A., & Gorzalka, B. B. (2012). Sex guilt mediates the relationship between religiosity and sexual desire in East Asian and Euro-Canadian college-aged women. *Archives of Sexual Behavior, 41*(6), 1485–1495.

CHAPTER 2

Hidden Disorder/Hidden Desire

Presentations of Low Sexual Desire in Men

Marta Meana and Eric T. Steiner

"**L**ow sexual desire remains the most mysterious of all the male sexual dysfunctions." With that pronouncement, Meana and Steiner proceed to suggest that the mystery revolves around two common phenomena: low desire being hidden under erectile difficulties or presentaton of low desire hiding actual desire that is being met outside of sex with the primary partner, or simply suppressed. In combination with a lack of evidence-based treatment for male HSDD other than testosterone replacement in hypogonadal men, these hidden aspects make for a significant assessment and treatment challenge. Within a multidisciplinary framework, Meana and Steiner outline approaches to both types of low desire presentations, drawing from "the sex therapy arsenal of cognitive-affective-behavioral and relationship skills-building techniques efficacious with other sexual problems." They also warn against damaging stereotypes about the imperturbability of male sexual desire and urge us to all take a closer look.

Marta Meana, PhD, is Professor of Psychology and Dean of the Honors College, University of Nevada, Las Vegas. She was the President of the Society for Sex Therapy and Research from 2011 to 2013 and an associate editor of the *Archives of Sexual Behavior* from 2010 to 2012. She is the editor of Springer's *Focus on Sexuality Research* book series and the author of over 70 peer-reviewed articles and book chapters.

Eric T. Steiner, PhD, is Assistant Professor of Psychology at National University in San Diego.

In Western culture and much of its academic literature, male sexual desire is assumed to be essentially uncomplicated: a simple biological urge seeking an outlet in a multi-layered social world that can thwart its easy release. Sexual desire in women, on the other hand, is characterized as complex, requiring a long list of arousal contingencies, mostly psychosocial in nature. This polarization is typified by Baumeister's (2000) statement that "women are the creatures of meaning . . . and men are the creatures of biology" (pp. 368–369). Assumptions aside, we know very little about sexual desire in men. In contrast, the past decade has witnessed an explosion of research on the nature of female sexual desire. Fueled by concerns that the high prevalence of low desire in women signaled a problem with existing diagnostic criteria for hypoactive sexual desire disorder (HSDD), theorists and researchers sought to investigate the nuances of women's desire that were unaccounted for therein (Meana, 2010). This effort has expanded our view of female sexual desire, but there has not been a commensurate effort to investigate the sexual desire of men. Some assumptions die hard. Some end up being true.

> That Friday morning, Maggie was delighted when Jason received a text canceling his weekend meeting in Chicago. Although they had not had sex for over a year, Maggie enjoyed her time with Jason and hated when he had business over the weekend. She was sad that he had lost all sexual desire (by his account) but had come to accept it. Both were in late middle age, and Maggie had finally decided that it shouldn't matter that much to her. She started unpacking his carry-on while he talked on the phone downstairs with his associate. Inside she found a box of condoms and Cialis.

Men presenting with low desire for sex as their primary complaint are not very common in clinical practice. Often coaxed into therapy by confused and hurt partners, some men reporting low sexual desire are actually fulfilling their desire in other ways (e.g., masturbation, extramarital affairs, Internet porn, paraphilias). In a considerable number of them, what presents as HSDD may actually be *hidden sexual desire disorder*. Regardless, the scarce data available indicate that the reasons for low sexual desire (with a current partner or anyone else) often involve a complex interaction of biological, psychological, relational, and sociocultural forces.

WHAT'S IN A NAME?:
DEFINING SEXUAL DESIRE PROBLEMS

Individual variation in the desire for sex is large, and one man's perceived low desire may be another's high. Primarily subjective in nature, definitions of desire problems tend to be mostly tautological. Low desire is classified as a sexual dysfunction in the *International Classification of Diseases* (ICD-10;

World Health Organization, 1992) and in the *Diagnostic and Statistical Manual of Mental Disorders* (DSM-IV-TR; American Psychiatric Association, 2000).

There are three criteria for a diagnosis of HSDD in DSM-IV-TR (American Psychiatric Association, 2000). The first requires a deficiency or absence of sexual fantasy and desire for sexual activity. Arguably, the definition of the disorder is no more descriptive than its name. The second criterion requires that there be associated *marked distress or interpersonal conflict*. Although there is controversy as to whether the distress criterion is justified (Althof, 2001), the point is moot from a clinical perspective. Only individuals who are upset or whose partners are upset seek treatment. The third criterion stipulates that low desire *not be better accounted for by a major psychiatric or medical condition, or by substance abuse*. This criterion is also of questionable clinical utility, as medical problems do not preclude the involvement of psychorelational factors amenable to treatment.

The diagnosis of HSDD in DSM-IV-TR is further subtyped as *lifelong or acquired, generalized or situational*, and due to *psychological factors or combined factors*. The lifetime-onset subtype has face validity and can be useful in determining whether the onset of HSDD coincides with potentially related life or health changes that could be targeted for intervention. The other two subtypes are more problematic. It is hard to determine whether low desire is situational or generalized when individuals cannot escape their situation without unacceptable consequences (e.g., a man who has lost desire for his wife but does not find it acceptable to test his desire under other circumstances—masturbation, pornography, or extramarital trysts). Finally, the causal subtype assumes the ability to distinguish psychological causes from physiological ones, a questionable assumption in many cases.

There have been no significant criteria changes for DSM-5 (American Psychiatric Association, 2013) diagnosis of HSDD in men. It is significant, however, that the diagnosis for men has been retained, whereas that for women has been merged with female sexual arousal and included in a new diagnosis called "sexual interest arousal disorder." This development is likely more reflective of the discrepancy in extant research for women and men than of gender differences in desire mechanisms.

REPORTING LOW DESIRE:
PREVALENCE AND ITS CONTINGENCIES

The number of men reporting episodes of low sexual desire is actually substantial; in many surveys it is the most prevalent male sexual complaint. A thoughtful review of epidemiological data, however, requires attention to four important specifiers: age and health complications, the distinction between sexual interest and sexual desire, symptom persistence, and associated distress. In summary, low sexual desire is more common in older men, with surveys that inquire about decreases in sexual *interest* rather than *desire* yielding significantly lower prevalence rates. Reports of low desire/interest also decrease as the persistence bar is raised (i.e., more men report low desire/interest lasting 1 month than 6 or more; lifelong lack of desire appears rare). Finally, associated distress remains largely unknown in men.

Although prevalence rates for low desire across studies have ranged from 0 to 40% depending on sample characteristics and methodology, recent reviews suggest a likely overall prevalence of low desire/interest in men between 15 and 25% (Brotto, 2010; Lewis et al., 2010). The extent to which the rates for low sexual desire/interest or decreases therein capture the prevalence of HSDD is unclear, though, as distress is rarely assessed. Perhaps this is a function of a sister assumption to the one about the imperturbability of male sexual desire—that a man with low desire must necessarily be distressed.

LACK OF TREATMENT SEEKING: WHERE ARE ALL THOSE MEN WITH LOW DESIRE?

The aforementioned prevalence estimates should result in a higher number of consultations than most clinicians report. There are multiple reasons why men may not seek help for perceived low desire. Older men or those with health problems may consider low desire normal under the circumstances. Men may also be hesitant to identify themselves as having a sexual dysfunction, as it impugns their masculinity in a culture that equates the latter with sexual virility. It is also possible that women are not as distressed as are men when partners experience a decrease in sexual desire, resulting in less interpersonal conflict and thus less urgency to seek help than when the woman is the partner lower in desire. The most likely explanation for the low rates of treatment seeking, however, is that men (and the research literature) are more focused on erections than on desire, despite the fact that erectile dysfunction (ED) may often be consequent to low desire. Research articles on erectile versus desire problems in men yield a 30:1 ratio.

COMORBIDITIES: IS IT A PROBLEM OF AROUSAL OR DESIRE? HIS OR THE PARTNER'S?

Sexual dysfunctions tend to co-occur (Fugl-Meyer & Fugl-Meyer, 2002), but clients generally present with the one they assume, accurately or not, to be primary. Despite the fact that both men and women find desire and arousal difficult to distinguish (Janssen, McBride, Yarber, Hill, & Butler, 2008), men are much more likely to present with arousal problems and women with desire concerns (e.g., Kedde, Donker, Leusink, & Kruijer, 2011). HSDD in men may thus often be hidden under ED, although there is very little data on comorbidity. One recent study, however, was successful in distinguishing HSDD in men independent of erectile dysfunction (DeRogatis et al., 2012).

Sexual dysfunctions in men also have a close association with men's perceptions of their partners' function (Lewis et al., 2010). This association can work in at least one of two ways. The partner's sexual dysfunction (e.g., pain with intercourse) can engender a loss of sexual desire in the man. Alternately, individuals with sexual difficulties can end up bonding as the dysfunction in one (e.g., HSDD in the man) happens to be "compatible" with the sexual dysfunction in the other (e.g., avoidance of sex in the partner with dyspareunia). This type of interdependency highlights the importance of treating couples, rather than individuals, whenever possible.

> After 5 weeks of cognitive-behavioral pain management treatment for dyspareunia, Kelly was elated to report that she and her husband, Rob, had had almost pain-free intercourse the night prior. Paradoxically, Rob was less than joyful, despite his apparently deep concern at the start of therapy about her inability to have intercourse. He later disclosed his fear that the near resolution of her problem would shine a spotlight on the fact that he did not really want to have sex very often.

WHY LOW DESIRE?: RISK FACTORS IN THE DEVELOPMENT OF SEXUAL DESIRE PROBLEMS

The interaction of biomedical, cognitive-affective, relational, and sociocultural dimensions is likely in most HSDD presentations. The longer the problem has persisted, the less likely it is that targeting one dimension exclusively will resolve problems in the others. The HSDD may have an originating factor (e.g., hypogonadism), but it may also have an equally powerful maintaining one (e.g., relationship conflict). Thus the simultaneous consideration of all potential risk factors is recommended, while remembering that risk factors are not necessarily causes. There are men in whom many of the following risk factors do not result in HSDD.

Biomedical Risk Factors

Age

Although age is accompanied by physiological changes (e.g., decreases in testosterone), health problems (e.g., neurological, cardiovascular), and medications (e.g., antihypertensives) that are likely to affect sexual function, age is more than a physiological phenomenon. It is also psychological and cultural. Older men are clearly at higher risk for the development of HSDD, but age should be considered holistically, as there are aspects (e.g., attitudes) that may be amenable to cognitive-behavioral intervention.

Hormones

Research on androgen replacement (in hypogonadal men) and suppression (in men with prostate hyperplasia) indicates that the effect of *testosterone* (T) on sexual desire in men is often direct, indirect, and dose-dependent. The administration of T to hypogonadal men generally increases sexual desire; it also results in improvements in mood and energy, which can augment desire (Corona, Rastrelli, Forti, & Maggi, 2011; Khera et al., 2011). However, the relationship between T and sexual function exists only below a certain T threshold (Isidori et al., 2005). The sexual desire levels of men with normal androgen levels do not increase as a function of T administration. T replacement is thus unlikely to be helpful to eugonadal men presenting with low desire. Although no treatment is without risk, the data increasingly indicate that T replacement in hypogonadal men is relatively safe. Some suggest that men on T replacement should follow the same screening recommendations for prostate cancer as those not on T replacement (Corona et al., 2011), whereas others recommend that prostate-specific antigen (PSA) be monitored in men over the age of 40 prior to T replacement and then 3, 6, and 12 months later with yearly screenings if no significant change is detected (Buvat et al., 2010). Rare though they are, chronic elevations of prolactin (PRL) have also been shown to have a negative impact on sexual desire in men, and, more important, they are associated with serious though treatable diseases (Buvat, 2003). Hyperprolactinemia (HPRL) has been linked to pituitary tumors and a variety of medications, including phenothiazines, tricyclic antidepressants, antiemetics, H2 blockers (for gastroesophageal reflux disease), and certain antihypertensives. High levels of *estrogens* and *cortisol* may also be associated with low desire in men, although these are rarely assessed in the first round of tests for what appears to be uncomplicated hypogonadism (Hackett, 2008; Kobori et al., 2009).

Illnesses and Medications

Illnesses that can affect sexual desire are legion, either as a function of pathophysiology or associated psychological effects. Renal failure, cardiovascular diseases, cancer, and substance dependence are among these, as are major depression or anxiety disorders. In addition, medications indicated for these problems can also have sexual side effects. Most commonly associated with low desire are selective serotonin reuptake inhibitors (SSRIs), prescribed primarily for depression and anxiety (Clayton & Balon, 2009).

Developmental and Cognitive-Affective Risk Factors

Psychological factors have been found to be stronger correlates of sexual desire in men than biomedical ones (e.g., Corona et al., 2004). Negative early life experiences (including sexual abuse) can shape attitudes toward sexuality and reactions to sexual difficulties. Family-of-origin messages about sexuality can also leave their mark, not uncommonly in the form of shame (Carvalho & Nobre, 2011). Cognitive interference with desire may consist of complex schema about male sexuality and how it "should" function, as well as more proximate distractions during sexual activity. Carvalho and Nobre (2011) found that lack of erotic thoughts during sex was statistically the strongest predictor of sexual desire in their sample of men. Attentional focus and performance anxiety have long been associated with low desire, although both may be more of an HSDD-maintaining factor than an originating one. Depressive and anxious mood undeniably interferes with desire in the majority of men, although a minority will engage in sexual activity to regulate negative moods (Bancroft et al., 2003). Most studies, however, show that men seeking help for sexual problems have higher levels of depression and anxiety and that depressed men recall the onset of their depression and desire problems to be approximately concurrent (Brotto, 2010).

Relational Risk Factors

Relationship factors feature prominently in men presenting with low desire in the context of a committed relationship (Corona et al., 2004). Lack of attraction to a partner is a difficult risk factor to target clinically. More amenable to intervention are low satisfaction with the quality of partnered sex or relationship conflict. Of particular relevance are lack of communication and intimacy, anger, hostility, dominance, and control in either member of the couple. Desire is often used as currency in maladjusted relationships, making sex the battleground for any number of nonsexual conflicts. Although noxious relationship dynamics are likely to result in sexual problems, the latter also occur in the context of healthy, loving relationships. It is common for desire to decrease over the length of a relationship, for sex to become routine over time, and for life stressors (e.g., parenting, work-related stress, conflicting schedules) to interfere with the vibrancy of sex (Sims & Meana, 2010). Fortunately, these risk factors are also amenable to intervention, and many long-term couples continue to desire each other and enjoy satisfying sex.

Sociocultural Risk Factors

Although most men are exposed to similar sociocultural risk factors, some may be particularly vulnerable to their negative effects. Male sexual socialization in contemporary Western culture sows the seeds for multiple problems by equating masculinity with sexual virility, depicting emotional expression as weak, and sexually objectifying women (Brooks & Elder, 2012). In addition, our culture offers unprecedented anonymous access to sexual stimuli (e.g., Internet pornography) that consist mostly of unrealistic depictions of sexual activity and idealized images of both male and female bodies. Masculinity ideology coupled with the persistent narrowing of what qualifies as sexually attractive provides fertile ground for vulnerable men to develop feelings of sexual inadequacy, to find their partners lacking, and to increasingly turn to sexual gratification that poses no aesthetic or interpersonal challenge.

ASSESSMENT: IS IT HSDD OR *HIDDEN* SEXUAL DESIRE DISORDER?

The assessment of HSDD presentations is optimized by a multidisciplinary strategy that combines (1) medical workups to rule out biomedical factors; (2) medical, developmental, sexual, and relationship history taking; (3) a detailed description of the presenting problem; (4) investigation of comorbid dysfunctions in the man and his partner; (5) an evaluation of the client's current relationship and sexual dynamics therein; and (6) patience for the potential disclosure of sexual secrets (e.g., lack of attraction to partner, extradyadic sexual fulfillment, paraphilias, same-sex preference, gender identity conflict) long after the initial assessment (Levine, Hasan, & Boraz, 2009). The disclosure of sexual secrets can be facilitated by interspersing couple sessions with individual ones, with clear rules about confidentiality.

In addition to the clinical interview, questionnaires can help assess and track treatment progress. The International Index of Erectile Function (IIEF; Rosen, Cappelleri, & Gendrano, 2002) is a validated measure that inquires about erectile function, orgasmic function, sexual desire, intercourse satisfaction, and overall satisfaction. Comorbid sexual dysfunction in a female partner can be assessed with the Female Sexual Function Index (FSFI; Rosen et al., 2000), which yields scores on desire, arousal, lubrication, orgasm, satisfaction, and pain. The Golombok–Rust Inventory of Sexual Satisfaction (GRISS; Rust & Golombok, 2007) has male and female versions that assess the quality of a couple's relationship, sexually and otherwise.

Depending on the medical history and a physician examination, laboratory tests may include fasting glucose and lipids, T (total and free), serum sex hormone-binding globulin, leutinizing hormone (LH), follicle-stimulating hormone (FSH), PRL, and thyroid function. Morning samples are preferred, as T is at its daytime high. Low T with high LH and FSH may indicate hypogonadism, whereas, if all three are low, a pituitary–hypothalamic disturbance (e.g., pituitary tumor) requiring treatment other than T replacement may be the culprit (Segraves & Balon, 2010).

Most cases that present as low desire will fall into one of four categories: (1) HSDD with significant biomedical involvement (e.g., hypogonadism, hyperprolactinemia, medications); (2) HSDD without biomedical involvement; (3) lack of desire for sex with a current partner—sexual desire is being fulfilled otherwise (e.g., masturbation, pornography, extra-marital affairs); (4) lack of desire for sex with a current partner—sexual desire is being suppressed. Teasing these apart can be difficult. Assessing readiness for change using motivational interviewing techniques (e.g, validating the client's reasons for being apprehensive about change, expressing empathy while pointing out discrepancies in the client's position, avoiding argumentation with client and demonstrating an understanding for resistance to change, and supporting self-efficacy while emphasizing that the client gets to choose what she or he wants with no judgment from the therapist) can indicate the presence of sexual secrets, uncover motivation discrepancies within the couple, and help align the pace of treatment to the client's stage of readiness (Miller & Rollnick, 2002).

TREATMENT/MANAGEMENT APPROACHES

The summary of recommendations from the 2009 International Consultation on Sexual Dysfunctions does not offer a differentiated treatment approach for the treatment of HSDD in men (Montorsi et al., 2010). An evidence-based approach to the specific management of sexual desire problems has to necessarily draw on the treatment outcome literature for comorbid dysfunctions (ED) and on nonspecific sex therapy research and clinical experience. As mentioned, there is likely to be a wide diversity in the type and number of influences on the desire of men presenting with HSDD or men in whom HSDD is comorbid with ED. Multidisciplinary assessment will determine the extent of the multidisciplinarity required in treatment, but it is likely that many men will require management on multiple fronts concurrently. Risk factors do not act on desire sequentially, thus their sequential targeting is unlikely to be as effective as a concurrent strategy.

Stage 1: Educate, Reduce Distress, Target Biomedical Influences

Most clients have little understanding of sexual function or ways in which physiology, psychology, relationships, and culture interact to affect it. In addition, there are persistent beliefs that can make men feel inadequate (e.g., they should always be ready for sex), as well as media- and pornography-propagated ideals (e.g., sex should be spontaneous) that are impossible to maintain (Zilbergeld, 1999). Education is the base from which to establish reasonable expectations, set realistic treatment goals, explore treatment options, and target cognitive distortions. Although some distress is necessary for client motivation, distress needs to be targeted early, as it interferes with desire and arousal. Instilling hope, normalizing, helping generate attainable goals focused on satisfaction rather than sexual frequency, and mediating the impact of the problem on the couples' nonsexual relationship can be useful distress-reduction strategies. Targeting biomedical influences will require coordination and collaboration with the appropriate treatment team health professionals.

Testosterone Replacement Therapy

HSDD in men with low testosterone (as a function of age or hypogonadism) is highly responsive to testosterone treatment (Khera et al., 2011). Although there is no definitive level of normal testosterone, there is general agreement that men with morning total testosterone levels consistently below 8 nmol/L (2.3 ng/mL or 230 ng/dL) are likely to benefit from testosterone replacement therapy (TRT). Administering T to men with HSDD who have normal total T levels greater than 12 nmol/L (3.5 ng/mL or 350 ng/dL) will likely have no effect on desire. In men whose total testosterone levels fall between 8 and 12 nmol/L, measuring free T may be helpful, with a lower limit of 225 pmol/L (65 pg/mL) generally accepted (Buvat et al., 2010). Effects appear to be contingent on maintaining a relatively constant blood level of T, which is facilitated by transdermal delivery (gels, patches, subcutaneous pellets). Although these are generally well tolerated and have lower adverse effects than injections or oral delivery methods, a conservative strategy would be to monitor for hepatotoxic T levels and PSA periodically. Men who continue to have erectile problems despite a return of sexual desire after TRT can be considered for combined TRT and phosphodiesterase type 5 (PDE-5) inhibitor therapy (Khera et al., 2011).

Treatment Involving Other Medical Conditions and/or Medications Affecting Desire

In cases of HPRL, treating the primary disorder (e.g., pituitary tumor) or replacing medication that increases PRL are the obvious strategies for the appropriate health professional. In cases of hypothyroidism, restoring thyroid function with medication has been shown to affect desire. If serotonin-acting antidepressants are suspected to be affecting desire, there are treatment options, including switching to antidepressants with fewer sexual side effects (e.g., nefazodone, mirtazapine, and bupropion) or reducing dosages (Segraves & Balon, 2010). For men with low T/hypogonadism and no psychosocial concerns, TRT may be sufficient to restore sexual desire and satisfaction. Recent research showed that TRT also had beneficial effects on couples' overall functioning (Conaglen & Conaglen, 2009). On the other hand, if low desire has been long-standing, it is likely to have left deleterious cognitive, affective, and relational traces that need addressing, even if the sex drive is restored.

Stage 2: Cognitive-Affective-Behavioral Therapy

Although there is precious little HSDD treatment outcome data for either men or women, there is evidence that treatment approaches combining cognitive, emotion-centered, and behavioral strategies, along with relationship skills building, may be effective in helping individuals and couples with difficulties, sexual and otherwise. There are also experienced sex therapists who claim success using any number or combination of the strategies that follow (e.g., Metz & McCarthy, 2010), ideally involving both members of the couple.

Cognitive Refocusing

Identifying and challenging maladaptive thoughts and restrictive sexual scripts that interfere with sexual desire and enjoyment is central. Men may present with an ideal of sex that neither they nor their partners are attaining, resulting in distressing thoughts about oneself, one's partner, and the relationship that can be inhibit desire and arousal. The use of sexual imagery and fantasy are other cognitive strategies commonly reported in the sex therapy literature on desire and arousal. Cognitively refocusing clients on sexual stimuli, either before or during sex, can have significant positive effects. Sexual self-concept is another important cognitive schema that might require intervention in men who have lost a sense of their virility.

Emotional Regulation

Some men and/or their partners will present with high levels of negative emotion about his lack of sexual desire, whereas others will suppress emotion for fear of its effect on the relationship. Neither scenario is helpful to the management of the problem. Developing affective awareness is as important as the modulation of emotions. HSDD cases characterized by emotionally focused coping can result in anger, hostility, and mood disturbances that can entrench the desire difficulty. Helping clients and partners modulate emotional reactivity can reduce stress and help them progress through treatment. Acceptance strategies (such as mindfulness) can be useful in this regard, but also in helping clients live with limitations that may not be within their control. Not all clients will be able to achieve the sexual function they wish they had or to achieve the desires of both partners equally. Learning to accept certain realities can have just as positive an impact as attempts to change what can be modified.

Stimulus Control and Behavioral Activation

By the time couples seek help for desire problems, their sexual interactions have often been disrupted on multiple levels. Sensate focus can act as the proverbial reset button that refocuses the couple on sensuality. Optimizing the timing and context of sexual interactions may seem obvious, but the literature shows that couples with busy lives tend to deprioritize sex and relegate it to contexts within which desire is likely to be low (e.g., at the end of the day when tired). In addition, couples with sexual problems are more likely to make timing errors, as frustration has set in and sexual demands can issue forth thoughtlessly or in anger. Expanding the sexual repertoire can also be helpful to couples whose sex has become mechanistic. The use of erotica can build desire, unless pornography use is one of the reasons underlying the low desire for a partner. Finally, healthy lifestyle changes may be helpful; of particular relevance are reducing stress, increasing exercise, smoking cessation, and decreasing alcohol use.

Relationship Skills-Building

Interventions range from targeting overall relational dynamics to specific directives for communication about sexual preferences. Relational conflict needs to be addressed first, as couples with low levels of trust and respect are unlikely to tolerate behavioral techniques to improve their sex life. Sound conflict resolution strategies revolve around taking responsibility rather than blaming, self-soothing rather than expecting one's partner to reduce one's anxiety, and taking one's ego out of the picture when considering a partner's dilemma (Schnarch, 2003). Disrupting the demand–withdrawal pattern of relating commonly witnessed in the context of HSDD can also be transforming. One partner insists on having his or her "needs" met, and the other reacts to this insistence by withdrawing. The more the latter withdraws, the more the former demands, and vice versa. On a less macro level, increasing affection, reactivating romantic ways of interacting, and enhancing communication skills can all work to build desire.

Can Hidden Sexual Desire Disorder Be Treated?

The strategies in Stage 2 can be applied concurrently with the treatment of biomedical factors or singularly in cases with no biomedical involvement. Things get more complicated if what looked like HSDD is actually lack of sexual desire for the partner or type of sex possible with that partner. A categorical lack of attraction, or even aversion, to a partner is difficult to change, and attempts can be very painful and damaging to both the man and his partner. There are two alternatives in such cases: either the person who is no longer attracted to his or her partner can try to recover that attraction without making the partner go through humiliating hoops, or the painful truth needs to be exposed so that the couple can make a decision. When the man's sexual preferences and/or identity (e.g., paraphilias, gender identity conflict, preference for gender opposite of partner) cannot be encompassed within the existing relationship, a similar, sensitively implemented exposition needs to occur. In these cases, the therapist is likely to be managing the fallout from the disclosure of the hidden desire and helping the couple negotiate a new direction. One exception is infidelity, in which desire may be reinstated if the couple is willing and able to overcome the crisis.

Treatment Summary

In summary, there is very little evidence-based treatment for male HSDD other than the administration of T to hypogonadal men. Treatment strategies are gleaned from a body of primarily clinically informed sex therapy literature that points in certain directions. First, assessment needs to be multidisciplinary so that treatment can be targeted concurrently at all implicated dimensions. Second, long-standing low desire is likely to have generated psychorelational problems not easily resolved by targeting the biomedical problem. Third, we have little choice but to treat nonbiomedical presentations of low desire with the sex therapy arsenal of cognitive-affective-behavioral and relationship skills-building techniques efficacious with other sexual problems. Finally, some presentations of low sexual desire in men may not be HSDD at all but desire that is being fulfilled outside of sex with the current partner. Figure 2.1 presents an assessment and treatment choice algorithm as explicated in this chapter.

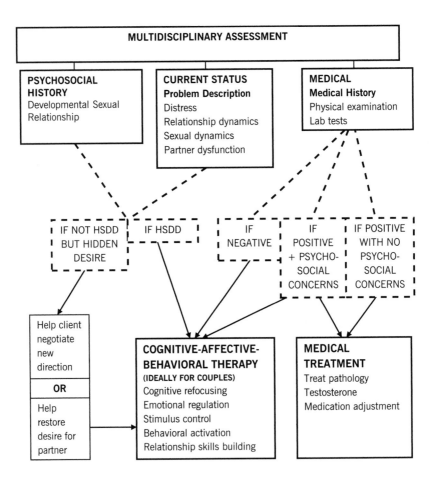

FIGURE 2.1. Presentation of male HSDD treatment algorithm.

CASE DISCUSSIONS

Case 1: The Hope and Hurt in Hidden Sexual Desire

Fifty-year-old Brad was a successful corporate lawyer who had been married to 45-year-old Stacey for 20 years. They had two boys under the age of 10, and Stacey was primarily a stay-at-home mom, although she ran a small landscaping consultant business from their home on a part-time basis. Their relationship appeared to have deteriorated significantly in the past 2 years, and they rarely had sex (she could recall three times in the past year). Stacey did most of the talking during that first session, while Brad insisted that she was exaggerating and that "things aren't that bad." She came across as angry, he as dismissive and annoyed by her. She had dragged him into therapy by threatening to leave if they did not do something to fix their relationship.

The marital conflict purportedly revolved around two issues, interpreted differently by each of them. Stacey complained about Brad's lack of attentiveness to her and their family life and about his lack of sexual desire for her. Brad complained that she was overly demanding and critical but conceded that he had in fact lost sexual desire in general. Brad seemed detached and self-involved, showing very little empathy for Stacey's distress during sessions. He worked long hours and was an avid runner, insisting on covering a large number of miles every day. Between work and the near-obsessive running, very little time was left for Stacey and the boys. Stacey, on the other hand, seemed unable to express anything without a caustic, hypercritical tone and black-and-white judgments. In terms of sexual desire, both agreed that he had close to none, but he refused to consult a physician, as he said he was perfectly healthy and did not want "to mess with hormones." He also denied in an individual session that he was fulfilling his sexual desire in other ways, including masturbation, which he claimed not to have engaged in for months.

Given their high level of relationship conflict, therapy first focused on the relationship, as it was unlikely they would be able to tolerate sex-focused interventions. With the goal of disrupting their maladaptive demand–withdrawal pattern, the therapy worked on shifting their focus from partner blame to personal responsibility for improving their own qualities as partners. Stacey committed herself to the effort and even signed up for anger-management classes at another venue. Brad's behavior-change efforts were more modest, but he appeared relieved at Stacey's diminished demands and calmer demeanor. There was definitely a marked improvement in their relationship. It was time to start addressing his lack of desire.

On the seventh session, Stacey came to therapy alone. She was distraught, and she was excited. They had just left a cinema the night prior when his cell phone rang, and something about the way he turned away from her to talk made her suspicious. Brad broke down and confessed to a 2-year affair with a 25-year-old law clerk, although he swore to end it and begged for forgiveness. She was deeply hurt but, paradoxically, excited to discover that he still had sexual desire that might be redirected toward her. Brad returned to therapy the week after, and Stacey was curiously more focused on reigniting their sex life than on punishing him or dwelling on the affair. In her new language of differentiation, she claimed that "I am owning wanting to stay married to him even if he had an affair, so what's the point of beating him up? It's my choice." Brad appeared somewhat listless but less resistant to therapy than he had been.

Although the infidelity was processed intermittently, they both wanted to focus on their sexual interaction. The expression of affection, sensate focus, romantic activation, and an emphasis on quality time and communication became the primary interventions. Although there was progress, Brad rarely initiated sex and appeared unenthusiastic during sexual encounters. His desire for Stacey was low. Slowly and painfully, she realized that he was no longer attracted to her and that, despite his fears about divorce and not living with his boys, their romance had ended. They decided to part ways. Stacey remained in therapy for another eight sessions to process the damage to her sense of self and to plan her new life. Brad moved in with the law clerk.

Comment

Working hard with a couple through relationship conflict and sexual dynamics only to discover in the end that one person is not attracted to the other is difficult for all involved. We all revel in the mystery of passion and chemical attraction until it results in a very hurt client, in a broken family, and in woefully ineffective therapeutic techniques rendered impotent by the inexplicability of desire. The case of Brad and Stacey reminds therapists that some problems of desire may not be amenable to intervention. On the other hand, cases such as these sometimes yield unexpected results. At the end of therapy, Stacey had become someone much more likely to make good relationship choices and much more likely to succeed in her next relationship. That was not the goal of therapy, but it was a welcome outcome.

Case 2: Love, Desire, and the Prostate

Fifty-four-year-old Charles and Betty had been married for 30 years and had 4 grown children and busy, fulfilling professional lives. Affluent and well known in the community for their charitable work, they were generally considered the perfect couple by all who knew them. The problem was that Charles and Betty had had an almost sexless marriage for the past 5 years, something that Betty had decided was no longer acceptable to her. Charles reluctantly agreed to engage in sex therapy for his lack of sexual desire.

Ten years earlier, Charles had been diagnosed with prostate cancer. Having had both parents die of cancer relatively young, the diagnosis had frightened Charles and sent him into an existential spin as he confronted his mortality. Although the prostate surgery had been successful at extracting the cancer, it had also left him with substantial erectile problems, in addition to a new sense of vulnerability. Papaverine injections made intercourse possible, but he hated injecting himself. Viagra worked but did not produce as rigid an erection as the injections and often left him with a serious headache. Slowly, Charles had started to initiate sex with Betty less frequently and had become less receptive to her advances. By the time they came to therapy, he claimed to feel no sexual desire at all and seemed somewhat hurt at Betty's insistence on restarting their sex life. Betty had been a trouper about the need for injections and Viagra. Neither bothered her, nor did the fact that the erections were never as rigid as they used to be. She felt perfectly comfortable working around all of that. What she could no longer tolerate was his lack of motivation to engage her sexually. The erectile complications and associated accoutrements were not about her; his not wanting to go to the trouble felt like it was.

An exploration of Charles's affect revealed that he had been deeply hurt about Betty's attitude toward the prostate cancer and the impact it had had on his sexual functioning. Charles had thought he might die, and Betty had treated the diagnosis as if it were "no more than a mosquito bite." This had made Charles feel unloved—she had not been there for him emotionally and, even worse, had made him feel like a baby for getting so worked up. When this was followed by Betty's annoyance at his squeamishness over the injections and his focus on his reduced rigidity, Charles was left feeling that Betty cared more about sex than about him. He had in the end lost sexual desire, but it wasn't because he did not find Betty attractive. It was because he needed to feel loved by Betty to feel desire, and he needed to feel manly, which neither Betty's no-nonsense attitude nor his erectile dysfunction made him feel.

Treatment involved building mutual affective awareness, tweaking sexual scripts, and activating different behaviors. Charles and Betty needed to nondefensively hear what each had experienced concerning the cancer threat and subsequent sexual difficulties, as well as what each had intended by their behavior. Betty's nonchalance, though insensitive, was a testament to how much she desired Charles, complications and all. Charles's narrow sexual script about masculinity and idealized sex was also targeted for modification. Finally, therapy focused on expanding their sexual repertoire, making it less penetration/rigidity focused, with an emphasis on sensuality and intimacy. Charles and Betty started having sex again. Their satisfaction was evident in their reports and in the way they related to each other as the therapy was terminated.

Comment

For all we read about love and relationships being central to women's sexual desire, this case illustrates that men's desire can also be deeply affected by relational factors and sexual self-concept. As men age and their desire and erectile function become less automatic, there is a "feminization" of male sexual desire wherein love, intimacy, trust, and self-esteem become increasingly important desire and arousal contingencies. It may be useful to advise women who have always assumed their male partner's desire to be imperturbable not to personalize changes that accompany age and health complications. The case of Charles and Betty also illustrates the primacy of a strong relationship in the prognosis for male HSDD.

The presentation of two cases in which the man had to be talked into therapy for his desire difficulties in no way implies that men with desire difficulties are never motivated to seek help. It illustrates that one of the strongest motivations for men to seek help for desire difficulties is the distress of their partners, much as in the case of women with HSDD (Maserejian et al., 2010).

CONCLUSIONS

Low sexual desire remains the most mysterious of all the male sexual dysfunctions. Rarely a presenting complaint in therapy, it is hard to know how many cases of low desire are hidden under ED complaints, which present primarily to physicians. Cases of PDE5 treatment-resistant ED may in fact be cases wherein desire was the primary problem. In addition, many presentations of male HSDD end up being cases wherein desire is actually intact but not viable within the client's current relationship and/or circumstances. All of this makes the assessment and therapy of male HSDD a tricky affair. The wisest approach is a multidisciplinary one that simultaneously leaves no stone unturned in assessment and throughout therapy (e.g., consideration of a wide variety of desire inhibitors or of alternate sources of sexual fulfillment) while dropping stereotypes about male sexual desire being imperturbable. Much like female sexual desire, male sexual desire is also affected by perceptions of love and trust and safety, increasingly so as men age.

Research is sorely needed for our understanding of sexual desire in men and its disturbances. We know more about ejaculation variations than about the motivational state that drives men to seek out or avoid sexual activity. The focus on physiological arousal has blinded researchers, clinicians, and the public to the fact that desire is an important part of the erection story. Desire is undoubtedly more elusive than erections; it is a construct rather than a measurement of girth. The purely subjective assessment of desire, however, encompasses the complex biological, psychological, relational, and sociocultural universe that makes human sexuality more than a simple drive. We seem to have understood the wisdom of that multidimensionality in our considerations of female sexuality. Although the story may be significantly different for men, it is time that we bring men's sexual desire out from the mechanistic cold into the fold of human complexity.

REFERENCES

Althof, S. (2001). My personal distress over the inclusion of personal distress. *Journal of Sex and Marital Therapy, 27*, 123–125.
American Psychiatric Association. (2000). *Diagnostic and statistical manual of mental disorders* (4th ed., text rev.). Washington, DC: Author.

American Psychiatric Association. (2013). *Diagnostic and statistical manual of mental disorders* (5th ed.). Arlington, VA: Author.

Bancroft, J., Janssen, E., Strong, D., Carnes, L., Vukadinovic, Z., & Long, J. S. (2003). The relation between mood and sexuality in heterosexual men. *Archives of Sexual Behavior, 32,* 217–230.

Baumeister, R. F. (2000). Gender differences in erotic plasticity: The female sex drive as socially flexible and responsive. *Psychological Bulletin, 126,* 347–374.

Brooks, G. R., & Elder, W. B. (2012). Sex therapy for men: Resolving false dichotomies. In P. Kleinplatz (Ed.), *New directions in sex therapy* (pp. 37–50). New York: Routledge.

Brotto, L. A. (2010). The DSM diagnostic criteria for hypoactive sexual desire disorder in men. *Journal of Sexual Medicine, 7,* 2015–2030.

Buvat, J. (2003). Hyperprolactinemia and sexual function in men: A short review. *International Journal of Impotence Research, 15,* 373–377.

Buvat, J., Maggi, M., Gooren, L., Guay, A. T., Kaufman, J., Morgentalier, A., et al. (2010). Endocrine aspects of male sexual dysfunctions. *Journal of Sexual Medicine, 7,* 1627–1656.

Carvalho, J., & Nobre, P. (2011). Predictors of men's sexual desire: The role of psychological, cognitive-emotional, relational, and medical factors. *Journal of Sex Research, 48,* 254–262.

Clayton, A. H., & Balon, R. (2009). The impact of mental illness and psychotropic medications on sexual functioning: The evidence and management. *Journal of Sexual Medicine, 6,* 1200–1211.

Conaglen, J. V., & Conaglen, H. M. (2009). The effect of treating male hypogonadism on couples' sexual desire and function. *Journal of Sexual Medicine, 6,* 456–463.

Corona, G., Mannucci, E., Petrone, L., Giommi, R., Mansani, R., Fei, L., et al. (2004). Psycho-biological correlates of hypoactive sexual desire in patients with erectile dysfunction. *International Journal of Impotence Research, 16,* 275–281.

Corona, G., Rastrelli, G., Forti, G., & Maggi, M. (2011). Update in testosterone therapy for men. *Journal of Sexual Medicine, 8,* 639–654.

DeRogatis, L., Rosen, R. C., Goldstein, I., Werneburg, B., Kempthorne-Rawson, J., & Sand, M. (2012). Characterization of hypoactive sexual desire disorder (HSDD) in men. *Journal of Sexual Medicine, 9,* 812–820.

Fugl-Meyer, A. R., & Fugl-Meyer, K. S. (2002). Sexual disabilities are not singularities. *International Journal of Impotence Research, 14,* 487–493.

Hackett, G. I. (2008). Disorders of male sexual desire. In D. L. Rowland & L. Incrocci (Eds.), *Handbook of sexual and gender identity disorders* (pp. 5–31). Hoboken, NJ: Wiley.

Isidori, A. M., Giannetta, E., Gianfrilli, D., Greco, E. A., Bonifacio, V., Aversa, A., et al. (2005). Effects of testosterone on sexual function in men: Results of a meta-analysis. *Clinical Endocrinology, 63,* 381–394.

Janssen, E., McBride, K. R., Yarber, W., Hill, B. J., & Butler, S. M. (2008). Factors that influence sexual arousal in men: A focus group study. *Archives of Sexual Behavior, 37,* 252–265.

Kedde, H., Donker, G., Leusink, P., & Kruijer, H. (2011). The incidence of sexual dysfunction in patients attending Dutch general practitioners. *International Journal of Sexual Health, 23,* 269–277.

Khera, M., Bhattacharya, R. K., Blick, G., Kushner, H., Nguyen, D., & Miner, M. (2011). Improved sexual function with testosterone replacement therapy in hypogonadal men: Real-world data from the Testim Registry in the United States. *Journal of Sexual Medicine, 8,* 3204–3213.

Kobori, Y., Koh, E., Sugimoto, K., Izumi, K., Narimoto, K., Maeda, Y., et al. (2009). The relationship of serum and salivary cortisol levels to male sexual dysfunction as measured by the International Index of Erectile Dysfunction. *International Journal of Impotence Research, 21,* 207–212.

Levine, S. B., Hasan, S., & Boraz, M. (2009). Male hypoactive sexual desire disorder. In R. Balon & R. T. Segraves (Eds.), *Clinical manual of sexual disorders* (pp. 161–184). Arlington, VA: American Psychiatric Publishing.

Lewis, R. W., Fugl-Meyer, K. S., Corona, G., Hayes, R. D., Laumann, E. O., Moreira, E. D., Jr., et al. (2010). Definitions/epidemiology/risk factors for sexual dysfunction. *Journal of Sexual Medicine, 7,* 1598–1607.

Maserejian, N. N., Parish, S., Shifren, J. L., Huang, L., Gerstenberger, E., & Rosen, R. R. (2010). Healthcare utilization in women diagnosed with hypoactive sexual desire disorder: Interim baseline results from the HSDD registry for women. *Journal of Women's Health, 19,* 2001–2009.

Meana, M. (2010). Elucidating women's (hetero)sexual desire: Definitional challenges and content expansion. *Journal of Sex Research, 47,* 104–122.

Metz, M. E., & McCarthy, B. W. (2010). Male sexuality and couple sexual health: A case illustration. *Journal of Family Psychotherapy, 21,* 197–212.

Miller, W. R., & Rollnick, S. (2002). *Motivational interviewing: Preparing people for change* (2nd ed.). New York: Guilford Press.

Montorsi, F., Adaikan, G., Becher, E., Giuliano, F., Khoury, S., Lue, T. F., et al. (2010). Summary of the recommendations on sexual dysfunctions in men. *Journal of Sexual Medicine, 7,* 3572–3588.

Rosen, R. C., Cappelleri, J. C., & Gendrano, N., III. (2002). The International Index of Erectile Function (IIEF): A state-of-the-science review. *International Journal of Impotence Research, 14,* 226–244.

Rosen, R., Brown, C., Heiman, J., Leiblum, S., Meston, C., Shabsigh, R., et al. (2000). The Female Sexual Function Index (FSFI): A multidimensional self-report instrument for the assessment of female sexual function. *Journal of Sex and Marital Therapy, 26,* 191–208.

Rust, J., & Golombok, S. (2007). *The handbook of the Golombok–Rust Inventory of Sexual Satisfaction (GRISS).* London: Pearson Assessment.

Schnarch, D. M. (2003). *Resurrecting sex: Solving sexual problems and revolutionizing your relationship.* New York: Harper Paperbacks.

Segraves, R. T., & Balon, R. (2010). Recognizing and reversing sexual side effects of medications. In S. B. Levine (Ed.), *Handbook of clinical sexuality for mental health professionals* (2nd ed., pp. 311–328). New York: Routledge.

Sims, K., & Meana, M. (2010). Why did passion wane?: A qualitative study of married women's attributions for declines in sexual desire. *Journal of Sex and Marital Therapy, 36,* 360–380.

World Health Organization. (1992). *Manual of the international statistical classification of diseases, injuries, and causes of death* (10th ed.). Geneva: Author.

Zilbergeld, B. (1999). *The new male sexuality.* New York: Bantam.

CHAPTER 3

Erectile Dysfunction
*Integration of Medical
and Psychological Approaches*

Raymond C. Rosen, Martin M. Miner,
and John P. Wincze

Being unable to get or maintain an erection can have a devastating effect on a man's self-esteem, his relationship, and his overall quality of life. Although the introduction of the PDE5 inhibitors such as Viagra and Cialis have promised a quick and easy cure, the reality is somewhat different. Many men fail to make adequate use of the medication or discontinue its use altogether. This may be true because interpersonal and psychological factors, long thought to be the cornerstone of a diagnosis of erectile dysfunction (ED), are given little attention by family practitioners, who are now the main prescribers of PDE5 medication.

In this chapter, Rosen, Miner, and Wincze advocate for an integrated model of medical and psychosocial interventions with "psychological and sex therapy approaches strongly emphasized." They critically review the available evidence and suggest that an integrated treatment approach is potentially superior to unimodal psychological or biological therapies. Future therapeutic directions that await empirical validation include the potential integration of cardiovascular risk prevention, lifestyle modification, and couple therapy approaches into the treatment for ED. A comprehensive approach of this type is likely to improve treatment adherence and outcome.

Raymond C. Rosen, PhD, is former Co-Director (with Sandra R. Leiblum) of the Sex and Marital Therapy Center of Robert Wood Johnson Medical School and Rutgers University. He also served as Chief Psychologist and Director of the Human Sexuality Program at Robert Wood Johnson Medical School from 1998 to 2006. Dr. Rosen has served as cochair of the first and second International Consultation in Sexual Medicine and also coedited the second and third volumes of *Principles and Practice of Sex Therapy.* He has served as a senior consultant to the U.S. Food and Drug Administration, the National Institutes of Health, other federal agencies, and to the pharmaceutical industry. Dr. Rosen has authored or edited nine books and more than 350 book chapters and peer-reviewed articles and has received multiple grants and awards. He is a member of several professional organizations and serves on the editorial boards of the *Archives of Sexual Behavior, Journal of Sexual Medicine, Menopause, Journal of Men's Health and Gender,* and the *Annual Review of Sex Research.* He is currently Chief Scientist at New England Research Institutes in Watertown, Massachusetts.

Martin M. Miner, MD, is Director of the Men's Health Center of The Miriam Hospital in Providence, Rhode Island, Clinical Associate Professor of Family Medicine and Urology at Warren Alpert Medical School of Brown University, and co-director of the Men's Health Center there. Active on several journal editorial boards, Dr. Miner also serves as a reviewer and has published extensively in the areas of erectile dysfunction, cardiovascular disease, benign prostatic hyperplasia, lower urinary tract symptoms, male sexuality, and hormone therapy for men. He has given numerous presentations in the United States and internationally, is active in several research studies on men's health, and is a consultant to the International Society of Sexual Medicine Consensus Panel.

John P. Wincze, PhD, is Associate Director of the Men's Health Center at The Miriam Hospital in Providence, Rhode Island, and Clinical Professor in the Department of Psychiatry and Human Behavior and in the Department of Psychology at Brown University. He has had more than 35 years of experience in the diagnosis and treatment of sexual problems and has published over 100 research papers, book chapters, and books in the area of sexual behavior. He has served as the head of the Psychology Licensing Board in the State of Rhode Island and is currently an Associate Editor of the *Journal of Sex Research.*

ED is the signature male sexual dysfunction in contemporary society, which has been the focus of intensive scientific and public interest and intense commercial activity over the past two decades. Since the approval in the U.S. of sildenafil (Viagra) in 1998, more than 100 million men worldwide have received prescriptions for phosphodiesterose type 5 (PDE5) inhibitors, countless websites have been disseminated, and an unknown number of men worldwide have been seen by physicians, pharmacists, or other health providers for ED. Defined as the inability to achieve or maintain erection sufficient for sexual activity, ED occurs in approximately 10% of men under 35 years of age and up to 50% or more of men over 60 (Feldman, Goldstein, Hatzichristou, Krane, & McKinlay, 1994; Panser et al., 1995; Rosen et al., 2004). In addition to being age-related, ED is associated with a wide array of medical and psychological risk factors (Feldman et al., 1994; Panser et al., 1995; Hall et al., 2009; Kupelian, Araujo, Chiu, Rosen, & McKinlay, 2010). It can have negative, or even in some cases devastating, effects on self-esteem, quality of life, and the man's partner relationship. Recent epidemiological studies have highlighted the association between ED and the broader indices of cardiovascular health and psychological well-being, suggesting that ED may be a harbinger or early warning marker for cardiovascular disease (CVD) and depression (Araujo et al., 2010; Inman et al., 2009; Kostis, Jackson, Rosen, & the Second Princeton Consensus Panel, 2005). At the same time, the availability of safe and effective oral therapies has led to a historically unprecedented number of men seeking treatment in the past two decades, with largely unknown consequences, positive or negative.

Evidence from epidemiological studies supports at least five broad observations:

1. ED is highly prevalent in aging men, affecting approximately 50% of all men older than 60. For many men, ED manifests first in their 40s and 50s but increases markedly in both prevalence and severity after age 60.
2. The degree of distress or bother associated with ED is inversely related to aging, as men older than 70 typically report a lesser degree of bother than their younger counterparts. This finding is consistent across studies. Consequently, distress and treatment seeking are usually higher in younger and middle-aged men and their partners, who are more likely to seek treatment overall.
3. The prevalence and incidence of ED are highly correlated with the presence of known risk factors and comorbidities. In particular, cardiovascular comorbidities (e.g., hypertension, hypercholesterolemia), diabetes mellitus, and the metabolic syndrome have all been associated with ED in multiple cross-sectional and longitudinal studies. Most recently, depression and lower urinary tract symptoms (LUTS) have been added to the list of significant medical comorbidities and risk factors.
4. Lifestyle factors, including smoking, obesity, and exercise, are also significant predictors of ED.
5. A complex and often interactive set of variables and determinants can lead to ED.

The following case vignette (Case 1) of a middle-aged man with ED and cardiovascular risk factors shows the interactive cycle of causes and consequences of ED in this man. The interaction of psychological causes in a younger man with ED is portrayed in Case 2 later in this chapter.

Case 1: ED in a 49-Year-Old Man

Bill K. was a 49-year-old, married stockbroker with a history of coronary artery disease and recent coronary bypass surgery. He had been married for the past 18 years and reported a satisfying sexual relationship with his wife for most of their relationship. The patient complained of increasing erection difficulties and loss of libido since undergoing coronary bypass surgery 2 years before. He was currently maintained on cholesterol-lowering and antihypertensive medications, in addition to intermittent use of benzodiazepines for anxiety. He reported increasing marital distress and was concerned that his wife might be having an affair with a colleague at work. The patient had experienced moderate success in achieving erection with sildenafil (100 mg) but had not attempted sexual intercourse with his wife for several months. His sexual desire was markedly reduced, and he noted that his wife was avoiding him sexually and emotionally. The patient felt anxious and helpless about his situation.

ED AND THE LINK TO CVD

Common risk factors for atherosclerosis are prevalent in patients with ED, and the risk of ED has been related to the number and severity of risk factors overall (Feldman et al., 1994; Bortolotti, Parazzini, Colli, & Landoni, 1997). In addition, the prevalence of ED is increased in patients with vascular comorbidities such as coronary artery disease (CAD; Solomon et al, 2003b; Kloner et al., 2003; Montorsi et al., 2003; Montorsi, Montorsi, & Schulman, 2003), diabetes (Bortolotti et al., 1997; Gazzaruso et al., 2004), cerebrovascular disease, hypertension, and peripheral arterial disease (Virag, Bouilly, & Frydman, 1985; Burchard et al., 2001). In fact, evidence is accumulating in favor of ED being viewed as a vascular disorder (Thompson et al., 2005; Schouten et al., 2008) or incipient vascular disorder in the majority of clinical patients (Inman et al., 2009; Nehra, Jackson, Miner, Billups, Burnett, et al., 2012).

Additionally, ED and CVD share a similar pathogenic involvement of the nitric oxide pathway leading to impairment of endothelium-dependent vasodilatation (early phase) and structural vascular abnormalities (late phase; Azadzoi & Goldstein, 1992). Thus ED may be considered as the clinical manifestation of a vascular disease affecting the penile circulation; likewise, angina pectoris is the clinical manifestation of a vascular disorder affecting coronary circulation.

Is ED a More Potent Predictor of CVD in the Younger (< Age 60) Male?

The concept of an increased relative cardiovascular burden or risk within patients with ED in the younger age group has been validated in a large Australian study, in which the incidence of atherosclerotic cardiovascular events in men less than 40 years of age with ED was shown to be *more than seven times* the incidence in a reference population representative of the general male population in Western Australia (Chew et al., 2010). Thus ED may be a potential marker for silent cardiovascular risk in younger men (Miner, 2009) and minorities (Billups, Blank, Padma-Nathan, Katz, & Williams, 2005), whose risk may be underestimated by traditional CVD risk factors. Although ED had little relationship to development of incident cardiac events in men age 70 years and older, it was associated with a *nearly 50-fold increase in the 10-year incidence in men 49 years and younger.*

DIAGNOSIS AND CLASSIFICATION OF ED

Diagnosis of ED has historically been based on the self-reported ability of the man to achieve and maintain erection sufficient for sexual performance (Lue et al., 2004; Hatzichristou et al., 2004). The disorder is further classified as organic or psychogenic, based on the presence of specific organic factors, including vascular, hormonal, or neurogenic determinants. If these factors are present to a significant degree, and if the patient's history is suggestive of a temporal association between onset of symptoms and the patient's medical condition, an organic diagnosis is suggested. Psychogenic ED has traditionally been used as a diagnosis of exclusion, which may be given in the absence of specific organic factors.

According to the DSM-5 (American Psychiatric Association, 2013) definition of erectile disorder, at least one of three symptoms (1, marked difficulty obtaining an erection; 2, marked difficulty maintaining an erection; 3, marked decrease in erectile rigidity) must have been present for a minimum duration of approximately 6 months and be expected on all or almost all (approximately 75–100%) occasions of sexual activity.

The third symptom mentioned (decrease in erectile rigidity) is new and has been added to the definition. The rationale provided does not specifically justify the new rigidity criterion, although this has been shown in multiple studies to correlate positively with the ability to achieve or maintain erection sufficient for sexual performance. As previously, DSM-5 recommends that the disorder be specified as lifelong versus acquired or generalized versus situational.

Additionally, it is important to include the presence of other male sexual dysfunction in the diagnosis. For example, recent studies have suggested that up to 30% of men with ED also report symptoms of premature ejaculation (Fisher et al., 2004). Rapid or premature ejaculation may develop as a secondary response to psychogenic ED or may precede the erection difficulty in some cases. In either event, the diagnosis should reflect the presence of concomitant ejaculatory and erection difficulty. In older men, it is not uncommon for men with ED to report loss of orgasm and ejaculation, as well as decreased sexual desire (Rosen et al., 2004). Again, these concomitant or comorbid symptoms of sexual dysfunction should be included in the differential diagnosis.

ETIOLOGY AND ASSESSMENT:
PATIENT EVALUATION IN THE POST-VIAGRA ERA

Along with new treatment approaches for ED, fundamental changes have occurred in the clinical assessment and evaluation of the disorder. Due in large part to the increasing management of ED by primary care physicians, in addition to the widespread use of PDE5 inhibitors, little attention is paid nowadays to taking detailed sexual histories or using specialized diagnostic testing (e.g. nocturnal penile tumescence, penile cavernosography). Medical or psychological testing for ED, once the mainstay of the diagnostic approach, is rarely used in most settings. Instead, focused symptom evaluation, along with the use of brief screening questionnaires, such as the International Index of Erectile Function (IIEF; Rosen et al., 2004), is the preferred approach in most primary care settings. In fact, *self-report of sexual symptoms is the cornerstone of ED assessment at the present time* (Hatzichristou et al., 2004). Although partner assessment is acknowledged as also important in most clinical guidelines and recommendations, partners are seldom included in the clinical evaluation in most medical settings. No studies have been performed on the relative contribution of partner involvement to ED treatment outcome, either.

Given the strong evidence of an association between ED and various medical risk factors (e.g., diabetes, coronary artery disease), recent guidelines have emphasized the importance of a comprehensive medical history and physical examination for all men with ED (Lue et al., 2004). The physical examination also provides an opportunity for patient education and reassurance regarding normal genital anatomy (Lue et al., 2004).

Selective laboratory testing is recommended in all cases. This includes investigation of the hypothalamic–pituitary–gonadal axis via assessment of androgenic status, particularly if sexual desire is reduced. There is disagreement about the relative value of the various testosterone assays, including total, free, and bioavailable testosterone (Qaseem et al., 2009). Standard serum chemistries, complete blood count (CBC), and lipid profiles may be of value and should be obtained if they were not performed in the past year. Finally, a serum prostate-specific antigen (PSA) test should be performed based on the patient's age and relative risk status, and certainly if the clinician suspects hypogonadism.

Specialized diagnostic procedures, such as nocturnal penile tumescence and rigidity (NPTR) testing or other specialized vascular or neurological procedures, may play a role in selected cases. For example, these procedures may be of value in evaluating young patients with pelvic or penile trauma who may be candidates for reconstructive vascular surgery. Patients with complicated diabetes or other endocrinopathies may benefit from further endocrinological studies. Patients with a history of cardiac disease or significant cardiovascular risk factors should be evaluated for potential cardiac risk associated with sexual activity. Consensus guidelines have been established for evaluating cardiac risks associated with sexual activity (DeBusk et al., 2000; Kostis et al., 2005)

Results of the initial evaluation and specialized testing should be carefully reviewed with the patient and the patient's partner, if possible, prior to initiating therapy. Potentially modifiable risk factors, such as cigarette smoking or alcohol abuse, should be addressed. Prescription drugs such as anti-hypertensives or antidepressants may be implicated in the patient's erectile difficulties and should be altered when medically indicated. Patients with specific endocrine deficiencies such as hypogonadism should be placed on hormone replacement therapy prior to initiation of direct therapies for ED. Additionally, sexual problems in the partner, such as a lack of lubrication, hypoactive sexual desire, or dyspareunia (painful intercourse), should be addressed. Patients and partners should be fully informed about the range of treatment options available, and the risks and benefits associated with each should be addressed.

Beyond the standard approach for medical evaluation of ED (Lue et al., 2004), several authors have recommended a combined medical–psychological approach to evaluation in all cases (Weeks & Gambescia, 2000; Wincze & Carey, 2001). An integrated approach to assessment has also been proposed by Althof and colleagues (2005), based on their comprehensive review of psychological and interpersonal factors in ED. Included in their model are the need for assessment of (1) patient factors, such as performance anxiety or sexual inhibition; (2) partner issues, such as low self-esteem or sexual performance problems; (3) quality of the overall relationship; and (4) sexual and contextual variables, such as financial stresses and family dysfunction. Each of these different areas of involvement is illlustrated in the following case study:

Case 2: A High School Student Complains of ED

Carl, at age 16, came to his primary care physician (Miner) complaining of erectile dysfunction. He was accompanied by his mother, who explained to the physician that Carl was very distraught over his problem and desperately wanted help. Carl stated that he had never had sexual relations with a girl but he knew that he had an erection problem because he was not getting erections "like [his] friends talked about." Also, he denied having any morning or nighttime erections, and he stated that during masturbation his erections were not as hard as they should be, although he was achieving orgasm and ejaculation. He stated that he had strong sexual desire for girls and had engaged in "heavy petting" but did not get firm erections.

In order to rule out any possible organic etiology contributing to Carl's erection problems, a number of tests were performed, including: hormone evaluation (total serum testosterone and bioavailable serum testosterone), doppler duplex ultrasound, and nocturnal penile tumescence (NPT). Carl was not taking any medications, and he was not being treated for any medical or psychological problems. All test results were in the normal range, and Carl was informed that his problem was most likely due to performance anxiety; he was referred to a clinical psychologist (Wincze). He was prescribed Cialis to help him when he got involved with another partner. It was explained that the Cialis could be used to help build his confidence but that it was not intended as a long-term solution.

Carl was seen alone for the psychological evaluation. He denied any past sexual abuse or trauma, but he stated that there was considerable tension in his home due to conflicts between his parents, who were planning to divorce. He denied any suicidal plans, but he stated that if his problem did not improve, he did not want to go through life not able to function with a girl. He denied any same-sex attractions and stated that he had had a number of sexual experiences with girls but would not let them touch his penis because he was too fearful that he would not get an erection.

The phenomenon of "performance anxiety" was explained to Carl, and it was emphasized that this was a common occurrence for males and that males of all ages could experience sexual problems. Carl did not have a girlfriend at the time he was seen; so it was explained to Carl that he should not avoid going out with girls but that he should look for girls whose personalities seemed very "easygoing." Carl was a good-looking boy who was athletic, and he felt he would have no trouble meeting girls who might be interested in him. It was also suggested that he should not get involved sexually with a girl until he felt very comfortable with her. The therapy plan was to continue meeting with Carl for support, and he was also encouraged to call for an appointment when he had questions or when he met a new girlfriend.

Carl was seen 2 weeks after his initial appointment, but he then missed a follow-up appointment and stopped attending therapy. Two years later (at age 18) Carl contacted the clinic again and was again complaining of erectile dysfunction. He was accompanied to the clinic by his mother, and he wanted his mother to attend the therapy session with him. His mother, who is a professional educator, was very concerned about Carl's frustration and anger over his problem. She explained that following his work-up 2 years previously, he had insisted on being brought to another physician for another evaluation. The results of this second evaluation also pointed to a psychogenic origin for Carl's erection difficulties. Carl was discouraged and did not want further help until more recently. Following this initial input from Carl's mother, she excused herself, and Carl was seen alone the remainder of the session.

Carl explained that he did have a steady girlfriend whom he had been going out with for over a year. They were sexual, and they were having intercourse. Carl said that his girlfriend was happy with their sexual relationship, but he felt his penis wasn't as hard as it should be and he did lose his erection on some occasions. He was very insistent that he had "tried everything" and "nothing worked." He did not want therapy; what he wanted was vasoactive injections. He had been given vasoactive injections as part of his medical work-up and he felt that this was the only solution.

Upon further questioning about what he felt might have caused the problem in the first place, he said, "I caused it myself by jelqing." He continued to explain that he felt that he had a small penis and he wanted to increase its size, so, he explored the Internet and found the "Jelqing" technique. In applying this technique to stretch his penis, he felt that he irreparably damaged his penis, which caused his erection difficulties. Following this disclosure, he agreed to continue in therapy to explore ways to address his problem.

Comment

This case illustrates that extreme concern over erectile functioning can occur at any age. Also, this case, as well as many more we have treated, illustrates the intensity with which an individual can hold onto a belief even in the face of contradicting evidence. In addition to the false belief about the etiology of his problem, Carl endorsed many other false beliefs about sexual functioning. He believed that a male should automatically obtain a full erection whenever he sees an attractive female, and he believed that a male should always be interested in sex.

When Carl initially came to the clinic for evaluation at age 16, he did not have a sexual partner. Because the therapy strategy to resolve an ED problem is greatly facilitated with the involvement of a supportive and informed partner, males presenting without partners are at a disadvantage. Nonetheless, even without a partner, specific issues and strategies can be addressed to better equip a male to resolve his problem. For example, addressing the following areas is helpful: common sexual misunderstandings, accurate and normative sexual information, performance anxiety, and selecting a compatible sexual partner.

In Carl's case, he was harboring a belief that he found very shameful; namely, that he had caused irreparable damage to himself by practicing "jelqing." The doctor's medical findings that there was nothing physically wrong with him were dismissed by Carl because "he knew what he had done to himself." His shame prevented him from sharing his secret with the doctors or with his mother. His shame and anxiety related to his sexual problem were no doubt exacerbated by his teenage insecurity and fear of peer ostracization if others should find out. When he finally revealed his secret, he put therapy in a position to address all of the issues contributing to his sexual problem.

CURRENT MEDICAL MANAGEMENT OF ED

Major changes have taken place in the assessment and treatment of ED since approval of sildenafil (Viagra) and two other PDE5 inhibitors, tadalafil and vardenafil (Cialis, Levitra), since 1998 (Rosen & McKenna, 2002; Rosen, 2005). The approval and availability of these three landmark drugs has greatly increased the number of men seeking treatment for ED and has significantly altered the medical and psychological management of the disorder.

Historically within the province of urologists and sex therapists, ED is now managed predominantly by primary care practitioners. Costly and potentially invasive diagnostic procedures such as penile cavernosography or caverno-sometry, once the mainstay of urological assessment of ED, are seldom performed nowadays. New management guidelines emphasize the need for a brief sexual and medical history and a focal physical examination. In reality, many middle-aged men with ED receive prescriptions for Viagra, Cialis, or Levitra with little or no medical or psychological evaluation. Further diagnostic studies are usually reserved for those patients who fail to respond to an initial trial of a PDE5 inhibitor (Lue et al., 2004).

Despite these important benefits, some disadvantages and risks associated with the widespread use of sildenafil have been identified. Although PDE5 inhibitors are generally safe and well tolerated, there may be specific medical risks for selected subpopulations. For example, concomitant nitrate use is a strong contraindication for all three current PDE5 inhibitors. Patients with high-risk cardiac conditions (e.g., unstable angina, recent myocardial infarction) may be at risk for sexual activity, although PDE5 use per se is not contraindicated in these patients (DeBusk et al., 2000; Kostis et al., 2005). Patients with sickle-cell disease or those using other erectogenic agents (e.g., intracorporal injections) may be at risk for priapism. Due to sildenafil's effects on phosphodiesterase enzymes in the eye, patients with opthalmological disorders (e.g., retinitis pigmentosa or nonarteric anterior ischemic optic neuropathy [NAION]) should be carefully evaluated prior to treatment with PDE5 inhibitors.

Although all three PDE5 inhibitors are effective in restoring erections in about 75% of men who use the drugs, differences have been observed in patient preferences or the pattern of side effects associated with the drugs. Some studies have suggested that sildenafil (Viagra) or vardenafil (Levitra) may be associated with a firmer or more satisfying erection, whereas other studies have suggested that tadalafil (Cialis) is preferred by many patients due to the longer lasting effects of the drug. One recent study, in particular, showed that the majority of patients preferred tadalafil due to the increased sense of spontaneity and reduced time pressure with this drug compared with sildenafil. Further studies are needed to confirm this finding.

Psychological Factors

Despite the efficacy and overall safety of PDE5 inhibitors (Padma-Nathan, 2003; Rosen & McKenna, 2002), increasing evidence suggests that a substantial proportion of men with ED discontinue treatment or fail to seek help. A recent large-scale, multinational study of more than 25,000 men in eight countries found that 58% of men with erection problems had discussed their problems with health professionals, although less than half of these men received prescriptions for sildenafil or other medication, and only 16% were continuing to use the drugs at the time of the study (Rosen et al., 2004). Multiple reasons were cited for the high rate of discontinuation, including lack of education or counseling from physicians, fear of side effects, partner concerns, and distrust of medications. Failed expectations may be another important reason for patient dropout from medical therapy, as many men or their partners are disappointed at the lack of change in the quality of the sexual relationship. For these reasons, the importance of combined medical and psychological treatment approaches has been emphasized.

Leiblum (2002), Perelman (2005), and others have noted additionally that success rates with PDE5 inhibitors may be significantly lower in couples who have experienced chronic sexual or marital conflict, lack of desire in one or both partners, or significant psychiatric illness in either partner. These individuals are generally excluded from clinical trials of sildenafil, and the efficacy of the drug in such cases is essentially unknown. PDE5s may also lose efficacy over time because of other factors, such as progression of the underlying disease state or development of tolerance to the pharmacological effects of the drug (El-Galley, Rutland, Talic, Keane, & Clark, 2001). Systematic trials of combination drug and sex therapy have not been performed to date. Despite their overall effectiveness in restoring erectile function for many men, PDE5 inhibitors should not be regarded as a panacea or "magic bullet" for achieving sexual happiness.

Whereas current management guidelines recommend sex or marital therapy (Althof et al., 2005; Lue et al., 2004) or the use of vacuum constriction devices (VCDs) as alternative first-line therapies, these are far less widely used at present than medications. The simplicity and ease of use of an oral medication are major advantages, particularly for primary care physicians with little training or interest in the management of sexual dysfunction. Referral to a sex therapist or mental health professional is only likely to occur when requested, when couples or psychological issues present a major obstacle to treatment, or when oral medications fail. Referrals for other urological treatments (e.g., intracorporal injection, penile implant surgery) are similarly reserved mostly for oral therapy failures nowadays.

PSYCHOSOCIAL ASSESSMENT
AND SEX THERAPY APPROACHES

The specific psychosocial therapy approach for ED is dependent on an understanding of all medical and nonmedical contributions to the problem. It is not a matter of which psychosocial therapy is most effective for treating ED, but rather it is a matter of which approach or approaches are most suitable for addressing the mosaic of contributions to a man's ED problem. The specific nonmedical approach, therefore, is dependent on a comprehensive assessment that identifies all factors contributing to the problem. Although a single factor may loom as the most likely contributor, more often than not there are two or more factors that may be contributing to a man's erection problem. In assessing ED, it is also especially important to identify the time line of the problem and consider *predisposing, precipitating,* and *maintaining* factors. Treatment may need to address all of the time-line factors or only one. For example, a precipitating factor for ED may have been a drinking experience, but the maintaining factor to be addressed is the performance anxiety.

The following model offers a conceptual strategy for a comprehensive assessment of all potential psychosocial contributions to ED. The model emphasizes a detailed consideration of three psychosocial areas: (1) self, (2) relationship/partner, and (3) environment.

The Assessment Model

Self

The self refers to all of the possible individual factors that a man experiencing ED is contributing to his sexual problem. Self-factors are considered separately from relationship/partner factors and environmental factors. In any of the three areas, there may be more than one factor contributing to the ED.

PERFORMANCE ANXIETY

Performance anxiety is the most common psychosocial factor and is inherent in most cases of ED. This term simply means a focus on performance rather than on the ongoing pleasure of sex. Because a man's penis (either flaccid or erect) is visible to both the man and his partner, the occurrence of an erection or lack of an erection is a known event. This increases the focus on performance for, men in a unique way that female partners do not usually experience. The word *anxiety* in this context is somewhat misleading. Early work that looked at anxiety and sexual arousal in women (Hoon, Wincze, & Hoon, 1977) and the subsequent work of Barlow and his associates with men (Barlow, Sakheim, & Beck, 1983; Cranston-Cuebas & Barlow, 1990) suggest that physiological concomitants of anxiety may be less important than the effects of performance demand or cognitive distraction.

Most men experiencing ED can readily identify the presence of performance anxiety. The assessment of performance anxiety is confirmed clinically if men are able to obtain erections under nonperformance situations such as during private masturbation to erotic stimulation, during sleep (confirmed by RigiScan assessment if a man is unaware of nocturnal erections), or during nondemand situations, such as when a female partner is menstruating and states she does not want intercourse. Men experiencing performance anxiety will report a focus on erections and a worry about erections during sexual activity; also, there is often a frequent visual or tactile checking of the penis.

COMORBID DISORDERS

Major mental health disorders such as depression, generalized anxiety, obsessive–compulsive disorder, posttraumatic stress disorder, and substance abuse may be so severe that the mere presence of these disorders may not only contribute to the ED but interfere with any therapeutic attempts to treat the ED. In most cases of ED, when a severe comorbid mental health disorder is present, therapy must first address the comorbid disorder before addressing the ED.

HISTORY OF NEGATIVE SEXUAL MESSAGES

In some men, ED is associated with a history of powerful negative sexual messages generated by family, culture, or religion. When this factor is present, men will experience a flood of guilt or negative thoughts associated with sexual activity that counteracts any positive sexual expression and leads to ED.

SEXUAL ABUSE OR TRAUMA

Men with a history of sexual or nonsexual trauma and abuse frequently present with loss of desire and/or difficulties in sexual performance. The degree of impairment varies widely depending on the extent and duration of the abuse.

GENDER IDENTITY, SEXUAL ORIENTATION, AND PARAPHILIA PROBLEMS

It is not unusual for some men to enter into sexual partnerships because of family expectations or social pressures in spite of a history of gender dysphoria, sexual orientation questions, or paraphilic desires. The rationalization is often that, once partnered, everything will work out. In fact, initial sexual relations in such cases often do work out (perhaps because novelty often contributes positively to sexual arousal), but, in long-term partnerships, ED may be subsequently experienced. In some cases, partners may initially accommodate a paraphilic desire but grow tired of this over time. When sex is attempted without the presence of paraphilic stimulation, ED occurs.

MISINFORMATION AND LACK OF SEXUAL SKILLS

Although there are some men who are sexual athletes, there are also men who are sexually unskilled. Men harboring sexual myths or misinformation who approach sex with an awkward narrow repertoire of sexual behaviors may be prone to ED. Some men, for example, may view foreplay as unnecessary or even as a weakness during sexual activity. Such views may inhibit adequate degrees of erotic input and result in ED. Comprehensive assessment must explore details about sexual behaviors and attitudes in men experiencing ED to identify any possible inhibitory factors.

Relationship/Partner

In many cases of ED, there are significant contributions associated with the dynamics of the relationship or specifically from the partner. In spite of partner-related contributions to ED, the focus of the problem may initially be presented as "the man's problem." When working with couples, assessment should be approached in the spirit of identifying contributions to the problem rather than assigning blame.

COUPLE CONFLICT

Interpersonal and couples issues play a major role in many, if not most, cases of erectile dysfunction. As noted by Masters and Johnson (1970), "there is no such thing as an uninvolved partner in any marriage in which there is some form of sexual inadequacy" (p. 2). Relationship conflicts may be a primary source of the sexual difficulty or may serve to exacerbate or maintain the male's inability to achieve adequate erections. Although the role of relationship factors is widely acknowledged in the clinical literature on the topic (e.g., Masters & Johnson, 1970; Kaplan, 1974; Leiblum & Rosen, 1991), relatively few studies have assessed the relationship between interpersonal distress and treatment outcome for ED. In an early study, sensate focus and graduated sexual stimulation techniques were evaluated in 36 couples presenting for treatment of psychogenic ED (Hawton, Catalan, & Fagg, 1992). The major determinant of treatment outcome in this study was the couples' ratings of marital communication prior to treatment. Couples with higher ratings of marital communication responded more rapidly and with better outcomes to the sex therapy interventions provided.

In addition to the paucity of outcome data, there is a lack of consensus regarding the choice of conceptual framework or intervention strategies for overcoming relationship conflicts in couples with ED. Thus some sex therapists have formulated couples issues from a psychodynamic perspective (e.g., Kaplan, 1974; Scharff, 1988; Levine, 1992); others have provided a cognitive-behavioral perspective (Wincze & Carey, 2001); still others have argued for a family systems approach (Verhulst & Heiman, 1979; LoPiccolo, 1992). This lack of agreement concerning theory and practice of couple therapy has impeded efforts to develop more standardized approaches for dealing with couples issues in ED. Rather, this essential aspect of treatment is often based upon an eclectic array of techniques and interventions.

COUPLE STRESS UNRELATED TO CONFLICT

In some cases, ED may be related to an overwhelming preoccupation with stress in a couple's life. A couple may get along well and love each other but be affected by serious problems, such as job loss, financial worry, a parent's failing health, or children's struggles. Although some couples are able to function sexually in spite of stress in their lives, many couples are not able to do so, and sexual relations end with ED.

LACK OF SEXUAL ATTRACTION TO A PARTNER

In some cases, the presence of ED is directly related to the lack of attraction that a man has toward his partner. The reason may be a history of conflict that has changed a man's perception of his partner, or it may be a partner's physical changes over time. Obesity and lack of personal care on the part of a partner are sometimes present in the dynamics of a couple's relationship as contributors to ED. Because of the sensitive nature of issues related to a partner's appearance, this is often a topic that is not openly discussed. As we discuss later, this is a prime reason that assessment interviews should be conducted separately for the man presenting with ED and his partner.

PARTNER-RELATED SEXUAL AND NONSEXUAL PROBLEMS

Men presenting with ED often ignore or diminish the impact that their partner's problems have on their ED. It is not at all unusual for a man presenting with ED to mention that his partner has never enjoyed sex, has never initiated sex, or has never been comfortable with sex. Although a partner's negative sexual attitude or limited sexual repertoire may not initially contribute to an ED problem, it may do so in the long run. In addition, a partner may have such severe mental health problems that there is an interference with sexual relations. A partner's severe depression, obsessive–compulsive disorder, or substance abuse can definitely inhibit sexual desire and behavior.

Environment

Therapists often make the false assumption that couples are having sex under favorable conditions and rarely ask about the specific environment or conditions under which sex usually occurs. An inquiry about the conditions under which sex occurs may identify interfering factors. Favorable conditions for sex usually include comfort, privacy, and relaxed time.

LACK OF COMFORT

Comfort includes not only the physical comfort of the bed or surface on which sex occurs but the general surroundings as well. Attempted sexual relations in the backseat of a car or in a bed with parents' pictures on the wall have been identified as contributors to ED in some of our patients.

LACK OF PRIVACY

Feelings of a lack of privacy have often been identified as factors contributing to ED in some of our patients. Worries about children or in-laws in the bedroom next door or in the house during sexual activity or worries about pets in the bedroom have all been mentioned as interfering factors. Architectural issues have also been identified in our patients, including lack of doors or glass doors on a bedroom.

LACK OF RELAXED TIME

Because of multiple responsibilities or commitments or because of demanding or incompatible work schedules, many couples are faced with conditions in which they have very little time with each other. One partner working a day shift and the other partner working a night shift or one partner traveling and coming home only on weekends severely limits favorable time for sexual relations. Couples in such situations often try to "take advantage of the time together" and engage in sexual activity whether they feel like it or not. It is not unusual that such conditions can contribute to ED.

Assessment Strategy

Men seeking professional help with sexual dysfunction generally and ED in particular typically present under three conditions: as single men without partners, as men with partners who are unavailable or uncooperative, and as men with partners who are available and cooperative. Whenever there is an available and cooperative partner, separate interviews are conducted to ensure conditions for full disclosure of all important factors and to evaluate each partner's perspective of the problem and each partner's medical, psychological, and sexual profile. The availability of a cooperative and available partner usually offers a more complete assessment and facilitates the therapy process.

Clinical Interview

With the preceding model in mind, psychological assessment of ED is accomplished primarily through a comprehensive interview that examines each of the possible contributing factors in the model. Confidentiality is assured to each separate partner so that the therapist can obtain important information that otherwise might not have been disclosed in the presence of a partner. For example, information related to masturbation practices, sexual relations with prostitutes, or sexual relations with another partner might not have been shared. This information, however, is clinically very important when attempting to understand the etiology and scope of the ED problem and when developing a treatment strategy. Assessment that reveals ED only with a partner but not in other circumstances would take a very different course than ED that occurs under all circumstances. When sexual or relationship secrets are revealed during partner assessment, the therapist faces a difficult challenge in how best to proceed.

Psychometrics

The use of psychometric instruments may be used as part of a comprehensive assessment strategy for ED. Valid and reliable instruments such as the Minnesota Multiphasic Personality Inventory (MMPI) may be used to evaluate the presence of comorbid disorders that may be contributing to the ED. The most widely used self-report scales for assessing erectile function directly are the International Index of Erectile Function (IIEF) (Rosen et al., 1997) and the Sexual Health Inventory for Men (SHIM) (Rosen, Cappelleri, Smith, Lipsky, & Pena, 1999), which are commonly used in both research and clinical settings. More specialized measures focus on rigidity and reliability of erection, including the validated Erection Quality Scale (EQS; Wincze et al., 2003; Wincze et al., 2004).

Sex Therapy and Integrated Treatment of ED

Treatment strategy is dependent on a comprehensive medical and psychosocial assessment. Depending on the exact nature of all of the factors in a particular case, treatment may focus entirely on medical factors, entirely on psychosocial factors, or on a combination of medical and psychosocial factors. Also, depending on the assessment findings, treatment may focus initially only on medical factors and subsequently on psychosocial factors, or simultaneously on both medical factors and psychosocial factors.

Because of all of the possible factors contributing to ED, there is no one prescription for treatment. Rather, there is a need to follow a pathway that addresses all factors contributing to the ED problem. Nonetheless, there are certain psychosocial approaches that present as part of most treatment protocols for men experiencing ED.

Sensate Focus

The sensate focus approach developed by Masters and Johnson (1970) is still a cornerstone of treatment for most cases of ED. The basic procedure asks a couple to have sexual relations without intercourse regardless of the man's erection. The procedure encourages couples to be orgasmic by any means other than intercourse. This procedure not only takes the focus off of the erection but introduces a novel approach and variety. Both of these elements are conducive to arousal. The goal of sensate focus is to focus on the moment and sensations rather than focusing on the outcome and performance. A therapist's suggestion, for example, to focus on the fragrance of your partner's hair, the feel of your partner's body helps to keep a man's mind in the moment. Couples are generally asked to repeat this exercise a number of times until there is a comfort with approaching sex and an achievement of being able to focus on the moment rather than the outcome. Most couples following this procedure will report experiencing erections within one or two sessions. Once erections are being achieved and comfort is present, then a therapist might suggest to the couple to include intercourse as an "option."

Cognitive-Behavioral Interventions

Cognitive interventions are used increasingly in the psychological treatment of erectile dysfunction. In particular, bibliotherapy and cognitive restructuring techniques are used to overcome sexual ignorance and to challenge the unrealistic sexual expectations that typically accompany ED (Wincze & Carey, 2001). We often recommend self-help books that address dysfunctional beliefs or other cognitive issues in men with ED (Alterowitz & Alterowitz, 2004; Wincze, 2009; Zilbergeld, 1992). Note that although the first book is oriented to prostate cancer survivors, the sections on cognitive issues are valuable and appropriate for all men with ED.

Men (and their partners) frequently harbor gross misconceptions regarding the basic mechanisms and processes of erectile function and causes of sexual dysfunction. The effects of illness and drugs, aging, and male–female differences in sexual response are additional common areas of ignorance. As noted by Zilbergeld (1992), men frequently subscribe to a fantasy-based model of sex, in which male performance is viewed as the cornerstone of every sexual experience and a firm erection is seen as the sine qua non of a satisfying sexual encounter. Sexual performance difficulties are often interpreted, according to this view, as a loss of masculinity or declining sexual interest in the partner.

Dysfunctional sexual beliefs and expectations are a potentially important focus for treatment. In an early study, elderly couples with a history of ED were randomly assigned to either an educational workshop program or a wait-list control condition (Goldman & Carroll, 1990). Posttreatment evaluations revealed a significant improvement in sexual knowledge and attitudes in the workshop participants, which was associated with increased sexual frequency and satisfaction. Educational interventions have recently been combined with medical therapies (Perelman, 2005), although the specific benefits of this combined approach need to be further evaluated.

Other authors have recommended that positive imagery training, either with or without masturbation, can assist in the development of sexual confidence and control (Rosen, Leiblum, & Spector, 1994; Zilbergeld, 1992). Again, these fantasy and masturbation exercises can be combined with use of oral medications, and clinicians frequently recommend use of PDE5 inhibitors initially with masturbation or fantasy to develop familiarity and comfort with the use of the drugs. On the other hand, Apfelbaum (2000) has cautioned that although sexual fantasies may be used by dysfunctional males to temporarily "bypass" a lack of arousal or interest in their partners, this solution is unlikely to be effective and may lead to a loss of sexual desire when used on a long-term basis.

Sexual Stimulation Techniques

It has often been noted that ED is most psychologically distressing for individuals or couples with limited sexual scripts and few alternatives to intercourse

(Zilbergeld, 1993; LoPiccolo, 1992; Gagnon, Rosen, & Leiblum, 1982; Leiblum & Rosen, 1991). In particular, performance demands and fear of failure are increased markedly for individuals or couples who lack alternative means of sexual satisfaction to penile–vaginal intercourse. For these individuals, the male's inability to achieve a firm and lasting erection typically results in a complete cessation of all sexual activity. This, in turn, may lead to diminished sexual desire in one or both partners and increased distance or conflict in the relationship (Leiblum & Rosen, 1991). A "vicious cycle" phenomenon frequently ensues, as the loss of sexual or affectionate interaction is associated with increased performance demands and interpersonal distress. In one early study, sexual communication training was found to be superior to sensate focus alone in the treatment of secondary erectile dysfunction (Takefman & Brender, 1984).

LoPiccolo (1992) has emphasized the critical role of the female partner's attitude toward nonintercourse forms of sexual stimulation. According to this author, the partner's willingness to be satisfied by manual or oral stimulation may be a critical determinant of treatment outcome in most cases of erectile dysfunction: "Far more effective than sensate focus in reducing performance anxiety is the patient's knowledge that his partner's sexual gratification does not depend on his having an erection. If the patient can be reassured that his partner finds their lovemaking highly pleasurable, and that she is sexually fulfilled by the orgasms he gives her through manual and oral stimulation, his performance anxiety will be greatly reduced" (LoPiccolo, 1992, p. 190). From this perspective, treatment is often focused on the sexual receptivity of the partner to nonintercourse forms of stimulation.

Elsewhere, a "sexual scripting" approach has been recommended for a variety of sexual performance difficulties, including ED (Gagnon, Rosen, & Leiblum, 1982; Rosen, Leiblum, & Spector, 1994). Essentially, this approach involves detailed assessment of both the performative, or overt, script between the partners and the ideal or imagined script of each individual partner. Performative scripts can be analyzed according to four major script dimensions: complexity, rigidity, conventionality, and satisfaction. In couples with chronic sexual dysfunctions, including ED, performative scripts typically become increasingly restricted, repetitive, and inflexible, with diminishing sexual satisfaction for either partner. Script restrictions may either precede the onset of a specific sexual problem or may develop as a consequence of the disorder (Leiblum & Rosen, 1991).

Case 3: Mr. and Mrs. E

John and Barbara were both 64 years old, had been married 40 years, and had two adult daughters. John was an employed professional white collar worker, and Barbara was employed part time in an office job. Both were college educated and were financially comfortable. John presented with a 10-year history of intermittent ED with his wife and a complaint of low desire. He also reported that he and Barbara had not had sex for 1 year. Recently, she was very angry because she discovered that John had been viewing pornography on the Internet. John reported that Barbara had considerable anger toward him and that they had a history of very poor communication. John also presented with a complicated medical history of untreated hypogonadism, hypertension, and dyslipidemia.

Barbara presented with a history of hypoactive sexual desire disorder, dyspareunia, and anger toward John. She was hurt by John's use of pornography and described herself as extremely sensitive to criticism and avoidant of conflict. Medically, Barbara presented with untreated type II diabetes, vaginal atrophy, and a past hysterectomy.

In a separate interview with John, he revealed that he was able to obtain an erection sufficient for penetration during masturbation to pornography, although the erection was not a completely full one. Both John and Barbara stated that they wanted to stay together, and both were willing to work together in therapy to improve their situation.

From the start of therapy both John and Barbara obtained medical treatment. John worked on diet changes and exercise, and treatment for hypogonadism was initiated. Barbara spent a week at a specialty clinic for diabetes and gained a great deal through the diabetic education and necessary diet changes. She also was seen by a gynecologist familiar with female sexual dysfunction and received treatment for vaginal atrophy.

Because the couple presented with a great deal of anger over pornography use, this issue was addressed initially and put into perspective in a way that was acceptable to both John and Barbara. They were each encouraged to see and appreciate the other's needs. In addition, it was necessary to also initially address communication issues through role playing with the therapist, as the couple's faulty communication was a continuing source of conflict. Focus on sexual issues in general and ED in particular was delayed until the medical issues, pornography issues, and communication issues were addressed and progress was made. The focus on sex began about 1 year after therapy was initiated and began with a more general focus on increasing intimacy. The couple were given assignments to arrange "date nights" and other intimacy exercises. After about 6 months of additional therapy, the couple reported spontaneous initiation of successful intercourse and success in achieving greater relationship intimacy.

Comment

This case illustrates an example of the type of complex cases that we see today. This type of complex case is a far cry from the more simplistic cases treated by Masters and Johnson in the early 1970s. This case is complicated by both the medical and psychosocial problems presented by both partners. It is also a case that illustrates the need to treat problems in sequence. The ED problem that was initially presented was not directly treated by psychological approaches until after a year of medical intervention and couple therapy. A key element in the successful treatment of this case was the motivation on the part of both John and Barbara to improve their situation. Blame was removed early on in therapy so that the couple could approach their mutual problem as "two adults working together." Sex was approached gradually, with an emphasis on building intimacy in terms of how the couple related to each other both verbally and physically. All intimacy was given value, and sexual intercourse was focused on as only one of many options to express intimacy.

CONCLUSIONS

Erectile dysfunction is a highly prevalent sexual disorder, with significant effects on mood, quality of life, and interpersonal relationships. Since the introduction of PDE5 inhibitors, approximately 100 million men worldwide have sought treatment for ED, and the drugs are now widely used as first-line therapy for ED, although many men fail to make adequate use of the medication. As described in this chapter, an integrated approach of medical and psychosocial interventions is feasible and potentially superior as an overall treatment approach. Psychological and sex therapy approaches are strongly emphasized in this model, either in conjunction with or as an alternative to medical therapies. Despite the overall safety and effectiveness of PDE5 inhibitors, many couples discontinue treatment for psychological and interpersonal reasons. This combined approach is intended to address these issues and to improve overall satisfaction with treatment.

Future directions for this area include the potential integration of cardiovascular risk prevention and lifestyle modification approaches, including weight loss and exercise, as adjunctive treatments for ED in men with both erection difficulties and major cardiovascular risk factors. The relative benefits and potential challenges in integrating couple therapy or treatment approaches involving partners of men with ED remains to be addressed. Finally, the impact of the new DSM-5 definition of ED and the inclusion of the penile rigidity criterion in particular remains to be evaluated.

REFERENCES

Alterowitz, R., & Alterowitz, B. (2004). *Intimacy with impotence (The couple's guide to better sex after prostate disease)*. Cambridge, MA: Da Capo Press.

Althof, S. E., Leiblum, S. R., Chevret-Measson, M., Hartman, U., Levine, S. B., McCabe, M., et al. (2005). Psychological and interpersonal dimensions of sexual function and dysfunction. *Journal of Sexual Medicine, 2,* 793–818.

American Psychiatric Association. (2013). *Diagnostic and statistical manual of mental disorders* (5th ed.). Arlington, VA: Author.

Apfelbaum, B. (2000). Retarded ejaculation: A much misunderstood syndrome. In R.

C. Rosen & S. R. Leiblum (Eds.), *Principles and practice of sex therapy* (3rd ed., pp. 205–241). New York: Guilford Press.

Araujo, A. B., Hall, S. A., Ganz, P., Chiu, G. R., Rosen, R. C., Kupelian, V., et al. (2010). Does erectile dysfunction contribute to cardiovascular disease risk prediction beyond the Framingham Risk Score? *Journal of the American College of Cardiology, 55,* 350–356.

Azadzoi, K. M., & Goldstein, I. (1992). Erectile dysfunction due to atherosclerotic vascular disease: The development of an animal model. *Journal of Urology, 147,* 1675–1681.

Barlow, D. H., Sakheim, D. K., & Beck, J. G. (1983). Anxiety increases sexual arousal. *Journal of Abnormal Psychology, 92,* 49–54.

Billups, K. L., Blank, A. J., Padma-Nathan, H., Katz, S., & Williams, R. (2005). Erectile dysfunction is a marker for cardiovascular disease: Results of the Minority Health Institute Expert Advisory Panel. *Journal of Sexual Medicine, 2,* 40–52.

Bortolotti, A., Parazzini, F., Colli, E., & Landoni, M. (1997). The epidemiology of erectile dysfunction and its risk factors. *International Journal of Andrology, 20,* 323–334.

Burchard, M., Burchard, T., Anastasiadis, A. G., Kiss, A. J., Shabsigh, A., & de La Taille, A. (2001). Erectile dysfunction is a marker for cardiovascular complications and psychological functioning in men with hypertension. *International Journal of Impotence Research, 13,* 276–281.

Chew, K. K., Finn, J., Stuckey, B., Gibson, N., Sanfilippo, F., Bremner, A., et al. (2010). Erectile dysfunction as a predictor for subsequent atherosclerotic cardiovascular events: Findings from a linked-data study. *Journal of Sexual Medicine, 7,* 192–202.

Cranston-Cuebas, M. A., & Barlow, D. H. (1990). Cognitive and affective contributions to sexual functioning. *Annual Review of Sex Research, 1,* 119–161.

DeBusk, R., Drory, Y., Goldstein, I., Jackson, G., Kaul, S., Kimmel, S., et al. (2000). Management of sexual dysfunction in patients with cardiovascular disease: Recommendations of the Princeton Consensus Panel. *American Journal of Cardiology, 86,* 175–181.

El-Galley, R., Rutland, H., Talic, R., Keane, T., & Clark, H. (2001). Long-term efficacy of sildenafil and tachyphylaxis effect. *Journal of Urology, 166,* 927–931.

Feldman, H. A., Goldstein, I., Hatzichristou, D. G., Krane, R. J., & McKinlay, J. B. (1994). Impotence and its medical and psychosocial correlates: Results of the Massachusetts Male Aging Study. *Journal of Urology, 151,* 54–61.

Fisher, W., Rosen, R., Eardley, I., Niederberger, C., Nadel, A., Kaufman, J., et al. (2004). The multinational men's attitudes to life events and sexuality (MALES) study phase II: Understanding PDE5 inhibitor treatment seeking patterns, among men with erectile dysfunction. *Journal of Sexual Medicine, 1,* 150–160.

Gagnon, J. H., Rosen, R. C., & Leiblum, S. R. (1982). Cognitive and social aspects of sexual dysfunction: Sexual scripts in sex therapy. *Journal of Sex and Marital Therapy, 8,* 44–56.

Gazzaruso, C., Giordanetti, S., De Amici, E., Bertone, G., Falcone, C., Geroldi, D., et al. (2004). Relationship between erectile dysfunction and silent myocardial ischemia in apparently uncomplicated type 2 diabetic patients. *Circulation, 110,* 22–26.

Goldman, A. S., & Carroll, J. L. (1990). Educational intervention as an adjunct to treatment of erectile dysfunction in older couples. *Journal of Sex and Marital Therapy*, 16, 127–141.

Hall, S. A., Kupelian, V., Rosen, R. C., Travison, T. G., Link, C. L., Miner, M. M., et al. (2009). Is hyperlipidemia or its treatment associated with erectile dysfunction?: Results from the Boston Area Community Health (BACH) Survey. *Journal of Sexual Medicine, 6*, 1402–1413.

Hatzichristou, D., Rosen, R., Broderick, G., Clayton, A., Cuzin, B., Derogatis, L., et al. (2004). Clinical evaluation and management strategy for sexual dysfunction in men and women. *Journal of Sexual Medicine, 1*, 49–57.

Hawton, K., Catalan, J., & Fagg, J. (1992). Sex therapy for erectile dysfunction: Characteristics of couples, treatment outcome, and prognostic factors. *Archives of Sexual Behavior, 21*, 161–176.

Hoon, P., Wincze, J., & Hoon, E. (1977) A test of reciprocal inhibition: Are anxiety and sexual arousal in women mutually inhibitory? *Journal of Abnormal Psychology, 86*, 65–74.

Inman, B. A., St. Sauver, J. L., Jacobson, D. J., McGree, M. E., Nehra, A., Lieber, M. M., et al. (2009). A population-based longitudinal study of erectile dysfunction and future coronary artery disease. *Mayo Clinic Proceedings, 84*, 108–113.

Kaplan, H. S. (1974). *The new sex therapy.* New York: Brunner/Mazel.

Kloner, R. A., Mullin, S. H, Shook, T., Matthews, R., Mayeda, G., Burstein, S., et al. (2003). Erectile dysfunction in the cardiac patient: How common and should we treat? *Journal of Urology, 170*, S46–S50.

Kostis, J. B., Jackson, G., Rosen, R., & the Second Princeton Consensus Panel. (2005). Sexual dysfunction and cardiac risk (the second Princeton Consensus Conference). *American Journal of Cardiology, 96*, 313–321.

Kupelian, V., Araujo, A. B., Chiu, G. R., Rosen, R. C., & McKinlay, J. B. (2010). Relative contributions of modifiable risk factors to erectile dysfunction: Results from the Boston Area Community Health (BACH) Survey. *Preventive Medicine, 50*, 19–25.

Leiblum, S. R. (2002). After sildenafil: Bridging the gap between pharmacologic treatment and satisfying sexual relationships. *Journal of Clinical Psychiatry, 63*, 17–22.

Leiblum, S. R., & Rosen, R. C. (1991). Couples therapy for erectile disorders: Conceptual and clinical considerations. *Journal of Sex and Marital Therapy, 17*, 147–159.

Levine, S. B. (1992). Intrapsychic and intrapersonal aspects of impotence: Psychogenic erectile dysfunction. In R. C. Rosen & S. R. Leiblum (Eds.), *Erectile disorders: Assessment and treatment* (pp. 198–225). New York: Guilford Press.

LoPiccolo, J. (1992). Postmodern sex therapy for erectile failure. In R. C. Rosen & S. R. Leiblum (Eds.), *Erectile disorders: Assessment and treatment* (pp. 171–197). New York: Guilford Press.

Lue, T., Giuliano, F., Montorsi, F., Rosen, R., Andersson, K. E., Althof, S., et al. (2004). Summary of the recommendations on sexual dysfunctions in men. *Journal of Sexual Medicine, 1*, 6–23.

Masters, W. H., & Johnson, V. E. (1970). *Human sexual inadequacy.* Boston: Little Brown.

Miner, M. (2009). Erectile dysfunction and the "window of curability": A harbinger of cardiovascular events [Editorial]. *Mayo Clinic Proceedings, 84*, 102–104.

Montorsi, F., Briganti, A., Salonia, A., Rigatti, P., Margonato, A., Macchi, A., et al.

(2003). Erectile dysfunction prevalence, time of onset and association with risk factors in 300 consecutive patients with acute chest pain and angiographically documented coronary artery disease. *European Urology, 44,* 360–365.

Montorsi, P., Montorsi, F., & Schulman, C. C. (2003). Is erectile dysfunction the "tip of the iceberg" of a systemic vascular disorder? [Editorial]. *European Urology, 44,* 352–354.

Nehra, A., Jackson, G., Miner, M., Billups, K. L., Burnett, A. L., Buvat, J., et al. (2012). The Princeton III Consensus recommendations for the management of erectile dysfunction and cardiovascular disease. *Mayo Clinic Procedures, 87*(8), 766–780.

Padma-Nathan, H. (2003). Efficacy and tolerability of tadalafil, a novel phosphodiesterase 5 inhibitor, in treatment of erectile dysfunction. *American Journal of Cardiology, 92*(Suppl. 1), 19M–25M.

Panser, L. A., Rhodes, T., Girman, C. J., Guess, H. A, Chute, C. G., Oesterling, J. E., et al. (1995). Sexual function of men ages 40 to 79 years: The Olmsted County Study of Urinary Symptoms and Health Status among Men. *Journal of the American Geriatric Society, 43,* 1107–1111.

Perelman, M. A. (2005). Psychosocial evaluation and combination treatment of men with erectile dysfunction. *Urologic Clinics of North America, 32,* 441–445.

Qaseem, A., Snow, V., Denberg, T. D., Casey, D. E., Jr., Forciea, M. A., Owens, D. K., et al. (2009). Hormonal testing and pharmacologic treatment of erectile dysfunction: A clinical practice guideline from the American College of Physicians. *Annals of Internal Medicine, 151,* 639–649.

Rosen, R. (2000). Integrating medical and psychological treatments for erectile dysfunction. In S. R. Leiblum & R. C. Rosen (Eds.), *Principles and practice of sex therapy.* New York: Guilford Press.

Rosen, R., & McKenna, K. (2002). PDE-5 inhibition and sexual response: Pharmacological mechanisms and clinical outcomes. *Annual Review of Sex Research, 13,* 36–88.

Rosen, R. C. (2005). Reproductive health problems in aging men. *Lancet, 366,* 183–185.

Rosen, R. C., Capelleri, J. C., Smith, M. D., Lipsky, J., & Penar, B. M. (1999). Development and evaluation of an abridged 5-item version of the International Index of Erectile Function (IIEF) as a diagnostic tool for erectile dysfunction. *International Journal of Impotence Research, 11,* 319–326.

Rosen, R. C., Fisher, W. A., Eardley, I., Niederber, C., Nadel, A., Sand, M., et al. (2004). The Multinational Men's Attitudes of Life Events and Sexuality (MALES) study: Prevalence of erectile dysfunction and related health concerns in the general population. *Current Medical Research and Opinion, 20,* 607–617.

Rosen, R. C., Leiblum, S. R., & Spector, I. (1994). Psychologically based treatment for male erectile disorder: A cognitive-interpersonal model. *Journal of Sex and Marital Therapy, 20,* 67–85.

Rosen, R. C., Riley, A., Wagner, H., Osterloh, I., Kirkpatrick, J., & Mishra, A. (1997). The International Index of Erectile Function (IIEF): A multi-dimensional scale for assessment of male erectile dysfunction (MED). *Urology, 49,* 822–830.

Rosen, R. C., Wing, R., Schneider, S., & Gendrano, N., III. (2005). Epidemiology of erectile dysfunction: The role of medical comorbidities and lifestyle factors. *Urologic Clinics of North America, 32,* 403–417.

Scharff, D. E. (1988). An object relations approach to inhibited sexual desire. In S. R.

Leiblum & R. C. Rosen (Eds.), *Sexual desire disorders* (pp. 45–74). New York: Guilford Press.

Schouten, B. W., Bohnen, A. M., Bosch, J. L., Bernsen, R. M., Deckers, J. W., Dohle, G. R., et al. (2008). Erectile dysfunction prospectively associated with cardiovascular disease in the Dutch general population: Results from the Krimpen Study. *International Journal of Impotence Research, 20*, 92–99.

Takefman, J., & Brender, W. (1984). An analysis of the effectiveness of two components in the treatment of erectile dysfunction. *Archives of Sexual Behavior, 13*, 321–340.

Thompson, I. M., Tangen, C. M., Goodman, P. J., Probatfield, J. L., Moinpour, C. M., & Coltsman, C. A. (2005). Erectile dysfunction and subsequent cardiovascular disease. *Journal of the American Medical Assocation, 294*, 2996–3002.

Verhulst, J., & Heiman, J. R. (1979). An interactional approach to sexual dysfunction. *American Journal of Family Therapy, 7*, 19–36.

Virag, R., Bouilly, P., & Frydman, D. (1985). Is impotence an arterial disorder?: A study of arterial risk factors in 440 impotent men. *Lancet, 1*(5422), 181–184.

Weeks, G. R., & Gambescia, N. (2000). *Erectile dysfunction: Integrating couple therapy, sex therapy and medical treatment.* New York: Norton.

Wincze, J. (2009). *Enhancing sexuality: A problem-solving approach to treating sexual dysfunction* (2nd ed.). New York: Oxford University Press.

Wincze, J. P., & Carey, M. P. (2001). *Sexual dysfunction: A guide for assessment and treatment* (2nd ed.). New York: Guilford Press.

Wincze, J., Rosen, R., Carsons, C., Korenman, S., Niederberger, C., Sadovsky, R., et al. (2004). Erection Quality Scale: Initial scale development and validation. *Urology, 64*, 351–356.

Wincze, J., Rosen, R., Korenman, S., Niederberger, C., Sadovsky, R., Carson, C., et al. (2003). Development and initial evaluation of the erection quality scale. *International Journal of Impotence Research, 15*, 179–180.

Zilbergeld, B. (1992). *The new male sexuality.* New York: Bantam Books.

Orgasm

CHAPTER 4

Orgasm Disorders in Women

Cynthia A. Graham

"Women clearly differ in how important orgasm is to their sexual satisfaction," Graham writes. She notes, however, that this difference may stem from how widely women vary in the ease and manner in which they experience orgasm. In general, most women find it easier to have an orgasm from self- as opposed to partner stimulation. Of those experiencing orgasmic difficulties, younger and older women are more frequently represented. Poor overall health and relationship difficulties are also associated with difficulty experiencing orgasm. These findings raise important questions: To what extent is a woman's difficulty experiencing orgasm during partnered sex due to an individual issue rather than a skills deficit on the part of her partner? Is orgasm a marker for relationship satisfaction? To what extent is experiencing orgasm a learned phenomenon? In response to these and other questions, Graham critically reviews the literature and neatly summarizes the requisite elements of a sensitive assessment of orgasmic difficulties. Although she acknowledges that directed masturbation remains a highly successful treatment approach, she advises that there is room for improvement. Medication and mindfulness are two of the options that are discussed as Graham makes the case for a more comprehensive treatment approach.

Cynthia A. Graham, PhD, is currently a Senior Lecturer in the Department of Psychology at the University of Southampton in the United Kingdom, a Research Fellow at The Kinsey Institute for Research in Sex, Gender, and Reproduction, and a Research Fellow at the Rural Center for AIDS/STD Prevention, Indiana University. She is Editor-in-Chief of the *Journal of Sex Research* and is an editorial board member for the *Journal of Sex and Marital Therapy* and the *International Journal of Sexual Health*. She is a Chartered Psychologist, an Associate Fellow of the British Psychological Society, a Fellow of the

Society for the Scientific Study of Sexuality, and was a member of the Sexual and Gender Identity Disorders Workgroup for DSM-5. She was elected President of the International Academy of Sex Research in 2009.

Although there is no universally accepted definition of orgasm (Mah & Binik, 2001), most proposed definitions incorporate both subjective experience and physiological changes. Unlike orgasm in the male, which is usually accompanied by ejaculation, there is no objective "marker" of orgasm in women, and there is no clear evidence that orgasm has a role to play in female reproductive fitness (Levin, 2011). Both the subjective experience of and the physiological changes associated with female orgasm are extremely varied (King, Belsky, Mah, & Binik, 2011; Meston, Levin, Sipski, Hull, & Heiman, 2004). Women also vary considerably in the age at which they first experience orgasm, the consistency with which they are able to reach orgasm, and the importance they attach to orgasm (Graham, 2010).

Medical and societal perspectives on female orgasm and about what constitutes a problem have shifted dramatically; the fact that we now recognize and treat lack of orgasm in women has been described as a "cultural accident" (Heiman, 2007). With very few exceptions (Brody, 2010), researchers and clinicians no longer make distinctions between "clitoral" and "vaginal" orgasms or consider orgasms achieved through one type of stimulation more or less "mature" or healthy than another (Laan & Rellini, 2011). Indeed, there is no clear evidence that orgasms can be reliably distinguished by the type or pattern of stimulation that is associated with them (Prause, 2011).

Women show wide variability in the type and intensity of stimulation that induces orgasm (American Psychiatric Association, 2013). Although orgasms are most commonly induced by genital stimulation, other types of nongenital stimulation, including imagery, can produce orgasms in some women (Komisaruk & Whipple, 2011). There is consistent evidence that women reach orgasm more easily by themselves than during partnered sexual activity (Laumann, Paik, & Rosen, 1999; Zietsch, Miller, Bailey, & Martin, 2011). Women who experience orgasm through clitoral stimulation but not during sexual intercourse do not meet *Diagnostic and Statistical Manual of Mental Disorders* (DSM-5) diagnostic criteria for female orgasmic disorder (FOD; American Psychiatric Association, 2013).

Orgasm problems most commonly present as delay or absence of orgasm, although a minority of women (6–15% in epidemiological surveys) report reaching orgasm too quickly (Laumann et al., 1999; Richters, Grulich, de Visser, Smith, & Rissel, 2003). The DSM classification of FOD (American Psychiatric Association, 2013) distinguishes between lifelong versus acquired subtypes (if the orgasm difficulties develop only after a period of normal functioning) and generalized versus situational subtypes (if the orgasm difficulties are limited to certain types of stimulation, situations, or partners) and includes a specification for a woman never having experienced an orgasm under any situation. Somewhat different terminology has been used in the clinical literature, in which "primary" anorgasmia (to refer to lifelong) and "secondary" (to denote situational or acquired orgasmic problems) have been used. Secondary FOD thus includes women who experience orgasm only during masturbation or only with specific sexual partners, as well as those who no longer experience orgasm at all but who have done so in the past. Secondary FOD is believed to be more common and more difficult to treat than primary FOD (Heiman, 2007).

EPIDEMIOLOGY

Determining the prevalence of female orgasmic problems is difficult, in part because the methods of evaluation and the time periods assessed have varied widely in epidemiological surveys (Graham, 2010). Moreover, although many researchers claim to have used standardized diagnostic criteria (e.g., DSM or *International Classification of Diseases and Related Health Problems* [ICD-10; World Health Organization, 1992]) to identify women with orgasmic disorders, few surveys have assessed the presence of clinically significant distress or the absence of other nonsexual mental disorders (both essential criteria for a DSM diagnosis of FOD). Although more recent surveys have included questions on distress regarding sexual difficulties (Bancroft, Loftus, & Long, 2003; Oberg, Fugl-Meyer, & Fugl-Meyer, 2004; Shifren, Monz, Russo, Segreti, & Johannes, 2008; Witting et al., 2008), these have still rarely assessed distress regarding *specific* sexual difficulties—for example, orgasmic problems.

It has been argued that the detailed clinical assessment needed to diagnose a sexual dysfunction cannot be undertaken by large-scale surveys (Graham & Bancroft, 2006). For example, in DSM-5 a diagnosis of FOD is not made if the orgasmic difficulties are considered the result of inadequate sexual stimulation, yet epidemiological surveys have rarely included assessment of the adequacy of sexual stimulation a woman receives. Although what constitutes "adequate" stimulation will vary across women (Brotto, Bitzer, Laan, Leiblum, & Luria, 2010) and is necessarily dependent to some extent on clinician judgment, establishing whether orgasmic problems are due to inadequate sexual stimulation remains a fundamental (albeit very difficult) task for the clinician (Laan & Rellini, 2011). The estimates from epidemiological surveys should therefore be seen as providing evidence on the prevalence of orgasmic difficulties or problems rather than on FOD or dysfunction (Richters et al., 2003).

In a review of the prevalence of female orgasmic problems reported in 11 surveys, all of which used nationally representative samples, Graham (2010) observed rates of between 3 and 34%. Considering the evidence on orgasmic disorder from European surveys, Fugl-Meyer and Fugl-Meyer (2006) concluded, "the prevalence . . . appears to vary so widely that at the moment there is no conclusive evidence" (p. 35). The few cross-cultural data available suggest even wider prevalence estimates; in the Global Survey of Sexual Attitudes and Behaviors (Laumann et al., 2005), the prevalence of "inability to reach orgasm" reported by women ranged from 17.7% (in northern Europe) to 41.2% (in Southeast Asia).

The duration of the symptoms, the length of the recall period, and whether distress concerning the orgasmic problem is assessed all affect prevalence rates of orgasmic difficulties (Graham, 2010; Hayes, Dennerstein, Bennett, & Fairley, 2008). A consistent finding has been that only about half of women who are unable to reach orgasm report associated distress (King, Holt, & Nazareth, 2007; Oberg et al., 2004; Shifren et al., 2008). In the United Kingdom National Survey of Sexual Attitudes and Lifestyles (NATSAL), although 14.4% of women reported orgasm problems that lasted at least 1 month, only 3.7% had persistent problems (defined as lasting at least 6 months in the previous year; Mercer et al., 2003). In a U.S. survey involving 31,581 women, although the age-adjusted prevalence of "low orgasm" was 21.8%, the prevalence of orgasm problems with associated distress was only 3.4% (Shifren et al., 2008). In another U.S. study, physical aspects of sexual response (including orgasm) were relatively weak predictors of distress, and only 30–50% of women (depending on age, with older women less distressed than younger women) who did not experience an orgasm reported marked distress about their sexual relationships (Bancroft et al., 2003).

Women clearly differ in how important orgasm is to their sexual satisfaction. In a U.S. national sample of heterosexual women ages 20–65 years, 29.1% rated having an orgasm as very or extremely important to their "sexual happiness" (in contrast, 83.2% rated feeling "emotionally close to my partner" as very or extremely important; Bancroft, Long, & McCabe, 2011). Laan and Rellini (2011) made the interesting suggestion that some women may report orgasms during partnered sex as being relatively unimportant because they do not consistently experience orgasms in this way and that women who reach orgasm more easily might also rate orgasm as more important.

Few surveys have assessed the prevalence of orgasm difficulties in older women, but these have suggested higher prevalence rates than in younger women (Heiman et al., 2011; Levine, Williams, & Hartmann, 2008; Lindau et al., 2007). In a nationally representative sample of 1,550 U.S. women ages 57–85 years, 34% of those who were sexually active reported anorgasmia for "several months or more" during the previous 12 months (Lindau et al., 2007). Even less is known about the frequency of orgasm problems experienced by younger women (i.e., those in late adolescence or early adulthood), but the limited data suggest that inability to orgasm is the most common persistent difficulty in this age group (O'Sullivan & Majerovich, 2008). Although the proportion of women who report having experienced orgasm does increase with age (Kinsey, Pomeroy, Martin, & Gebhard, 1953), there have been conflicting findings on the association between age and orgasm problems. Some studies have reported that younger women had a greater likelihood of orgasmic difficulties than older women (Laumann et al., 1999), others have found no relationship between age and orgasm problems (Oberg et al., 2004), and some have reported that older women were more likely to report inability to reach orgasm than younger women (Richters et al., 2003). Kinsey et al. (1953) estimated that approximately 9% of women did not experience orgasm through their lifetimes. Although the prevalence of orgasm difficulties is difficult to ascertain, clinic-based studies most often cite orgasm problems as the second most common presenting complaint in women (with low sexual interest as the most frequent; Robinson, Munns, Weber-Main, Lowe, & Raymond, 2011). It has been suggested that women with orgasm problems present less frequently now than when sex therapy was first introduced in the 1970s (Heiman, 2007; Robinson et al., 2011).

Factors that have been consistently associated with the likelihood of a woman experiencing orgasm difficulties include poor physical and mental health (Bancroft et al., 2003; Laumann et al., 1999; Richters et al., 2003) and relationship difficulties/partner variables (Goldhammer & McCabe, 2011; Kelly, Strassberg, & Turner, 2004). Witting et al. (2008) investigated sexual function, compatibility with partner, and sexual distress in a population-based Finnish sample of 5,463 women. Orgasm dysfunction decreased with age and with relationship length. All of the partner-compatibility items (too little foreplay; poor communication; partner more interested in sex than you are; you and/or your partner cannot do things "the right way" during sexual activity; you and/or your partner have sexual needs that you/he do not want to satisfy; partner is unattractive; partner has erection problems; partner has problems with early ejaculation) were associated with orgasm dysfunction. All partner-compatibility items (in particular, poor communication) were significantly associated with distress about sex.

There is evidence of a high degree of comorbidity between FOD and other sexual difficulties, particularly problems with arousal, vaginal dryness, and sexual desire (Basson, 2002; Fugl-Meyer & Fugl-Meyer, 2002; Nobre, Pinto-Gouveia, & Gomes, 2006). On the basis of this comorbidity, as well as the overlap between women's experiences of sexual arousal and sexual desire (Brotto, 2010; Graham, 2010), some have argued that we should consider reconceptualizing orgasmic problems not as a separate discrete category but as more of a "global" or arousal-related problem (Basson, 2002; Hartmann, Heiser, Ruffer-Hesse, & Kloth, 2002). These suggestions are highly relevant to the merging of the categories of desire and arousal disorders in DSM-5 (Brotto, 2010; Graham, 2010).

ASSESSMENT AND DIAGNOSTIC ISSUES

Assessment Issues

In identifying whether a problem is primarily orgasmic, it is important to first establish that sexual arousal has occurred. Details about sexual repertoire during partnered sex, in particular the adequacy of stimulation received from a partner, and information about a partner's sexual functioning should be obtained. It is also important to keep in mind that some women are unsure whether or not they have experienced an orgasm. Heiman (2007) suggested that an agreed-upon subjective definition of orgasm was an important starting point in assessment.

Comorbidity of sexual difficulties in partners is common. There is some evidence, for example, that women are more likely to experience orgasm difficulties when their male partners have premature ejaculation (Hobbs, Symonds, Abraham, May, & Morris, 2008). When one partner receives individual therapy for a sexual problem, there is often also improvement in sexual functioning in the other partner (Heiman et al., 2007).

Although there are now a number of validated psychometric instruments designed to assess women's sexual functioning and although almost all of these include questions on orgasm, most clinicians would not use these in place of a detailed, broad-based clinical interview (Brotto et al., 2010). For women in a relationship, interviews should ideally be conducted with both partners, separately and together, and the aim should be to try to establish predisposing, precipitating, and maintaining factors for the orgasm difficulties. Possible contributing biological, psychosocial, and contextual factors (including cultural and religious beliefs/values) should all be explored. History of physical illness, surgery, and medical use should be carefully assessed (see Brotto et al., 2010, for a comprehensive list of factors typically included in an assessment).

Questions about attitudes toward masturbation and masturbation history should be included, including the type of stimulation used during masturbation. As is discussed later, masturbation is an important component in most treatment approaches for FOD. Clinicians should, however, be sensitive to the fact that sometimes for cultural and religious reasons some women will not be open to engaging in masturbation. Although gender differences in sexual attitudes and behavior are narrowing, women are still less likely to masturbate than men and report engaging in masturbation less frequently (Petersen & Hyde, 2011). Kinsey and colleagues' interview data suggested that women who masturbated to orgasm before marriage were more likely to reach orgasm during intercourse with their husbands than women who had never masturbated (Kinsey et al., 1953).

Also relevant to assess are expectations that a woman (and her partner) hold about female orgasm. In a qualitative study of women ages 19–60 years, the participants expressed a strong desire to experience orgasm through heterosexual intercourse in order to please their partners (Nicolson & Burr, 2003). Many individuals adhere to rigid sexual scripts dictating that women should orgasm before their male partner and that men are responsible for "bringing" their female partners to orgasm (Muehlenhard & Shippee, 2010). The strong media messages about the importance of orgasm for women may also engender unrealistic expectations and pressure on women to have orgasms.

As discussed earlier, the presence of a woman's distress about experiencing infrequent or absent orgasm should be carefully assessed. In a U.K. study of women attending general practice clinics, although 18% of the women met ICD-10 criteria for orgasmic dysfunction, only 8% met criteria and also perceived that they had a sexual problem. An even smaller proportion (5%) met diagnostic criteria and reported that their anorgasmia was a "somewhat" or "very" distressing problem (King et al., 2007). One study that focused on predictors of women's distress about their "own sexuality" or about their sexual relationship found that orgasmic frequency was not a significant predictor of distress; the best predictors were measures of general emotional well-being and the woman's emotional relationship with the partner during sexual activity (Bancroft et al., 2003).

For a clinician seeing women presenting with acquired orgasmic difficulties, one crucial task of assessment is to consider to what extent a change in the woman's experience of orgasm is an understandable, and perhaps even adaptive, response to adverse conditions in her life or in her relationship (Graham & Bancroft, 2009). The "three windows approach" (Bancroft, 2009) provides a useful framework to assess this. Through the first window (the "current situation"), the clinician considers to what extent various factors in the woman's current relationship and life might be relevant to the orgasmic difficulty. Are there circumstances present that would be *expected* to have an impact on the woman's ability to experience orgasm? If so, then this may suggest the presence of an adaptive inhibition of sexual response (Bancroft et al., 2003) rather than a sexual "dysfunction." Amanda, a 35-year-old married woman with three young children, including 18-month-old twins, came to therapy with problems reaching orgasm, Although she had been able to experience orgasm throughout most of her 10-year marriage to Tim, a 40-year-old lawyer, she had found it increasingly difficult to do so over the past 6 months. Initial assessment uncovered a number of factors that might be relevant. After almost 2 years on maternity leave, Amanda had recently returned to work full time. Tim contributed little to the child-care and the housework, and Amanda had become increasingly resentful about this, particularly as her job, as a marketing manager in a bank, was quite stressful and she often returned home exhausted. Two months before attending therapy, Tim's parents had come to stay with the couple for an extended (4-week) visit, which increased the workload for Amanda (as well as her resentment and fatigue).

Through the second window ("vulnerability of the individual"), the woman's sexual history is examined, as well as her propensity to become sexually inhibited. There is considerable individual variation in the extent to which women's ability to experience sexual arousal and pleasure is affected by factors such as negative sexual experiences, anxiety, and other factors. Although inhibition of sexual response is most often adaptive, high levels of sexual inhibition may be associated with increased vulnerability to experiencing sexual problems (Bancroft, 2009). There is some evidence that women who score high on measures of inhibition "proneness" are more likely to report orgasm difficulties (Sanders, Graham, & Milhausen, 2008). Other relevant factors to assess through this second window are the need to maintain self-control (e.g., a fear of "letting go" sexually), negative attitudes toward sexuality and/

or about one's body, and the presence of dysfunctional sexual beliefs (Nobre & Pinto-Gouveia, 2006). A woman's feelings about her body and about her genitals should be explored. There is evidence that a more positive genital self-image is positively associated with a woman's having ever experienced orgasm, both during masturbation and from receiving cunnilingus (Herbenick & Reece, 2010). Returning to the case of Amanda, assessment through the second window revealed another possible etiological factor underlying her orgasm difficulties. She had long-standing issues with her body image, dating back to adolescence when she was diagnosed with bulimia nervosa. Although she was now a normal weight, she still had a fear of becoming overweight and had found the weight gain during her last pregnancy difficult to cope with. She also mentioned that during sexual activity, she was quite self-conscious about her stretch marks and avoided certain positions in which she felt that she looked "fat."

Finally, through the third window ("health-related factors") the clinician considers various health-related factors that can influence sexual functioning. These include current mental and physical health and sexual side effects of medication. In the case of Amanda, the clinician needed to consider whether another relevant factor might have been the initiation of oral contraceptives (OC) 6 months before she presented for therapy. Although most of the research on OC-related sexual side effects relates to sexual interest, there is some evidence that orgasm frequency might decline in women using OCs (Battaglia et al., 2012).

Diagnostic Issues

The first inclusion of FOD in the DSM was in the third edition of the manual (DSM-III; American Psychiatric Association, 1980), in which it was labeled "inhibited female orgasm." In DSM-IV and DSM-IV-TR (American Psychiatric Association, 1994, 2000), the disorder was renamed FOD, but the essential feature of the disorder remained a recurrent and persistent delay in or absence of orgasm following a normal sexual excitement phase. The major change from DSM-III to DSM-IV was the inclusion of the distress criterion, by which the symptoms were required to cause marked distress or interpersonal difficulty.

Regarding FOD, there are two substantive changes in the DSM-5 criteria (American Psychiatric Association, 2013) compared with DSM-IV-TR (American Psychiatric Association, 2000). The first change is that specific cutoff criteria for both duration and frequency of symptoms are provided. "Recurrent and persistent" were not clearly operationalized in DSM-IV-TR, and, as discussed previously, the prevalence of mild, transient orgasmic difficulties is considerably higher than that of persistent, severe problems (Graham, 2010). To avoid pathologizing normal variations in orgasmic functioning, the DSM-5 criteria (for all of the sexual dysfunctions) include the requirement that symptoms be present for a minimum duration of approximately 6 months and be experienced on all or almost all (approximately 75–100%) occasions of sexual activity. The second change relates to Criterion A, which now requires a marked degree of at least one of two symptoms: delay in, or absence of, orgasm or reduced intensity of orgasmic sensations. The justification for the addition of the intensity symptom is that clinically it is not uncommon to find women reporting reduced orgasmic intensity, particularly in association with some types of neurological disease or medication use (Basson, 2002). The revised criteria reflect the fact that orgasm is not an "all or nothing" phenomenon and that diminished intensity of orgasm may be a problem for some women (Graham, 2010). When Jennifer, a 50-year-old woman, had completed a course of chemotherapy treatment for breast cancer, she was relieved to discover that her interest in, and overall enjoyment of, sexual activity with her husband had not diminished. She did, however, notice a marked reduction in the intensity of the orgasms she experienced and presented for therapy with this complaint.

The reference in DSM-IV-TR to the orgasm difficulty occurring following a normal excitement phase has not been retained in the DSM-5 criteria, for several reasons. First, this statement has caused considerable confusion among clinicians and researchers, as it suggested that a diagnosis of female sexual arousal disorder (FSAD) would preclude a diagnosis of FOD; in fact, the DSM-IV-TR text included a clear statement that both diagnoses can be made. Second, in practice clinicians (and indeed women themselves) find it difficult or even impossible to establish whether a "normal excitement phase" has occurred (Laan & Rellini, 2011). The phrase "normal excitement phase" also suggests a linear, universal model of sexual response in women, which recent research does not support (Graham, 2010).

The requirement that the orgasm problem cause distress was retained (Criterion B), as was Criterion C, which states that a diagnosis of FOD would be made only if the symptoms in Criterion A are not better explained by a nonsexual mental disorder, by the effects of a substance (e.g., a drug of abuse, a medication), by another medical condition, or by significant relationship distress or other significant stressors.

Regarding the possible impact of the changes in diagnostic criteria introduced in DSM-5, there has been little discussion in the literature about the likely impact of the changes in diagnostic criteria for FOD (in contrast with other diagnostic categories such as female sexual interest/arousal disorder (SIAD; DeRogatis et al., 2010). Because the major change for FOD is that specific duration and severity criteria are required for a diagnosis, one possible outcome is that fewer women will be diagnosed with acquired FOD (the severity and duration criteria would have no impact on lifelong FOD, given that women with this diagnosis have never experienced an orgasm). Given the evidence on the variability in women's experiences of orgasm and the high prevalence of short-term fluctuations in orgasmic functioning, raising the threshold for diagnosis of FOD seems justified. Although the impact of the DSM-5 changes for FOD will be apparent only after the criteria are in use by clinicians (unfortunately, American Psychiatric Association field trials for the sexual dysfunctions were not funded), the rationale for the changes was based on research evidence, as well as on long-standing critiques of the DSM-IV criteria (Graham, 2010).

ETIOLOGY

Many possible etiological factors are relevant to orgasmic dysfunction, but in many cases, the etiology remains unclear, even after detailed assessment. One likely reason for this is that we still have limited understanding of the mechanisms underlying female orgasm (Bancroft, 2009). In most women with FOD, the causes of orgasm difficulties are also likely to be multifactorial.

Psychosocial Factors

Although a wide range of psychological factors, such as anxiety and distraction, can all potentially influence women's experience of orgasm, there is a great deal of individual variability in the likelihood that women are affected by these. For example, although there is evidence that a history of sexual abuse or rape is associated with orgasmic difficulties, this is not always the case (Rellini & Meston, 2007), and we understand little about why individual women vary in this respect. One recent study has suggested that the tendency to avoid interpersonal closeness and emotional involvement may mediate the relationship between lower orgasmic functioning and a history of childhood sexual abuse (Staples, Rellini, & Roberts, 2012).

Although, historically, certain personality factors have been linked to orgasmic difficulties (e.g., "histrionic traits" in DSM-III; American Psychiatric Association, 1980), there is limited evidence for associations between orgasmic ability and personality traits (American Psychiatric Association, 2013; Mah & Binik, 2001). One U.K. twin study that investigated personality factors and their association with female coital orgasmic frequency reported that introversion, emotional instability, and "not being open to new experiences" were related to orgasmic infrequency (Harris, Cherkas, Kato, Heiman, & Spector, 2008). In contrast, in a recent study of Australian twins, although orgasm rates in women showed substantial heritability, they were phenotypically and genetically independent of 19 other traits assessed, including extraversion and neuroticism (Zietsch et al., 2011).

Communications about sex and communication deficits within couples have been suggested as etiological factors in the development of orgasm problems. Although some research has suggested problematic communication patterns in couples in which the female partner has FOD (Kelly et al., 2004), it is not clear whether the communication problems were a cause or an effect of the orgasmic difficulties.

Fear of losing control is another oft-cited etiological factor for orgasmic difficulties. Apart from Fisher's (1973) detailed early studies of women with low and high orgasmic "attainment," however, there has been little empirical study of this. The need to maintain self-control may be particularly important in women with primary anorgasmia or those who are able to experience orgasm during masturbation but not during sexual activity with a partner.

Physiological Factors

A wide range of physical illnesses, neurological and gynecological conditions, and medications can impair orgasmic functioning (Basson & Weijmar Schultz, 2007; West, Vinikoor, & Zolhoun, 2004). Conditions such as multiple sclerosis, thyroid problems, arthritis, pelvic nerve damage from radical hysterectomy, and spinal cord injury have all been associated with FOD (Bancroft, 2009; Shifren et al., 2008). Women with vulvovaginal atrophy are more likely to report orgasm difficulties than women without this condition (Levine et al., 2008). Menopausal status has not been consistently associated with the likelihood of orgasm problems (Avis, Stellato, Crawford, Johannes, & Longcope, 2000).

Selective serotonin reuptake inhibitors (SSRIs) are known to delay or inhibit orgasm in women, affecting between 30 and 60% of individuals taking them (Montgomery, Baldwin, & Riley, 2002). There have been many attempts to reverse these side effects using various other medications but with limited effectiveness, particularly for women (for a review, see Bancroft, 2009).

APPROACHES TO TREATMENT

Psychological Treatments

A number of psychological approaches have been used to treat FOD, including psychodynamic, cognitive-behavioral, and systems theory approaches (Heiman, 2007). The focus in this chapter is on cognitive-behavioral treatments (CBT), as these have received the most empirical support.

Cognitive-Behavioral Approaches

Cognitive-behavioral approaches include directed masturbation (DM; sometimes called "guided masturbation"), communication skills training, sensate focus (SF) exercises, sex education, Kegel exercises, and systematic desensitization. Of these, DM has received the most support, particularly for women with primary anorgasmia, although it is often combined with other methods, such as SF.

Introduced in the 1970s, DM comprises a program of education, followed by exercises involving self-exploration and self-pleasuring (Heiman & LoPiccolo, 1988). Early phases of the program focus on the woman carrying out "solo" homework exercises, first involving nongenital touching and then gradually progressing to genital stimulation (sometimes incorporating a vibrator). Later phases include guidance on how to transfer orgasmic experiences to partnered sexual activity. DM has been evaluated in individual, couple, group, and bibliotherapy formats, although few studies have compared the effectiveness of these different modalities. Heiman (2002) concluded that there was sufficient evidence that DM (either alone or in combination with SF) met American Psychological Association criteria for a "well established," empirically supported treatment for primary anorgasmia and as a "probably efficacious" treatment for secondary anorgasmia. More recently, Ter Kuile, Both, and van Lankveld (2012) reviewed nine randomized controlled trials and concluded that following DM (delivered in either an individual or couple format), 60–90% of women with primary anorgasmia were able to experience orgasm during masturbation and a slightly lower proportion (33–85%) became orgasmic during partnered sexual activity. The authors concluded that for women with primary FOD, DM is the treatment of choice; for women with secondary FOD, although DM may be helpful, additional techniques, such as communication training, may be more valuable.

SF exercises, consisting of a graded series of touching exercises, from nongenital to genital, can be used in either an individual or couple context. These can reduce the "genital focus" and goal-directed nature of the sexual activity evident in many women presenting with orgasmic problems. In a number of controlled studies, DM in combination with SF was more effective than SF alone (Heiman, 2002). Very few studies have assessed the use of SF alone, and in general little research has evaluated the effectiveness of different components of multimodal treatment packages (Ter Kuile et al., 2012). Regarding other behavioral techniques, such as systematic desensitization, communication skills training, and Kegel exercises, there is no empirical evidence that they are effective treatments for primary or secondary anorgasmia when used on their own, although they can be useful adjuncts to DM.

A smaller number of treatment outcome studies have evaluated cognitive-behavioral approaches that incorporate a more explicit focus on changing maladaptive cognitions that may be affecting orgasmic functioning. In one such study, involving 10 sessions of sexual skills training, anxiety reduction techniques, and cognitive retraining, therapy was successful for 80% of the female participants with anorgasmia (McCabe, 2001).

The coital alignment technique (CAT) is a coital position designed to increase clitoral stimulation during vaginal intercourse. There is some evidence from controlled studies of women with primary anorgasmia that it might be effective (Pierce, 2000), although some of these studies included components of DM as well as CAT, and all had small sample sizes.

Recently, mindfulness techniques, based on Eastern techniques designed to increase nonjudgmental, "present moment" awareness, have been used in therapy for women with problems related to desire, arousal, and orgasm. Although to date there have been no controlled trials of mindfulness as a treatment for FOD, uncontrolled studies suggest that this approach has promise as an adjunct to CBT (Laan, Rellini, & Barnes, 2013).

Pharmacological and Medical Treatments

There are currently no approved pharmacological treatments for women with FOD. In a recent review of treatments for FOD, the authors concluded, "data support several potential treatments such as bupropion, sildenafil, estrogen, and testosterone" (Ishak, Bokarius, Jeffrey, Davis, & Bakhta, 2010, p. 3254). However, because of the lack of clinical trials that have evaluated these treatments in women with FOD, all of the studies included in this review involved women with *other* sexual disorders (e.g., FSAD, hypoactive sexual desire disorder).

Clinical trials of the use of testosterone patches as a treatment for women with low sexual desire have reported significant increases in orgasm frequency compared with placebo (e.g., Davis et al., 2008), but again none of these studies included women with primary orgasm complaints. Similarly, although several studies have investigated the effects of tibolone, a synthetic steroid, on sexual functioning in postmenopausal women and have reported improvements in orgasmic functioning (Ziaei, Moghasemi, & Faghihzadeh, 2010), none of these have sampled women with FOD.

There has been one randomized, placebo-controlled trial of sildenafil for women with sexual side effects related to SSRI use. At baseline 98.7% of the women reported marked delay in orgasm; sildenafil was associated with significant improvement in orgasmic functioning compared with placebo (Nurnberg et al., 2008).

Nutritional supplements such as ArginMax, which contains L-arginine, ginseng, and ginkgo, have been heavily marketed as "natural" sexual enhancement products, but there have only been two controlled studies of their efficacy in improving orgasmic functioning. In one randomized, placebo-controlled trial in pre-, peri-, and postmenopausal women, ArginMax had no significant effect on orgasm frequency (Ito, Polan, Whipple, & Trant, 2006). Another study investigated the effect of administration of ginkgo biloba extract on women with arousal and/or sexual desire problems (Meston, Rellini, & Telch, 2008). Compared with placebo, there were no positive effects of the active treatment on orgasmic functioning (or on arousal, desire, or lubrication).

The Eros clitoral therapy device is an FDA-approved, prescription-only vacuum therapy device designed to enhance clitoral blood flow and improve sexual arousal in women with sexual problems. The only published evidence that the device improves ability to achieve orgasm comes from uncontrolled studies involving small samples of women (Billups et al., 2001).

Summary

To summarize, cognitive-behavioral approaches, in particular DM, either alone or in combination with other techniques such as SF, remain the treatment of choice for most cases of female orgasmic difficulty. This is in line with recent "standard operating procedures" put forward by the International Society of Sexual Medicine, which recommended DM in conjunction with other interventions, such as sex education, anxiety reduction techniques, and CBT, as the main therapeutic tool in FOD (Laan et al., 2013). There has been very little research that has evaluated pharmacological or hormonal treatments in women diagnosed with FOD, and there are currently no empirically supported pharmacological or hormone treatments for female orgasmic problems. Figure 4.1 presents a treatment choice algorithm for FOD.

As discussed earlier, the etiology of FOD is often multifactorial. For example, SSRI-related side effects may be partially responsible for initiating an orgasm problem, but psychological and relationship factors may contribute to maintenance of the problem. Even where a clinician does not have the opportunity to work as part of a multidisciplinary team, it is important in clinical assessment and management of women with sexual problems that there is an understanding by the clinician not only of physical mechanisms but also of psychological and sociocultural factors.

In the following section, two clinical examples are presented, both involving CBT treatment with couples in which the female partner presented with orgasmic difficulties—one a case of lifelong anorgasmia and the other of situational anorgasmia.

CASE DISCUSSIONS

Case 1

Ellen was a 28-year-old woman who had married Brian, age 32, a year previously. She had had several sexual relationships before, but this was the first relationship that she had wanted to result in marriage. In general, the couple was very close and expressed a lot of affection.

Recently Brian had been asking Ellen why she didn't experience an orgasm when they had sex. She had found this difficult to discuss. In fact, she had had no problem reaching orgasm during masturbation on her own and first experienced orgasm in this way when she was 16. However, she had always used a particular technique that involved lying on top of something that would produce pressure on her clitoris and moving her body around. She had never described this to any of her sexual partners and had always been vague about her orgasms, though not denying that she had experienced them.

Ellen referred herself to a female sex therapist without telling Brian. She wanted to find out what sort of help might be available. The therapist asked her in detail about how she stimulated herself sexually and what various methods she had tried. She had not tried using a vibrator. She was then asked how she would feel telling Brian about these experiences. She would find it difficult, she explained, because she thought she was in some way abnormal, and she was worried about how he would react. The therapist then asked Ellen to describe what happened when they were having sex. Ellen typically found the physical contact pleasurable and enjoyed stimulating Brian sexually and giving him pleasure. She would get sexually aroused when Brian caressed

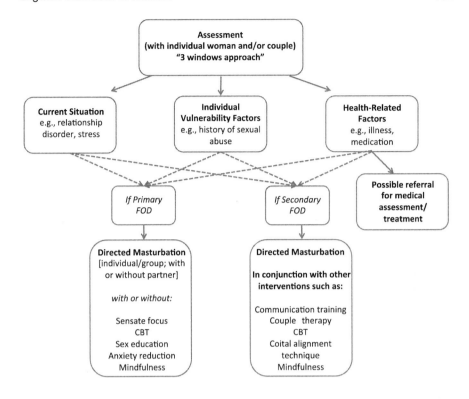

FIGURE 4.1. Treatment algorithm for FOD.

her around her genitalia, and his natural tendency was to proceed to vaginal intercourse as the next step in giving her, as well as himself, more pleasure and eventually orgasm. Although Ellen enjoyed the sensation of having him inside her, in particular the closeness and intimacy involved, she did not get as much sexual pleasure as when Brian was directly stimulating her genitalia, particularly her clitoris. Also, the "vaginal insertion" phase was typically short, because Brian would soon ejaculate.

The therapist came to the conclusion that the next appropriate step would be to start couple therapy. First, she wanted to reassure Ellen that there was nothing abnormal about her own method of achieving orgasm. Women varied substantially in what type of stimulation suited them best. There was no reason why Ellen should not incorporate her method of stimulation into her lovemaking with Brian, though they might need to experiment a bit. The idea of incorporating a vibrator into the process might be worth considering. However, the first step would be to explain to Brian what worked for her, and the therapist could help this process by assuring Brian that there was nothing abnormal about Ellen's pattern of stimulation. It was, however, made clear to Ellen that this would be a gradual process. The therapist would need to meet Brian and check with him as to how he would feel about engaging in sex therapy. She would check as to whether Brian had any particular concerns, including any about his own sexual responsiveness.

Both Brian and Ellen were motivated to engage in therapy together. The therapist first made clear that this would be a gradual process, in which the therapist would set clear limits to what the couple could do in the period between each therapy session, and that for the first few sessions, this would not involve genital stimulation of either partner (SF, stages 1 and 2). It was explained that this phase was often helpful in uncovering important issues about the relationship that may need to be dealt with first.

The couple agreed to accept this approach, and the first therapy appointment was arranged. This involved the usual assignments of avoiding any genital contact, but each partner in turn would focus on touching the other's body, initially to find ways of enjoying the touch, and subsequently to give pleasure to the person being touched. Ellen and Brian reported reasonable success with these assignments, with each being able to indicate what they liked and avoiding what they didn't like. They also recognized, somewhat to their surprise, the extent to which each enjoyed being the "toucher."

The next crucial step was to gradually include genital touching in these sessions, with each taking her or his turn. By this time it had become easier for Ellen to talk about her particular needs, and these were discussed and their "normality" emphasized at the treatment session before starting the genital touching (SF stage 3). This stage started off reasonably well, with pleasure being experienced and expressed. At the next treatment session, the therapist talked further about Ellen's particular needs and encouraged her to try using a part of Brian's body, perhaps his thigh, to rub her clitoris against. Much to Ellen's relief, Brian expressed interest in her doing this. The couple was also encouraged to obtain a vibrator and to both try using this as a form of stimulation (SF Stage 4). They were reminded that they had not yet reached SF Stage 5, when vaginal intercourse was added to the agenda.

There was good progress; the vibrator enabled both of them to experience orgasm in the presence of the other, and on another session, Ellen achieved orgasm rubbing on Brian's thigh. They were now allowed to incorporate vaginal intercourse, with the understanding that the thigh rubbing or vibrator could be used after a period of vaginal intercourse if either partner wanted to.

This successful outcome reflected the basically satisfactory relationship that existed between Ellen and Brian; that there were no major relationship hurdles to be overcome. The main issue was for Ellen to be open about her needs, and the gradual approach involved in this type of sex therapy paved the way for her.

Case 2

Anne was a 26-year-old woman who had recently started her first "steady" sexual relationship with Colin, a 29-year-old man. She had had three previous sexual partners, though the relationships were short-lived, and the sexual activity involved was not particularly enjoyable for her. With Colin she had found sexual contact to be pleasurable, and she had enjoyed giving him sexual pleasure. But Anne had never experienced an orgasm. Colin asked her about this and expressed concern that she seemed unable to have this experience. Anne decided to seek professional advice and made an appointment with a female sex therapist.

Anne reported no real history of masturbation. She had made some attempts at genital stimulation, but these didn't go very far. She described a long-standing anxiety about "letting herself go" sexually, most obviously in a relationship context. What would happen if she lost control? A key factor in Anne's history was her being sexually abused at the age of 12 by her 16-year-old brother. He had started to caress her, and she found this pleasurable and exciting, then he proceeded to rape her, which she found painful and extremely traumatic emotionally. No one else found out about this, and her account to the therapist was the first time she had spoken to anyone about it. After she recovered from the initial shock and came to realize, even though she was not to blame, how "sinful" this event was, she started to worry about the fact that initially she had found the encounter enjoyable. Thus the fear of "letting herself go" sexually was established.

As she progressed through adolescence, Anne emerged as a sexually attractive young woman. Men often showed interest in her, and, on the face of it, the idea of having a sexual relationship with a man, being married, and having a child all appealed to her. But underlying this was a fear of losing control of herself sexually.

The therapist reached the conclusion that Anne should first be treated on an individual basis, before looking at how she was faring in her relationship with Colin. It was explained to Anne that "fear of losing control" or "letting herself go" is commonly experienced by women. The key process is to establish a relationship with someone whom you trust and with whom it is safe to "let yourself go." In fact this is a particular aspect of human sexuality: The ability to "lose control" in front of another person and to remain safe and secure is a powerful factor in establishing intimacy (Bancroft, 2009). The most important and striking form of "loss of control," for both women and men, is experiencing orgasm. For a moment you are out of control (what Kinsey et al., 1953, likened to an epileptic fit), though overall it is a pleasurable experience.

The primary objective of the individual therapy was to enable Anne to experience orgasm on her own. It was, of course, possible that she might fall into the 9% of women that Kinsey et al. (1953) concluded were never able to experience orgasm. On the other hand, her history suggested a marked inhibitory factor, with the possibility that if the inhibitory component could be lessened in therapy, orgasm would occur.

There were two components to this therapy: working out suitable behavioral goals for her to work toward on her own and exploring, as she worked toward these goals, her feelings about her sexuality and the impact of her childhood abuse experience. Behaviorally, Anne was asked to go through an SF program, similar to that used for couples, in which within defined limits she explored how to touch herself. Initially, this involved only nongenital parts of her body. If she started to feel any pleasant sensation, what was her emotional reaction to it? Gradually, she reported positive responses, first to nongenital touching and later to genital touching. The latter, in particular, tended to make her feel anxious. This anxiety was discussed. Why should she feel anxious doing this to herself? To some extent the therapist needed to counter her traditional attitudes about masturbation being sinful, making the important point that masturbation is a crucial way for a woman to learn about her own sexuality and to enable her to effectively be involved in a sexual relationship.

With genital self-stimulation Anne made some progress, though not to the point of orgasm. She was starting to feel more comfortable about these sexual sensations and to feel that she was not in danger of losing control because of them. Anne was then asked to try a vibrator. She was apprehensive but willing. Initially she was asked to use the vibrator on nongenital parts of the body. Her experience with this was that the effects could vary from the pleasurable to the uncomfortable, depending on how the vibrator was applied. Then she tried the vibrator on her clitoris. This initially made her anxious, because the resulting sensations were intense. But the therapist reassured her and reminded her that inducing an orgasm in the privacy of her home would be completely safe.

Eventually, the vibrator induced an orgasm. Anne was somewhat shocked; this was an intense, unusual experience, but quite enjoyable. The therapist then encouraged her to continue using both self-touch and the vibrator two or three times a week for the next month. So far all of this was outside her relationship with Colin. She continued to elicit pleasurable orgasms using the vibrator, though not every time, and was feeling less anxious and less worried about "losing control." The therapist then suggested that Anne talk to Colin about what the therapy had involved. If he reacted in a positive way (which he did), then she could discuss bringing self-touch and vibrator stimulation into her lovemaking sessions with him, guiding him to follow some of the ways that she had learned to stimulate herself. She should not expect to experience an orgasm during vaginal intercourse but might do so either before or after. Anne did well over the next few weeks, gradually finding herself free from fear of losing control in the presence of Colin and able to enjoy orgasms in his presence.

CONCLUSIONS

The approaches taken in both of the preceding cases involved the use of a cognitive-behavioral approach with two couples presenting with fairly straightforward sexual difficulties. The same type of approach, suitably adapted, can be adopted with clients presenting with more complex, or comorbid, sexual problems. The successful outcomes highlight the importance of a careful assessment and of tailoring the approach used to the needs of the particular couple. For example, in the case involving Anne and Colin, individual sessions were first arranged with Anne, and only later were conjoint sessions held. For women presenting with primary anorgasmia, therapy may often (but not always) proceed in this way, with the initial goal being for a woman to reach orgasm on her own.

This chapter highlights how female orgasm in many ways remains an enigma. However, although basic research into the central mechanisms underlying orgasm in women is required, there is a pressing need for further treatment outcome studies, particularly of psychological therapies, but also of pharmacological treatments. Only with additional research on both types of treatment will we be able to develop effective integrated treatments.

It is now 20 years since Hawton (1992) questioned whether sex therapy research had "withered on the vine." Since then there has been a paucity of psychological treatment outcome studies, particularly on treatments for arousal, desire, and orgasm disorders in women, whereas there is now an abundant literature on trials of potential pharmacological treatments for these disorders (Ishak et al., 2010). As Heiman (2002) commented, the tendency to neglect the importance of evidence for psychological treatments is "troubling and a poor reflection on the field overall at a time when female (and male) sexual functioning could benefit from (a) more research on both psychologic and physiologic treatments and (b) a pursuit of comparison and combination studies of each treatment category." (p. 449)

ACKNOWLEDGMENT

I thank John Bancroft for his help in providing the clinical examples and for his feedback on drafts of the chapter.

REFERENCES

American Psychiatric Association. (1980). *Diagnostic and statistical manual of mental disorders* (3rd ed.). Washington, DC: Author.

American Psychiatric Association. (1994). *Diagnostic and statistical manual of mental disorders* (4th ed.). Washington, DC: Author.

American Psychiatric Association. (2000). *Diagnostic and statistical manual of mental disorders* (4th ed., text rev.). Washington, DC: Author.

American Psychiatric Association. (2013). *Diagnostic and statistical manual of mental disorders* (5th ed.). Arlington, VA: Author.

Avis, N. E., Stellato, R., Crawford, S., Johannes, C., & Longcope, C. (2000). Is there an association between menopause status and sexual functioning? *Menopause*, 7, 297–309.

Bancroft, J. (2009). *Human sexuality and its problems* (3rd ed.). Edinburgh, UK: Churchill Livingston/Elsevier.

Bancroft, J., Loftus, J., & Long, J. S. (2003). Distress about sex: A national survey of women in heterosexual relationships. *Archives of Sexual Behavior, 32,* 193–208.

Bancroft, J., Long, J. S., & McCabe, J. (2011). Sexual well-being: A comparison of U.S. Black and White women in heterosexual relationships. *Archives of Sexual Behavior, 40,* 725–740.

Basson, R. (2002). Are our definitions of women's desire, arousal, and sexual pain disorders too broad and our definition of orgasmic disorder too narrow? *Journal of Sex and Marital Therapy, 28,* 289–300.

Basson, R., & Weijmar Schultz, W. (2007). Sexual sequelae of general medical disorders. *Lancet, 369,* 350–352.

Battaglia, C., Battaglia, B., Mancini, F., Busacchi, P., Paganotto, M. C., Morotti, E., & Venturoli, S. (2012). Sexual behavior and oral contraception: A pilot study. *Journal of Sexual Medicine, 9,* 550–557.

Billups, K. L., Berman, L., Berman, J., Metz, M. E., Glennon, M. E., & Goldstein, I. (2001). A new non-pharmacological vacuum therapy for female sexual dysfunction. *Journal of Sex and Marital Therapy, 27,* 435–441.

Brody, S. (2010). The relative benefits of different sexual activities. *Journal of Sexual Medicine, 7,* 1336–1361.

Brotto, L. A. (2010). The DSM diagnostic criteria for hypoactive sexual desire disorder in women. *Archives of Sexual Behavior, 39,* 221–239.

Brotto, L. A., Bitzer, J., Laan, E., Leiblum, S., & Luria, M. (2010). Women's sexual desire and arousal disorders. *Journal of Sexual Medicine, 7,* 586–614.

Davis, S. R., Moreau, M., Kroll, R., Bouchard, C., Panay, N., Gass, M., et al. (2008). Testosterone for low libido in postmenopausal women not taking estrogen. *New England Journal of Medicine, 359,* 2005–2017.

DeRogatis, L. R., Laan E., Brauer, M., van Lunsen, R.H.W., Jannini, E., Davis, S. R., et al. (2010). Responses to the proposed DSM-V changes. *Journal of Sexual Medicine, 7,* 1998–2014.

Fisher, S. (1973). *The female orgasm.* New York: Basic Books.

Fugl-Meyer, A. R., & Fugl-Meyer, K. S. (2006). Prevalence data in Europe. In I. Goldstein, C. M. Meston, S. R. Davis, & A. M. Traish (Eds.), *Women's sexual function and dysfunction: Study, diagnosis and treatment* (pp. 34–41). Abingdon, Oxon, UK: Taylor & Francis.

Fugl-Meyer, K., & Fugl-Meyer, A. R. (2002). Sexual disabilities are not singularities. *International Journal of Impotence Research, 14,* 487–493.

Goldhammer, D. L., & McCabe, M. (2011). A qualitative exploration of the meaning and experience of sexual desire among partnered women. *Canadian Journal of Human Sexuality, 20,* 19–29.

Graham, C. A. (2010). The DSM diagnostic criteria for female orgasmic disorder. *Archives of Sexual Behavior, 39,* 256–270.

Graham, C. A., & Bancroft, J. (2006). Assessing the prevalence of female sexual dysfunction with surveys: What is feasible? In I. Goldstein, C. M. Meston, S. R. Davis, & A. M. Traish (Eds.), *Women's sexual function and dysfunction: Study, diagnosis and treatment* (pp. 52–60). Abingdon, Oxon, UK: Taylor & Francis.

Graham, C. A., & Bancroft, J. (2009). The sexual dysfunctions. In M. Gelder, J. Lopez-Ibor, N. Andreasen, & J. Geddes (Eds.), *New Oxford textbook of psychiatry* (2nd. ed., pp. 821–831). Oxford, UK: Oxford University Press.

Harris, J. M., Cherkas, L. F., Kato, B. S., Heiman, J. R., & Spector, T. D. (2008). Normal variations in personality are associated with coital orgasmic infrequency in heterosexual women: A population-based study. *Journal of Sexual Medicine*, 5, 1177–1183.

Hartmann, U., Heiser, K., Ruffer-Hesse, C., & Kloth, G. (2002). Female sexual desire disorders: Subtypes, classification, personality factors and new directions for treatment. *World Journal of Urology, 20,* 79–88.

Hawton, K. (1992). Sex therapy research: Has it withered on the vine? *Annual Review of Sex Research, 3,* 49–72.

Hayes, R. D., Dennerstein, L., Bennett, C. M., & Fairley, C. K. (2008). What is the "true" prevalence of female sexual dysfunctions, and does the way we assess these conditions have an impact? *Journal of Sexual Medicine, 5,* 777–787.

Heiman, J. R. (2002). Psychologic treatments for female sexual dysfunction: Are they effective and do we need them? *Archives of Sexual Behavior, 31,* 445–450.

Heiman, J. R. (2007). Orgasmic disorders in women. In S. R. Leiblum (Ed.), *Principles and practice of sex therapy* (4th. ed., pp. 84–123). New York: Guilford Press.

Heiman, J. R., Long, J. S., Smith, S. N., Fisher, W. A., Sand, M., S., & Rosen, R. C. (2011). Sexual satisfaction and relationship happiness in midlife and older couples in five countries. *Archives of Sexual Behavior, 40,* 741–753.

Heiman, J. R., & LoPiccolo, J. (1988). *Becoming orgasmic: A sexual and personal growth program for women* (Rev. ed.). New York: Simon & Schuster.

Heiman, J. R., Talley, D. R., Bailen, J. L., Oskin, T. A., Rosenberg, S. J., Pace, C. R., et al. (2007). Sexual function and satisfaction in heterosexual couples when men are administered sildenafil citrate (Viagra) for erectile dysfunction: A multicentre, randomised, double-blind, placebo-controlled trial. *BJOG: An International Journal of Obstetrics and Gynaecology, 114,* 437–447.

Herbenick, D., & Reece, M. (2010). Development and validation of the Female Genital Self-Image Scale. *Journal of Sexual Medicine, 7,* 1822–1830.

Hobbs, K., Symonds, T., Abraham, L., May, K., & Morris, M. F. (2008). Sexual dysfunction in partners of men with premature ejaculation. *International Journal of Impotence Research, 20,* 512–517.

Ishak, W. W., Bokarius, A., Jeffrey, J. K., Davis, M. C., & Bakhta, Y. (2010). Disorders of orgasm in women: A literature review of etiology and current treatments. *Journal of Sexual Medicine, 7,* 3254–3268.

Ito, T. Y., Polan, M. L., Whipple, B., & Trant, A. S. (2006). The enhancement of female sexual function with ArginMax, a nutritional supplement, among women differing in menopausal status. *Journal of Sex and Marital Therapy, 32,* 369–378.

Kelly, M. P., Strassberg, D. S., & Turner, C. M. (2004). Communication and associated relationship issues in female anorgasmia. *Journal of Sex and Marital Therapy, 30,* 263–276.

King, M., Holt, V., & Nazareth, I. (2007). Women's views of their sexual difficulties: Agreement and disagreement with clinical diagnoses. *Archives of Sexual Behavior, 36,* 281–288.

King, R., Belsky, J., Mah, K., & Binik, Y. (2011). Are there different types of female orgasm? *Archives of Sexual Behavior, 40,* 865–875.

Kinsey, A. C., Pomeroy, W. B., Martin, C. E., & Gebhard, P. H. (1953). *Sexual behavior in the human female*. Philadelphia: Saunders.

Komisaruk, B. R., & Whipple, B. (2011). Non-genital orgasms. *Sexual and Relationship Therapy, 26,* 356–372.

Laan, E., & Rellini, A. H. (2011). Can we treat anorgasmia in women? The challenge to experiencing pleasure. *Sexual and Relationship Therapy, 26,* 329–341.

Laan, E., Rellini, A. H., & Barnes, T. (2013). Standard operating procedures for female orgasmic disorder: Consensus of the International Society for Sexual Medicine. *Journal of Sexual Medicine, 10*, 74–82.

Laumann, E. O., Nicolosi, A., Glasser, D. B., Paik, A., Gingell, C., Moreira, E., et al. (2005). Sexual problems among women and men aged 40–80 years: Prevalence and correlates identified in the Global Study of Sexual Attitudes and Behaviors. *International Journal of Impotence Research, 17*, 39–57.

Laumann, E. O., Paik, A., & Rosen, R. C. (1999). Sexual dysfunctions in the United States: Prevalence and predictors. *Journal of the American Medical Association, 281*, 537–544.

Levin, R. J. (2011). The human female orgasm: A critical evaluation of its proposed reproductive functions. *Sexual and Relationship Therapy, 26*, 301–314.

Levine, K. B., Williams, R. E., & Hartmann, K. E. (2008). Vulvovaginal atrophy is strongly associated with female sexual dysfunction among sexually active post-menopausal women. *Menopause, 15*, 661–666.

Lindau, S. T., Schumm, L. P., Laumann, E. O., Levinson, W., O'Muircheartaigh, C. A., & Waite, L. J. (2007). A study of sexuality and health among older adults in the United States. *New England Journal of Medicine, 357*, 762–774.

Mah, K., & Binik, Y. M. (2001). The nature of human orgasm: A critical review of major trends. *Clinical Psychology Review, 21*, 823–856.

McCabe, M. (2001). Evaluation of a cognitive behavior therapy program for people with sexual dysfunction. *Journal of Sex and Marital Therapy, 27*, 259–271.

Mercer, C. H., Fenton, K. A., Johnson, A. M., Wellings, K., Macdowall, W., McManus, S., et al. (2003). Sexual function problems and help seeking behaviour in Britain: National probability sample survey. *British Medical Journal, 327*, 426–427.

Meston, C. M., Levin, R. J., Sipski, M. L., Hull, E. M., & Heiman, J. R. (2004). Women's orgasm. *Annual Review of Sex Research, 15*, 173–257.

Meston, C. M., Rellini, A. H., & Telch, M. J. (2008). Short- and long-term effects of ginkgo biloba extract on sexual dysfunction in women. *Archives of Sexual Behavior, 37*, 530–547.

Montgomery, S. A., Baldwin, D. S., & Riley, A. (2002). Antidepressant medications: A review of the evidence for drug-induced sexual dysfunction. *Journal of Affective Disorders, 69*, 119–140.

Muehlenhard, C. L., & Shippee, S. K. (2010). Men's and women's reports of pretending orgasm. *Journal of Sex Research, 47*, 552–567.

Nicolson, P., & Burr, J. (2003). What is "normal" about women's (hetero)sexual desire and orgasm?: A report of an in-depth interview study. *Social Science and Medicine, 9*, 1735–1745.

Nobre, P. J., & Pinto-Gouveia, J. (2006). Dysfunctional sexual beliefs as vulnerability factors for sexual dysfunction. *Journal of Sex Research, 43*, 68–75.

Nobre, P. J., Pinto-Gouveia, J., & Gomes, F. A. (2006). Prevalence and comorbidity of sexual dysfunctions in a Portuguese clinical sample. *Journal of Sex and Marital Therapy, 32*, 173–182.

Nurnberg, H. G., Hensley, P. L., Heiman, J. R., Croft, H. A., Debattista, C., & Paine, S. (2008). Sildenafil treatment of women with antidepressant-associated sexual dysfunction. *Journal of the American Medical Association, 300*, 395–404.

Oberg, K., Fugl-Meyer, A. R., & Fugl-Meyer, K. S. (2004). On categorization and quantification of women's sexual dysfunctions: An epidemiological approach. *International Journal of Impotence Research, 16*, 261–269.

O'Sullivan, L. F., & Majerovich, J. (2008). Difficulties with sexual functioning in a sample of male and female late adolescent and young adult university students. *Canadian Journal of Human Sexuality, 17*, 109–121.

Petersen, J. L., & Hyde, J. S. (2011). Gender differences in sexual attitudes and behavior: A review of meta-analytic results and large datasets. *Journal of Sex Research, 48*, 149–165.

Pierce, A. P. (2000). The coital alignment technique (CAT): An overview of studies. *Journal of Sex and Marital Therapy, 26*, 257–268.

Prause, N. (2011). The human female orgasm: Critical evaluations of proposed psychological sequelae. *Sexual and Relationship Therapy, 26*, 315–328.

Rellini, A., & Meston, C. (2007). Sexual function and satisfaction in adults based on the definition of child sexual abuse. *Journal of Sexual Medicine, 4*, 1312–1321.

Richters, J., Grulich, A. E., de Visser, R. O., Smith, A. M. A., & Rissel, C. E. (2003). Sexual difficulties in a representative sample of adults. *Australian and New Zealand Journal of Public Health, 27*, 164–170.

Robinson, B. E., Munns, R. A., Weber-Main, A. M., Lowe, M. A., & Raymond, N. C. (2011). Application of the sexual health model in the long-term treatment of hypoactive sexual desire and female orgasmic disorder. *Archives of Sexual Behavior, 40*, 469–478.

Sanders, S. A., Graham, C. A., & Milhausen, R. R. (2008). Predicting sexual problems in women: Relevance of sexual inhibition and sexual excitation. *Archives of Sexual Behavior, 37*, 241–251.

Shifren, J. L., Monz, B. U., Russo, P. A., Segreti, A., & Johannes, C. B. (2008). Sexual problems and distress in United States women. *Obstetrics and Gynecology, 112*, 970–978.

Staples, J., Rellini, A. H., & Roberts, S. P. (2012). Avoiding experiences: Sexual dysfunction in women with a history of sexual abuse in childhood and adolescence. *Archives of Sexual Behavior, 41*, 341–350.

Ter Kuile, M. M., Both, S., & van Lankveld, J. J. D. M. (2012). Sexual dysfunctions in women. In P. Sturmey & M. Hersen (Eds.). *Handbook of evidence-based practice in clinical psychology: Vol. II. Adult disorders* (pp. 413–436). Hoboken, NJ: Wiley.

West, S. L., Vinikoor, L. C., & Zolhoun, D. (2004). A systematic review of the literature on female sexual dysfunction prevalence and predictors. *Annual Review of Sex Research, 15*, 40–172.

Witting, K., Santtila, P., Varjonen, M., Jern, P., Johansson, A., von der Pahlen, B., & Sandnabba, K. (2008). Female sexual dysfunction, sexual distress, and compatibility with partner. *Journal of Sexual Medicine, 5*, 2587–2599.

World Health Organization. (1992). *ICD-10: International Statistical Classification of Diseases and Related Health Problems* (10th ed.). Geneva, Switzerland: Author.

Ziaei, S., Moghasemi, M., & Faghihzadeh, S. (2010). Comparative effects of conventional hormone replacement therapy and tibolone on climacteric symptoms and sexual dysfunction in postmenopausal women. *Climacteric, 13*, 147–156.

Zietsch, B. P., Miller, G. F., Bailey, M., & Martin, N. G. (2011). Female orgasm rates are largely independent of other traits: Implications for "Female Orgasmic Disorder" and evolutionary theories of orgasm. *Journal of Sexual Medicine, 8*, 2305–2316.

CHAPTER 5

Treatment of Premature Ejaculation

Psychotherapy, Pharmacotherapy, and Combined Therapy

Stanley E. Althof

Althof remarks: "These days, delaying men's ejaculatory latency is relatively straightforward; however, restoring men's sexual confidence and reversing the impact on the relationship is more complicated." Althof observes that treatment options for men suffering from premature ejaculation (PE) have expanded from the early days of sex therapy in which behavioral interventions such as stop–start or the squeeze technique predominated. Psychopharmacological interventions are now quite often used, alone or in conjunction with behavioral techniques. This change reflects an understanding that rapid ejaculation may not simply be the result of faulty learning or unfortunate early life experiences but may stem from a biological vulnerability. Despite our increasing knowledge concerning the biological underpinnings of PE, Althof asserts that sex therapy is more relevant now than ever. He notes that the psychological impact of PE on a man, his partner, and their relationship may be very damaging. PE can make sexual intimacy a frustrating experience for the woman and a humiliating one for the man. Anxiety, which maintains the pattern of rapid ejaculation, may lead to the development of other sexual problems, including erectile dysfunction, and may not abate with medication alone. Choosing the right combination of medication and individual and couple therapy is key to treatment success. And yet despite all the reasons for optimism Althof still cautions "that we cannot help everyone."

112

Stanley E. Althof, PhD, is the Executive Director of the Center for Marital and Sexual Health of South Florida and Professor Emeritus at Case Western Reserve University. Dr. Althof is a clinical psychologist who specializes in both male and female sexual problems, as well as relationship issues. Dr. Althof has served as the President of both the Society for Sex Therapy and Research (SSTAR) and the International Society for Women's Sexual Health (ISSWSH). He is currently a Board Member of the Sexual Medicine Society of North America. Dr. Althof is an accomplished speaker on sexual problems of men and women and has over 100 peer-reviewed publications.

The landscape has dramatically changed for patients seeking treatment for premature ejaculation (PE). Prior to the mid-1990s, psychotherapy or behavioral treatment was considered to be the treatment of choice for this distressing sexual dysfunction. By 1995, clinicians began successfully experimenting with the off-label administration of selective serotonin reuptake inhibitors (SSRIs) to delay ejaculatory latency (Waldinger, Zwinderman, Schweitzer, & Olivier, 2004). Over the past 7 years, dapoxetine, a novel, short-acting SSRI, received medical approval in several countries, but not the United States. Other compounds are in various stages of development, but as of this writing, none have received approval.

Given the efficacy and relative safety of the off-label treatments, some clinicians may perceive psychotherapy/behavior therapy for rapid ejaculation as an obsolete and antiquated intervention. On the contrary, psychotherapy and a combination of medical treatment and psychotherapy remain more relevant than ever. These days delaying men's ejaculatory latency is relatively straightforward, however, restoring men's sexual confidence and reversing the impact on the relationship is more complicated (Althof, 2005).

Psychotherapy remains useful either in its traditional form as the sole intervention for men or couples with rapid ejaculation or, in an updated rendering, as an integral aspect of a combined medical and psychological intervention (Althof, 2003, 2005; Althof et al., 2010)

WHAT'S IN A NAME?: DEFINING PE

Several definitions of PE exist, having been crafted by various professional organizations and/or individuals (American Psychiatric Association, 2000; Masters & Johnson, 1970; Metz & McCarthy, 2003; Waldinger, Hengeveld, & Zwinderman, 1998; World Health Organization, 1994). The major criticisms of the existing definitions include their failure to be evidence based, lack of specific operational criteria, excessive vagueness, and reliance on the subjective judgment of the diagnostician. Nonetheless, three common constructs underlie most definitions of PE: (1) a short ejaculatory latency; (2) a lack of perceived self-efficacy or control about the timing of ejaculation; and

(3) distress and interpersonal difficulty (related to the ejaculatory dysfunction).

Because of the discontent with the existing definitions, as well as pressure from the regulatory agencies concerning the inadequacy of the PE definitions, the International Society for Sexual Medicine (ISSM) convened a meeting of experts to review the evidence-based literature and to develop a definition grounded in clearly definable scientific criteria (McMahon et al., 2008). After carefully reviewing the literature, the committee proposed that lifelong PE is

> A male sexual dysfunction characterized by ejaculation which always or nearly always occurs prior to or within about one minute of vaginal penetration, and the inability to delay ejaculation on all or nearly all vaginal penetrations, and negative personal consequences, such as distress, bother, frustration and/or the avoidance of sexual intimacy. (McMahon et al., 2008)

The definition applies only to intravaginal sexual activity. It does not define PE in the context of other sexual behaviors or men having sex with men. Additionally, the Committee concluded that there are insufficient published objective data to propose a new evidence-based definition of acquired PE, although it believed that the proposed criterion for lifelong PE might be applied to acquired PE as well.

DSM-5 (American Psychiatric Association, 2013) has accepted the ISSM definition, adding that the dysfunction needs to be present for at least 6 months and occur in 75% of sexual intercourse events. Overall, I am pleased to see DSM-5 moving away from its previous definition to a more evidence-based criterion set. The subtypes of lifelong and acquired PE have also been retained and may prove useful in selecting appropriate treatment interventions.

"Lifelong" PE characterizes a man who has always struggled with the dysfunction, whereas "acquired" refers to an individual who previously had the ability to control ejaculation but who later developed the dysfunction. Approximately two-thirds of men with PE have the lifelong form, and one-third have the acquired type. It may turn out that a subgroup of lifelong rapid ejaculators have a biological vulnerability, but not those with acquired symptoms (Cooper, Cernoskey, & Colussi, 1993; Gospodinoff, 1989).

Case Vignette

Larry, a 58-year-old attorney in his second marriage, typified men with lifelong rapid ejaculation. He described never being able to last more than 15 seconds with any sexual partner. He had tried masturbating prior to lovemaking, excessively drinking alcohol, and distracting himself with nonsexual thoughts. He had read books about premature ejaculation and diligently practiced the stop–start exercises to no avail. This "disability" was a great source of shame for him, and he felt it had greatly interfered in his relationships prior to marriage and in both of his marriages. His wife, Dana, was supportive and praised Larry for going "all out to please her after his orgasm." They appeared to have a good relationship, and neither partner had significant psychological problems. They had come for consultation after reading that SSRIs were helpful to men with rapid ejaculation. He seemed like an ideal candidate for pharmacotherapy and did well with it.

Acquired PE calls upon the clinician to explore the forces that generated the new symptom, which may reflect recent psychosocial stressors or be a consequence of an illness (prostatitis, hyperthyroidism), medication, or surgery. For instance, acquired rapid ejaculation may be a consequence of erectile failure. Men with ED develop performance anxiety regarding their erectile reliability, hurry intercourse, and are at risk to develop PE.

DSM-IV-TR (American Psychiatric Association, 2000) also instructs clinicians to designate whether the PE is generalized or specific. "Generalized" refers to a man who manifests the conditions with all partners, whereas in the specific type the man has a variable pattern of normal ejaculation with some partners and rapid ejaculation with others. A specific pattern would strongly suggest that psychological factors are responsible for the rapid ejaculation. It is not uncommon for men to report a greater ejaculatory latency during masturbation than during partner sexual behaviors. However, the longer latency with masturbation does not by itself constitute a specific form of PE, especially if the man reports rapid ejaculation with all sexual partners.

Case Vignette

Jay, a 6'2" well-muscled, 30-year-old, never-married Marine sought consultation because he had developed rapid ejaculation with his new partner of 6 weeks. Jay prided himself on his masculinity and said he could not understand why this was happening to him now.

There was a bragging quality to Jay as he detailed his sexual history. He had slept with many women and had never suffered from rapid ejaculation. Most of his prior relationships were of relatively brief duration. Jay enjoyed being single and sleeping around.

The essential question in my mind was what was different now. With some embarrassment Jay revealed that he was intimidated by his new partner. She was a beautiful, successful woman, the CEO of a small corporation, and he felt "dominated" by her. I asked if he had ever been in a relationship with any other woman in which he felt dominated. At first he said no, then he laughed and recalled that many years ago there was such a woman, and, yes, he also suffered from rapid ejaculation with her. We immediately knew which issue to focus on.

Anteportal ejaculation is the term for men who ejaculate prior to vaginal penetration and is considered the most severe form of PE. Such men or couples typically present when they are having difficulty conceiving children.

It is estimated that 5% of men with lifelong PE suffer from anteportal PE (Pagani, Rodrigues, Torselli, & Genari, 1996; Waldinger, Rietschel, Nothen, Hengeveld, & Olivier, 1998)

Although they are not evidence based, Waldinger proposed two additional "subtypes" for men who are distressed about their ejaculatory function but do not meet the ISSM criterion for PE (Waldinger, 2008). These subtypes should be considered provisional; however, they accurately characterize many men who do not qualify for the diagnosis of PE and are asking for help. These two subtypes are termed "natural variable PE" and "premature-like ejaculatory dysfunction." Natural variable PE is characterized by early ejaculations that occur irregularly and inconsistently with a subjective sense of diminished control. This subtype is not considered a sexual dysfunction or psychopathology but rather a normal variation in sexual performance.

Premature-like ejaculatory dysfunction is characterized by (1) subjective perception of consistent or inconsistent rapid ejaculation during intercourse; (2) preoccupation with an imagined early ejaculation or lack of control of ejaculation; (3) actual intravaginal ejaculation latency time (IELT) in the normal range or even of longer duration (i.e., an ejaculation that occurs after 5 minutes); (4) ability to control ejaculation (i.e., to withhold ejaculation at the moment of imminent ejaculation) may be diminished or lacking; and (5) the preoccupation is not better accounted for by another mental disorder (Waldinger, 2008).

Case Vignette

George, a 35-year-old single auto worker, came in asking for a drug to prolong his ejaculatory latency. His girlfriend was complaining that he ejaculated too quickly and that she was unable to reach orgasm. Upon inquiry George stated that his IELT was 20 minutes. I was astounded that he believed he had rapid ejaculation. He was obviously distressed and hurt by his girlfriend's comments and very much wanted to please her.

I asked how long he thought the average man lasted during intercourse. Forty minutes, he responded. He said the guys at work talked about intercourse that lasted between 30 and 60 minutes. He had difficulty believing me when I told him that the average man lasted between 5 and 10 minutes. He was not relieved to hear me say that he did not have rapid ejaculation. He still wanted to know how he could prolong his ejaculation and was upset that we were not willing to give him medication. I urged him to consider coming to see me with his girlfriend but was not surprised that he did not follow through.

This vignette highlights the not infrequently seen dynamic of women who blame men for their struggles with orgasm or sexual pain. On the other hand, George's girlfriend may have held false beliefs about how easily and regularly women achieve orgasm with intercourse.

PREVALENCE

Most articles on rapid ejaculation begin by asserting that it is the most common male sexual dysfunction, affecting approximately one in three men. Several recent cross-sectional, international, epidemiological studies support the 20–30% prevalence figure for this disorder (Jannini & Lenzi, 2005; Laumann et al., 2005; Rosen, Porst, & Montorsi, 2004).

All these studies, however, have employed patient self-report or patient dissatisfaction with rapidity of ejaculation during intercourse rather than a diagnosis by a trained clinician. Reporting dissatisfaction with ejaculatory latency or labeling oneself as premature is not the same as meeting any of the published criterion sets, even the much-criticized DSM-IV-TR (American Psychiatric Association, 2000) definition. It may indeed be a problem for the individual; he may, however, not have a sexual dysfunction (recall the description of premature-like ejaculatory syndrome). In my opinion, these figures are likely to be an overestimate of the true prevalence of rapid ejaculation.

The prevalence of any disorder can be significantly changed by modifying its definition. With the adoption of the DSM-5 (American Psychiatric Association, 2013) definition of PE, with its approximately 1-minute IELT criterion, the prevalence of PE will be greatly reduced.

Is PE a Disorder of the Young?

It has always been assumed that rapid ejaculation is a dysfunction of the young, with diminishing prevalence with age. This notion presumes that with age men habituate to the exciting sexual sensations or that there is a slowing of the ejaculatory reflex. This long-held belief was recently challenged by publication of two datasets demonstrating that the prevalence of premature/rapid ejaculation was constant across age groups ranging from 18 to 70 (Laumann, Paik, & Rosen, 1999; Rosen et al., 2004). These studies are limited because they did not follow men longitudinally to assess changes in IELT with age. Nonetheless, it appears that the belief that the prevalence of PE diminishes with age is not supported by current data. From a cross-sectional perspective, PE appears to affect a broader age range of individuals than ED, and the prevalence of PE appears to be higher than that of ED in any given age bracket studied.

ETIOLOGY

For years the prevailing opinion was that rapid ejaculation was a psychological or learned condition. However, a series of biological investigations has begun to unravel the physiological underpinnings of the ejaculatory process, leading theorists to speculate about organic contributions to this disorder (Gospodinoff, 1989; Grenier & Byers, 1997; Metz & McCarthy, 2003).

At this juncture, unlike in erectile dysfunction, in which a coherent story of smooth muscle relaxation/contraction mediated by nitric oxide has been elucidated, the pathophysiology of PE remains incomplete and yet to be determined.

Even if we were able to unequivocally state that a man's PE was due to exclusively biological factors, he would still manifest a psychological response that would worsen the condition. Additionally, his partner is also likely to be psychologically affected by the dysfunction, even if the condition might be due exclusively to organic factors.

The most promising biological etiologies include the role of serotonin receptors, an individual's genetic predisposition, hyperthyroidism, prostatitis, and increased penile sensitivity or nerve conduction abnormalities. However, none of these mechanisms account for more than a small percentage of men with PE.

In support of the serotonin receptor hypothesis, based on studies of rodents, Waldinger, Berendsen, Blok, Olivier, and Holstege (1998) report that activation of the 5-HT_{2C} receptor delays ejaculation whereas activation of the 5-HT_{1A} receptor speeds up ejaculation. Assuming congruency between rodent and human neuroreceptors, Waldinger, Berendsen, et al. (1998) speculate that rapid ejaculation may be understood as a hypofunction of the 5-HT_{2C} receptor or a hyperfunction of the 5-HT_{1A} receptor. Because of safety concerns, this work cannot at present be performed on humans, so it remains only a highly intriguing theory.

The genetic hypothesis of PE was first formed by Bernhard Schapiro in 1942, who described how some family members of men with PE also have PE (Schapiro, 1943). Many years later Waldinger, Berendsen, et al. (1998) hypothesized that both the IELT and lifelong PE for some men are genetically determined. Like Schapiro, Waldinger (Waldinger, Rietschel, Nothen, Hengeveld, & Olivier, 1998) also found a high prevalence of PE among first-degree male relatives of Dutch men with lifelong PE. Additionally, a genetic study of 1,196 Finnish male twins between the ages of 33 and 43 years (Jern et al., 2007) suggested that genetics accounts for 28% of the variance, with no shared environmental variance (0%) and 72% nonshared environmental variance. One possible interpretation of these findings is that genetic influences may create a diathesis or predisposition in some men to ejaculate prematurely.

Endocrine control of the ejaculatory reflex is still not completely clarified (Corona et al., 2011). There is evidence to indicate a link between depression, serotonin, and thyroid hormones. Carani reported that 50% of men with hyperthyroidism had PE and, when successfully treated, the prevalence of PE fell to 15% (Carani, Isidori, & Granata, 2005).

Regarding the heightened penile sensitivity and/or nerve conduction hypothesis, the findings of several studies have been contradictory. Some support this notion; others show no relationship between PE and either heightened penile sensitivity or rapidity of the bulbocavernosus reflex (Fanciullacci, Colpi, Beretta, & Zanollo, 1988; Gospodinoff, 1989; Mirone et al., 2001).

Psychological Theories

There are multiple psychological explanations as to why men develop PE. Unfortunately, none of the theories evolve from evidence-based research; rather, they are the products of thoughtful synthesis by clinicians from several schools of thought. Although untested, the theories are thought provoking and have been helpful to clinicians over the years.

In 1927, Karl Abraham, a German psychoanalyst, speculated that PE is due to a combination of the man's unconscious hostile feelings toward women and his passive pleasure, as a child, in losing control of his urination (passive urethral eroticism), which in adulthood transforms itself into his passive pleasure in giving up control of ejaculation. Thus ejaculation into the woman's vagina was equated with "soiling" or "debasing" her. The man takes his sexual pleasure, unconsciously soils her, and in so doing deprives her of sexual pleasure. Simultaneously he gives himself over to the passive pleasure of letting go of his ejaculation without any attempt to control his sexual excitement or delay ejaculation (Abraham, 1927).

A second psychoanalytic explanation focuses on the man's unresolved excessive narcissism during infancy, which results in his placing exaggerated importance on his penis. This hypothesis might explain the selfishness observed in some rapid ejaculators who seem unconcerned with pleasuring their partners.

In 1943, Bernard Schapiro introduced the notion that PE was a psychosomatic disorder. In his view, premature ejaculation is a bodily symptom that expresses the man's psychological conflict, akin to psychosomatic explanations for headache, backache, and stomach pain. In his view, because men with PE had "weakened" genitourinary systems, they became rapid ejaculators rather than expressing their psychological conflict through another organ system (e.g., headache; Schapiro, 1943).

Psychodynamic theorists consider anxiety to be the primary etiological agent in precipitating the symptom of rapid ejaculation. However, anxiety is not a singular concept; it is employed to characterize at least three different mental phenomena. Anxiety may refer to (1) a phobic response, such as being fearful (i.e., afraid of the dark, wet, unseen vagina); (2) an affect, the end result of conflict resolution in which two contradictory urges are at play (i.e., the man is angry at his partner but feels guilty about directly expressing his hostility); or (3) anticipatory anxiety, commonly referred to as performance anxiety, in which preoccupation with sexual failures and poor performance leads to deteriorating sexual function and avoidance of future sexual interactions.

Conceptualizing PE in more of a behavioral-learning perspective, Masters and Johnson (1970) emphasized the concept of "early learned experience." By reviewing the case histories of men with PE, Masters and Johnson noted that many men described first sexual experiences characterized by haste and nervousness, for example, making love in the backseat of an automobile or an encounter with a prostitute. Masters and Johnson speculated that based on their initial experiences the men became conditioned to ejaculate rapidly.

Kaplan (1989) considered "lack of sexual sensory awareness" to be the immediate, here-and-now cause of rapid ejaculation. She believed that men fail to develop sufficient feedback regarding their level of sexual arousal. Such men experience themselves as going from low levels of arousal to ejaculation without any awareness.

The Role of Performance Anxiety

Performance anxiety per se does not generally cause the initial episode of rapid ejaculation; however, it is pernicious in maintaining the dysfunction. By the time patients present for psychological intervention, the initial precipitating event often is obscured because of the intensity of the man's performance anxiety. A further complication of performance anxiety is that it distracts the man from focusing on his level of arousal, rendering him helpless to exert voluntary control over sexual arousal and ejaculation. In fact, men believe that focusing on their level of arousal will only cause them to ejaculate even more rapidly.

IMPACT ON THE MAN AND THE COUPLE

Premature ejaculation affects both individual and relationship quality of life (QOL). Qualitative research showed that the majority of men with PE (68%) report a decrease in sexual self-confidence. Moreover, half of the single men describe either avoidance of relationships or reluctance to establish new relationships. Men in relationships report distress at not satisfying their partners, with some worrying that their partners would be unfaithful to them because of their PE.

Embarrassment regarding discussing PE was the primary reason for not consulting a physician, cited by 67% of respondents. Interestingly, almost half thought no treatment existed (47%).

Hartmann, Schedlowski, and Kruger (2005) characterize men with PE as preoccupied with thoughts about controlling their orgasm, with anxious anticipation of a possible failure, with thoughts about embarrassment and about keeping their erections. In contrast, they found that functional men focused on sexual arousal and sexual satisfaction.

Intimacy is also affected in men with PE. Men with PE scored lower on all aspects of intimacy (emotional, social, sexual, recreational, and intellectual) and had lower QOL (lower levels of satisfaction in all areas) than sexually functional men (McCabe, 1997).

PE also has a negative effect on the partner's QOL. A recent study showed a relationship between PE and lower partner sexual satisfaction in heterosexual couples (Byers & Grenier, 2003). Partners are not just distressed because of the quality of the man's sexual performance; they are also upset because the condition and the man's associated distress often lead to a rapid and unwanted interruption of intimacy. Women are also angry with their partners with PE because they do not feel that their concerns have been genuinely "heard" by the men nor that they are unwilling to "fix" the problem. Men likewise believe that their partners do not understand the degree of frustration and humiliation that they routinely experience. This disconnection between the men and their partners is the basis for considerable relationship tension. Thus, for men in stable relationships, PE should be recognized as a couple's issue. All these studies suggest that the psychosocial impact of PE on the patient and partner has profound psychosocial consequences.

EVALUATION

Although clinicians conceptually separate evaluation and treatment processes, patients do not. For them the "cure" begins with the first encounter. The patient is, of course, correct; the attentive therapist is aware that the psychotherapeutic relationship and all its transference ramifications are initiated with the first handshake and entry into the consulting room.

Attend to the Therapeutic Relationship before Attending to the Data

The establishment of a respectful, comfortable, and healing relationship with the patient(s) is the primary goal of the evaluation session. Too often the secondary goal of gathering data displaces the more human process of relating to one another. The man and his partner are likely to be anxious and uncomfortable; they are about to share aspects of their intimate life with a stranger.

Talking about sexual matters does not come naturally to most people. The therapist must first set them at ease before progressing into the more difficult material. When couples seem ready to work, one can ask, "What brings you in?" Others may need more soothing, so asking, "How is it for you to come in today and talk with me?" may be helpful. For the very anxious patient, it may be advisable to start by asking, "Did you have any trouble finding the office?"

Look for Early Resistance

Infrequently, even when the presenting problem is sexual, there are first meetings at which sexual issues are not discussed. This is significant and challenges the therapist to assess whether the resistance belongs to the patient or to the therapist. I still recall my reluctance to ask an elderly European gentleman about his sexual life because he very much reminded me of my father. Unknowingly, I was avoiding taking a sexual history. At 15 minutes into the hour this man asked, "So, when are you going to ask me about sex?" He was right. I laughed to myself, recognizing the countertransference, and was able to proceed.

Patients' reluctance to share sexual material may arise from a number of factors. The old analytic maxim "resistance before conflict" is good advice. Inquiry should shift from descriptions of the couple's sexual life to understanding what prevents the man or woman from discussing this subject.

In most ordinary clinical interviews, sociocultural and religious prohibitions against talking about sexual life are encountered. These include: "In our family, such matters were never discussed" and "I grew up thinking it was wrong to talk about sex with anyone." Sometimes the gender of the interviewer is the focus of the resistance. "I can't talk about this with a male/female doctor." Acknowledging the patient's discomfort and giving permission and reassurance often overcomes resistance stemming from these sources. If the therapist's gender continues to be an unyielding source of resistance, referral should be made to a colleague of the opposite gender.

Patients' expectations regarding treatment also contribute to resistance. Couples do not know what to expect. Some are afraid that the therapist will physically examine them or watch them engage in sexual behavior. Others may have concerns about the therapist being sexual with them or asking them to engage in sexual behaviors that they consider unconventional.

The Secret: The Pitfalls from Collusion

A stronger, more persistent source of resistance initially stems from patients' reluctance to reveal aspects of their lives that are embarrassing, shameful, or hurtful to themselves or their partners. These secrets kept from the therapist may have their origins in fragments of traumatic childhood sexual experiences, awareness of unconventional fantasies, extramarital relationships, or conflictual young adult life events that have not been shared with others, such as the suicide of a brother, periods of sexual promiscuity, a visit to a prostitute, having been raped, or a homosexual encounter.

Some patients rationalize that these events, feelings, or fantasies are unrelated to the current problem and therefore do not need to be shared. Conversely, others are keenly aware of the impact of the secrets on their psychological and sexual lives but lack sufficient trust, courage, or motivation to address these problematic life dilemmas.

Honesty between patient and therapist is the cornerstone of treatment. Conscious avoidance and withholding of information compromises the therapeutic process. My current policy is not to begin couple treatment if one partner asks me not to talk about a relatively current and important issue, for example, a 2-year affair that ended 2 months before. I have less difficulty agreeing to maintain a secret such as "Twenty years ago, on an out-of-town business trip, I had a one-night affair." My rationale is that I do not see a brief, remote affair as necessarily relevant and that disclosure of the event to the partner may prove to be more destructive than helpful.

Assessment: What to Ask

Each therapist needs to develop his or her style and method of assessing PE. What follows is my method. Figure 5.1 offers an assessment and treatment algorithm that readers might find helpful.

If the man with PE is in a relationship, I generally ask to see the couple together and the man and woman alone separately. Partners are not always initially willing to be part of the process. In that situation, I see the man alone. I begin by asking a patient when the PE began and whether there was ever a time when he had control over ejaculation. I chart the course of the problem and ask specifically about average IELT, degree of voluntary control, distress, and sexual satisfaction. I want to know why he or they have chosen to seek treatment at this point in time and what prevented them from seeking consultation previously.

I move on to take a sexual history to identify whether there are any coexisting sexual dysfunctions and to learn whether the patient has PE with all partners or only specific partners. Then I ask the patient to recount in detail a recent sexual encounter. This helps to clarify the degree of performance anxiety, the narrowness or broadness of his sexual repertoire, his cognitions and affect, what happens after he ejaculates, and the responses of the partner to his dysfunction. I attempt to ascertain whether he attends to or has an awareness of his level of sexual arousal. I inquire as to the strategies he has employed to delay ejaculation and whether or not they were successful. I also ask if he was previously in psychotherapy and what that experience was like for him. From a medical standpoint, I ask about health issues inquiring about prostatitis and hyperthyroidism, specifically in acquired PE.

The next portion of the assessment focuses on his interpersonal relationship and the impact of PE on the couple's sexual and nonsexual intimacy and overall relationship. Questions about the partner are broached, such as the following: Does she suffer from any sexual dysfunctions? Does she engage in strategies to help delay his rapid ejaculation, or does she seem to encourage his ejaculating rapidly? Is she willing to participate in treatment? These questions allow the therapist to form preliminary judgments regarding the partner's willingness to help with treatment versus her potential to sabotage it.

Lastly, I try to ascertain the patient's interpersonal style, psychological comorbidities, and limitations or strengths regarding treatment. All this data should help me to develop preliminary hypotheses as to the predisposing, precipitating, maintaining, and contextual factors and what resistances might interfere with treatment (McCabe et al., 2009).

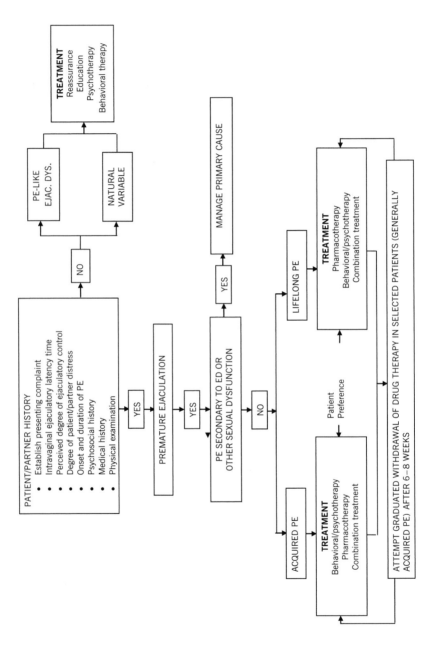

FIGURE 5.1. Algorithm for the management of PE. Reprinted with permission from D. Rowland.

THE FIRST DECISION: INDIVIDUAL OR COUPLE TREATMENT, PHARMACOTHERAPY, OR COMBINED PSYCHOLOGICAL–PHARMACOLOGICAL THERAPY

The evaluation concludes with the therapist offering the patients his or her understanding of the issues and treatment recommendations. There are several distinct possibilities: individual therapy for one or both partners, conjoint or couple treatment, pharmacotherapy alone, or combined pharmacological and psychological treatment.

It seems odd that combined pharmacological and psychological treatment of sexual problems has not established itself as a mainstream intervention for either mental health clinicians or sexual health physicians who treat sexual problems (e.g., urologists or family practice physicians). Generally, mental health clinicians offer psychological interventions, and medical practitioners offer pharmacological treatment. Studies on combined medical and psychological therapy all demonstrate that combined treatment is superior to medical treatment alone (Li, Zhy, Xu, Sun, & Wang, 2006; Steggall, Fowler, & Pryce, 2008; Tang, Ma, Zhao, Liu, & Chen, 2004; Yuan, Dai, Yang, Guo, & Liang, 2008). What follows is a discussion of psychotherapy alone, pharmacological treatment alone, and combined therapy.

When to Offer What

Psychotherapy alone is best reserved for men and couples for whom the precipitating and maintaining factors are clearly psychological and the psychosocial obstacles are too great to surmount with pharmacotherapy alone. Examples of these psychosocial obstacles include: (1) patient variables, such as the degree of performance anxiety or presence of depression; (2) partner issues, such as how she copes with the sexual dysfunction or whether his rapid ejaculation obscures her sexual dysfunction; (3) interpersonal nonsexual variables, such as a chronically unsatisfying relationship; (4) contextual variables, including lack of privacy; and (5) each partner's expectations from treatment (e.g., "he should last 20 minutes because it takes me that long to have an orgasm").

Individual psychotherapy is the default choice for single men not in relationships. In addition to treating the sexual dysfunction, therapy must address these men's often-seen reluctance to enter into new relationships for fear of humiliating themselves and disappointing the woman. Psychotherapy can only go so far without the presence of a partner. For these men, treatment is sometimes divided into two phases: treatment when there is no partner and later resumption of treatment when they establish a new relationship.

For men in relationships, individual psychotherapy is recommended when the psychological variables supporting the dysfunction are thought to be more intrapsychic than interpersonal, for example, fear of penetrating a dark, wet, warm vagina or excessive fear of or hostility to women. These are generally products of unresolved childhood issues that continue to interfere in the man's adult sexual life. Individual psychotherapy may also be the treatment of choice when the relationship is deemed too chaotic or unworkable or when the partner refuses to participate. Individual treatment in these situations is of course limited given the limitations of the interpersonal environment.

Conjoint psychotherapy is recommended for men with either lifelong or acquired forms of PE in which both partners are relatively psychologically healthy and motivated to pursue treatment. Ideally, the precipitating and maintaining factors can be elucidated, the impact of the dysfunction on both partners can be clarified, and interventions directed at him, her, and both of them can be initiated.

Pharmacotherapy alone is recommended when the man has severe lifelong premature ejaculation, is sexually experienced, is in a satisfying relationship, and has reasonable expectations regarding treatment outcome. These men must understand that pharmacotherapy alone will not "cure" the problem; the rapid ejaculation will return as soon as they stop taking the medication. They must therefore be willing to continue on the medication for the foreseeable future.

Combined therapy offers the best of both worlds (Althof, 2003, 2005, 2006; Perelman, 2003, 2006). Pharmacotherapy will rapidly delay ejaculation and allow the man to regain some sexual confidence. Psychotherapy will help the man or couple maximize gains from pharmacotherapy. It seeks to help men and couples overcome the psychosocial obstacles that interfere with making effective use of the pharmacological intervention. The man can be taught to attend to sensations rather than fear his arousal. He can learn to pace his arousal and expand his sexual repertoire without fear that it will lead to rapid ejaculation. In time, he can be slowly weaned from pharmacotherapy and implement what he has learned in psychotherapy. Not all men will be able to give up the pharmacological intervention; some, however, will be pleased that "on their own" they have triumphed over adversity.

PSYCHOTHERAPY ALONE

Present-day psychotherapy for rapid ejaculation is an integration of psychodynamic, systems, behavioral, and cognitive approaches within a short-term psychotherapy model (Althof, 2005; Kaplan, 1989; Levine, 1992; Masters & Johnson, 1970; McCarthy, 1990; Metz & McCarthy, 2003; Semans, 1956; Zilbergeld, 1992). The guiding principles of treatment are to learn to control ejaculation while understanding the meaning of the symptom and the context in which it occurs. Psychotherapy and behavioral interventions improve ejaculatory control by helping men and couples to: (1) learn techniques to control and/or delay ejaculation, (2) gain confidence in their sexual performance, (3) lessen performance anxiety, (4) modify rigid sexual repertoires, (5) surmount barriers to intimacy, (6) resolve interpersonal issues that precipitate and maintain the dysfunction, (7) come to terms with feelings or thoughts that interfere with sexual function, and (8) increase communication. Psychodynamically oriented therapists view the dysfunction as a metaphor through which the couple is trying to simultaneously conceal and express conflicting aspects of themselves or the relationship. In symbolic terms, the dysfunction contains a compromised solution to one of life's dilemmas.

Alternatively, behavior therapists understand the dysfunction as a conditioned response or a maladaptive response to interpersonal or environmental occurrences. They provide exercises known as stop–start or the squeeze technique as homework to help the man comfortably attend to his sensations and learn to pace his arousal. I find a modified stop–start method (detailed later in the chapter) much more effective than the squeeze technique because it does not require withdrawal from the vagina, and squeezing too hard can be painful for the man.

Men fear focusing on their sexual excitement, believing it will cause them to ejaculate even more quickly. They attempt to diminish or limit their sexual excitement by resorting to wearing multiple condoms, applying desensitization ointment to the penis, repeatedly masturbating prior to intercourse, not allowing partners to stimulate them, or distracting themselves by performing complex mathematical computations while making love. These tactics, however creative, curtail the pleasures of lovemaking and are generally unsuccessful. These men typically describe themselves as having two points on their subjective excitement scale—no excitement and the point of ejaculatory inevitability. They fail to focus on their arousal and are unable to perceive or linger in midrange sexual excitement. In treatment, men are instructed to focus on their sexual arousal. By utilizing graduated behavioral exercises, they are taught to identify and become familiar with intermediate levels of sexual excitement. Successively, beginning with masturbation and moving progressively through foreplay and intercourse, they master the ability to linger in this range, thereby delaying ejaculation. A more detailed description of the stop–start technique is given in David and Trish's upcoming vignette.

In addition to teaching the men sexual skills and resolving the interpersonal and intrapsychic issues related to rapid ejaculation, it is also helpful to address the cognitive distortions that help maintain the dysfunction. Rosen, Leiblum, and Spector (1994), in discussing erectile dysfunction, list eight forms of cognitive distortion that may interfere with sexual function. These forms of distortion are just as applicable to rapid ejaculation and include: (1) all-or-nothing thinking ("I am a complete failure because I come quickly"); (2) overgeneralization ("If I had trouble controlling my ejaculation last night, I won't be able to this morning"); (3) disqualifying the positive ("My partner says our lovemaking is satisfying because she doesn't want to hurt my feelings"); (4) mind reading ("I don't need to ask, I know how she felt about last night"); (5) fortune-telling ("I am sure things will go badly tonight"); (6) emotional reasoning ("Because a man feels something is true, it must be"); (7) categorical imperatives ("should," "ought to," and "must" dominate the man's cognitive processes); and (8) catastrophizing ("If I fail tonight my girl-friend will dump me").

Psychoeducational interventions also aim to rework the behavioral reper-toire of the man or couple, referred to as their sexual script (Gagnon, Rosen, & Leiblum, 1982). Self-help books, such as that by Metz and McCarthy (2003), may prove helpful to men either by themselves or as a supplement to treatment. Men with rapid ejaculation limit foreplay because they fear becom-ing too excited. By modifying rigid and narrow scripts, therapists may help couples establish a more satisfying sexual life.

Resistance

No therapy ever progresses without some resistance on the part of the patient or couple. It is to be expected. Resistance seeks to keep the status quo. It is not easy for patients to give up comfortable, yet maladaptive, behaviors. But with confrontation, interpretation, and gentle humor patients can be encouraged to relinquish resistance and "try on" new behavioral and interpersonal routines.

Case Illustrations of Psychotherapy

What follow are two vignettes that characterize different aspects of psycho-logical treatment. The first portrays a middle-aged couple who both were motivated and committed to overcoming his rapid ejaculation. The second vignette describes a complicated drama in which rapid ejaculation was the least of this couple's problems.

Case 1: David

David, a 45-year-old married antique dealer with lifelong rapid ejaculation, came for consultation at the urging of his wife, Trish. She had become increas-ingly frustrated with the lack of intimacy in their marriage and was totally "disgusted" with the quality of their sexual life. She was tired of hearing him apologize after ejaculating and simply wanted him to do something, anything, to fix it.

In conjoint treatment, David sheepishly admitted that he was afraid of vaginas. He joked about being "a real Freudian case." He wasn't exactly sure why he developed this fear, but he never felt comfortable with the warmth and wetness of Trish's vagina. He was glad that he could finally talk about this hidden fear, and over time it dissipated. Trish was surprised; this was a part of David she didn't know. It precipitated intense anger at David, which expressed itself in demeaning and excessively critical comments. This resistance gave way to my interpretation that her anger served as an obstacle to David's shar-ing his subjective life with her. I also spoke about zones of privacy and that none of us can ever know the other completely.

Conjoint treatment had four initial foci: (1) talking with David regarding his fear of vaginas, (2) instructing him on how to focus in on his arousal and control it, (3) addressing the relational and intimacy issues, and (4) decreasing her level of anger.

I suggested that they temporarily suspend attempts at intercourse. They were both agreeable to this. Trish talked about feeling simultaneously angry at all the years David did nothing and happy that he was finally addressing the problem.

In terms of behavioral exercises, we began with an updated version of stop–start in which I asked David to imagine sexual arousal on a scale from 0 to 10, where 9 is a point of ejaculatory inevitability. I explained to him that I wanted to teach him to linger in the midrange of excitement, somewhere between 5 and 7. I asked him to go home and masturbate, imagining his arousal on the 0–10 scale. When he reached 6 he was to stop and allow his arousal to dissipate to a 3 or 4. Then he was to start masturbating again and stop at 6. I told him to do this four times before allowing himself to ejaculate. He was to practice these exercises at least four times per week.

After several weeks of talking about his fears, abstaining from intercourse, and practicing masturbating to midlevel arousal, we moved on to having Trish masturbate him to midranges of arousal. She was told to manually or orally stimulate him until he asked her to stop. David's task was to concentrate on his level of arousal and ask Trish to stop when he reached a 6. Then, as he had previously, he was to allow his excitement to diminish and allow it to build up to 6 several times before achieving orgasm. Trish was a supportive and committed partner and understood the purpose of the exercise. She was told that she could ask David to pleasure her in any noncoital fashion. She did so on several occasions.

Following David's mastering his excitement with manual or oral stimulation, I suggested that the couple have 2 minutes of intercourse without thrusting. This was a test to see whether David's fear of the wet and warm vagina would interfere with his ability to concentrate on arousal. I urged David not to apologize should he ejaculate, but rather to hold Trish and continue being emotionally intimate with her. Trish greatly appreciated this suggestion. David did surprisingly well; he ejaculated only once out of six attempts and remembered not to apologize. The couple moved on to have intercourse with thrusting, and again David was instructed to stop the exciting movements when he reached a level of 6 on the 0–10 arousal scale. He was to follow the same pattern of stopping, allowing his arousal to diminish and then resuming thrusting until he reached 6. They were to do this several times before he could ejaculate.

All along we had also been discussing how they could deepen their level of intimacy. David's fears and Trish's anger were identified as roadblocks to intimacy. With a little help from me, as they worked together on the sexual problem, each was able to be more intimate with the other. Within 4 months, David had achieved moderate to good control, and both felt that their relationship had significantly improved. I continued to see them every 4 months for 2 years to ensure that they sustained their gains.

Case 2: Ken

Ken, a self-centered, 26-year-old, married stockbroker sought treatment for lifelong rapid ejaculation. He took no responsibility for his dysfunction, projecting the blame to his wife, Mia, for being too attractive. He harshly reproached her, saying, "You get me too excited." In addition to his conspicuous narcissism, he also was severely compulsive, having to change his underwear and shower several times daily. He dismissed my suggestion to consider taking SSRI medication that could simultaneously diminish his compulsivity and delay ejaculatory latency. He insisted that he did not need any psychotropic medication.

The marital climate was dominated by his jealousy of Mia's professional success. Mia was depressed and overwhelmed; her mother had recently passed away, and she had two young boys under age 3.

None of my interventions were successful. Ken refused medication, and Mia had little energy available to devote to conjoint therapy. The couple never made time to complete behavioral assignments; they wanted a quick, simple fix to all their problems. After 6 weeks we mutually agreed to terminate.

Interestingly, Mia came to my office 8 years later complaining of anorgasmia. Now divorced and thriving professionally, she was a single mother of two young preteen boys. She described the painful process of her marriage disintegrating as she helplessly watched Ken spiral downward professionally, propelled by his cocaine abuse and sexual addiction to prostitutes. Whether true or not, Ken told her that he never ejaculated rapidly with prostitutes, only with her.

Mia continued in treatment for approximately a year and a half. She had begun a new relationship and was afraid of allowing herself to be vulnerable to another man. Her sexual symptom served to create distance and protect her from feeling too close to her boyfriend.

Psychotherapy Outcome Studies

Evidence-based medicine has become the gold standard for judging the efficacy of psychological or medical interventions. Studies at the highest level require moderate to large sample sizes with designs being randomized, placebo-controlled, double-blinded, and with 6-month to 1-year follow-up data. Sex therapy treatment outcome studies can be characterized as uncontrolled, unblinded trials; few meet the requirements for high-level evidence-based studies. The literature consists of reports on small to moderately sized cohorts of participants who received different forms of psychological interventions with limited or no follow-up. In most studies, active treatment was not compared with placebo, control, or wait-list groups. With few exceptions, the quality of the PE treatment outcome studies is inadequate.

Masters and Johnson (1970) reported on 186 men who were seen in their quasi-residential model utilizing multiple treatment modalities, including the squeeze technique, sensate focus, and individual and conjoint therapy, as well as sexual skills and communication training. They reported "failure rates" of 2.2% and 2.7% immediately posttherapy and at 5-year follow-up, respectively. Never before or since has any clinical center been able to replicate either the initial or posttreatment efficacy rates reported by Masters and Johnson. For example, only 64% of men in Hawton and colleagues' (Hawton & Catalan, 1986; Hawton, Catalan, & Fagg, 1992) studies and 80% of Kaplan's (1983) cohort were characterized as successful in overcoming rapid ejaculation immediately posttherapy.

In a recent study, De Carufel and Trudel (2006) demonstrated an eightfold increase in IELT among men treated with behavioral techniques compared with a wait-list control condition. The participants maintained their gains at the 3-month follow-up and reported increased sexual satisfaction in addition to the gains in IELT. This is one of the few high-quality PE treatment outcome studies.

The majority of studies with long-term follow-up noted a tendency for men to suffer relapses. In writing about the problem of relapse in treating all forms of sexual dysfunction, Hawton et al. (1992) reported that recurrence of or continuing difficulty with the presenting sexual problem was commonly being reported by 75% of couples; this caused little to no concern for 34%. Patients indicated that they discussed the difficulty with the partner, practiced the techniques learned during therapy, accepted that difficulties were likely to recur, and read books about sexuality. In spite of the decrease in IELT over time, patient sexual satisfaction remained very high!

The concept of relapse prevention has begun to be incorporated into sex therapy. McCarthy (1993), in discussing relapse prevention, suggests that therapists schedule periodic "booster" or "maintenance" sessions following termination. Patients remark that knowing that they will be seen again in 6 months keeps them on target, because they know they will have to "report" on their progress. The follow-up sessions can also be used to work out any "glitches" that have interfered with their progress.

PHARMACOTHERAPY

There are presently two methods of pharmacological treatment of rapid ejaculation: (1) both daily and "as-needed" dosing schedules of SSRIs or clomipramine (a tricyclic antidepressant), and (2) topical administration of prilocaine/lidocaine.

Dapoxetine has received approval for the treatment of PE in over 30 countries, but not in the United States. It is a rapid-acting and short-half-life SSRI with a pharmacokinetic profile suggesting a role as an on-demand treatment for PE (Buvat, Tesfaye, Rothman, Rivas, & Giuliano, 2009; Hellstrom et al., 2005; McMahon et al., 2009; Pryor et al., 2006). No drug–drug interactions associated with dapoxetine, including phosphodiesterase inhibitor drugs, have been reported. In clinical trials, dapoxetine 30 mg or 60 mg taken 1–2 hours before intercourse is more effective than placebo from the first dose, resulting in a 2.5–3.0-fold increases in IELT, increased ejaculatory control, decreased distress, and increased satisfaction. Dapoxetine was comparably effective in men with both lifelong and acquired PE. Treatment-related side effects were uncommon and dose-dependent and included nausea, diarrhea, headache, and dizziness. There was no indication of an increased risk of suicidal ideation or suicide attempts and little indication of withdrawal symptoms with abrupt dapoxetine cessation (Levine, 2006).

Off-label treatment with the SSRIs paroxetine (Paxil), sertraline (Zoloft), and fluoxetine (Prozac) and the tricyclic antidepressant clomipramine (Anafranil) has been successfully employed to treat rapid ejaculation. It is believed that all have similar mechanisms of action. The dose range for each drug is paroxetine: 20–40 mg; clomipramine, 12.5–50 mg; sertraline, 50–200 mg; and fluoxetine, 20–40 mg. Ejaculation delay is observed within the first week and tends to improve over several weeks. Side effects from these medications are dose-related and include fatigue, yawning, nausea, gastrointestinal upset, and excessive sweating. There is some controversy over whether these medications cause impulsive behaviors and increased suicidal ideation. Given the seriousness of these side effects, patients on pharmacotherapy for rapid ejaculation should be closely monitored. Although infrequent, some men report diminished libido and erectile dysfunction after starting on these medications. Side effects are seen in the first week but generally diminish over the course of 2–3 weeks. Finally, these drugs should not be abruptly discontinued. Doing so may lead to an unpleasant "withdrawal syndrome" (Althof et al., 2010).

Greater success has been achieved with daily dosing than with "as-needed" schedules. However, men prefer "as-needed" schedules for several reasons, including cost and convenience, and because sexual activity for most men is not a daily event.

The use of topical local anesthetics such as lidocaine and/or prilocaine as a cream, gel, or spray is well established and is moderately effective in delaying ejaculation. PSD502 is a lidocaine–prilocaine spray currently in clinical trials. Trial results indicated that the treated group reported a 6.3-fold increase in IELT and associated improvements in self-administered questionnaire measures of control and sexual satisfaction (Dinsmore et al., 2007). Because of the unique formulation of the compound, there were minimal reports of hypoethesias and transfer to the partner. Other topical anesthetics are associated with significant penile hypoanesthesia and possible transvaginal absorption, resulting in vaginal numbness and resultant female anorgasmia unless a condom is used.

There are reports that PDE5 inhibitors can also be of benefit to men with rapid ejaculation (Aversa et al., 2011). There is controversy over whether or not they truly benefit men with rapid ejaculation.

COMBINED PSYCHOLOGICAL–
PHARMACOLOGICAL THERAPY

The psychological aspects of a combined psychological–pharmacological treatment are different from those of psychotherapy alone. Such interventions are more directive, advice oriented, educational, and technique focused. They target the psychosocial obstacles created after the onset of the dysfunction, such as avoidance of foreplay, restrictive sexual patterns that are resented by partners, and unwillingness to discuss the problem, which itself creates a barrier. The goals of combined therapy include (1) identifying and working through the resistance to medical intervention that leads to premature discontinuation, (2) reducing or eliminating performance anxiety, (3) helping the patient to gain sexual confidence, (4) understanding the context in which men and couples make love, and (5) helping patients to modify maladaptive sexual scripts.

Combined treatment may be especially helpful when the treatment effects of pharmacotherapy are modest. By lessening the psychosocial obstacles that interfere with treatment and offering patients methods to delay ejaculation, the impact of pharmacotherapy can be enhanced.

Case Illustration of Combined Therapy

Rick, a 27-year-old male, had been married to Laura for 3 years. He described a lifelong history of PE. They had significant marital discord focusing on his lack of vocational success and his involvement with a quasi-cult-like group. Laura had become increasingly angry at his lack of success and time devoted to this group, as well as having an unsatisfying sexual life.

Rick was asking for medication to help his PE. Because of the significant marital discord, we recommended combination pharmacological and psychological therapy. He received 20 mg of paroxetine, which was slowly increased to 40 mg, and both partners were seen in weekly conjoint psychotherapy. Our rationale was to demonstrate to both partners rapid success in delaying ejaculation while we focused on their interpersonal issues.

Rick looked to the cult-like group for support and affirmation because he was feeling badly about himself, his vocational failures, and the marriage. Laura was angry at the increasing distance between them and his downward spiraling.

Rick and Laura used the conjoint sessions to discuss their disappointments and also practiced the graduated stop–start technique. After 3 months Rick's IELT had quadrupled, sex was more frequent, and he terminated his involvement in the group. Laura's anger had dissipated, and she was satisfied with the progress in their sexual life.

After 4 months we began to slowly decrease the dose of paroxetine but reminded Rick about attending to his level of excitement. At 6 months he was taking 10 mg of paroxetine and was able to maintain his increase in IELT. Rick felt more confident in general and was looking to change careers. Laura was supportive of his career change and feeling better about their marriage.

CONCLUSIONS

In spite of our most diligent efforts, it is not possible to help all individuals who present for treatment of rapid ejaculation. For some, none of the interventions—psychotherapy alone, pharmacotherapy alone, or combined treatment—overcome early trauma, the aftermath of years of destructive interactions, or limited psychological resources in the man or the couple.

There are instances in which patients achieve profound psychological gains, yet their control over ejaculation does not improve. Similarly, the man may demonstrate significantly improved IELT, yet the relationship issues remain.

Psychotherapy and pharmacotherapy have their limitations. We cannot help everyone; not all patients want their problem resolved. Some patients may do better with another therapist or a physician, but there are some who will not benefit from any treatment. At these times, the therapist should discuss the limitations of his or her method of intervention and discuss any and all other reasonable options for ejaculatory delay. Although these cases are discouraging, in general the majority of men and couples achieve modest gains sexually, psychologically, and relationally in treatment.

REFERENCES

Abraham, K. (1927). *Selected papers*. London: Hogarth Press.

Althof, S. (2003). Therapeutic weaving: The integration of treatment techniques. In S. Levine, C. Risen, & S. Althof (Eds.), *Handbook of clinical sexuality for mental health professionals* (pp. 359–376). New York: Brunner Routledge.

Althof, S. (2005). Psychological treatment strategies for rapid ejaculation: Rational, practical aspects and outcome. *World Journal of Urology, 23*(2), 89–92.

Althof, S. (2006). Sex therapy in the age of pharmacotherapy. *Annual Review of Sex Research*, 116–132.

Althof, S., Abdo, C., Dean, J., Hackett, G., McCabe, M., McMahon, C., et al. (2010). International Society for Sexual Medicine Guidelines for the Diagnosis and Treatment of PE. *Journal of Sexual Medicine, 7*, 2847–2969.

American Psychiatric Association. (2000). *Diagnostic and statistical manual of mental disorders* (4th ed,, text rev.). Washington, DC: Author.

American Psychiatric Association. (2013). *Diagnostic and statistical manual of mental disorders* (5th ed.). Arlington, VA: Author.

Aversa, A., Francomano, D., Bruzziches, R., Natali, M., Spera, G., & Lenzi, A. (2011). Is there a role for phosphodiesterase type-5 inhibitors in the treatment of premature ejaculation? *International Journal of Impotence Research, 23*, 17–23.

Buvat, J., Tesfaye, F., Rothman, M., Rivas, D. A., & Giuliano, F. (2009). Dapoxetine for the treatment of premature ejaculation: Results from a randomized, double-blind, placebo-controlled phase 3 trial in 22 countries. *European Urology, 55*(4), 957–967.

Byers, S., & Grenier, G. (2003). Premature or rapid ejaculation: Heterosexual couples' perception of men's ejaculatory behavior. *Archives of Sexual Behavior, 32*(3), 261–270.

Carani, C., Isidori, A. M., & Granata, A. (2005). Multicenter study on the prevalence of sexual symptoms in male hypo- and hyperthyroid patients. *Journal of Clinical Endocrinology and Metabolism, 90*, 6472–6479.

Cooper, A., Cernoskey, Z., & Colussi, K. (1993). Some clinical and psychometric characteristics of primary and secondary premature ejaculators. *Journal of Sex and Marital Therapy, 8*, 276–288.

Corona, G., Jannini, E. A., Lotti, F., Boddi, V., De Vita, G., Forti, G., et al. (2011). Premature and delayed ejaculation: two ends of a single continuum influenced by hormonal milieu. *International Journal of Andrology, 34*(1), 41–48.

De Carufel, F., & Trudel, G. (2006). Effects of a new functional sexological treatment for premature ejaculation. *Journal of Sex and Marital Therapy, 32*, 97–114.

Dinsmore, W. W., Hackett, G., Goldmeier, D., Waldinger, M., Dean, J., Wright, P., et al. (2007). Topical eutectic mixture for premature ejaculation (TEMPE): A novel aerosol-delivery form of lidocaine-prilocaine for treating premature ejaculation. *British Journal of Urology International, 99*(2), 369–375.

Dresser, M. J., Desai, D., Gidwani, S., Seftel, A., & Modi, N. B. (2006). Dapoxetine, a novel treatment for premature ejaction, does not have pharmacokinetic interactions with phosphodiesterase-5 inhibitors. *International Journal of Impotence Research, 18*, 104–110.

Fanciullacci, F., Colpi, G., Beretta, G., & Zanollo, A. (1988). Cortical evoked potentials in subjects with true premature ejaculation. *Andologia, 20*, 326–330.

Gagnon, J., Rosen, R., & Leiblum, S. (1982). Cognitive and social aspects of sexual dysfunction: Sexual scripts in sex therapy. *Journal of Sex and Marital Therapy, 8*, 44–56.

Gospodinoff, J. (1989). Premature ejaculation: Clinical subgroups and etiology. *Journal of Sex and Marital Therapy, 15*, 130–134.

Grenier, G., & Byers, S. (1997). Rapid ejaculation: A review of conceptual, etiological, and treatment issues. *Archives of Sexual Behavior, 24*, 447–472.

Hartmann, U., Schedlowski, M., & Kruger, T. H. (2005). Cognitive and partner-related factors in rapid ejaculation: Differences between dysfunctional and functional men. *World Journal of Urology, 23*(2), 93–101.

Hawton, K., & Catalan, J. (1986). Prognostic factors in sex therapy. *Behavior Research and Therapy, 24*, 377–385.

Hawton, K., Catalan, J., & Fagg, J. (1992). Sex therapy for erectile dysfunction: Characteristics of couples, treatment outcome, and prognostic factors. *Archives of Sexual Behavior, 21*, 162–175.

Hellstrom, W. J., Althof, S., Gittelman, M., Streidle, C., Ho, K. F., Kell, S., et al. (2005). Dapoxetine for the treatment of men with premature ejaculation (PE): Dose-finding analysis. *Journal of Urology, 173*(4), 238.

Jannini, E. A., & Lenzi, A. (2005). Ejaculatory disorders: Epidemiology and current approaches to definition, classification and subtyping. *World Journal of Urology, 23*(2), 68–75.

Jern, P., Santtila, P., Alanko, K., Harlaar, N., Johansson, A., von der Pahlen, B., et al.

(2007). Premature and delayed ejaculation: Genetic and environmental effects in a population-based sample of Finnish twins. *Journal of Sexual Medicine, 4,* 1739–1749.

Kaplan, H. S. (1983). *The evaluation of sexual disorders: Medical and psychological aspects.* New York: Brunner/Mazel.

Kaplan, H. S. (1989). *How to overcome premature ejaculation.* New York: Brunner/ Mazel.

Laumann, E., Nicolosi, A., Glasser, D., Paik, A., Gingell, C., Moreira, E., et al. (2005). Sexual problems among women and men aged 40–80 years: Prevalence and correlates identified in the Global Study of Sexual Attitudes and Behaviors. *International Journal of Impotence Research, 17,* 39–57.

Laumann, E., Paik, A., & Rosen, R. (1999). Sexual dysfunction in the United States: Prevalence and predictors. *Journal of the American Medical Association, 281,* 537–544.

Levine, L. (2006, November). *Evaluation of withdrawal effects with dapoxetine in the treatment of premature ejaculation (PE).* Poster presented at the meeting of the SMSNA.

Levine, S. B. (1992). *Sexual life: A clinician's guide.* New York: Plenum.

Li, P., Zhy, G., Xu, P., Sun, J., & Wang, P. (2006). Interventional effect of behavioral psychotherapy on patients with premature ejaculation [Chinese]. *Zhonghua Nan Ke Xue, 12,* 717–719.

Masters, W., & Johnson, V. (1970). *Human sexual inadequacy.* Boston: Little, Brown.

McCabe, M. (1997). Intimacy and quality of life among sexually dysfunctional men and women. *Journal of Sex and Marital Therapy, 23,* 276–290.

McCabe, M., Althof, S. E., Assalian, P., Chevret-Measson, M., Leiblum, S. R., Simonelli, C., et al. (2009). Psychological and interpersonal dimensions of sexual function and dysfunction. *Journal of Sexual Medicine, 7*(1, Pt. 2), 327–336.

McCarthy, B. (1990). Cognitive-behavioral strategies and techniques in the treatment of early ejaculation. In S. Leiblum & R. Rosen (Eds.), *Principles and practice of sex therapy: Update for the 1990s* (pp. 141–167). New York: Guilford Press.

McCarthy, B. (1993). Relapse prevention strategies and techniques in sex therapy. *Journal of Sex and Marital Therapy, 19,* 142–147.

McMahon, C., Kim, S., Park, N., Chang, C., Rivas, D., Tesfaye, F., et al. (2009). Treatment of premature ejaculation in the Asia–Pacific region: Results From a phase III double-blind, parallel-group study of dapoxetine. *Journal of Sexual Medicine, 7,* 256–268.

McMahon, C. G., Althof, S. E., Waldinger, M. D., Porst, H., Dean, J., Sharlip, I. D., et al. (2008). An evidence-based definition of lifelong premature ejaculation: Report of the International Society for Sexual Medicine (ISSM) ad hoc committee for the definition of premature ejaculation. *Journal of Sexual Medicine, 5*(7), 1590–1606.

Metz, M., & McCarthy, B. (2003). *Coping with premature ejaculation: How to overcome PE, please your partner, and have great sex.* Oakland, CA: New Harbinger.

Mirone, V., Longo, N., Fusco, F., Mangiapia, F., Granata, A., & Perretti, A. (2001). Can the BC reflex evaluation be useful for the diagnosis of primary premature ejaculation? *International Journal of Impotence Research, 13,* S47.

Pagani, E., Rodrigues, O., Torselli, M., & Genari, D. (1996). Characterization of 305 men with complaints of premature ejaculation. *International Journal of Impotence Research, 8,* 172.

Perelman, M. (2003). Sex coaching for physicians: Combination treatment for patient and partner. *International Journal of Impotence Research, 15,* S67–S74.

Perelman, M. (2006). A new combination treatment for premature ejaculation. A sex therapist's perspective. *Journal of Sexual Medicine, 3,* 1004–1012.

Pryor, J. L., Althof, S. E., Steidle, C., Rosen, R. C., Hellstrom, W. J., Shabsigh, R., et al. (2006). Efficacy and tolerability of dapoxetine in treatment of premature ejaculation: An integrated analysis of two double-blind, randomised controlled trials. *Lancet, 368*(9539), 929–937.

Rosen, R., Leiblum, S., & Spector, I. (1994). Psychologically based treatment for male erectile disorder: A cognitive-interpersonal model. *Journal of Sex and Marital Therapy, 20,* 67–85.

Porst, H., Montorsi, F., Rosen, R., Gaynor, L., Grupe, S., & Alexander, J. (2007). The premature ejaculation prevalence and attitudes (PEPA) survey: A multinational survey. *European Urology, 51,* 816–823.

Schapiro, B. (1943). Premature ejaculation: A review of 1130 cases. *Journal of Urology, 50,* 374–379.

Semans, J. (1956). Premature ejaculation. *Southern Medical Journal, 49,* 352–358.

Sigmond, S. T., Roblin, D., Hart, K., & Althof, S. (2003). How does premature ejaculation affect a man's life. *Journal of Sex and Marital Therapy, 29,* 361–370.

Steggall, M., Fowler, C., & Pryce, A. (2008). Combination therapy for PE: Results of a small-scale study. *Sex and Relationship Therapy, 23,* 365–376.

Tang, W., Ma, L., Zhao, L., Liu, Y., & Chen, Z. (2004). Clinical efficacy of Viagra with behavior therapy against premature ejaculation [Chinese]. *Zhonghua Nan Ke Xue, 10,* 366–367.

Waldinger, M. (2008). Premature ejaculation: Different pathophysiologies and etiologies determine its treatment. *Journal of Sex and Marital Therapy, 34,* 1–13.

Waldinger, M., Berendsen, H. H., Blok, B. F., Olivier, B., & Holstege, G. (1998). Premature ejaculation and serotonergic antidepressants-induced delayed ejaculation: The involvement of the serotonergic system. *Behavioral Brain Research, 92,* 111–118.

Waldinger, M., Hengeveld, M. W., & Zwinderman, A. (1998). An empirical operationalization study of DSM-IV diagnostic criteria for premature ejaculation. *International Journal of Psychiatry in Clinical Practice, 2,* 287.

Waldinger, M., Rietschel, M., Nothen, N., Hengeveld, M. W., & Olivier, B. (1998). Familial occurrence of primary premature ejaculation. *Psychiatric Genetics, 8,* 37–40.

Waldinger, M. D., Zwinderman, A. H., Schweitzer, D. H., & Olivier, B. (2004). Relevance of methodological design for the interpretation of efficacy of drug treatment of premature ejaculation: A systematic review and meta-analysis. *International Journal of Impotence Research, 16*(4), 369–381.

World Health Organization. (1994). *International classification of diseases and related health problems* (10th ed.). Geneva, Switzerland: Author.

Yuan, P., Dai, J., Yang, Y., Guo, J., & Liang, R. (2008). A comparative study on treatment for premature ejaculation: Citalopram used in combination with behavioral therapy versus either citalopram or behavioral therapy alone [Chinese]. *Chinnese Journal of Andrology, 22,* 35–38.

Zilbergeld, B. (1992). *The new male sexuality.* New York: Bantam Books.

CHAPTER 6

Delayed Ejaculation

Michael A. Perelman

"**D**elayed ejaculation (DE) is probably the least common, and least under-stood of the male sexual dysfunctions," this chapter begins. In fact, delayed ejaculation is often misdiagnosed or at least misunderstood by clinicians, many of whom do not fully grasp the interpersonal and psychological distress caused by this relatively rare condition. According to Perelman, a key factor for understanding many men with DE is that the reality of partnered sex pales in comparison with the intensity of technique and fantasy occurring during masturbation. This conceptualization highlights the importance of taking a thorough sexual history, including specific questions about the method of masturbation. Improving communication and increasing sexual satisfaction during partnered sex are keys to treatment success. DE may be similar to hypoactive sexual desire in men, in that the sexual problem is a manifestation of a preference for some other type sexual activity rather than partnered sex. In the case of DE, this preference is associated with a style of masturbation and accompanying fantasy with which partnered sex does not compete.

Michael A. Perelman PhD, is Clinical Professor of Psychiatry, Reproductive Medi-cine, and Urology at the Weill Medical College of Cornell University in New York City. He is the Co-Director of the Human Sexuality Program, Payne Whitney Clinic of the New York Presbyterian Hospital. Dr. Perelman has served on several professional society boards of directors and is currently the Past President of the Society for Sex Therapy and Research (SSTAR). He has been elected a Fellow of both the Sexual Medicine Soci-ety of North America (SMSNA) and the International Society for the Study of Women's Sexual Health (ISSWSH). The American Association of Sex Educators, Counselors, and Therapists (AASECT) certify him as a sex therapy diplomate, supervisor, sex educator, sex counselor, and continuing education provider and recently honored him with the 2012 Award for Professional Standard of Excellence.

Delayed ejaculation (DE) is probably the least common and least understood of the male sexual dysfunctions (MSDs). A man diagnosed with DE finds it difficult or impossible to ejaculate *and* experience orgasm. This diagnosis requires distress about the symptom(s), adequate sexual stimulation, and a conscious desire to achieve orgasm. Failure to ejaculate may occur during masturbation or partner manual, coital, or anal stimulation. Men with DE usually have no difficulty attaining or maintaining erections.

Confusion about nosology has been the case historically for the full spectrum of male orgasm and ejaculatory disorders, from premature ejaculation (PE) through various diminished ejaculatory disorders (DEDs; Perelman, McMahon, & Barada, 2004). Nomenclature misunderstanding is in part related to the fact that ejaculation and orgasm usually occur simultaneously, despite being separate physiological phenomena. Orgasm is usually coincident with ejaculation but is a central sensory event that has significant subjective variation. In the fifth edition of the American Psychiatric Association's *Diagnostic and Statistical Manual of Mental Disorders* (DSM-5; American Psychiatric Association, 2013), the condition is labeled "delayed ejaculation" instead of the imprecise "male orgasmic disorder" or the pejorative "retarded ejaculation." The definition requires one of two symptoms: either a marked delay in or a marked infrequency or absence of ejaculation on 75–100% of occasions for at least 6 months. The DSM-IV (American Psychiatric Association, 2000) subtype (due to psychological or combined factors) has been eliminated; however, delayed ejaculation is still characterized in DSM-5 as lifelong or acquired and generalized or situational.

Although this chapter focuses on DE, there are other DEDs or alterations of ejaculation and/or orgasm that include anejaculation, painful ejaculation, and retrograde ejaculation. DED also encompasses reductions in volume, force, sensation of ejaculation, and the rarer postorgasmic illness syndrome (POIS; Perelman et al., 2004). These distinctions are important for sex therapists because the specificity of the patient's complaint affects both the treatment provided and the medical understanding needed to coordinate with the patient's physician(s). A man's psychological reaction to real anatomical changes, even when minor, may affect his experience of orgasm. For instance, transurethral procedures causing retrograde ejaculation should not be casually dismissed, whether or not this probable side effect was discussed in advance of surgery—especially if it was not. Finally, even slight changes in semen volume might alter orgasm in a manner that is very "real" for some men. A man taking an antidepressant who is suffering from DE requires a different treatment approach than does a patient whose orgasm and ejaculation are "weaker" when taking a 5-alpha reductase inhibitor (5 αRI) for alopecia.

Men with DE typically report less coital activity, higher levels of relationship distress, sexual dissatisfaction, lower subjective arousal, anxiety about their sexual performance, and were general health issues than sexually functional men (Abdel-Hamid & Saleh, 2011; Rowland, van Diest, Incrocci, & Slob, 2005). The psychological and interpersonal impact of DE is often not appreciated by clinicians, who sometimes misperceive and fail to diagnose this condition. Some partners enjoy the extended intercourse; however, they eventually may experience pain, injury, and/or distressing questions (e.g., "Does he really find me attractive?"). Although initially blaming themselves, partners might become angry at the often misguidedly perceived rejection. Some men will fake orgasm to avoid an anticipated negative reaction. Distress is often greatest when conception "fails," yet fear of pregnancy leads some men to avoid dating or to avoid sex altogether (Corona et al., 2006; Perelman, 2004).

DE prevalence rates in the literature are low, rarely exceeding 3% (Laumann, Paik, & Rosen, 1999; Rowland, Keeney, & Slob, 2004). The intravaginal ejaculatory latency time (IELT) distribution curves recently used to characterize and define PE can assist in understanding DE prevalence (McMahon et al., 2008). Male IELT exhibits a skewed distribution in PE, with men ejaculating more rapidly than women tend to reach orgasm (Patrick et al., 2005; Waldinger, McIntosh, & Schweitzer, 2009). Segraves (2010) pointed out the difficulty in both diagnosis and the ensuing confusion about prevalence rates when depending *only* on IELT duration data. The concept of "control" does not correlate perfectly with IELT and is, of course, mitigated by volition (Jern, Gunst, Sandqvist, Sandnabba, & Santtila, 2011). Some men with an IELT of 20 minutes may deliberately delay their ejaculation, whereas others might be distressed over not ejaculating after 10 minutes, especially if their partners are "already done."

DE has been seen as a clinical rarity since the beginning of sex therapy. Yet DE rates will likely rise secondary to demographics and our male population's age-related ejaculatory decline (Perelman, 2003a). DE rates will also rise due to increased use of 5 αRI (Rowland, 2006) and the widespread use of selective serotonin reuptake inhibitors (SSRIs; Georgiadis, Reinders, Van der Graaf, Paans, & Kortekaas, 2007). Despite rates remaining low relative to other MSDs, many men do suffer from DE.

ETIOLOGY

Neither pathophysiology nor psychogenic etiology should be assumed without both medical investigation and a focused psychosexual history. Of course, biogenic and psychogenic etiologies are neither independent nor mutually exclusive. Genetically predetermined ejaculatory thresholds have a prodigious impact on ejaculatory ease and latency time and are distributed in a manner similar to a number of other human characteristics (Perelman, 2009; Waldinger, 2011). However, human experience is better explained when one postulates that such thresholds predetermine a range of response, a "scattercloud" rather than a "trigger point." The timing of a particular ejaculation would be the result of a variety of psychosocial, cultural, and behavioral (PSCB) factors that influence the biologically predetermined range (Perelman & Rowland, 2006). This integrated biological and PSCB model would account for the variation in latencies between men and the intraindividual range of each man. This multilayered conceptualization is different from current animal models that postulate an exclusive neurobiological threshold model, as well as different from the early "psychological" theories described next (Olivier et al., 2011). A bio-psychosocial-cultural model explains the variation, both between and within given individuals, and provides a better theoretical model (Perelman & Rowland, 2006).

PSYCHOLOGICAL AND BEHAVIORAL MODELS

Early psychodynamic explanations saw DE as an outgrowth of psychic conflicts suggesting malingering, unconscious, and unexpressed anger, whereas other theorists suggested that men with DE are "unwilling" to receive pleasure. Some dynamic theorists ascribe fear: of semen loss; of female genitals; of hurting the partner through ejaculation; and of "defiling" the partner. Clinicians from various theoretical persuasions note pregnancy concerns among men with DE and also observe how referrals may be tied to a female partner's wish to conceive (Althof, 2012; Perelman & Rowland, 2006). Masters and Johnson (1970) first suggested an association between DE and religion; for a few men, orthodox beliefs limit the experience needed to learn how to ejaculate and thus normal function is inhibited.

Other factors associated with partnered sex that contribute to DE include anxiety, lack of confidence, and poor body image (Perelman & Rowland, 2006). Anxiety draws the man's attention away from erotic cues that enhance arousal and can interfere with genital stimulation sensation, resulting in insufficient excitement for climax, even if erection is maintained. Apfelbaum (2000) considers DE to be a desire disorder specific to partnered sex, believing that these men prefer sex with themselves rather than partnered sex. Apfelbaum suggests that a couple may interpret the man's erectile response as erroneous evidence that he is sufficiently aroused to attain orgasm (Apfelbaum, 2000). Perelman later posited that inadequate arousal was probably responsible for increased anecdotal reports of DE when men used oral medications for erectile dysfunction (ED) (Perelman, 2003a). Those men did not experience sufficient erotic excitement before and during coitus to reach orgasm, believing their erections indicated sexual arousal when they primarily indicated vasocongestive success.

Perelman identifies three factors highly associated with DE: higher frequency of masturbation (more than three times per week); idiosyncratic masturbatory style, and a disparity between the reality of sex with a partner compared with preferred sexual fantasies during masturbation (Perelman, 2002, 2005). While preparing this chapter, I reviewed 175 records from my practice of men ages 18–90 diagnosed with DE over the last 20 years. Almost 90% of these men could orgasm relatively easily with masturbation, and coital anorgasmia was almost exclusively the primary diagnosis. Although DE is correlated with high-frequency masturbation, the most frequent behavioral factor causing DE is an "idiosyncratic masturbatory style," which I define as a technique not easily duplicated by the partner's hand, mouth, or vagina. Specifically, many men with DE engage in self-stimulation that is striking in terms of the speed, pressure, intensity, duration, and the "spot" focused upon to produce an orgasm (Perelman, 2005). In fact, some of these men will report penile irritation and erythema secondary to their masturbatory pattern (Abdel-Hamid & Saleh, 2011; Perelman, 2001). Almost universally, these men fail to communicate their stimulation preferences to their partners (or to previous doctors) because of shame or embarrassment. The disparity between the reality of sex with their partners and the sexual fantasies (whether or not unconventional) they prefer to use during masturbation is another cause of DE (Perelman, 2001). That disparity takes many forms, such as partner attractiveness, body type, sexual orientation, and the specific sex activity performed (Perelman, 2002; Rowland et al., 2004).

BIOLOGICAL MODELS

In some instances, a somatic condition accounts for DE, as any procedure or disease that disrupts sympathetic or somatic innervation to the genital region has the potential to interfere with ejaculation and orgasm. Thus spinal cord injury, multiple sclerosis, pelvic-region surgery, severe diabetes, alcoholic neuropathies, hormonal abnormalities, and medications that inhibit α-adrenergic innervation of the ejaculatory system are associated with DE (Master & Turek, 2001; Vale, 1999; Witt & Grantmyre, 1993). Comprehensive lists of agents causing ejaculatory delay are available and include many antihypertensive antiadrenergic agents and antidepressants, as well as antipsychotic drugs (Segraves, 2010; Perelman et al., 2004).

Low penile sensitivity, often associated with aging (Paick, Jeong, & Park, 1998; Rowland, 1998) may exacerbate difficulty reaching orgasm, but it is not usually a primary cause. Variability in the sensitivity of the ejaculatory reflex may be a factor. Recently, Waldinger and Schweitzer (2005) advocated for an etiology based on appreciating orgasmic disorders as neurobiological variants of a "normal" ejaculatory distribution curve. This view is derived from animal studies (primarily male rat latencies; Pattij et al., 2005), as well as studies demonstrating similar (albeit skewed) distribution curves for a random population of men from different countries (Waldinger et al., 2009). IELT reflects genetic biological variability, and diagnosable orgasmic disorders are primarily deviations from "normal" behavior. However, ejaculatory latency is an endpoint consequence that is also determined by a range of PSCB factors, not just a genetically determined biological set point.

Dichotomizing etiology, diagnosis, and treatment into classifications such as psychogenic and biological are too categorical. Genetic predispositions affect the typical speed and ease of ejaculation for any particular organism; however, many of these components are influenced by past experiences and present context (Perelman, 2006b). The most useful approach to understanding human responses is to integrate—rather than isolate—the biological and PSCB components. The goal is identifying peripheral and/or central orgasmic elements that contribute to each man's varied response.

Our understanding of the biology of male orgasmic processes is increasing markedly but remains limited; for instance, even the male refractory period is poorly characterized (Paduch, Bolyakov, Beardsworth, & Watts, 2010). "Normal" male orgasm is refractory subsequent to the previous ejaculation, yet refractory latency increases for men secondary to surgical, medical, or pharmaceutical complications. Given new data showing that cognitive processes can affect neurotransmitters, distinctions between psychology and biology are clearly less binary than many previously presumed (Etkin, Pittenger, Polan, & Kandel, 2005). Delayed ejaculation is best understood as an endpoint response that represents the interaction of biological, psychological, social, and cultural factors.

EVALUATION AND DIAGNOSIS

The evaluation of DE focuses on uncovering potential physical and learned causes of the disorder. The Sexual Tipping Point® (STP) model offers a clinically useful heuristic for conceptualizing the role both biogenic and PSCB factors play in determining the etiology of MSDs generally, and DE in particular (Perelman, 2009). The STP is the characteristic threshold for an expression of a sexual response for any individual, which may vary dynamically within and between sexual experiences. The specific threshold for the sexual response is determined by these multiple factors for any given moment or circumstance, with one factor or another dominating as others recede in importance. Every man, whether he experiences a "normal" ejaculatory latency or delayed ejaculation, has a multidimensional, predetermined "ejaculatory tipping point" (EjTP; Perelman, 2006a). Appropriate assessment appreciates the interdependent influence of these factors on the endpoint dysfunction for each man (see Figures 6.1 and 6.2).

It is frequently useful for a urologist to conduct a genitourinary examination and medical history that may identify physical anomalies, as well as contributory neurological and endocrinological (especially androgen levels) factors (Corona et al., 2012). Attention should be given to identifying reversible urethral, prostatic, epididymal, and testicular infections. Finally, with secondary DE in particular, adverse pharmaceutical side effects—most commonly from serotonin-based prescriptions—should be ruled out.

A focused psychosexual evaluation is critical and typically begins by differentiating this MSD from other sexual problems and reviewing the

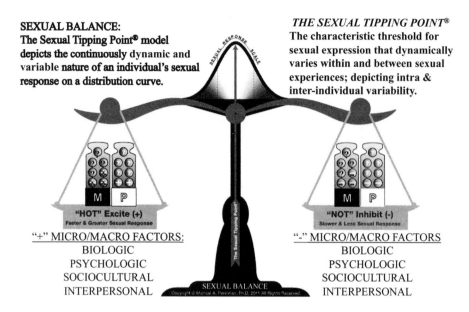

SEXUAL BALANCE:
The Sexual Tipping Point® model depicts the continuously dynamic and variable nature of an individual's sexual response on a distribution curve.

THE SEXUAL TIPPING POINT®
The characteristic threshold for sexual expression that dynamically varies within and between sexual experiences; depicting intra & inter-individual variability.

"HOT" Excite (+)
Faster & Greater Sexual Response

"NOT" Inhibit (-)
Slower & Less Sexual Response

"+" MICRO/MACRO FACTORS:
BIOLOGIC
PSYCHOLOGIC
SOCIOCULTURAL
INTERPERSONAL

SEXUAL BALANCE
Copyright © Michael A. Perelman, Ph.D. 2011 All Rights Reserved

"-" MICRO/MACRO FACTORS
BIOLOGIC
PSYCHOLOGIC
SOCIOCULTURAL
INTERPERSONAL

FIGURE 6.1. The multifactorial etiology of sexual function and dysfunction: Sex is always both mental and physical; the mental factors can turn you on as well as turn you off, and the same is true of physical factors. Copyright 2013 MAP Educational Fund and adapted for use with permission.

conditions under which the man is able to ejaculate. The problem's developmental course should be noted, including variables that improve or worsen performance (particularly those related to psychosexual arousal). What distinguishes sex therapists from all other health care providers is our comfort using highly detailed and specific sexual language. Perceived partner attractiveness, the use of fantasy during sex, anxiety surrounding coitus, and masturbatory patterns all require exploration. For instance, the patient should be asked: (1) "What is the frequency of your masturbation?"; (2) "How do you masturbate?"; (3) "In what way does the stimulation you provide yourself differ from your partner's stimulation style, in terms of speed, pressure, etc.?"; (4) "Have you communicated your preference to your partner(s), and if so, what was their response?" Additional questions can be asked to give greater specificity to the putative role of masturbation in the disorder and to clarify other relevant etiological factors. If orgasmic attainment was possible previously, life events and circumstances temporally related to orgasmic cessation should be reviewed. Events in question may include pharmaceuticals, illness, or a variety of psychological stressors. A therapist should investigate previous treatment approaches, including the use of herbal therapies, home remedies, and so forth. Information regarding the partner's perception of the problem

Represents: Mental & Physical "Causes"

 Represents: Factors

Represents: Positive (+) or Negative (-) Factors,

Represents: Currently Unknown (?) Factors,
hopefully to be discovered in the future.

Adding the factors results in a dynamic representation of an individual's sexual response at any moment in time; the SEXUAL TIPPING POINT is displayed on a normal distribution curve, incorporated into a balance scale.

Neutral   Hot   Not

FIGURE 6.2. Key to the Sexual Tipping Point model. Copyright 2013 MAP Educational Fund and adapted for use with permission.

and her satisfaction with the relationship may help. Sexual and relationship inventories in general, and even ones specific to ejaculation, such as the Male Sexual Health Questionnaire (MSHQ), improve research methodology but provide only limited diagnostic enhancement (Rosen et al., 2004; Wei, Dunn, Litwin, Sandler, & Sanda, 2000).

TREATMENT

Discussion of a potential biological predisposition is helpful in reducing patient and partner anxiety and mutual recriminations while improving therapeutic alliance (Perelman, 2004, 2005). Masters and Johnson (1970) first advocated specific exercises when treating DE. Current approaches usually emphasize integrating a behavioral masturbatory retraining within a nuanced sex therapy (Apfelbaum, 2000; Masters & Johnson, 1970; Perelman, 2003b, 2006a; Sank, 1998). Masturbation can serve as rehearsal for partnered sex. By informing the patient how his masturbation conditioned his response, stigma is minimized and partner cooperation can be evoked. Of course, masturbation retraining is only a means to an end; the goal of therapy for DE is evoking higher levels of psychosexual arousal within a mutually satisfying experience.

It is useful to help men with primary DE identify their sexual arousal preferences through self-exploration and stimulation. Masturbation training is similar to models described for women, but the use of vibrators, often recommended by urologists, is rarely needed (Perelman, 2006a). Masturbation exercises progressing from neutral to pleasurable sensations (without orgasm) remove the "demand" aspects of performance (Apfelbaum, 2000). Fantasizing can help block thoughts that might otherwise interfere with arousal. Some men with DE manifest an overeagerness to "please" that must be addressed. In general, a clinician should validate (not encourage) an autosexual orientation when encountering it in a man, as this helps remove the stigma that DE is a form of withholding from a partner. General anxiety-reduction techniques may also be helpful in treating some men with DE. Finally, couple therapy, when appropriate, involves encouraging the man and his partner to share their sexual preferences so that both their needs are met.

Lack of adequate stimulation was the salient variable for the first couple I treated for DE over 30 years ago. A very young and sexually naïve Orthodox Jewish couple presented with a symptom of primary DE, which interfered with their religiously mandated desire for a large family. The cause was a complete lack of stimulation, as the couple would lie quietly together during coitus, waiting for his ejaculation to occur. Once informed of the need for friction and the benefit of movement, a pregnancy soon ensued, and they now have eight children (Perelman, 1994). Although education is a necessary part of therapy, it is almost never sufficient in and of itself.

Therapy for secondary DE shares similarities with treatment for primary DE. However, the patients with secondary DE should be counseled to suspend masturbatory activity temporarily and limit orgasmic release to their desired goal activity, that is, coital orgasm. Reducing or discontinuing both masturbation (typically for 14–60 days) and (usually) noncoital orgasm evokes patient resistance. The clinician needs to provide support to ensure adherence to this suspension. Depending on motivation level, masturbation interruption must sometimes be compromised and negotiated. A man who insists upon continuing to masturbate might be encouraged to alter style ("switch hands") and to approximate the stimulation likely to be experienced through manual, oral, or vaginal stimulation by his partner (Perelman & Rowland, 2006). In addition to suspending noncoital orgasmic release, the patient should use fantasy and bodily movements during coitus that approximate the thoughts and sensations experienced in masturbation. Single men should use condoms during masturbation to rehearse "safe sex." Sexual fantasies may be realigned so that thoughts experienced during masturbation better match those occurring during coitus. Efforts to increase the arousing capacity of the partner by reducing the disparity between the man's fantasy and the actuality of sex with his partner may be useful. Significant disparity tends to characterize more severe and recalcitrant DE and relationship problems, with consequently poorer prognosis (Perelman, 2001).

TREATMENT OUTCOME

To date there is no evidence for a pharmaceutical demonstrating anything beyond anecdotal success in decreasing ejaculatory latency, and there is no approved drug treatment for DE. Researchers have explored "antidotes" such as yohimbine, cyproheptadine, and bupropion, among others; however, this research was typically confined to animal experiments (Carro-Juareza & Rodriguez-Manzo, 2003) or focused on antidepressant-induced DE (Clayton et al., 2004; McCormick, Olin, & Brotman, 1990). There is some limited support for the use of bupropion, but a recent study concludes that the drug seems to be of only limited benefit (Abdel-Hamid & Saleh, 2011). Clearly further trials are needed.

Unlike urologists, some sex therapists report good success rates when treating DE (Masters & Johnson, 1970; Perelman & Rowland, 2006); yet these results should be viewed as exploratory, albeit encouraging. Althof (2012) notes the difficulty in evaluating sex therapy treatment outcomes, because the published studies use small samples, uncontrolled, nonrandomized methodologies, and lack validated outcome measures. Disparity between the results of different professionals may well reflect clinically different treatment populations. Only well-designed multicenter clinical trials will establish an answer. In the meantime, the two cases that follow demonstrate how a sex therapist can effectively support mutual sexual harmony and satisfaction with couples suffering from DE.

CASE DISCUSSIONS

Case 1

George (53) had become less attracted to Janice (52) but wanted the coitus with orgasm that once characterized their sex life. He did not wish to "hurt" Janice by discussing his diminished attraction. He suffered from "metabolic syndrome" and was hypogonadal. Coital activity had gradually disappeared. He had masturbated to "help fall asleep" at least two to three times per week since adolescence. He now needed greater pressure, speed, and focused attention on "sensitive parts" to orgasm with masturbation. His physician, presuming he had ED, took a brief sex history and obtained a testosterone level. The doctor gave sildenafil samples (with limited instruction) and told George not to worry. Returning for follow-up, George said, "The pills I took 15 minutes before sex did not work; soon after penetration, I lost my erection." When he lost his erection, the couple argued. The physician attributed George's remaining problems to his low testosterone level and prescribed a topical androgen gel. George telephoned the physician 4 weeks later and indicated that "the gel had not helped," and the physician reportedly told him it was "in his head" and suggested a sex therapist, referring him to me. George wanted treatment and had "no patience for lengthy 'shrinking' or touchy-feely stuff." Problems with the patient's sexual script and the earlier treatment were apparent. Coital intercourse with his spouse was no longer arousing. George reported, "It felt like work." Detailed inquiry revealed that his wife's vagina felt "slack." Was the sildenafil ineffective, or was his hypogonadal status the key factor, despite the gel normalizing his T levels? These and other issues were not likely to become clear, even with the most exact testing. Problems with his physician's treatment plan were summarized in a manner to generate hope. George was enlisted in developing a new plan. He agreed to stop masturbating until he was able to have coitus with orgasm on three successive occasions with his wife. This goal was arbitrary but generated by the patient himself and therefore useful, as discontinuing masturbation is difficult to motivate. He continued using both the sildenafil and the testosterone his physician prescribed. Proper instructions for using the PDE5 were given, and George was educated about men's need for greater stimulation with aging. He asked for more direct penile touching from his wife and complimented her improved technique. George preferred a coital position different from the female-superior posture they previously used. Conveniently, Janice agreed, as the earlier position was uncomfortable after her recent knee surgery. Male-superior coitus allowed him to control the angle and pace of thrusting. George was instructed to close his eyes and fantasize about whatever "worked best." Initially guilty for thinking of someone other than Janice, he was reassured that he could open his eyes at the moment of orgasm, and that could become his new fantasy. He was instructed to move inside her in a manner that duplicated (as closely as possible) the sensations he preferred during masturbation. He was reassured that once his capacity was restored, if Janice had any concerns, the couple could be seen together, and he could learn additional techniques. Earlier he declined couple counseling, as reportedly they both felt "it was his problem." The whole notion of treatment format is complex, but couple cooperation is the key to good treatment, not necessarily the couple's mutual attendance in the clinician's office (Perelman, 2003b).

It took 10 weekly sessions for him to reach his goal of three successive coital experiences. Before reintroducing masturbation, he was weaned from sildenafil. For a couple of months, he split the sildenafil into smaller pieces, until he "forgot" to take it at all! The couple experienced a "second honeymoon," and Janice was thrilled with his increased interest in sex with her. George was advised to use the sildenafil as needed during future periods of either physical or emotional stress. With his physician's guidance he could wean himself on and off the drug as the situation warranted. He was advised about the possibility of age-associated symptoms and offered coping strategies. George began masturbating again but limited the speed and pressure to what he experienced inside his wife's vagina. Suggestions were provided to help him relax in advance of bedtime. He declined a referral to a sleep specialist. At 2-year follow-up he was still masturbating as a soporific periodically; however, the frequency was self-titrated to monthly to ensure that it would not interfere with the now again preferred coitus.

Partner issues affect males' ejaculatory interest and capacity, but two require special attention: fertility and resentment. The pressure of a woman's "biological clock" is often an initial treatment driver. The woman—and often the man—usually resist(s) intrusions on their plan to conceive. If the therapist suspects the patient's DE is related to fear of conception, he or she should inquire about the patient's ability to experience ejaculation with and without contraception. Such a "test" serves as a powerful diagnostic indicator. If the DE occurs only during "unprotected" sex, the therapist can assume that conception is a primary concern. The therapist must then find an acceptable way to refocus the treatment temporarily on the issues responsible for the patient's ambivalence. Resolving those issues typically requires individual work with the man and occasionally with the partner. Fortunately, the high levels of motivation that usually characterize fertility-related cases improve prognosis.

Case 2

James, a 34-year-old lawyer, was referred to his urologist for infertility treatment by his wife's gynecologist. James and Joan (32) had been married 4 years, had failed to conceive, and did not want to wait to pursue infertility treatment. James reported difficulty with ED and DE over the previous months. His urologist diagnosed a testicular transposition, noting that James's right testis was behind the left. Also observing James's severely scarred frenulum, the urologist recommended circumcision, as well as correction of the transposition. Surgery was scheduled in 3 months, during James's upcoming vacation. A varicocelectomy was also discussed due to a palpable varicocele. Another urologist reconfirmed the surgical recommendations. The varicocelectomy recovery period would have delayed potential conception by approximately 6 months. The urologist prescribed tadalafil and, in his referral note, suggested that couple treatment might help minimize the impact of the delays caused by the surgery.

The couple was first evaluated individually, followed by a conjoint session. They were in love and eager for a child. Each feared he or she had "caused the infertility." James suggested that his ED might be related to both work stress and the performance pressure he felt when Joan was ovulating.

Although these issues exacerbated the problem, it was clear from the history that there was another reason for James's DE. He preferred masturbation to coitus, and he did this at high frequency and in an idiosyncratic manner (due to early injury). He had torn the frenulum of his penis (secondary to penile adhesions of his uncircumcised penis) during an adolescent coital experience. Subsequently, any time he attempted coitus, his penis would bleed, and he had pain. He developed an intense fear of hurting himself during coitus and avoided it. Unfortunately, he never discussed this with any of his physicians, nor did they ask him direct questions about his sexual response. These critical facts emerged in his first session. The challenge was helping him feel safe sharing this information with his wife, as he felt ashamed. Based on her first consultation, it was clear that she would be supportive. She was relieved to understand why this man she loved seemed to avoid sex. He was a gentle and generous lover, and she was content with their sex life but wanted a baby.

The sex therapy expanded his repertoire of orgasmic variability, and within 90 days of beginning treatment Joan became pregnant. James would have willingly suffered to impregnate her, but of course that was not necessary. General sex education, counseling, and some sex therapy exercises were provided. He first stopped masturbating and later altered his style and frequency. He was instructed to move his body during coitus in a manner as to not hurt himself and instead enhance both his own and his partner's pleasure. After the pregnancy, the urologist performed a circumcision so that James would not have to be so precise in his movements and the likelihood of pain could be reduced. Finally, after the birth of their child, the urologist performed the varicocelectomy, which did benefit the quality, quantity, and motility of James's sperm (which were indeed subnormal despite the successful pregnancy). E-mail follow-up included thanks and the baby's first-birthday photo! A recent follow-up 2 years later informed me that Joan was pregnant with their second child.

Fertility-related or not, anger toward the partner is an important causal factor and must be ameliorated through individual and/or conjoint consultation. Anger acts as a powerful anti-aphrodisiac, and although some men avoid sexual contact entirely when angry, others attempt to perform, only to find themselves modestly aroused and unable to function. The man's assertiveness should be encouraged, but the therapist should also remain sensitive and responsive to the impact of change on the partner, as well as to alterations in the couple's equilibrium.

As treatment progresses, interventions may be experienced as mechanistic and insensitive to the partner's needs and goals. In particular, many women respond negatively to an impression that the man is essentially masturbating himself with her body, as opposed to engaging in connected lovemaking. This perception is exacerbated when men need pornography to distract themselves from negative thoughts in order to function. Indeed, because these men are sometimes disconnected emotionally from their partners, the therapist must help the partner become comfortable with the idea of postponing greater intimacy. Once the patient is functional, the therapist can encourage a man toward greater sensitivity. Alternatively, both partners may be disconnected from each other but otherwise in a valued stable relationship. The therapist must support the patient's goals but not push the man (or couple) unnecessarily toward a preordained concept of success. Here, the concept of "good enough sex" provides guidance (Metz & McCarthy, 2007).

Not all cases treated resolve themselves so easily. Often, an orgasm with coitus is obtained but is not preferred in reality. These men will frequently need support from the therapist to express their preference for noncoital orgasms, especially when their coital orgasms were less satisfactory and obtained only by painstaking effort. However, therapists who readily negotiate compromises with a couple whose female partner prefers noncoital stimulation should recognize the parallel with men suffering from coital DE. Therapists must assess their own prejudices and assist couples in identifying workable sexual scripts regardless of gender. Yet for some men with DE, partner psychopathology, values regarding pornography, and relationship issues may predetermine failure.

Often the most difficult cases are men suffering sexual sequelae subsequent to prostate cancer, whether treated surgically, medically, or with radiation. In these cases vibratory devices become desirable, as greater stimulation is required secondary to the damage caused by the cancer treatments. Devices for this purpose are being evaluated by urologists (Nelson, Ahmed, Valenzuela, Parker, & Mulhall, 2007; Tajkarimi & Burnett, 2011). Sex therapists should focus on the many patients who are often disheartened by their sexual side effects secondary to prostate cancer treatments, even when the patient received proper informed consent guidance from their physician in advance of that treatment (Perelman, 2008). Yet sex therapists may find themselves humbled when rehabilitating a response that is severely anatomically limited. As one man treated for post-prostatectomy orgasmic change said, "it used to feel like a jet engine . . . it became a 'paperclip' after surgery. You've got me back to a prop plane, and that is what I need to live with." Certainly, the greater the anatomical damage, the more psychotherapy facilitates adjustment to the loss rather than restoration of function. Of course, when less information has been provided to the patient regarding potential adverse side effects of treatment, the matter becomes even more complex and difficult to manage.

CONCLUSIONS

In summary, high-frequency idiosyncratic masturbation, combined with fantasy–partner disparity, often predisposes men to experience problems with arousal and ejaculation. An integrated and individually nuanced sex therapy that is derived from an appreciation of multidimensional etiology and supports multidisciplinary cooperation is the optimal treatment today (see Figure 6.3). Should a safe and effective drug become available, a major paradigm shift toward combining drugs and sex therapy when treating DE will occur, as happened when PDE5's became available to treat ED. Better understanding of the ejaculatory process may lead to pro-ejaculatory drugs (most likely dopaminergic), but there will always be a role for sex therapy.

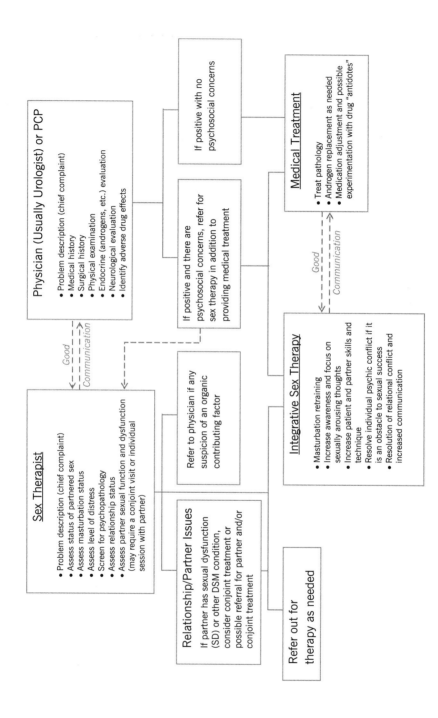

FIGURE 6.3. DE treatment algorithm.

Physician (Usually Urologist) or PCP
- Problem description (chief complaint)
- Medical history
- Surgical history
- Physical examination
- Endocrine (androgens, etc.) evaluation
- Neurological evaluation
- Identify adverse drug effects

If positive with no psychosocial concerns

If positive and there are psychosocial concerns, refer for sex therapy in addition to providing medical treatment

Medical Treatment
- Treat pathology
- Androgen replacement as needed
- Medication adjustment and possible experimentation with drug "antidotes"

Sex Therapist
- Problem description (chief complaint)
- Assess status of partnered sex
- Assess masturbation status
- Assess level of distress
- Screen for psychopathology
- Assess relationship status
- Assess partner sexual function and dysfunction (may require a conjoint visit or individual session with partner)

Good Communication

Refer to physician if any suspicion of an organic contributing factor

Relationship/Partner Issues
If partner has sexual dysfunction (SD) or other DSM condition, consider conjoint treatment or possible referral for partner and/or conjoint treatment

Refer out for therapy as needed

Integrative Sex Therapy
- Masturbation retraining
- Increase awareness and focus on sexually arousing thoughts
- Increase patient and partner skills and technique
- Resolve individual psychic conflict if it is an obstacle to sexual success
- Resolution of relational conflict and increased communication

Good Communication

152

REFERENCES

Abdel-Hamid, I., & Saleh, E. (2011). Primary lifelong delayed ejaculation: Characteristics and response to bupropion. *Journal of Sexual Medicine, 8*, 1772–1779.

Althof, S. (2012). Psychological interventions for delayed ejaculation/orgasm. *International Journal of Impotence Research, 24*(4), 131–136.

American Psychiatric Association. (2000). *Diagnostic and statistical manual of mental disorders* (4th ed., text rev. ed.). Washington, DC: Author.

American Psychiatric Association. (2013). *Diagnostic and statistical manual of mental disorders* (5th ed.). Arlington, VA: Author.

Apfelbaum, B. (2000). Retarded ejaculation: A much-misunderstood syndrome. In S. R. Lieblum & R. C. Rosen (Eds.), *Principles and practice of sex therapy* (2nd ed., pp. 205–241). New York: Guilford Press.

Carro-Juareza, M., & Rodriguez-Manzo, G. (2003). Yohimbine reverses the exhaustion of the coital reflex in spinal male rats. *Behavioral Brain Research, 141*(1), 43–50.

Clayton, A. H., Warnock, J. K., Kornstein, S. G., Pinkerton, R., Sheldon-Keller, A., & McGarvey, E. L. (2004). A placebo-controlled trial of bupropion SR as an antidote for selective serotonin reuptake inhibitor-induced sexual dysfunction. *Journal of Clinical Psychiatry, 65*(1), 62–67.

Corona, G., Jannini, E., Lotti, F., Boddi, V., De Vita, G., Forti, G., et al. (2012). Premature and delayed ejaculation: Two ends of a single continuum influenced by hormonal milieu. *International Journal of Andrology, 34*, 41–48.

Corona, G., Mannucci, E., Petrone, L., Fisher, A., Balercia, G., De Scisciolo, G., et al. (2006). Psychobiological correlates of delayed ejaculation in male patients with sexual dysfunctions. *Journal of Andrology, 27*(3), 453–458.

Etkin, A., Pittenger, C., Polan, J., & Kandel, E. R. (2005). Toward a neurobiology of psychotherapy: Basic science and clinical applications. *Journal of Neuropsychiatry and Clinical Neurosciences, 17*, 145–158.

Georgiadis, J., Reinders, S., Van der Graaf, F., Paans, A., & Kortekaas, R. (2007). Brain activation during human male ejaculation revisited. *NeuroReport, 18*(6), 553–557.

Jern, P., Gunst, A., Sandqvist, F., Sandnabba, N. K., & Santtila, P. (2011). Using ecological momentary assessment to investigate associations between ejaculatory latency and control in partnered and non-partnered sexual activities. *Journal of Sex Research, 48*(4), 316–324.

Laumann, E., Paik, A., & Rosen, R. (1999). Sexual dysfunction in the United States: Prevalence and predictors. *Journal of the American Medical Association, 281*(6), 537–544.

Master, V., & Turek, P. (2001). Ejaculatory physiology and dysfunction. *Urologic Clinics of North America, 28*(2), 363–375.

Masters, W., & Johnson, V. (1970). *Human sexual inadequacy.* Boston: Little, Brown.

McCormick, S., Olin, J., & Brotman, A. (1990). Reversal of fluoxetine-induced anorgasmia by cyproheptadine in two patients. *Journal of Clinical Psychiatry, 51*(9), 383–384.

McMahon, C., Althof, S., Waldinger, M., Porst, H., Dean, J., Sharlip, I., et al. (2008). An evidence-based definition of lifelong premature ejaculation: Report of the International Society for Sexual Medicine (ISSM) ad hoc committee for the definition of premature ejaculation. *Journal of Sexual Medicine, 5*(7), 1590–1606.

Metz, M. E., & McCarthy, B. W. (2007). The "good-enough sex" model for couple sexual satisfaction. *Sexual and Relationship Therapy, 22*(3), 351–362.

Nelson, C., Ahmed, A., Valenzuela, R., Parker, M., & Mulhall, J. (2007). Assessment of penile vibratory stimulation as a management strategy in men with secondary retarded orgasm. *Urology, 69*(3), 552–556.

Olivier, B., Chan, J. S., Snoeren, E. M., Olivier, J. D., Veening, J. G., Vinkers, C. H., et al. (2011). Differences in sexual behaviour in male and female rodents: Role of serotonin. *Current Topics in Behavioral Neurosciences, 8*, 15–36.

Paduch, D., Bolyakov, A., Beardsworth, A., & Watts, S. (2010). Factors associated with ejaculatory and orgasmic dysfunction in men with erectile dysfunction: Analysis of clinical trials involving the phosphodiesterase type 5 inhibitor tadalafil. *BJU International, 109*, 1060–1067.

Paick, J., Jeong, H., & Park, M. (1998). Penile sensitivity in men with premature ejaculation. *International Journal of Impotence Research, 10*(4), 247–250.

Patrick, D., Althof, S., Pryor, J., Rosen, R., Rowland, D., Ho, K., et al. (2005). Premature ejaculation: An observational study of men and their partners. *Journal of Sexual Medicine, 2*(3), 358–367.

Pattij, T., de Jong, T. R., Uitterdijk, A., Waldinger, M. D., Veening, J. G., Cools, A. R., et al. (2005). Individual differences in male rat ejaculatory behaviour: Searching for models to study ejaculation disorders. *European Journal of Neuroscience, 22*(3), 724–734.

Perelman, M. (1994). The urologist and cognitive behavioral sex therapy. *Contemporary Urology, 6*, 27–33.

Perelman, M. (2001). Integrating sildenafil and sex therapy: Unconsummated marriage secondary to ED and RE. *Journal of Sex Education and Therapy, 26*, 13–21.

Perelman, M. (2002). FSD partner issues: Expanding sex therapy with sildenafil. *Journal of Sex Marital Therapy, 28*(Suppl, 1), 195–204.

Perelman, M. (2003a). Regarding ejaculation, delayed and otherwise [Letter to the editor]. *Journal of Andrology 24*(4), 496.

Perelman, M. (2003b). Sex coaching for physicians: Combination treatment for patient and partner. *International Journal of Impotence Research, 15*(Suppl. 5), S67–S74.

Perelman, M. (2004). Retarded ejaculation. *Current Sexual Health Reports, 1*, 95–101.

Perelman, M. (2005). Idiosyncratic masturbation patterns: A key unexplored variable in the treatment of retarded ejaculation by the practicing urologist [Abstract]. *Journal of Urology, 173*(4), 340.

Perelman, M. (2006a). Editorial comment on the Nelson, C. J., et al. "Assessment of penile vibratory stimulation as a management strategy in men with secondary retarded orgasm." *Urology, 69*(3), 555–556.

Perelman, M. (2006b). A new combination treatment for premature ejaculation: A sex therapist's perspective. *Journal of Sexual Medicine, 3*(6), 1004–1012.

Perelman, M. (2008). Post-prostatectomy orgasmic response. *Journal of Sexual Medicine 5*(1), 248–249.

Perelman, M. (2009). The Sexual Tipping Point: A mind/body model for sexual medicine. *Journal of Sexual Medicine, 6*(3), 629–632.

Perelman, M., McMahon, C., & Barada, J. (2004). Evaluation and treatment of the ejaculatory disorders. In T. Lue (Ed.), *Atlas of male sexual dysfunction* (pp. 127–157). Philadelphia: Current Medicine.

Perelman, M., & Rowland, D. (2006). Retarded ejaculation. *World Journal of Urology, 24*(6), 645–652.

Rosen, R. C., Catania, J., Pollack, L., Althof, S., O'Leary, M., & Seftel, A. D. (2004). Male Sexual Health Questionnaire (MSHQ): Scale development and psychometric validation. *Urology, 64*(4), 777–782.

Rowland, D. (1998). Penile sensitivity in men: A composite of recent findings. *Urology, 52*(6), 1101–1105.

Rowland, D. (2006). Neurobiology of sexual response in men and women. *CNS Spectrums, 8*(Suppl. 9), 6–12.

Rowland, D., Keeney, C., & Slob, A. (2004). Sexual response in men with inhibited or retarded ejaculation. *International Journal of Impotence Research, 16*(3), 270–274.

Rowland, D., van Diest, S., Incrocci, L., & Slob, A. (2005). Psychosexual factors that differentiate men with inhibited ejaculation from men with no dysfunction or another sexual dysfunction. *Journal of Sexual Medicine, 2*(3), 383–389.

Sank, L. (1998). Traumatic masturbatory syndrome. *Journal of Sex and Marital Therapy, 24*(1), 37–42.

Segraves, R. (2010). Considerations for a better definition of male orgasmic disorder in DSM-V. *Journal of Sexual Medicine, 7*(2, Pt. 1), 690–695.

Tajkarimi, K., & Burnett, A. (2011). The role of genital afferents in the physiology of the sexual response and pelvic floor function. *Journal of Sexual Medicine, 8,* 1299.

Vale, J. (1999). Ejaculatory dysfunction. *BJU International, 83*(5), 557–563.

Waldinger, M., McIntosh, J., & Schweitzer, D. (2009). A five-nation survey to assess the distribution of the intravaginal ejaculatory latency time among the general male population. *Journal of Sexual Medicine, 6*(10), 2888–2895.

Waldinger, M., & Schweitzer, D. (2005). Retarded ejaculation in men: An overview of psychological and neurobiological insights. *World Journal of Urology, 23*(2), 76–81.

Waldinger, M. D. (2011). Toward evidence-based genetic research on lifelong premature ejaculation: A critical evaluation of methodology. *Korean Journal of Urology, 52*(1), 1–8.

Wei, J. T., Dunn, R. L., Litwin, M. S., Sandler, H. M., & Sanda, M. G. (2000). Development and validation of the Expanded Prostate Cancer Index Composite (EPIC) for comprehensive assessment of health-related quality of life in men with prostate cancer. *Urology, 56*(6), 899–905.

Witt, M., & Grantmyre, J. (1993). Ejaculatory failure. *World Journal of Urology, 11*(2), 89–95.

Pain

CHAPTER 7

Genital Pain in Women and Men

It Can Hurt More Than Your Sex Life

Sophie Bergeron, Natalie O. Rosen,
and Caroline F. Pukall

The experience of genital pain during intercourse is extremely distressing to both the sufferer and her or his partner, who may feel confused, guilty, sympathetic, and/or deprived. The consequences of this problem extend beyond sexual intercourse and affect individual psychological heath, as well as relationship satisfaction. "Our clinical experience suggests that dyspareunia is not a condition that can be treated successfully by any single health professional." This conclusion reached by Bergeron, Rosen, and Pukall is a sobering reminder that dyspareunia is a complex set of problems that requires multidisciplinary assessment and treatment. They point out that sex therapists are ideally positioned to coordinate treatment efforts. Traditionally, medically oriented treatment interventions are delivered in a linear fashion, from the least (e.g., topical creams) to the most invasive (e.g., surgery) and risk-laden options. However, in reviewing the treatment literature for dyspareunia, the authors note that when multiple interventions targeting different etiological mechanisms are delivered simultaneously rather than sequentially, treatment may be more efficient, effective, and engaging for patients, their partners, and the treating professionals. Bergeron and colleagues point out that cognitive-behavioral sex therapy/pain management is an empirically validated noninvasive therapeutic option and is likely a good starting point in the multimodal management of dyspareunia. They also point out new research concerning genital pain in men, suggesting that the idea of dyspareunia as a "woman's problem" may not be accurate.

Sophie Bergeron, PhD, is an Associate Professor of Psychology at Université de Montréal. She is the author and coauthor of numerous articles, chapters, and conference presentations on the topics of dyspareunia and vulvodynia. Dr. Bergeron's research focuses on the treatment outcome of dyspareunia, as well as on the role of psychosocial variables in the experience of sexual pain, with an emphasis on romantic relationship factors. Her work has led to the development and empirical validation of a cognitive-behavioral group intervention for women with dyspareunia. She has served on the Executive Committee of the Society for Sex Therapy and Research and is on the editorial board of *Archives of Sexual Behavior.*

Natalie O. Rosen, PhD, is an Assistant Professor in the Department of Psychology and Neuroscience at Dalhousie University and a Registered Clinical Psychologist. Dr. Rosen's research focuses on the role of interpersonal factors in the experience of vulvo-dynia and associated disruptions to couples' sexual, psychological, and relationship functioning. She also studies genito-pelvic pain and sexuality in women and couples during pregnancy and postpartum. She received the 2014 President's New Researcher Award from the Canadian Psychological Association for her early career achievements. She is on the editorial board of the Archives of Sexual Behavior.

Caroline F. Pukall, PhD, is a Professor in the Department of Psychology at Queen's University and the Director of the Sex Therapy Service at the Psychology Clinic. Dr. Pukall received the Department of Psychology Teaching Award in 2011. Her research focuses on vulvodynia (i.e., chronic genital pain in women), sexual difficulties (e.g., sexual arousal issues, vaginismus), women's health issues, and same-sex relationships. Her work is funded by several organizations, including the Canadian Institutes of Health Research and the National Vulvodynia Association. Dr. Pukall is an Associate Editor for the *Journal of Sexual Medicine* and is on the editorial board of several journals, including *Archives of Sexual Behavior.*

"Will I ever enjoy sex?"; "Is there something physically, psychologically, and sexually wrong with me?"; "Do I still love my partner?"; "Is the pain all in my head?"; "Am I still a woman?"; "Can my relationship survive this?" Most women and men who suffer from genital pain will ask themselves questions such as these as they struggle to understand and cope with this distressing problem, which negatively affects their sexuality and romantic relationship.

Nearly all health professionals have seen a woman or a couple who suffers from genital pain, whether they know it or not. Estimates of the prevalence of genital pain range from 6.5% to 45% in older women and from 14 to 34% in younger women (van Lankveld et al., 2010). Further, 20% of sexually active adolescent girls reported vulvovaginal pain during intercourse lasting more than 6 months (Landry & Bergeron, 2011).

Genital pain, often causing dyspareunia (painful intercourse), can result from underlying physical pathologies such as endometriosis, interstitial cystitis, lichen sclerosis, and other genital infections (e.g., candidiasis, herpes, bacterial vaginosis) but also from events such as childbirth and menopause. Genital pain can also fall under the general term of *vulvodynia*—which is characterized by a burning pain for which there are no relevant physical findings. The International Society for the Study of Vulvovaginal Disease (ISSVD) classifies vulvodynia into two symptom presentations: localized, which involves a portion of the vulva, and generalized, which involves the entire vulva (Moyal-Barracco & Lynch, 2004). The most common subtype of localized vulvodynia is provoked vestibulodynia (PVD), characterized by a burning pain that is elicited via pressure to the vulvar vestibule or attempted vaginal penetration in sexual and nonsexual contexts. Some women report suffering from pain located deeper in the vaginal canal, which often manifests as deep dyspareunia. Unfortunately, little research has been conducted with this population in order to accurately describe the condition, and the involvement of mental health professionals has been limited. The information presented in this chapter, however, is likely still pertinent for women experiencing deeper vaginal/pelvic pain.

Despite strong arguments in favor of a pain conceptualization (Binik, 2010), DSM-5 (American Psychiatric Association, 2013) has retained dyspareunia in the category of sexual dysfunction. Furthermore, dyspareunia and vaginismus have been collapsed into a single diagnostic entity called *genitopelvic pain/penetration disorder,* due to considerable overlap between the two conditions. The diagnostic criteria for this new disorder include difficulty with at least one of the following: (1) experiencing vaginal penetration; (2) pain with vaginal penetration; (3) fear of vaginal penetration or of pain during vaginal penetration; (4) pelvic floor muscle dysfunction. The change emphasizes the multidimensional aspects of genital pain.

ASSESSMENT

A study found that only 60% of women who reported chronic genital pain sought treatment, and 40% of those women never received a diagnosis (Harlow, Wise, & Stewart, 2001). This finding highlights the importance of routinely inquiring about genital pain. Direct questions are often necessary, as many women will not volunteer information about sexual problems (Lindau, Anderson, & Gavrilova, 2007).

> During her annual visit to her gynecologist, Sandy complained about her menopausal symptoms. She did not mention pain during intercourse, but when her physician asked about it, she began crying and said that it was what bothered her the most about the hormonal changes and how much this was taking a toll on her sex life with her husband.

Assessment and diagnosis of dyspareunia should include the organic, cognitive, affective, behavioral, and interpersonal factors that may be involved in the onset and persistence of genital pain. Creating an open, validating, and nonjudgmental context for the assessment is essential.

The psychosocial assessment should begin with a detailed evaluation of the pain, including (1) properties of the pain, such as onset, temporal pattern, pain duration, location (superficial or deep), quality, and severity; (2) factors that may ameliorate or exacerbate the pain; (3) interference of the pain and other comorbid issues (e.g., other sexual problems, relationship and/or psychological distress); (4) personal explanations for the pain; and (5) previous treatment attempts and outcomes. It is important to ask about genital pain during nonsexual activities (e.g., urination, tampon use), which will demonstrate an understanding of whether the pain influences other aspects of women's lives. Next, a sexual history should include the woman's sexual activities, both partnered and unpartnered; prior sexual experiences; and the impact of the pain on sexual desire, arousal, orgasmic capacity, and frequency of intercourse, as well as sexual satisfaction.

The final component is an assessment of the cognitive, affective, behavioral, and interpersonal dimensions of the pain in both the woman and her partner, if she is in a relationship. Several important cognitive distortions may play a role in genital pain and in treatment outcomes, including catastrophizing, hypervigilance, and pain self-efficacy (i.e., the belief in one's ability to control the pain). Affective reactions, such as fear of pain and heightened anxiety or depression, are also common. These responses likely contribute to the extensive avoidance, which can go beyond vaginal intercourse, seen in many women and couples. Finally, how the pain affects relationship dynamics, as well as how relationship factors may affect the pain and sexual impairment, need to be carefully assessed. These factors may include partners' responses to the pain that are solicitous ("Are you okay? Any pain?"), negative ("It doesn't hurt—it's all in your head!") or facilitative ("Let's try a sexual activity that is not painful for you"), as well as the degree of emotional self-disclosure about the pain and subsequent validating and invalidating partner reactions. As the following vignette illustrates, sometimes the difficulty involves misinterpreted communication:

> Nancy, a young woman in her twenties, had been experiencing dyspareunia for the last 3 years. In therapy, she and her partner explored the different ways in which they communicate about the pain. Nancy revealed that when John said, during sex, "It's been so long," it made her feel inadequate and was experienced as pressure to engage in intercourse. John was in fact trying to express how much he enjoys his intimacy with her. However, John was empathic to Nancy's distress and did not invalidate her take on their interaction. He subsequently was able to find other ways to convey his pleasure to Nancy.

Standardized self-report questionnaires (e.g., Female Sexual Function Index: Rosen et al., 2000; McGill Pain Questionnaire: Melzack, 1975) may complement, but should never replace, a thorough psychosocial assessment. These measures may be useful for making comparisons with clinical norms or to assist in tracking treatment progression.

A physician or gynecologist knowledgeable about genital pain should take a medical history and conduct a gynecological examination. The examination should include a cotton-swab test, which consists of palpating different areas of the vulva and asking the woman to rate the intensity of the pain (e.g., on a scale from 0–10), as well as vaginal and cervical cultures to exclude infection-related pain. If possible, careful palpation of the uterus and adnexae using a small speculum and/or a transvaginal sonographic assessment may be performed for deep genitopelvic pain (van Lankveld et al., 2010).

ETIOLOGY OF GENITAL PAIN

Historically, genital pain has been considered to be a consequence of either physical factors or psychological and sexual difficulties, despite recent research and theorizing suggesting that these two perspectives can and should be combined. We have proposed an integrated model taking into account the interdependency of biopsychosocial factors in genital pain and its associated impairments.

Biomedical Factors

A number of biomedical risk factors have been found to be more common in women with genital pain than in controls, including: early puberty and pain with first tampon use, vulvovaginal and urinary tract infections, early and prolonged use of oral contraceptives, nociceptor proliferation and sensitization, and lower touch and pain thresholds (see van Lankveld et al., 2010). A recent study using a mouse model of PVD showed that recurrent yeast infections can cause persistent vulvar pain by replicating important features of human PVD such as allodynia (Farmer et al., 2011). These findings suggest that both peripheral and central mechanisms play an etiological role in genital pain.

Studies investigating pelvic floor muscle (PFM) dysfunction indicate that abnormalities of the PFM while at rest, including hypertonicity and poor muscle control, hypersensitivity, and increased mucosal sensitivity, may close the vaginal hiatus and thus interfere with penetration. Women may also exhibit a defensive reaction of the PFM during attempted vaginal penetration. A vicious cycle involving the pain and further muscle dysfunction makes it difficult to identify cause and effect and is complicated by the involvement of psychosocial factors.

Cognitive, Affective, and Behavioral Factors

A recent study found that adolescent girls suffering from genital pain reported experiencing more sexual abuse, as well as a greater fear of physical abuse, than those who did not report genital pain (Landry & Bergeron, 2011). Further, a population-based study of adult women found that sexual, physical, and psychological abuse was linked to a four- to sixfold increased risk of genital pain in adulthood (Harlow & Stewart, 2005). Additional factors that predict greater pain intensity, sexual impairment, or both include pain catastrophizing, fear of pain, hypervigilance to pain, lower self-efficacy, negative attributions about the pain, and anxiety (Desrochers, Bergeron, Landry, & Jodoin, 2008).

Current cross-sectional study designs do not allow us to identify whether psychosocial factors precede the pain experience or whether the pain intensity heightens these factors and leads women to avoidance. A useful model, borrowed from the pain literature, is that of fear avoidance. According to this model, an initial pain experience, possibly caused by an injury, may be interpreted as threatening (catastrophizing), leading to fear of pain and to avoidant behaviors, which in turn lead to hypervigilance followed by disability (sexual dysfunction) and disuse (potential reduction of the sexual repertoire) (Vlaeyen & Linton, 2000).

Interpersonal Factors

There appear to be no differences in self-reported dyadic adjustment and no association between dyadic adjustment and pain in women with dyspareunia (Smith & Pukall, 2011). Nonetheless, recent studies have found that attachment orientation, attributions, and partner responses were associated with pain intensity and psychosexual functioning (see Bergeron, Rosen, & Morin, 2011; Smith & Pukall, 2011).

Expressions of pain may evoke empathic responses or assistance or may maximize proximity to the partner. Partner responses to the pain may in turn reinforce and perpetuate the pain experience. In women with PVD, more highly solicitous partner responses were associated with greater pain during intercourse, and this association was mediated by greater catastrophizing. More solicitous and less negative partner responses were also associated with more sexual satisfaction in women. Facilitative partner responses, in which the partner encourages the woman's efforts at coping with the pain, were associated with decreased pain and increased sexual satisfaction. Facilitative responses may allow couples to focus on less painful activities and on the emotional benefits of sexual activity.

MALE DYSPAREUNIA

In contrast to the large literature devoted to dyspareunia in women, there is relatively little coverage of male dyspareunia. What exists suggests that males can suffer from various conditions affecting their pelvic and genital organs, leading to localized or generalized pain during nonsexual and/or sexual activities, such as erection and ejaculation. The prevalence of male dyspareunia is unclear, but data suggest that it ranges from 5 to 15% (e.g., Clemens, Meenan, O'Keeffe Rosetti, Gao, & Calhoun, 2005).

DSM-IV-TR's (American Psychiatric Association, 2000) definition of dyspareunia applies to males and females; however, there has been much more evolution in the term as it relates to females (see Binik, 2010). Although several research groups have made great strides in the domain of male dyspareunia recently, the diagnosis of male dyspareunia has been excluded from DSM-5 (American Psychiatric Association, 2013) because of lack of sufficient data.

Therefore one needs to look elsewhere for an empirically based definition of male dyspareunia. The most recent term, urologic or urological chronic pelvic pain syndrome (UCPPS), describes a variety of urogenital pain symptoms due to different conditions such as chronic pelvic pain syndrome (CPPS; recurrent idiopathic pelvic pain), interstitial cystitis, and other issues (Shoskes, Nickel, Rackley, & Pontari, 2009). Shoskes and colleagues have proposed that each patient with UCCPS has different etiological mechanisms, disease characteristics, symptom constellations, and progression pathways that should be described in a clinical phenotyping classification system called UPOINT. It details the dimensions that need to be evaluated by the physician: urinary, psychosocial, organ-specific, infection, neurological/systemic, and tenderness. Evaluating each dimension by using a thorough clinical assessment consisting of a physical examination, standard investigations, validated questionnaires, and additional testing if necessary can lead to the recommendation of specific therapies. For example, if tenderness of skeletal muscles is predominant, pelvic and/or general physiotherapy exercises would be recommended. Unfortunately, the issue of comorbid sexual difficulties—including erectile dysfunction and premature ejaculation—is not a formal part of the UPOINT system, but such concerns should be assessed thoroughly in order to provide a patient with a comprehensive treatment plan.

Interestingly, patterns of sensitivity, pelvic floor muscle function, and neural activation and structure in males with UCCPS closely mirror findings in women with PVD (e.g. Davis, Morin, Binik, Khalifé, & Carrier, 2011). This information may lead to a new understanding of the factors involved in the development and maintenance of male dyspareunia and may provide support for a novel reconceptualization of UCCPS similar to what has happened in the domain of female dyspareunia in DSM-5 (2013).

Another condition that males can experience is anodyspareunia, recurrent or persistent anal pain experienced by the receptive partner in anal intercourse. Prevalence rates range from 12 to 14% in men who have sex with men (Damon & Rosser, 2005).

APPROACHES TO TREATMENT

Treatment interventions for dyspareunia are multiple and target different hypothesized etiological mechanisms. They are generally delivered in a linear fashion, beginning with purportedly less invasive, safer options followed by more risk-laden modalities such as surgery, depending on the subtype of genital pain and patient preference. This approach is based on clinical observations and, when possible, empirical evidence.

Medical Options

Women with dyspareunia often consult their family physicians in their initial help-seeking attempts and thus often receive a medical intervention, which includes topical applications, oral medications and, as a last resort, surgery. In recent years, the most frequently prescribed topical medication has been lidocaine, a local anesthetic. Two prospective studies in women with PVD were promising (Zolnoun, Hartmann, & Steege, 2003; Danielsson, Torstensson, Brodda-Jansen, & Bohm-Starke, 2006); however, they lacked placebo conditions. Nevertheless, lidocaine is well tolerated by patients and more studied than other topical options.

Oral medications are widely recommended by physicians and are empirically validated for the treatment of neuropathic pain, although not yet for vulvodynia. Two studies have examined prospectively the effectiveness of low-dose tricyclic antidepressants in mixed groups of women with vulvodynia. In a sample of 83 women, Reed (2006) found that 59% improved by more than 50%. Foster et al. (2010) conducted a randomized, placebo-controlled trial that showed that oral desipramine and lidocaine did not yield greater pain reductions than placebo, although all conditions resulted in significant pre- to posttreatment improvements. Given that most medical options do not provide optimal results, some physicians have traditionally turned toward surgery as the next step.

Vestibulectomy has been the most studied treatment for PVD. Recent publications continue to support the positive outcome of this surgical excision, with success rates of 65–70% or higher (Landry, Bergeron, Dupuis, & Desrochers, 2008). Because research concerning vestibulectomy has many methodological limitations, some clinicians warn that it should be recommended only after failure of more conservative options. Others claim that this cautionary statement is not justified by data. The ideal study to solve this controversy empirically would be to compare vestibulectomy with sham surgery, although this type of design is fraught with ethical issues.

We conducted a randomized treatment outcome study of PVD comparing vestibulectomy, group cognitive-behavioral sex therapy/pain management (CBT), and electromyography (EMG) biofeedback (Bergeron, Binik, Khalifé, Pagidas, Glazer, et al., 2001; Bergeron, Khalifé, Glazer, & Binik, 2008). Although all three treatments yielded significant improvements at posttreatment and at 6-month follow-up on pain during intercourse, vestibulectomy resulted in approximately twice the pain reduction of the two other treatments. At the 2.5-year follow-up, vestibulectomy remained superior to the other conditions in its impact on pain during the cotton-swab test but was equal to group CBT for pain during intercourse. Overall, these results suggest that vestibulectomy is a safe and efficacious treatment for

PVD, although, at long-term follow-up, no better than CBT. Hence, within a multimodal treatment approach, nonsurgical interventions are recommended first.

Pelvic Floor Physical Therapy

Glazer, Rodke, Swencionis, Hertz, and Young (1995) were the first to apply EMG biofeedback training to the treatment of dyspareunia. In a retrospective study, they found that half of 33 patients with mixed vulvodynia reported pain-free intercourse. In their randomized trials, both Bergeron, Khalifé, Glazer, and Binik (2008) and Danielsson et al. (2006) showed significant pre- to posttreatment changes in pain and sexual function in women assigned to the biofeedback condition, although they did not differ significantly from CBT or topical lidocaine.

Some have argued that pelvic floor physical therapy might be a more optimal modality, as it includes but is not limited to EMG biofeedback. Physical therapy also involves education about the role of the pelvic floor musculature in the maintenance of dyspareunia, as well as manual and insertion techniques. Bergeron et al. (2002) carried out a retrospective study of 35 women with PVD who had taken part in pelvic floor physical therapy. Self-reported pain during intercourse and gynecological examinations was significantly reduced pre- to posttreatment, and significant increases in frequency of intercourse, sexual desire, and sexual arousal were reported. Recently, in a prospective study involving 11 women with PVD, Gentilcore-Saulnier, McLean, Goldfinger, Pukall, and Chamberlain (2010) demonstrated that a physical therapy program led to a significant reduction in pain during vaginal palpation. Further, participants reported significant decreases in pain during intercourse and during a gynecological examination, as well as improved overall sexual function (Goldfinger, Pukall, Gentilcore-Saulnier, McLean, & Chamberlain, 2009).

Studies to date suggest that pelvic floor physical therapy, including biofeedback, represents a promising option for treating genital pain, although randomized controlled trials are lacking. Moreover, there is an emerging trend toward combining physical therapy and sex therapy as a first-line intervention in a multidisciplinary approach to treatment, and patients often feel more comfortable with this option than with psychotherapy alone.

Cognitive–Behavioral Sex Therapy/Pain Management

Despite their widespread use in the multimodal treatment of other chronic pain syndromes and their similar or superior success rates as compared with medical interventions, sex therapy and pain management are largely absent from treatment recommendations published in the medical literature. These interventions generally focus on reducing pain, restoring sexual function, and improving the romantic relationship by targeting the thoughts, emotions, behaviors, and couple interactions associated with the experience of dyspareunia. The first stage of treatment typically involves psychoeducation about a multidimensional view of pain and its negative impact on sexuality, including the role of psychological factors in the maintenance and exacerbation of the pain and ensuing sexual difficulties. Self-exploration of the genitals in order to localize the pain and the use of a pain diary are generally introduced at this stage. The second stage focuses on reducing maladaptive coping strategies such as catastrophizing, hypervigilance to pain, avoidance, and excessive anxiety, while increasing such adaptive strategies as approach behaviors, self-assertiveness, reconnecting with the partner through nonsexual physical and emotional intimacy, expanding the sexual repertoire to steer the focus away from intercourse, and facilitating experiences of desire, arousal, and sexual intimacy for both partners.

Bergeron, Khalifé, Glazer, and Binik (2008) investigated the efficacy of a combination of group cognitive-behavioral sex therapy and pain management (CBT) in two different randomized studies of women with PVD. In the first study, described previously in the subsection on medical options, participants who received CBT reported significant improvements in pain at a 6-month follow-up and, at a 2.5-year follow-up, were equivalent to women having undergone a vestibulectomy with respect to pain experienced during intercourse. In another study (Bergeron, Khalifé, & Dupuis, 2008), participants were randomly assigned to either a corticosteroid cream condition or to group CBT for a 13-week treatment period. At posttreatment, women in the CBT condition were significantly more satisfied with their treatment, displayed significantly less pain catastrophizing, and reported significantly better global improvements in pain and sexual functioning than women assigned to the topical application condition. These findings suggest that CBT may yield a positive impact on more dimensions of PVD than does a topical treatment. In a randomized clinical trial involving a mixed group of 50 women with vulvodynia, Masheb, Kerns, Lozano, Minkin, and Richman (2009) also found that CBT resulted in significantly greater reductions in pain and improvements in sexual function than supportive psychotherapy. In summary, studies focusing on CBT show that it is an empirically validated noninvasive therapeutic option and may be a good starting point in the multimodal management of dyspareunia.

Alternative Treatments

Other attempts at pain relief in women with dyspareunia have been explored. Hypnotherapy and acupuncture were the focus of two prospective pilot studies, showing that participants experienced the treatments as positive and saw improvements in pain and sexuality (Landry et al., 2008). Considering that hypnosis and acupuncture appear to be devoid of adverse effects and are successfully used in the treatment of other pain problems, more rigorous studies are warranted.

Summary

In conclusion, studies focusing on the treatment of dyspareunia involve several methodological flaws, including lack of control groups, poor specification of outcome, nonstandardized treatment protocols, rudimentary or absent pain and sexual function measurement, and short follow-ups. Although there is still a pressing need for randomized controlled clinical trials, it is noteworthy that sex therapy/pain management is the most empirically validated intervention to date, which is at odds with its lack of visibility in treatment algorithms. Unfortunately, although many psychological interventions involve the significant other, no treatment outcome research has focused on couple therapy. Despite the high number of medical options, only vestibulectomy has demonstrated efficacy. Moreover, in line with a biopsychosocial model of dyspareunia, it is unlikely that any single modality will have a positive impact on all aspects of the condition, which underlines the importance of adopting a multidisciplinary, multimodal treatment approach.

A MULTIDISCIPLINARY MODEL OF CARE FOR DYSPAREUNIA: PROMISES AND PITFALLS

In parallel with accumulating evidence suggesting the involvement of multiple etiological pathways, a multidisciplinary model of care has now been espoused by most experts in the field (Goldstein, Pukall, & Goldstein, 2009), as per the recommendations of the Third International Consultation on Sexual Medicine for women's sexual pain disorders (van Lankveld et al., 2010). Advantages of this model—especially when interventions are applied in a combined rather than sequential fashion—include a speedier treatment process, less resistance to any one single modality, more engaged patients and health professionals, increased coherence among the various physicians and therapists involved, and, last but not least, multiple dimensions of dyspareunia being targeted simultaneously. This multidisciplinary model is reflected in a recent excellent self-help book (Goldstein, Pukall, & Goldstein, 2011) and in the information provided by the National Vulvodynia Association (2013), a patient advocacy group. In particular, sex therapists are well positioned to coordinate treatment efforts and to provide education about pain and sexual function, as well as interactions therein. The broad range of interventions they offer can contribute to reduce pain, psychological distress, and relationship difficulties, in addition to improving sexual function and adherence to other treatment regimens. A key to the success of working in a multidisciplinary fashion lies in challenging patients' assumptions about their pain being entirely physical or psychological. Until they adopt a multifactorial view of their problem, it remains difficult to develop a strong therapeutic alliance and to work collaboratively, irrespective of the type of treatment or health professional. One of the ways to achieve this is to provide education about the interdependency of biomedical, cognitive, affective, behavioral, and relationship factors in the onset and maintenance of dyspareunia.

CASE DISCUSSION: MULTIMODAL TARGETED GROUP INTERVENTION FOR PVD

We advocate that, where possible, women participate in an empirically supported group cognitive-behavioral pain management and sex therapy program such as the manualized treatment developed by Bergeron, Binik, and Larouche (2001). In those situations in which a group is not possible, we believe that the essential elements of the treatment program can be delivered in individual therapy. The advantage of a group is that it reduces shame and the stigma often felt by women with dyspareunia. The group also serves as a powerful motivating force for its members.

Group Members and Assessment

The group we are describing involved 8 women between the ages of 23 and 51 years. All had been diagnosed with dyspareunia, some lifelong, others acquired. All the women were currently in heterosexual relationships. We will follow the progress of Anita, a 34-year-old woman who lived with her husband of 8 years. She spontaneously began experiencing pain during intercourse 7 years ago. She had suffered in silence for several years until her husband confronted her about the lack of sex and intimacy in their lives. It was then that Anita realized that she had been avoiding not only sex but any alone time with her husband, fearing that it would or could lead to sex. Anita talked to her gynecologist, who diagnosed her with PVD and referred her to the group.

Overview of Treatment

The treatment consisted of 10 sessions, 1.5 hours each, over 13 weeks and focused on topics such as psychoeducation; the multidimensional view of pain; impact of pain on sexuality; genital self-exploration; increasing sexual desire, arousal, and assertiveness; cognitive restructuring; role of avoidance; partners' responses to the pain; and communication skills. A very important element of the group therapy experience was the opportunity that the women had to meet other women who struggled with the same issues. As Anita put it, "I always felt a bit of a freak—I mean 14-year-olds could do something I couldn't. I was a little worried about the group at first, but everyone is so, well, normal. It's a relief."

One of the first instructions given in the group was for the women to complete pain diaries, documenting their pain duration and intensity, pain-related thoughts, feelings, and behaviors, sexual response, and coping efforts in response to both sexual and nonsexual stimuli. It was explained to the women that the pain diaries would help them identify patterns of responses to the pain, including how their pain is affected by events in their lives. Anita was concerned that doing the pain diary would make her focus too much on the pain, which she generally tried not to think about. When asked whether this might be a helpful strategy, she ruefully agreed that, because avoidance did not work, she would try the pain diaries. In group, the women shared their pain diaries, which helped in clarifying their triggers for varying intensity of pain. For example, Anita found that if her husband was acting "amorously" toward her during the day, she anxiously anticipated sex, and her pain was more intense than it was if her husband "surprised" her by asking for sex. Simultaneously, group sessions focused on giving women the skills to alleviate pain. These skills were taught in the group with instructions given to practice at home. These skills included relaxation strategies (e.g., diaphragmatic breathing, progressive muscle relaxation), PFM exercises (Knight & Shelly, 2008), and vaginal dilation. PFM exercises, such as Kegels, helped the women to increase awareness and improve relaxation of the musculature that circles the vagina and urethra and to use these skills during sexual activity to reduce pain. Vaginal dilation involves gently and slowly inserting a finger or other dilator into the vagina, usually coupled with relaxation, in order to break the association between having something in the vagina and pain. Women also practiced cognitive restructuring, which helps reduce the impact of anxiety-provoking, maladaptive thoughts. For example, Anita noted in her pain diary the following thoughts about sex with her husband: "I can't do this" and "this [my PVD] is unfair to my husband." These thoughts resulted in anxious anticipation of pain and decreased her sexual desire and arousal. She learned to replace these thoughts with more realistic, coping thoughts, such as "intercourse may be painful, but I can do other things that are more pleasurable" and "my husband would say that this [PVD] is not my fault and he loves me." Anita happily reported to the group at the next meeting that by replacing these thoughts she had had less pain when having intercourse with her husband. She found it particularly helpful to use cognitive restructuring *before* intercourse because it helped focus her attention toward the more pleasurable aspects of being intimate with her husband. Anita's success encouraged other women in the group to practice cognitive restructuring.

Several members of the group who had lifelong dyspareunia were very reluctant to do the vaginal dilation exercises. Having a mixed group of women (those with lifelong and acquired dyspareunia) was helpful because many of the women who had previous experience with pain-free intercourse and genital touching were able to draw on these past experiences to help them with the dilation exercises. The group dynamic was supportive and empowering in that each woman's success prompted others to push themselves a little bit more. For example, the first time it was assigned, Anita did not do the dilation exercises. She sat quietly in the subsequent group as the other women discussed their attempts. The next week Anita talked about feeling bad that she had not done the exercises and that hearing about how others dealt with their fear encouraged her to try out the dilation. Happily, Anita was able to identify ways she could insert her finger without causing pain.

Partners were invited to attend the eighth session. This session encouraged partners to express their needs, frustrations, and the impact of pain on their sex lives and relationships. It also included a discussion of partner responses to the pain. For example, the difference between solicitous partner responses, which encourage avoidance (e.g., ending all sexual activity or being overly attentive to the pain), and facilitative partner responses, which encourage adaptive coping (e.g., suggesting nonpainful sexual activities, expressing enjoyment during sex), were highlighted. Finally, some basic communication strategies, tailored to sex and PVD, were practiced in the session. Michael, Anita's husband, clearly fell in the solicitous-partner category. He said that he could not imagine doing anything that would cause Anita pain, let alone get pleasure from something that caused her pain. He felt the same way about her anxiety, so that when he noticed Anita feeling anxious about sex, he would immediately back off and tell her it was "Okay, we don't have to do this. I can wait until this gets better." For her part, Anita thought that Michael was an incredibly supportive and understanding partner. Of course, 7 years later, Michael was feeling hopeless, and it was clear that both were colluding in a pattern of avoidance. In group, it was explained to couples that partner responses to pain and to anxiety about pain should be different. It helped Michael to know that he could be encouraging Anita not to be fearful rather than, as he previously thought, telling her to experience pain so that he could have pleasure. Michael learned to say things like "I'm really happy that we are doing this [being sexually intimate]" and "why don't we switch to a different position/activity that feels good for both of us?"

Couples were given *sensate focus* exercises as homework to aid in identifying their sexual needs. They involve three progressive steps in which partners take turns giving and receiving massage or touch: (1) nonerotic (nongenital) massage, (2) massage that includes genital touching but focuses on sensations and arousal rather than orgasm or performance, and (3) erotic touching for sexual pleasure. After trying the first step, Anita said that Michael was happy to be involved in the homework and that they felt it improved their intimacy. She said it was extremely helpful that intercourse was "off the table," because it reduced her anxiety and helped them focus more on the pleasurable sensations. All the women agreed that having other ways to satisfy their own and their partner's sexual desires was both a relief and a bit exciting. Anita said she felt "sexy" again for the first time in a long time.

Couple work continued, with the women bringing exercises home to do with their partners. One exercise was to do the vaginal dilation exercise using the partner's finger, with the pace and angle of insertion guided by the woman. Again, Anita did not do the exercise the first time it was assigned, and again she sat quietly in group while the other women discussed their progress. Anita's avoidance was rooted in her fear that, if she put significant effort into this treatment and her pain did not improve, then she would lose hope of ever being pain free. She was confronted with the possible outcomes if she continued to avoid treatment—that is, she could be fairly certain that nothing would improve. When Anita did finally do the exercise with Michael, he was able to practice his facilitative responding. On two of the insertions Anita experienced pain, and they stopped; on one she experienced no pain; and on a fourth attempt she experienced pain, but she did some cognitive restructuring—"It's okay, Michael loves me, we can do other things if this hurts"—as well as some deep breathing, and they tried again with success. This same strategy was employed in graduated steps until by the end of group Anita had been able to have intercourse with discomfort but not pain. She enjoyed the sexual experience in its entirety and felt confident that one day, if she continued to use the coping skills she learned, she would be able to have pain-free intercourse.

Some, but not all, of the women fared as well as Anita. Of the 8, Anita and two other woman were able to have intercourse with no or little pain. Two women had been able to do the dilation exercises with their partners' fingers and reported experiences of heightened sexual desire and arousal at various points during treatment but still had significant pain during sex. One woman dropped out because she felt the group was not helping her. One woman did not report any significant improvement in her genital pain, but she had not sufficiently practiced many of the coping tools. She felt more satisfied sexually, which she attributed to her and her partner focusing more on nonpenetrative sexual activities. The remaining woman said that she felt overwhelmed by the treatment program and frequently withdrew by not doing any homework or missing a session. Her most significant outcome was admitting that she had some control over improving her pain and sex life should she choose to do so in the future.

CONCLUSIONS

Our clinical experience suggests that dyspareunia is not a condition that can be treated successfully by any single health professional. Unfortunately, there is very little research evaluating a multimodal approach to the treatment of dyspareunia, although the outcome appears very positive (e.g. Spoelstra, Dijkstra, van Driel, & Weijmar Schultz, 2011). These promising findings point toward the need for more empirical work aimed at validating an integrated approach to care for this highly prevalent women's sexual health issue.

Groups may be particularly beneficial for women who have been recently diagnosed and for those who are not dealing with serious additional psychological (e.g., depression) or relationship (e.g., separation or divorce) difficulties. For some women, the group treatment may be sufficient to provide them with the tools to continue progressing on their own. However, many women will require additional treatment following the group, such as couple therapy to deal with relational components of the pain and/or individual therapy to address deeper psychological issues (e.g., history of sexual abuse).

REFERENCES

American Psychiatric Association. (2000). *Diagnostic and statistical manual of mental disorders* (4th ed., text rev.). Washington, DC: Author.

American Psychiatric Association. (2013). *Diagnostic and statistical manual of mental disorders* (5th ed.). Arlington, VA: Author.

Bergeron, S., Binik, Y. M., Khalifé, S., Pagidas, K., Glazer, H. I., Meana, M., & Amsel, R. (2001). A randomized comparison of group cognitive-behavioral therapy, surface electromyographic biofeedback, and vestibulectomy in the treatment of dyspareunia resulting from vulvar vestibulitis. *Pain, 91,* 297–306.

Bergeron, S., Binik, Y. M., & Larouche, J. (2001). *Treatment manual for cognitive-behavioral group therapy with women suffering from dyspareunia.* Unpublished treatment manual. McGill University Health Centre, Montréal, Canada.

Bergeron, S., Brown, C., Lord, M. J., Oala, M., Binik, Y. M., & Khalifé, S. (2002). Physical therapy for vulvar vestibulitis syndrome: A retrospective study. *Journal of Sex and Marital Therapy, 28,* 183–192.

Bergeron, S., Khalifé, S., & Dupuis, M.-J. (2008, March). *A randomized comparison of cognitive-behavioral therapy and medical management in the treatment of provoked vestibulodynia.* Paper presented at the annual meeting of the Society for Sex Therapy and Research, Chicago, IL.

Bergeron, S., Khalifé, S., Glazer, H. I., & Binik, Y. M. (2008). Surgical and behavioral treatments for vestibulodynia: Two-and-one-half year follow-up and predictors of outcome. *Obstetrics and Gynecology, 111,* 159–166.

Bergeron, S., Rosen, N. O., & Morin, M. (2011). Genital pain in women: Beyond interference with intercourse. *Pain, 152,* 1223–1225.

Binik, Y. (2010). The DSM diagnostic criteria for dyspareunia. *Archives of Sexual Behavior, 39,* 292–303.

Clemens, J. Q., Meenan, R. T., O'Keeffe Rosetti, M. C., Gao, S. Y., & Calhoun, E. A. (2005). Incidence and clinical characteristics of National Institutes of Health Type III prostatitis in the community. *Journal of Urology, 174,* 2319–2322.

Damon, W., & Rosser, B. R. (2005). Anodyspareunia in men who have sex with men: Prevalence, predictors, consequences and the development of DSM criteria. *Journal of Sex and Marital Therapy, 31,* 129–141.

Danielsson, I., Torstensson, T., Brodda-Jansen, G., & Bohm-Starke, N. (2006). EMG biofeedback versus topical lidocaine gel: A randomized study for the treatment of women with vulvar vestibulitis. *Acta Obstetricia et Gynecologica Scandinavica, 85,* 1360–1367.

Davis, S. N. P., Morin, M., Binik, Y. M., Khalifé, S., & Carrier, S. (2011). Use of pelvic floor ultrasound to assess pelvic floor muscle function in urological chronic pelvic pain syndrome in men. *Journal of Sexual Medicine, 8,* 3173–3180.

Desrochers, G., Bergeron, S., Landry, T., & Jodoin, M. (2008). Do psychosexual factors play a role in the etiology of provoked vestibulodynia? A critical review. *Journal of Sex and Marital Therapy, 34,* 198–226.

Farmer, M. A. Taylor, A. M., Bailey, A. L., Tuttle, A. H., MacIntyre, L. C., Milagrosa, Z. E., et al. (2011). Repeated vulvovaginal fungal infections cause persistent pain in a mouse model of vulvodynia. *Science Translational Medicine,* 3(101), 101ra91.

Foster, D. C., Kotok, M. B., Huang, L. S., Watts, A., Oakes, D., Howard, F. M., et al. (2010). Oral desipramine and topical lidocaine for vulvodynia: A randomized controlled trial. *Obstetrics and Gynecology, 116,* 583–593.

Gentilcore-Saulnier, E., McLean, L., Goldfinger, C., Pukall, C. F., & Chamberlain, S. (2010). Pelvic floor muscle assessment outcomes in women with and without provoked vestibulodynia and the impact of a physical therapy program. *Journal of Sexual Medicine, 7,* 1003–1022.

Glazer, H. I., Rodke, G., Swencionis, C., Hertz, R., & Young, A. W. (1995). Treatment of vulvar vestibulitis syndrome with electromyographic biofeedback of pelvic floor musculature. *Journal of Reproductive Medicine, 40,* 283–290.

Goldfinger, C., Pukall, C. F., Gentilcore-Saulnier, E., McLean, L., & Chamberlain, S. (2009). A prospective study of pelvic floor physical therapy: Pain and psychosexual outcomes in provoked vestibulodynia. *Journal of Sexual Medicine, 6,* 1955–1968.

Goldstein, A., Pukall, C., & Goldstein, I. (2011). *When sex hurts: A woman's guide to banishing sexual pain.* Philadelphia, PA: DaCapo Press.

Goldstein, A. T., Pukall, C. F., & Goldstein I. (2009). *Female sexual pain disorders: Evaluation and management.* Oxford, UK: Wiley-Blackwell.

Harlow, B. L., & Stewart, E. G. (2005). Adult-onset vulvodynia in relation to childhood violence victimization. *American Journal of Epidemiology, 161,* 871–880.

Harlow, B. L., Wise, L. A., & Stewart, E. G. (2001). Prevalence and predictors of chronic lower genital tract discomfort. *American Journal of Obstetrics and Gynecology, 185,* 545–550.

Knight, S. J. M., & Shelly, E. R. (2008). Assessment and treatment of pelvic pain. In J. Haslam & J. L. Laycock (Eds.), *Therapeutic management of incontinence and pelvic pain* (pp. 241–247). New York: Springer.

Landry, T., & Bergeron, S. (2011). Biopsychosocial factors associated with dyspareunia in a community sample of adolescent girls. *Archives of Sexual Behavior, 40,* 877–889.

Landry, T., Bergeron, S., Dupuis, M.-J., & Desrochers, G. (2008). The treatment of vestibulodynia: A critical review. *The Clinical Journal of Pain, 24,* 155–171.

Lindau, S. T., Gavrilova, N., & Anderson, D. (2007). Sexual morbidity in very long-term survivors of vaginal and cervical cancer: A comparison to national norms. *Gynecologic Oncology, 106,* 413–416.

Masheb, R. M., Kerns, R. D., Lozano, C., Minkin, M. J., & Richman, S. (2009). A randomized clinical trial for women with vulvodynia: Cognitive-behavioral therapy vs. supportive therapy. *Pain, 141,* 31–40.

Melzack, R. (1975). The McGill Pain Questionnaire: Major properties and scoring methods. *Pain, 1,* 277–299.

Moyal-Barracco, M., & Lynch, P. J. (2004). 2003 ISSVD terminology and classification of vulvodynia: A historical perspective. *Journal of Reproductive Medicine, 49,* 772–777.

National Vulvodynia Association. (2013). *Treatment.* Retrieved from *www.nva.org/treatment.html.*

Reed, B. D. (2006). Vulvodynia: Diagnosis and management. *American Family Physician, 73,* 1231–1238.

Rosen, R., Brown, C., Heiman, J., Leiblum, S., Meston, C., Shabsigh, R., et al. (2000). The Female Sexual Function Index (FSFI): A multidimensional self-report instrument for the assessment of female sexual function. *Journal of Sex and Marital Therapy, 26,* 191–208.

Shoskes, D. A., Nickel, J. C., Rackley, R. R., & Pontari, M. A. (2009). Clinical phe-
    notyping in chronic prostatitis/chronic pelvic pain syndrome and interstial cysti-
    tis: A management strategy for urologic chronic pelvic pain syndromes. *Prostate
    Cancer and Prostatic Diseases, 12,* 177–183.
Smith, K. B., & Pukall, C. F. (2011). A systematic review of relationship adjustment
    and sexual satisfaction among women with provoked vestibulodynia. *Journal of
    Sex Research, 48,* 166–191.
Spoelstra, S. K., Dijkstra, J. R., van Driel, M. F., & Weijmar Schultz, W. C. (2011).
    Long-term results of an individualized, multifaceted, and multidisciplinary ther-
    apeutic approach to provoked vestibulodynia. *Journal of Sexual Medicine, 8,*
    489–496.
van Lankveld, J. J., Granot, M., Weijmar Schultz, W. C., Binik, Y. M., Wesselmann,
    U., Pukall, C. F., et al. (2010). Women's sexual pain disorders. *Journal of Sexual
    Medicine, 7,* 615–631.
Vlaeyen, J. W., & Linton, S. J. (2000). Fear-avoidance and its consequences in chronic
    musculoskeletal pain: A state of the art. *Pain, 85,* 317–332.
Zolnoun, D. A., Hartmann, K. E., & Steege, J. F. (2003). Overnight 5% lidocaine
    ointment for treatment of vulvar vestibulitis. *Obstetrics and Gynecology, 102,*
    84–87.

CHAPTER 8

Lifelong Vaginismus

Moniek M. ter Kuile and Elke D. Reissing

Ter Kuile and Reissing reject the DSM-IV definition of vaginismus with its central criterion of vaginal muscle spasm. Instead, they present a conceptualization of lifelong vaginismus as a vaginal penetration phobia. This reconceptualization is based on the fear-avoidance model of chronic pain: "The basic tenet of the model is that catastrophic thinking about vaginal penetration and/or a catastrophic interpretation of a negative experience with penetration will give rise to vaginal penetration-related fear. To cope with fear, a woman may avoid all activities related to vaginal penetration. . . . " The treatment implications of this reconceptualization are dramatic. They imply that the traditional Masters and Johnson vaginal dilatation therapy may be inadequate, as it does not sufficiently expose the woman to the phobic stimulus (vaginal penetration) while preventing avoidance. Instead, ter Kuile and Reissing adapt for vaginismus the highly effective paradigm for phobias of prolonged exposure. The result is therapist-aided prolonged *in vivo* exposure. The therapist encourages, guides, and reduces avoidance while the woman performs all insertions. Given professional caveats for psychologists directing such *in vivo* genital exposure, this intervention should occur in a medical setting and include the partner. If the strikingly effective initial results for this intervention are confirmed, then *in vivo* exposure may become a treatment breakthrough for vaginismus.

Moniek M. ter Kuile, PhD, is an associate professor in the Department of Gynaecology of Leiden University Medical Center in the Netherlands. She is registered as a health care psychologist and clinical psychologist by the Dutch Ministry of Health. She is a supervisor of clinical trainees for the Dutch Association for Behavioral and Cognitive Therapy (VGCT) and the Dutch Society of Sexology (NVVS).

Elke D. Reissing, PhD, CPsych, is professor at the School of Psychology and director of the Human Sexuality Research Laboratory at the University of Ottawa in Canada.

She is the supervisor for sex therapy training at the Centre for Psychological Services and Research and has a private practice serving mostly women with vulvo-vaginal pain and vaginismus.

Eva, 27 years old, 3 years married to Rob, was referred by her general practitioner with the complaint that sexual intercourse had never been possible; attempts resulted in pain and significant fear and were typically avoided.

DESCRIPTION OF THE PROBLEM

In line with current nosology, Eva would be diagnosed with lifelong vaginismus, which is defined in DSM-IV-TR (American Psychiatric Association, 2000) as an involuntary contraction of the vaginal musculature that interferes with coitus. However, the focus on vaginal spasm as the key diagnostic criterion has not been supported empirically (Reissing, Binik, Khalifé, Cohen, & Amsel, 2004). An international consensus committee had suggested revised criteria that are more reflective of the clinical presentation of vaginismus: "persistent difficulties to allow vaginal entry of a penis, a finger, and/or any object, despite the woman's expressed wish to do so. There is variable involuntary pelvic muscle contraction, (phobic) avoidance and anticipation/fear/experience of pain" (Basson et al., 2003). In response to the lack of empirical support for the DSM diagnostic criteria and the persistent difficulties in clearly differentiating vaginismus from dyspareunia, the two sexual pain disorders in DSM-IV-TR have been merged into a new DSM-5 (American Psychiatric Association, 2013) disorder called "genito-pelvic pain/penetration disorder" (GPPPD; Binik, 2010).

Vaginismus can be either lifelong or acquired. In acquired vaginismus, a woman who was able to experience intercourse is no longer able to do so. She may be unable or unwilling to continue experiencing pain associated with intercourse. In acquired vaginismus, the interference with intercourse may be the result of pain (e.g., due to vulvodynia). Shared etiology makes it difficult to differentiate acquired vaginismus from dyspareunia, and treatment described for dyspareunia may be more effective (see Bergeron, Rosen, & Pukall, Chapter 7, this volume). The treatment approach described here can be helpful for women with acquired vaginismus in which fear and avoidance of penetration have become central and interfere with treatment approaches used for dyspareunia. In this chapter, however, we focus on women with lifelong vaginismus who have never been able to experience complete vaginal intercourse and who demonstrate marked fear and avoidance of vaginal penetration. Hence, unless otherwise specified, in this chapter we refer to lifelong vaginismus as "vaginismus."

PREVALENCE AND INCIDENCE

Epidemiological studies often subsume vaginismus in more generalized questions about pain with intercourse, resulting in few accurate prevalence estimates. The best estimates of reported rates vary between 0.4 and 6.0% (e.g., Christensen et al., 2011). In more sexually conservative cultures, significantly higher prevalence rates have been observed (e.g., Yasan & Gurgen, 2009).

ETIOLOGY

Research on the etiology of vaginismus is lacking, and no definite cause has been identified. Conservative and religious attitudes, lack of sex education, sexual abuse, and relationship factors have all been reported as potential causal variables; however, none have been confirmed empirically (e.g., van Lankveld, et al., 2010). A somatic explanation for lifelong vaginismus is found very infrequently (0–5%) and can include hymeneal or vaginal abnormalities. Research shows that many women diagnosed with vaginismus also experience vulvar pain. This vulvar pain is typically diagnosed as provoked vestibulodynia but may also be the result of pelvic muscle tension and/or lack of sexual arousal and lubrication.

Three lines of inquiry into the etiology of vaginismus have emerged as promising in the past decade.

Pelvic Floor Muscle Involvement

Seven studies have assessed pelvic muscle activity with a surface electromyography (EMG), vaginal probe or needle EMG, and pelvic muscle palpation by trained physical therapists (Binik, 2010). There is some indication of differences in resting muscle tone and in response to contraction–relaxation instructions among women with vaginismus or dyspareunia and control participants without pain. However, at this point, no consistent differences have been established. It has been suggested that increased pelvic muscle tension and/or contractions are a "general" protective mechanism in response to potential threat for all women (van der Velde, Laan, & Everaerd, 2001); women with vaginismus show this specific defense reflex in response to potential vaginal penetration (Shafik & El-Sibai, 2002).

Sexual and Psychological Factors

Vaginismus is classified as a sexual dysfunction; however, little information is available on sexual function and response in sufferers. Whereas some women report few sexual problems if vaginal penetration is not anticipated or attempted, others find their sexual function significantly compromised (e.g., van Lankveld et al., 2010). Women with vaginismus appear to respond differently to erotic stimuli, reporting more thoughts about negative consequences of intercourse, and demonstrate increased negative affective appraisal of vaginal penetration. For example, elevated fears of injury and losing control, as well as negative self- and genital image, worries about genital incompatibility, and disgust have been reported (e.g., Borg, de Jong, & Weijmar Schultz, 2010; Reissing, 2012; Klaassen & ter Kuile, 2009). Despite the negative affect and cognitions to sexual stimuli, thermographically measured sexual arousal while watching erotic films depicting vaginal penetration or other sexual activities remains intact in women suffering from vaginismus (Cherner & Reissing, 2013).

Fear–Avoidance Model of Vaginismus

The fear-avoidance model of vaginismus (FAM-V; see Figure 8.1) is based on the fear-avoidance model for chronic pain (Vlaeyen & Linton, 2000). This model provides an explanation of why vaginal penetration problems develop in some women who experience anxiety and/or pain with attempts at vaginal penetration (Reissing, 2009; ter Kuile, Both, & van Lankveld, 2010).

The basic tenet of the model is that catastrophic thinking about vaginal penetration and/or a catastrophic interpretation of a negative experience with penetration will give rise to vaginal penetration-related fears. To cope with fear, a woman may avoid all activities related to vaginal penetration or she may be hypervigilant to stimuli that are related to her specific fearful thoughts (e.g., pain, genital incompatibility). The latter can result in an exaggerated attention to physical sensations and increased anxiety that facilitates the experience of pain during attempted vaginal penetration. These attempts are met with defensive pelvic muscle contractions. Increased muscle tone, along with lack of sexual arousal and lubrication, result in further pain. The inability to "achieve" penetration in turn contributes to negative experiences and confirms negative expectations, thereby further exacerbating and perpetuating the vicious cycle of vaginismus. Vaginismus, as conceptualized by

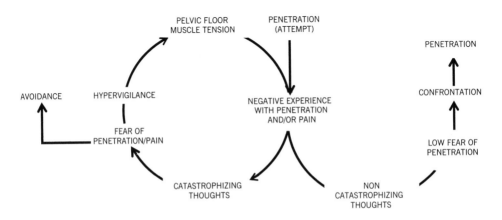

FIGURE 8.1. Fear-avoidance model of vaginismus (FAM-V).

the FAM-V model, may be akin to a specific phobia. As with the treatment of phobias, exposure to the feared object or situation is essential in overcoming the phobia. The goals for treatment in lifelong vaginismus are to reduce catastrophization, to promote a decrease in avoidance, and to increase positive experiences with vaginal penetration. This direct confrontation and disconfirmation of penetration-related fears results in breaking the cycle of vagnismus.

ASSESSMENT

The current lack of universally agreed-upon and empirically supported diagnostic criteria complicates the assessment of vaginismus. In our clinical practice, the components that constitute the FAM-V guide us in a comprehensive assessment of all aspects related to the patient's vaginal penetration problem.

Ruling Out Organic and Psychological Comorbidity

We recommend a consultation with a gynecologist to rule out hymeneal and vaginal pathology that could interfere with vaginal penetration and to educate the woman about her anatomy. Whenever possible, it is preferable that the examination be carried out by a health care professional familiar with genital pain and penetration problems. A visual inspection of the external genitalia is typically sufficient in revealing pathology. Patient preparation is central to an educational pelvic examination (EPE) to avoid further distress. To facilitate the EPE, the patient is informed of what to expect, reassured that no vaginal insertion will be attempted, invited to be an active participant (e.g., holding a mirror to observe the exam), and reminded that she can terminate the exam whenever she wishes. Instructions on coping with fear and anxiety can be very helpful (e.g., breathing techniques). In our experiences, almost all women can tolerate an examination with good preparation. For many, a successful gynecological examination is reassuring, eliminates fears about physical pathology, and represents an important first step in overcoming their problems.

Psychological concerns may need to be addressed prior to treatment. Although there is no evidence that women with vaginismus demonstrate worse psychological adjustment, problems such as untreated trauma, affective disorders, significant couple conflict, or a partner's sexual problem can interfere with treatment. A brief, structured interview and the use of self-report questionnaires (e.g., Outcome Questionnaire [OQ-45], Lambert et al., 1996; Dyadic Adjustment Scale, Busby, Christensen, Crane & Larson, 1995; or the Achenbach System of Empirically Based Assessment (ASEBA) family of scales, *www.aseba.org*) can be very useful in determining when a referral for psychological counseling should precede treatment for vaginismus.

Eva's physical examination was limited to a visual inspection of her external genitalia, and no pathology was noted. She was quite anxious in anticipation of the examination but put at ease by the process of the EPE. No mental health concerns were noted during her interview, and she reported no sexual abuse.

Severity of Vaginal Penetration Problems and Treatment Motivation

Eva, like most other woman with lifelong vaginismus, had also never been able to insert a finger or tampon or to have a pelvic exam with finger or speculum insertion. She and her husband were very anxious that "physical causes" were making vaginal penetration impossible and colluded in avoiding attempts. This was their first attempt at formal treatment, and both were very hopeful of overcoming the problem in order to be able to conceive children.

Treatment motivation is particularly important in overcoming vaginismus because fear and avoidance need to be countered with significant commitment to therapy. Discussion of previous failed attempts and partner collusion can shed further light on avoidance behaviors that can compromise therapy. In addition, it appears that for some women, the desire to conceive a child is the foremost treatment goal, and additional goals regarding overall sexual function may not be considered relevant. It may be useful for some women to be provided with information on self-insemination and guidance in selecting a midwife or obstetrician with an understanding of vaginismus.

Catastrophizing Cognitions and Penetration–Related Fears

The FAM-V suggests that catastrophizing cognitions typically result in specific, penetration-related fears. The most common penetration-related fears are that penetration is impossible because of a small vagina or pathology and/or will be exceedingly painful. Eva initially indicated that she desired nothing more than being able to experience intercourse, but her inability to insert a tampon led her to believe that her vagina could not possibly accommodate a penis. Her belief of genital incompatibility may have led her to fear that intercourse would be impossible or very painful. The Vaginal Penetration Cognition Questionnaire (VPCQ; Klaassen & ter Kuile, 2009) can be used to assess vaginal penetration cognitions.

Avoidance/Hypervigilance

In the FAM-V the driving force is the avoidance of vaginal penetration, which eliminates the possibility of confrontation and disconfirmation of catastrophic cognitions. While the woman is avoiding intercourse, she is temporarily stepping out of the FAM-V, which serves to negatively reinforce the cycle; that is, if she is not attempting vaginal penetration, she experiences no symptoms. The occasional attempt is accompanied by significant fear and hypervigilance for dreaded emotions or experiences (e.g., loss of control, pain). Invariably the attempt ends in failure and disappointment. Importantly, the negative experience of a failed attempt further perpetuates and exacerbates the vicious cycle of the FAM-V.

> Eva's husband colluded with her in avoiding intercourse. He had observed her difficulties and shared her fears about physiological pathology. He cared for his wife and wanted to avoid the negative emotional fallout. They had been married for 3 years but could barely remember attempts at intercourse. However, Eva and Rob did not avoid sexual intimacy but explicitly agreed that vaginal penetration would not be attempted.

Marked Tensing or Tightening of the Pelvic Floor Muscles

Pelvic reactivity is an important component in the FAM-V because of its potential of maintaining and exacerbating the vicious cycle by making attempts at penetration painful and impossible. At this point, it is not clear whether women with vaginismus are able to provide reliable information on the presence or severity of their pelvic floor muscle tone and/or reactivity. Gynecologists may observe reactive pelvic muscles, and observations from the partner can be helpful. Questions about micturition and/or defecation problems can also be revealing and indicative of more chronic and severe tonicity. Some women may benefit from a formal assessment by a physical therapist with experience in pelvic floor problems. In the absence of resources for assessment by allied health care professionals, therapists can help clients increase proprioception and accuracy of self-assessment by practicing contract–release exercises using a mirror.

> Eva displayed an elevated degree of pelvic reactivity during the EPE but reported no micturition or defecation problems.

Additional Consideration in the Assessment for Exposure Therapy: Vasovagal Syncope

Although most women with vaginismus respond with increased autonomic arousal upon exposure to the feared penetration stimulus, 5–10% have a unique pattern of responding. This consists of a diphasic response in which heart rate and blood pressure increase briefly and then suddenly drop. This is accompanied by feelings of dizziness and can result in fainting. The term "vasovagal syncope" has been used to describe this phenomenon, and it has been reported in patients with blood, injection, and injury phobias (Barlow, 2002). In our clinical experience, patients who respond to attempted penetration with a diphasic response typically have a history of fainting upon exposure to other feared cues. Briefly verifying such experiences is useful in the development of the treatment plan.

Eva recalled experiencing fainting spells when exposed to blood and injections, and she was very afraid that she could faint during the gynecological examination.

APPROACHES TO TREATMENT

Medical Treatment

Different forms of medical treatments have been used to address vaginismus. These include surgical interventions to remove the hymen or to enlarge the introitus, injections of botulinum toxin, application of topical anesthetic creams, and the use of anxiolytic medication. However, no evidence of the effectiveness of these treatments is available from controlled studies (e.g., van Lankveld, et al, 2010).

Pelvic Floor Physical Therapy

Referrals for physical therapy (PT) appear to be increasingly common, but specific treatment techniques and therapy course and outcome are currently uncertain because women with vaginismus are typically excluded from outcome studies evaluating PT for sexual pain disorders. A retrospective study demonstrated positive treatment outcome with interventions similar to those used in treatment of vulvodynia but with significantly longer treatment duration (Reissing, Armstrong, & Allen, 2013). Prospective, controlled studies including women with lifelong vaginismus specifically are urgently needed to elucidate whether PT is a promising therapy option.

Psychological Treatment

Anxiety-reduction techniques, along with gradual exposure to vaginal penetration, are frequently applied in the treatment of vaginismus and form the core element of treatment, which typically includes a range of other interventions, such as cognitive restructuring, education, and sex therapy (Melnick, Hawton, & McGuire, 2012).

The first randomized controlled trial (RCT) investigated 117 women with lifelong vaginismus assigned to cognitive-behavioral therapy (CBT) either in group or bibliotherapy format or to a wait-list control group (van Lankveld et al., 2006). After receiving either treatment format for 3 months, 18% of the treated participants had successfully attempted intercourse, compared with none in the wait-list group. CBT did not produce changes in subjective reports of sexual functioning of participants or their partners. Successful treatment outcome was partly mediated by a reduction of "fear of coitus" and of avoidance behavior. Consequently, it was hypothesized that the effectiveness of treatment could be enhanced by focusing more explicitly and systematically on exposure to the stimuli that are feared.

To test this hypothesis, a prolonged, therapist-aided exposure treatment was developed (ter Kuile et al., 2009). Exposure at the hospital was self-controlled, (patient performed vaginal penetration exercises), facilitated by a female therapist, consisted of a maximum of three 2-hour sessions per week, and followed up with exercises at home. Of the 10 participants, 9 reported intercourse following treatment, and, for 5, intercourse was possible within the first week of treatment. Exposure was successful in decreasing fear and negative penetration beliefs and treatment gains were maintained at 1-year follow-up. Recently, these results were replicated in a multicenter, wait-list RCT including 70 women with lifelong vaginismus (ter Kuile, Melles, de Groot, Tuijman-Raasveld, & van Lankveld, 2013). Following treatment, 89% of the participants could experience intercourse and reported decreases in negative penetration beliefs and sexual distress. For most (90%), intercourse was possible within the first 2 weeks of treatment after an average of 2.5 hours of exposure at the hospital. The ability to experience intercourse did not result in complete sexual rehabilitation for 50% of participants. All couples who were able to experience intercourse at 3 months' follow-up were offered three sessions of sex therapy aimed at increasing overall sexual function and pleasure. More than 40% chose additional sex therapy. At the 1-year follow-up, the large reduction in symptoms related to vaginismus, negative penetration beliefs, and sexual distress obtained after exposure treatment remained. However, other aspects of sexual function (e.g., desire, orgasm) did not improve, and there were no indications that the extra sessions of sex therapy affected treatment outcome in the long term.

Current State of Knowledge

The treatment success of recent exposure-type treatments is significantly greater than that of therapies that combine multiple treatment techniques. Although it is potentially promising, not enough information is available to evaluate the effectiveness of physical therapy. We posit that treatment success can be significantly increased by directly focusing on confronting vaginal penetration-related fear via *in vivo* exposure.

In Vivo Exposure Therapy for Lifelong Vaginismus

We have previously suggested a conceptualization of lifelong vaginismus as a penetration phobia. Specific phobias are one of the best understood psychological disorders, with considerable treatment success using *in vivo* exposure to feared objects and situations (e.g., Barlow, 2002). Therapist-aided exposure results in fewer avoidance behaviors and greater reduction of fear compared with treatment with less therapist involvement. A critical component of exposure is that the duration of the session has to be long enough (2–3 hours) to disconfirm a priori catastrophic expectations and to consolidate such learning. It is generally accepted that massed, *in vivo* exposure (i.e., over several consecutive days) is more effective for fear reduction than spaced exposure (i.e., one weekly session). Exposure in a variety of locations and situations to a variety of stimuli can reduce the rate of relapse. Furthermore, there are indications that including the partner can improve outcome (e.g., Barlow, 2002). *In vivo* exposure for vaginismus can be therapist assisted or carried out in the home setting. Therapist-aided exposure has a number of advantages over home-based exposure only. The initial exposure session takes place in a professional setting with a knowledgeable therapist, increasing the woman's feelings of reassurance. The role of the therapist is to guide the woman (and her partner) through the difficulty of approaching the penetration-related fears, to manage the associated intense fear, and to encourage nonavoidance. The therapist can actively assist the couple in learning how to best practice exposure at home and support the couple in overcoming difficulties as they occur. Exposure treatment carried out at home is a possible alternative, but the role of the therapist is crucial in focusing the couple on confronting avoidance, managing anticipatory anxiety, and practicing massed exposure. Our recommendations concerning exposure therapy for vaginismus are as follows:

1. Exposure is carried out *in vivo*, and the duration of the practice is long enough to disconfirm a priori catastrophic expectations.
2. Exposure is practiced with varied stimuli (fingers, own or partner's; dilators; tampon; penis).
3. Exposure is practiced in varied situations (e.g., different positions, locations, with and without partner, with and without sexual arousal).
4. If possible, the partner is always included in treatment. The partner's role is to assist the woman in reducing avoidance and to encourage her during exposure exercises.
5. During the therapist-aided exposure session, insertion is carried out by the woman.
6. The role of the therapist is to coach the woman and her partner to manage fear and avoidance and to prepare for home exercises.

Multidisciplinary Treatment of Lifelong Vaginismus

The treatment of vaginismus is best carried out in a multidisciplinary context, with all members of the treatment team sharing the conceptualization of vaginismus and the treatment plan. It is essential to rule out organic pathology; however, we believe the value of the gynecologist on a multidisciplinary team goes well beyond this task. The educational pelvic examination can be a first step in overcoming vaginismus by presenting an opportunity for education on vulvovaginal structures, reproductive health, and physiological capacity for intercourse. The educational role can also be assumed by a pelvic-floor-expert physical therapist who can also assist the patient to increase proprioception of her pelvic floor muscles. Clinical psychologists who are trained in the basic principles of exposure are best equipped to accompany the couple during exposure treatment. A number of professional caveats face psychologists work-ing with therapist-aided, *in vivo* exposure in vaginismus (e.g., seminudity, cli-ent practicing vaginal penetration in the presence of the therapist), and we recommend that therapist-aided exposure be carried out in a medical setting.

CASE DISCUSSION

After a clinical intake interview and external gynecological examination, it was recommended that Eva and Rob start with therapist-aided exposure treatment. Massed exposure is emotionally intense, and homework assignments are time-consuming. Therefore, we generally recommend that couples take time off from work in the week following the first exposure session. In our clinical experience, practice of relaxation exercises prior to *in vivo* exposure did not contribute to treatment process and outcome; therefore, specific relaxation exercises prior to exposure were not included in the treatment protocol. During the therapist-aided session, however, relaxation and/or breathing instruction can be sug-gested by the therapist (for the treatment manual, see ter Kuile et al., 2007).

Prior to the first exposure session, Eva and Rob attended an information session discussing the following topics: (1) the rationale of exposure treat-ment for vaginismus (using the FAM-V); (2) what to expect during exposure therapy; (3) the nature and frequency of homework exercises; (4) Rob's par-ticipation at the hospital and his active involvement in the exercises at home; and (5) the development of a hierarchy of fear- and tension-eliciting vaginal penetration stimuli to use during exposure (tampon, finger[s], penis with and without movement). Eva expected that the most fearful step would be penetra-tion, regardless of who would insert a dilator or finger and whether or not there was movement. The goal of the exposure sessions at the hospital was self-insertion of a dilator or fingers that was slightly larger than the circumfer-ence of the erect penis of her partner.

The Therapist-Aided Exposure Session

A brief conversation at the beginning of the exposure session indicated that, as expected, both partners were very nervous. It had been established in the assessment that Eva was at risk for experiencing feelings of dizziness and that she was afraid of fainting. Therefore, she was instructed to drink two glasses of water before the session to prevent loss of blood pressure. In response to dizziness, she was instructed to briefly stop the exercises and tense the muscles of her body to raise blood pressure. "Applied tension" has been demonstrated as an effective intervention in patients with blood phobia (e.g., Barlow, 2002). Care is also taken to arrange the gynecological examination chair or table in a fashion that does not interfere with the exercises and so that, should the woman faint, a fall can be prevented.

The therapist and Rob stood beside the chair, and all were able to see the vaginal penetration exercises by means of a handheld mirror. Eva began by touching her vulva with her fingers and spreading her labia minora. As expected, she felt increasingly dizzy when touching (and seeing) her vulva and vaginal entrance. The therapist instructed Eva to use applied tension and moved the chair to a more horizontal position. Within a couple of minutes she was able to compensate for the decrease in blood pressure and continue the exercises. She was very relieved that she mastered this step. She subsequently proceeded with the gradual insertion of one finger using lubricant. Eva was inclined to withdraw her hand immediately whenever she had unpleasant feelings or sensations. Rather than avoiding these feelings, she was encouraged to hold her finger still and to describe sensations and feelings she was experiencing. Unpleasant sensations disappeared within a few seconds. The experience of increasing anxiety, being able to tolerate the feelings, and the subsequent decrease in anxiety was described as "surprising" and increased Eva's confidence that she would be able to handle more exposure exercises.

She was encouraged to move her finger gently, which she experienced without much anxiety. As she did not experience any feelings of dizziness at this phase of the exposure exercises, the chair was moved back to the original position, allowing for practice in different positions. Quite soon she was able to insert two fingers. Eva was surprised by her progress in disconfirming her penetration-related fears that vaginal penetration was impossible and painful. She experienced some pain when she moved her fingers, but the pain subsided when she focused on a gentle down-bearing pressure in her pelvic area. Next, she practiced the same steps in squatting, sitting, and standing positions, first with her finger and then with different-sized dilators. She experienced a precipitous rise in anxiety and intense desire to terminate the session when inserting the largest dilator. She was encouraged to focus on the sensations she felt, to describe her discomfort, and to stay still and practice relaxation with diaphragmatic breathing. Negative sensations subsided gradually, and she felt significant joy and pride at her success in sustaining and reducing heightened anxiety. After 1.5 hours of practice, she was able to insert a vaginal probe of 12 cm circumference and three of her fingers; the ultimate goal of 12 cm was achieved and exceeded. To conclude, she practiced with a lubricated tampon, which she was able to insert without problems.

During the postexposure conversation, Eva stated that she was extremely relieved and very satisfied with the results she had achieved. The experience of vaginal penetration with very little pain and using a dilator that was slightly larger than her husband's penis directly disconfirmed her fears. She described the experience of unpleasant feelings and sensations disappearing gradually if she did not stop the exercise but talked about her experience while trying to relax her body as the most important step for her ("This is a huge discovery for me!"). Rob felt reassured that vaginal penetration was possible without pain and felt empowered to assist Eva actively in home exercises. They went home with instructions to repeat the exercises the same day using plenty of lubricant. Progressive steps for Rob during homework exercises included: (1)

inserting his fingers (one, two, or three); (2) touching the entrance to Eva's vagina with his erect penis without penetration; (3) inserting his erect penis without thrusting; and (4) inserting his penis with thrusting.

Following the Therapist–Aided Exposure *In Vivo* Session

Eva and Rob had an appointment at the outpatient clinic 2 days later, during which they related that practicing at home had gone well. Rob could easily insert two fingers, but his third was more difficult. His penis could be inserted halfway, but it felt awkward because they struggled to find a comfortable position. The therapist and the couple concluded that no further exposure sessions at the hospital were necessary while daily home exercises continued. During the third appointment, the couple reported that intercourse was possible and painless. Eva's menstruation had started, and when she tried to insert a tampon, she nearly fainted and experienced heightened anxiety. Rob stayed calm, reminded Eva of the applied tension exercise to manage her dizziness, and suggested that Eva insert the tampon while lying on her back. She followed these steps for a couple of days, and every day tampon insertion became easier. Managing and overcoming this challenge was an important step for Eva and Rob and increased their confidence that they had the necessary tools to handle any future challenges.

During the 6- and 12-week consultations, Eva and Rob reported that sexual intercourse was still possible but not pleasant. The arousal created during foreplay decreased as soon as penetration was attempted. Three additional sessions were planned focusing on maintenance of sexual arousal during penetration. Eva chose to practice alone initially by allowing arousal to build with clitoral stimulation and then inserting a finger or a small vibrator. During the third consultation, she recounted that she was able to move the vibrator intravaginally and was able to facilitate orgasm. The couple encountered more difficulty when practicing together. Eva appeared to be hypervigilant to unexpected movement from her husband, which prompted a decrease in arousal. They believed, however, that they could progress further without additional sessions. During a final appointment a year following treatment, the couple was satisfied with their sex life, stating that sexual intercourse was arousing and pleasant for both if they used the woman-superior position. Other positions still elicited a decline in sexual arousal. Nevertheless, the couple stated that they were very satisfied with the results achieved, and treatment was concluded.

Evaluation

In line with research findings, the couple was able to experience a first intercourse within the first week of exposure therapy. Overall, 10 sessions were necessary to achieve the desired treatment outcome of pain-free, pleasurable intercourse; only one of these sessions involved a therapist-aided exposure session at the hospital.

What can be said about possible mediating influences on the effects of treatment? According to the FAM-V model, the penetration-related fears are maintained in women with vaginismus because avoidance prevents disconfirmation of the catastrophic beliefs. By directly reducing avoidance and increasing successful penetration behaviors, fears are disconfirmed; catastrophization is reduced and eventually eliminated. In the case of Eva and Rob, beliefs about vaginal pathology, genital incompatibility and expectation of pain were progressively disconfirmed by "normal" findings with the gynecological examination and the ability to insert dilators or fingers with little and later no pain during exposure exercises. Reduction of catastrophizing resulted in a reduction of fear, and avoidance behaviors as a coping strategy were no longer necessary. *In vivo* exposure results in intense anxiety and negative emotions; nonetheless, the rewards to the patient(s) in terms of pride, sense of achievement, and empowerment are highly beneficial. Eva and Rob described experiences in the exposure session as "a discovery" and "changing their views on vaginal penetration." Subsequent massed exposure at home consolidated and expanded on the successful experiences of the therapist-assisted exposure session. Rob was quite effective in helping Eva through a critical moment when a new penetration experience (tampon) briefly reversed treatment gains, which further empowered the couple to manage possible future challenges.

CONCLUSIONS

In this chapter we focused on women with lifelong vaginismus who have never been able to experience complete vaginal intercourse and who demonstrate marked fear and avoidance of vaginal penetration. Recent treatment outcome reports are in line with research suggesting that lifelong vaginismus may be more akin to a penetration phobia. We can assume with a good degree of confidence at this point that focusing treatment on fear and avoidance behaviors will result in a significant decrease of negative penetration beliefs and fears, in turn resulting in successful intercourse for nearly all women with lifelong vaginismus. However, the experience of intercourse does not automatically imply that penetration is also pleasurable. Future research has to investigate which additional treatment interventions may be helpful to improve overall sexual function and pleasure. Finally, it is currently unclear to what degree women with acquired vaginismus or dyspareunia could benefit from exposure therapy and how or whether the treatment protocol would need to be adjusted.

In general, a significant paucity of research for *lifelong* vaginismus has to be noted. Only recently have researchers attended to possible differences between women who develop an inability to experience intercourse, typically in response to dyspareunia, and those women who have never been able to experience intercourse. The combination of vaginismus and dyspareunia into GPPPD for DSM-5 (American Psychiatric Association, 2013) is empirically based and in line with the available research on the overlap and/or continuity on various symptom dimensions between the two penetration-related problems. However, in view of the relative neglect of lifelong vaginismus in the empirical literature thus far, it can be argued that not enough information is available to conclude that both problems are indeed the same disorder. A combination of vaginismus and dyspareunia, at this point, carries the risk of extinguishing the recently nascent empirical research interest in lifelong vaginismus which may—or may not—demonstrate lifelong vaginismus as a distinct clinical affliction requiring differential treatment recommendations.

REFERENCES

American Psychiatric Association. (2000). *Diagnostic and statistical manual of mental disorders* (4th ed., text rev.).Washington, DC: Author.

American Psychiatric Association. (2013). *Diagnostic and statistical manual of mental disorders* (5th ed.). Arlington, VA: Author.

Barlow, D. H. (2002). *Anxiety and it disorders: The nature and treatment of anxiety and panic* (2nd ed.). New York: Guilford Press.

Basson, R., Leiblum, S., Brotto, L., Derogatis, L., Fourcroy, J., Fugl-Meyer, K., et al. (2003). Definitions of women's sexual dysfunction reconsidered: Advocating expansion and revision. *Journal of Psychosomatic Obstetrics and Gynecology, 24*, 221–229.

Binik, Y. M. (2010). The DSM diagnostic criteria for vaginismus. *Archives of Sexual Behavior, 39*, 278–291.

Borg, C., de Jong, P. J., & Weijmar Schultz, W. W. (2010). Vaginismus and dyspareunia: Automatic vs. deliberate disgust responsivity. *Journal of Sexual Medicine, 7*, 2149–2157.

Busby, D. M., Christensen, C., Crane, D. R., & Larson, J. H. (1995). A revision of the Dyadic Adjustment Scale for use with distressed and non-distressed couples: Construct hierarchy and multidimensional scales. *Journal of Marital and Family Therapy, 21*, 289–308.

Cherner, R. A. & Reissing, E. D. (2013). A psychophysiological investigation of sexual response in women with lifelong vaginismus. *Journal of Sexual Medicine, 10(5)*, 1291–1303.

Christensen, B. S., Gronbaek, M., Osler, M., Pedersen, B. V., Graugaard, C., & Frisch, M. (2011). Sexual dysfunctions and difficulties in Denmark: Prevalence and associated sociodemographic factors. *Archives of Sexual Behavior, 40*, 121–132.

Klaassen, M., & ter Kuile, M. M. (2009). The development and initial validation of the Vaginal Penetration Cognition Questionnaire (VPCQ) in a sample of women with vaginismus and dyspareunia. *Journal of Sexual Medicine, 6*, 1617–1627.

Lambert, M. J., Burlingame, G. M., Umphress, V., Hansen, N. B., Vermeersch, D. A., Clouse, G. C., et al. (1996). The reliability and validity of the Outcome Questionnaire. *Clincal Psychology and Psychtherapy, 3*, 249–258.

Melnick, T., Hawton, K., & McGuire, H. (2012). Interventions for vaginismus. *Cochrane Database of Systemic Reviews, 12*.

Reissing, E. D. (2009). Vaginismus: Evaluation and management. In A. T. Goldstein, C. F. Pukall, & I. Goldstein (Eds.), *Female sexual pain disorders: Evaluation and management* (pp. 229–234). Oxford, UK: Wiley-Blackwell.

Reissing, E. D. (2012). Consultation and treatment history and causal attributions in an online sample of women with lifelong and acquired vaginismus. *Journal of Sexual Medicine, 9,* 251–258.

Reissing, E. D., Armstrong, H. L., & Allen, C. (2013). Pelvic floor physical therapy for women with lifelong vaginismus: A retrospective chart review and interview study. *Journal of Sex and Marital Therapy, 39,* 1–15.

Reissing, E. D., Binik, Y. M., Khalifé, S., Cohen, D., & Amsel, R. (2004). Vaginal spasm, pain, and behavior: An empirical investigation of the diagnosis of vaginismus. *Archives of Sexual Behavior, 33,* 5–17.

Shafik, A., & El-Sibai, F. (2002). Study of the pelvic floor muscles in vaginismus: A concept of pathogenesis. *European Journal of Obstetrics, Gynecology, and Reproductive Biology, 105,* 67–70.

ter Kuile, M. M., Both, S., & van Lankveld, J. J. D. M. (2010). Cognitive-behavioral therapy for sexual dysfunctions in women. *Psychiatric Clinics of North America, 33,* 595–610.

ter Kuile, M. M., Bulte, I., Weijenborg, P. T. M., Beekman, A., Melles, R., & Onghena, P. (2009). Therapist-aided exposure for women with lifelong vaginismus: A replicated single-case design. *Journal of Consulting and Clinical Psychology, 77,* 149–159.

ter Kuile, M. M., Melles, R., Groot, H. E., Tuijnman-Raasveld, C. C., & van Lankveld, J. J. D. M. (2013). Therapist-aided exposure for women with lifelong vaginismus: A randomized waiting-list controlled trial of efficacy. *Journal of Consulting and Clinical Psychology.*

ter Kuile, M. M., Weijenborg, P. T. M., Beekman, A., Groot, H. E., Tuijnman-Raasveld, C. C., van Lankveld, J. J. D. M., et al. (2007). *Treatment manual, therapist-aided exposure for women with lifelong vaginismus.* Retrieved from *www/mmterkuile.nl.*

van der Velde, J., Laan, E., & Everaerd, W. (2001). Vaginismus, a component of a general defensive reaction. An investigation of pelvic floor muscle activity during exposure to emotion-inducing film excerpts in women with and without vaginismus. *International Urogynecology Journal and Pelvic Floor Dysfunction, 12,* 328–331.

van Lankveld, J. J. D. M., Granot, M., Schultz, W. C. M. W., Binik, Y. M., Wesselmann, U., Pukall, C. F., et al. (2010). Women's sexual pain disorders. *Journal of Sexual Medicine, 7,* 615–631.

van Lankveld, J. J. D. M., ter Kuile, M. M., de Groot, H. E., Melles, R., Nefs, J., & Zandbergen, M. (2006). Cognitive-behavioral therapy for women with lifelong vaginismus: A randomized waiting-list controlled trial of efficacy. *Journal of Consulting and Clinical Psychology, 74,* 168–178.

Vlaeyen, J. W. S., & Linton, S. J. (2000). Fear-avoidance and its consequences in chronic musculoskeletal pain: A state of the art. *Pain, 85,* 317–332.

Yasan, A., & Gurgen, F. (2009). Marital satisfaction, sexual problems, and the possible difficulties on sex therapy in traditional Islamic culture. *Journal of Sex and Marital Therapy, 35,* 68–75.

PART II

SEX THERAPY FOR OTHER SEXUAL DISORDERS

CHAPTER 9

The Paraphilias

An Experiential Approach to "Dangerous" Desires

Peggy J. Kleinplatz

Paraphilias are typically treated today via cognitive-behavioral and/or pharmacological therapy aimed at controlling or reducing the frequency and intensity of atypical sexual behaviors and their corresponding sexual urges. Indeed, controlling (if not eliminating) unusual sexual interests is often the wish of the client or couple, as deviant interests often wreak havoc on their lives and in the extreme can result in legal difficulties and incarceration. Kleinplatz reviews the gaps in our knowledge of the paraphilias and cautions against filling in these gaps with moral judgments. Indeed, she raises the question as to whether these diverse sexual interests have much in common other than their presumed low prevalence. Whereas forensic psychology addresses criminal and coercive paraphilias, sex therapy could, but has not, adequately addressed treatment of non-coercive paraphilias. In this chapter, Kleinplatz argues that Experiential Psychotherapy, which focuses on effecting substantive personality change rather than overt behavior, may be an effective strategy for treating the paraphilias.

Peggy J. Kleinplatz, PhD, is Professor of Medicine and Clinical Professor of Psychology at the University of Ottawa. She is a clinical psychologist, Certified in Sex Therapy, Sex Education and as a Diplomate in and Supervisor of Sex Therapy. She is currently Chair of Ethics and former Chair of Certifications for the American Association of Sexuality Educators, Counselors and Therapists. Dr. Kleinplatz has edited three books, most recently *New Directions in Sex Therapy: Innovations and Alternatives* (Routledge, 2012), winner of the AASECT 2013 Book Award. Her clinical work focuses on eroticism and transformation. Her current research focuses on optimal sexuality, with a particular interest in sexual health in the elderly, disabled, and marginalized populations.

In this chapter, I present a survey of the literature on the paraphilias, offer a clinical illustration, and discuss the outcome of a clinical case against the backdrop of the predominant paradigms. The difficulty is that much of the literature in this area is geared toward readers working with forensic populations rather than for sex therapists. In addition, the methods, goals, and outcomes are focused on reducing recidivism rather than on the kinds of personal development valued by psychotherapists. Please bear with me as I move across different domains, suggesting the application of an established clinical model, that is, Experiential Psychotherapy, for an innovative use by sex therapists in working with atypical sexual desires.

In attempting to provide an overview of the paraphilias, a major obstacle is that the literature in the area is divided across professional (and other) lines. It appears in three different domains: First, the large forensic literature on sex offenders is focused on controlling the paraphiliac's behavior, distinguishing or determining commonalities among deviant behavioral patterns; on reducing recidivism or at least predicting recidivism rates accurately; and on protecting the public from the sex offender (Laws & O'Donohue, 2008). Second, the scarce sex therapy literature discusses the etiology and meaning of unusual sexual desires, classification of sexual variations, the possibility of comorbid disorders, whether or not the paraphilias are subject to change, and, almost parenthetically, the relative *absence* of patients and their lack of motivation for treatment (Darcangelo, 2008; Hucker, 2008: Krueger, 2009b; Lussier & Piché, 2008; Morin & Levenson 2008). A third and growing domain is in the literature among those who are aroused by consensual albeit unconventional sexual activities. This literature is mostly oriented toward education and support of sexual minority community members and advocacy in the face of uncomprehending, judgmental and downright hostile mental health professionals and an adversarial legal system. Within this literature, the entire enterprise of trying to diagnose, classify, and control sexual behavior among consenting adults is seen as morally rather than scientifically based and is thus ethically dubious. None of these vantage points is especially friendly toward the major concerns of the other domains, which makes an integrated perspective on the paraphilias rather challenging.

This chapter calls for a review of the empirically based treatment literature. That would require accurate information on the prevalence of the paraphilias, how to classify and conceptualize them, how to assess them, what the goals of treatment ought to be, what the treatments consist of, and how to assess effective outcome of treatments for the paraphilias. It might also be nice to know what causes the paraphilias. Unfortunately, there is little information in some of these areas and even less consensus on the rest.

WHAT ARE THE PARAPHILIAS?

By definition, paraphilias are unusual sexual interests. The DSM-IV-TR (American Psychiatric Association, 2000) listed the paraphilias as follows: voyeurism, exhibitionism, frotteurism, pedophilia, fetishism, sexual sadism, sexual masochism, and transvestic fetishism. A ninth category, paraphilia not otherwise specified (NOS), is a grab-bag category for an unlimited assortment of other sexual proclivities, most of which will probably never appear in the clinical or research literature. The paraphilias tend to be divided in terms of coercive or illegal (i.e, voyeurism, exhibitionism, frotteurism, pedophilia) versus the non-coercive paraphilias (i.e., fetishism, consensual sexual sadism and masochism, transvestism).

The professional literature on the paraphilias is limited by uncertainty as to what they are, how many there are, and what their frequency might be. The category comprises sexual proclivities listed together only by virtue of being relatively uncommon. It is clear that some are unusual (e.g., pedophilia, frotteurism) and others are downright rare (e.g., apotemnophilia), but we do not even have accurate data on just how atypical they are. A recent German population sample found that 62.4% of men reported sexual arousal to at least one of the DSM-IV-TR paraphilias, indicating that the presence of paraphilic desires may be far more common than previously believed (Ahlers, 2011). Frequency estimates are also compromised by the fact that most people who have unusual sexual interests do not have only one sexual proclivity, unusual or otherwise (Langevin, Lang, & Curnoe, 1998). Of course, prevalence estimates are also limited by the reluctance of individuals who have been pathologized, criminalized, and otherwise marginalized to report their conduct to the authorities. The only consistent element across the literature is the notion that the large majority of paraphiliacs are male.

Outside the forensic or clinical literature, one can learn about the astonishingly broad variety of unusual sexual interests in the community via the Internet (e.g., by visiting *Fetlife.com*, a social networking site for the "kink" world). As of February, 2012 Fetlife listed 1,243,518 members, who shared 5,604,935 pictures and 47,191 videos, participated in 1,734,663 discussions in 37,801 groups, were going to 5,070 upcoming events, and reading 597,138 blog posts. Or as it states on the opening page of the Fetlife website, "Welcome to kinky heaven!"

CONCEPTUALIZATION AND CLASSIFICATION

Newring, Wheeler, and Draper (2008, p. 301) have observed, "Before we can treat 'it,' we need to know what 'it' is, or whether 'it' is worth a diagnostic label." A review of the literature indicates precisely how arbitrary classification of the paraphilias has been over the last 50 years or so. Sexual deviations have been listed and removed from the DSM across successive editions (Moser

& Kleinplatz, 2005). The social rather than empirical basis for classification of "deviant" sexuality was most notoriously exemplified by the early inclusion of homosexuality and subsequent removal in 1973. The current list has shifted repeatedly. The question of whether or not the paraphilias necessarily constitute a disorder at all remains controversial.

As for theoretical conceptions of the paraphilias, our understanding is even more limited. The forensic practitioner is not especially concerned with how to conceive of the origins and meaning of sexual variations. The average sex therapist may have been trained in psychodynamic, behavioral, and biological theories of psychopathology but generally is unlikely to be seeing patients who present for treatment of atypical sexuality. The literature is filled with references to the paraphilias overall, making statements that are not particularly useful to either set of practitioners. As described by Darcangelo (2008, p. 115), "Many studies draw conclusions about paraphilias in general, rather than differentiating among the various types of paraphilias. Given the considerable overlap among paraphilias, this is not too surprising." On the other end are clinicians or researchers who have a specific interest in a particular paraphilia, for example, fetishism or frotteurism. However, that literature tends to be sparse, and there is no way of knowing to what extent our understanding of the frotteur can be extrapolated and applied to understanding of the fetishist. If researchers agree that it is difficult to even estimate the prevalence rates for the various paraphilias (e.g., Lussier & Piché, 2008), the consensus in the literature is that it is more complex to imagine a cohesive conceptualization of the paraphilias. Much of the literature on sexual deviance is focused on pedophilia, rape, and exhibitionism (Laws & O'Donohue, 2008). All three of these associated behaviors are illegal, although rape is not currently listed as a paraphilia in DSM-5 (American Psychiatric Association, 2013). The other paraphilias are "orphans" with little funding for research into their prevalence, conceptualization, or treatment. In other words, the focus is on criminality rather than psychopathology, which are hardly synonymous. Thus our knowledge of the paraphilias is limited by the bifurcation by which professionals are assigned to deal with which "disorder," making it impossible to discern whether we are even talking about one kind of phenomenon or a variety of discrete phenomena.

If it is difficult to disentangle sexual deviance, illegal behavior, and psychopathology, any attempt to understand atypical sexuality is further hampered by the lack of theoretical integrity or even appropriate empirical measures for sexual normalcy (Kleinplatz & Moser, 2005; Moser & Kleinplatz, 2005). As the situation is described in Laws and O'Donohue's review, "There are no well-corroborated accounts of the psychopathology involved in the paraphilias. In addition, too little is known about 'normal' sexuality and sexual development. Thus, again, there are gaps in what constructs ought to be measured" (2008, p. 6).

In addition to disciplinary divisions, public opinion plays a role in classification and conceptualization of the paraphilias. Depending on which particular paraphilia is under discussion, the lay public reactions vary from "Throw those perverts in prison and throw away the key" to "Let's castrate them all" to "Why does anybody care what a bunch of consenting adults do in the privacy of their own homes?" Both professionals and the public react quite differently to those who sexually abuse children—whether or not they actually are pedophiles—as compared with cross-dressers at home, whether or not they are diagnosable as transvestic fetishists. In addition, community groups have taken stands on the consequences of being diagnosed as pathological in terms of social stigma. Parents who have lost custody disputes or individuals who have lost their jobs or civil rights due to DSM diagnoses object strongly to the diagnosis of paraphilia, particularly given that most paraphilias cause no distress or dysfunction. Most conspicuously, BDSM activists object to receiving any kind of diagnosis for behavior that is judged as pathological based on social prejudice as opposed to empirical evidence (Kleinplatz & Moser, 2004; Moser & Kleinplatz, 2005; Nichols, 2006; Reiersøl & Skeid, 2006). Krueger (2009a) reports that in over 400,000,000 visits to primary care physicians in the United States, not one case was diagnosed of Sexual Sadism or Sexual Masochism. Such evidence, the controversy about DSM classification, and the lack of compelling empirical evidence for pathologizing atypical sexuality per se have had an impact on classification and conceptualization of the paraphilias.

DSM-5

DSM-5 redefines the concept of paraphilia as "any intense and persistent sexual interest other than sexual interest in genital stimulation or preparatory fondling with phenotypically normal, consenting adult human partners" (Blanchard, 2009a). This definition advances a conceptualization for the paraphilias that was missing in the DSM-IV. Blanchard notes that its main advantage is replacing a definition by concatenation (i.e., listing) with a definition by exclusion. For better or for worse, it makes it decidedly clear that our professional conception of sexuality is still focused on activities directed between the legs and that whatever deviates from that goal is construed as abnormal.

Although the main advantage of this new DSM-5 definition is the umbrella description of the paraphilias, the specifying of abnormal behaviors listed in the DSM-IV-TR paraphilia section remains. In addition, according to the DSM-5 website, two new paraphilia categories were proposed in 2009: "coercive paraphilic disorder" and "pedohebephilia" to replace and expand the pedophilia category. See Quinsey (2009), Blanchard (2009b), and Blanchard, Lykins, Wherrett, Kuban, Cantor, et al. (2009) respectively, for a description of these proposals. Neither of these new categories was retained in DSM-5.

Most important, DSM-5 accepted Blanchard's proposal (Blanchard, 2009a, 2009b) to differentiate between the designation of paraphilia as a proclivity versus as a disorder:

Paraphilias are not *ipso facto* psychiatric disorders. We are proposing that the DSM-V make a distinction between *paraphilias* and paraphilic *disorders*. A paraphilia by itself would not automatically justify or require psychiatric intervention. A *paraphilic disorder* is a paraphilia that causes distress or impairment to the individual or harm to others. One would *ascertain* a paraphilia (according to the nature of the urges, fantasies, or behaviors) but *diagnose* a paraphilic disorder (on the basis of distress and impairment). In this conception, having a paraphilia would be a necessary but not a sufficient condition for having a paraphilic disorder (Blanchard, 2009b).

THE ORIGINS OF DESIRE(S)

This still leaves some sexologists and lay people with the question "Why does that turn them on?" as opposed to the more fundamental question of why anything might turn anyone on. The traditional, etiological discourse has focused on the cause(s) of unusual sexual interests, whether explained in terms of psychodynamic, behavioral, or other theories of psychopathology that explore developmental factors in the origins of unusual sexual proclivities. In recent years, the evolutionary discourse has supplanted the etiological discourse. That is, the evolutionary discourse defines normal sexuality in terms of purpose (i.e., propagation of the species), with sexual psychopathology defined in terms of deviating from the presumably biologically driven correct purpose of sexual behavior (see Cantor, Chapter 10, for a discussion of the biological basis of pedophilia). Such literature tends to investigate physiological markers of atypical sexuality among sex offenders (e.g. left-handedness, brain injury, neuropsychological profiles, functional asymmetry [e.g., Blanchard, Cantor, & Robichaud, 2006]). Even within this body of research, there is no consistent evidence for a distinct biological basis for the paraphilias (Cantor, 2012). But the focus remains on the atypical, as though we need to explain (away) divergent sexuality with no need to even notice our corresponding lack of understanding of normative sexual inclinations.

In the 1980s, Money contributed the theory of "lovemaps," a construct intended to describe the origins of all sexual desire (1986). Money hypothesized that early sexual interactions (e.g., childhood sex play acting as a rehearsal for adult sexual expression) create a mental template during a child's vulnerable periods, at approximately age 8. These become imprinted and later manifest in adult sexual expression. Prevention, prohibition, or other interference can cause the developmental process to go awry, thus resulting in "vandalized lovemaps," that is, the paraphilias.

Freund (1990) conceptualized the paraphilias as "courtship disorders," while Blanchard describes them as erotic target location errors (Freund & Blanchard, 1993). The former refers to the inability to engage in the appropriate behaviors leading to heterosexual intercourse, whereas the latter refers to an incorrect object choice, which should be an adult, heterosexual partner. Both presuppose a correct sequence and ultimate objective for sexual relations.

ASSESSMENT

It is commonly known that a significant proportion, and perhaps most, of patients referred for the assessment of paraphilia are referred as a result of committing a criminal sexual offense. Assessment of the paraphilias is complicated not only by the factors mentioned earlier but also by methodological and ethical considerations in evaluating sex offenders. Those who undergo assessment or treatment procedures in compliance with court orders or in an effort to reduce their sentences may not be motivated to be honest. The clinicians conducting the assessment for sentencing or for risk of recidivism upon release are acting in society's best interests but do not necessarily represent the best interests of the individual being evaluated. One way of circumventing self-report biases and aiming for objectivity has been the use of phallometric testing. However, there are serious reservations about the reliability, validity, and lack of standardization in phallometry (Darcangelo, Hollings, & Paladino, 2008, p. 122).

As for the individuals with various paraphilias who are unlikely to seek therapy in any case, there is even less literature on assessment of them. The general recommendations are for assessment via clinical interview with a detailed developmental and sexual history, as well as the history of the problem. In particular, clinicians are advised to determine whether the individual would even qualify for diagnosis at all, based on the existence of distress or lack thereof and social, occupational, or interpersonal impairment. There are mixed recommendations as to the value of psychometric measures. For example, Krueger and Kaplan (2008, p. 154) state, "Generally speaking, individual clinicians should review available instruments and alternatives, and decide for themselves what would be most useful." That is, there is no set of "best practices" or preferred assessment tools available in the literature for such evaluations (cf. Hucker, 2008; Mann, Ainsworth, Al-Attar, & Davies, 2008; Newring et al., 2008). Laws and O'Donohue (2008) recognize the need for effective assessment tools in their comprehensive review of the literature but report concerns about accuracy, validity, and reliability in current assessment of the paraphilias. Clinicians are advised to be attentive to any signs of neurological deficits, to enquire as to history of head injuries and drug use, and to consider possible referral for neuropsychological assessment. These recommendations are more likely to appear in the literature on pedophilia and exhibitionism than in the literature on cross-dressing or masochism.

It is unfortunate that the literature on assessment of the non-coercive paraphilias is so vague and sparse, given that individuals or couples in which one or both have unusual—and sometimes discrepant—sexual interests do occasionally appear in our offices. For example, patients often present with difficulties with arousal or desire in a particular relationship that upon enquiry are related to different conceptions of sexuality; these differences are often distinguished by divergent sexual fantasies, some of which may be atypical. Experienced sex therapists recognize that sexual fantasies often cause shame and guilt and are shrouded in secrecy, even when the fantasy content is nor-mophilic, not to mention when it is unusual. It is helpful to treat the desire *discrepancy* rather than focusing on the atypical nature of the sexual desires, particularly when the individuals do not conceive of the nature of the sexual desires as requiring treatment (Kleinplatz & Moser, 2004; Nichols, 2006).

Perhaps one reason for the dearth of literature on the paraphilias in psy-chotherapy practice is the discomfort among clinicians in dealing with atypi-cal sexuality per se, as well as the potential for assessment and treatment to result in legal entanglements (e.g., court testimony). Although the clinician's reluctance is understandable, for those who are willing to expand practice in this area, it is recommended that they consult with skilled forensic sexologists to learn how to navigate through legal complexities. Therapists who recognize their own squeamishness in dealing with atypical sexuality may wish to seek supervision to process countertransference issues. It is also advisable that cli-nicians educate themselves about alternate sexual expression and familiarize themselves with local community resources and support groups.

TREATMENT

During the 1970s and 1980s, the cognitive-behavioral approaches to treat-ment for the paraphilias predominated. They attempted to control and reduce the unacceptable behavior and corresponding urges. Over the past 30 years, the literature has reflected the growing prominence of pharmacologi-cal approaches in treating sexual difficulties in general and paraphilic sexual behavior in particular.

The paraphilias qualify for treatment only when they involve distress and dysfunction—and a patient. In the sex *therapy* literature, there is lit-tle discussion in recent years of how to treat the non-coercive paraphilias, presumably at least partially because individuals with unusual sexual pro-clivities do not present for treatment of them. When sexuality has become the clinical focus of interest, the goal is increasingly to reduce distress (and sometimes the resulting dysfunction) caused by stigma rather than to treat the paraphilia per se (Kleinplatz & Moser, 2004; Moser & Kleinplatz, 2002; Nichols, 2006). Individuals can reduce feelings of being alienated and ashamed by joining support groups (e.g., for cross-dressers), educational and advocacy groups, or social groups for like-minded individuals (e.g., the BDSM "munch," a social opportunity to meet others interested in BDSM at a restaurant, outside a sexual environment). These may include opportuni-ties for meeting prospective sexual partners. All manner of options exist in online groups.

Although there are numerous single-case reports, there is a dearth of ran-domized controlled trial (RCT) literature on treatment of the paraphilias out-side the forensic literature. First, obviously, for ethical reasons, RCT designs are not advisable for paraphilias when there are concerns about public safety.

Second, although individuals with unusual sexual interests may appear in our offices (e.g., BDSM), given that these desires are not intended to be the focus of treatment (Kleinplatz & Moser, 2004; Nichols, 2006), the literature on "treatment" outcome is necessarily limited.

Of the individuals with a paraphilia that causes concern to society, many will not wish treatment. According to Morin and Levenson (2008, p. 101), "Sex offenders do not often choose therapy; therapy is chosen for them. The most skilled therapist, using the most effective techniques, will not change an individual who is not motivated to change." Obviously, there are ethical considerations in "offering" treatment to those who do not wish treatment except when the incentive is to stay out of or be released from prison. Conversely, contrary to the panic (and wording) in many news stories, not all pedophiles will ever act on their desires, and many, if not most, cases of child sexual abuse are committed by adults whose primary erotic arousal is to adults. Pedophiles may seek therapy to deal with their attractions to minors without any legal requirement or implications.

The predominant sex offender treatment programs at present consist of pharmacological intervention—specifically, the anti-androgens in combination with the SSRIs, for example, medroxyprogesterone acetate or cyproterone acetate with fluoxetine. This is referred to in the popular press as "chemical castration." It is generally recommended that this be combined with cognitive-behavioral therapy (CBT; Briken & Kafka, 2007; Guay, 2009), often including social skills training and relapse prevention. Symptoms are controlled for only as long as the patient remains medicated. There is no cure; rather, the hope is for rehabilitation. That is, the predominant treatments do not attempt to change the nature of the individual's desires but rather their intensity and frequency and his or her ability to act on them.

A few of the sex offender treatment programs reject the traditional relapse prevention model and are supplemented by community support available to the sex offender upon his or her release (Marshall, Marshall, Serran, & O'Brien, 2011). The Circles of Support and Accountablity (COSA) program, pioneered in Ontario, makes extensive use of volunteer and professional supports and shows significant promise for reducing recidivism (Wilson, Cortoni, & McWhinnie, 2009).

There is much controversy as to whether the existing interventions are effective. The outcome data are described as dismal, discouraging, inconsistent, and contradictory (Corabian, Dennett, & Harstall, 2011; Hanson, Bourgon, Helmus, & Hodgson, 2009). The same complications that contaminate the initial assessment reappear in the outcome literature. Although some clinician/researchers are optimistic about the salutary effects of treatment on sex offenders (e.g., Fedoroff & Marshall, 2010; Marshall & Marshall, 2010; Marshall et al., 2011), others are less impressed. Some believe that treatment of sex offenders could actually make matters worse (Rice, 2010; Seto et al., 2008). A series of review articles on the treatment of the paraphilias cites reports of patient noncompliance, high dropout rates, long-term treatment failures, and the need for treatment to continue indefinitely, if not for life (Gijs, 2008; Greenfield, 2006; Guay, 2009).

Given the need for long-term use of these medications in sex offenders, it is striking that few articles identify reduction in sexual desire, arousal, response, and functioning as "unwanted" or "significant side effects." On the contrary, such outcomes are seen as indications of treatment effectiveness. The fact that sexual pleasure is hard to relinquish does not seem to be a consideration. By contrast, Guay (2009) reviews the many adverse physical and sexual effects of these drugs, pointing out the need for better tolerated medications.

THE EXPERIENTIAL MODEL

An alternative approach originates in Experiential Psychotherapy (Mahrer, 1996/2004, 2002, 2011). It was developed over a 40-year period using extensive psychotherapy-process research on the world's largest psychotherapy tape library, representing master clinicians of every orientation. The objective in developing Experiential Psychotherapy was to establish methods intended to bring about substantive personality change rather than aiming for treatment of specific DSM disorders (Mahrer, 1996/2004a, 2004b). Although this model has not commonly been applied in treatment of the paraphilias (with certain exceptions; e.g., Kleinplatz, 2006, 2012; Kleinplatz & Krippner, 2005; Mahrer, 2012), its potential effectiveness in dealing with sexual problems, given its goals, methods, and so forth, makes it especially useful for sex therapy in general and for unusual sexual behaviors in particular (Kleinplatz, 1998, 2004, 2007, 2010; Mahrer & Boulet, 2001). It is likely to be brief psychotherapy and, therefore, time- and cost-effective. This approach can also be used for individual, marital/couple, and group therapy.

Experiential Psychotherapy (Mahrer, 1996/2004a) is unique, brings about fundamental change relatively quickly, and may seem intimidating to those unfamiliar with this approach. It does not aim to treat symptoms, problems, or conditions (Mahrer, 1996/2004a) but instead uses the presenting problem as an opportunity for qualitative change. The goals are for the client to integrate whatever is deepest within, thereby becoming a "qualitatively new person," and for the client to be free of any painful feelings that were present at the outset (Mahrer, 1996/2004a, pp. 81–82). In other words, the goal of Experiential Psychotherapy is to allow the individual to fulfill—rather than contain—his or her sexual and other potentials. Although there is no attempt to target behaviors—sexual or otherwise, deviant or normophilic—when fundamental personality change is effected, the results are manifest in sexual and other desires, wishes, fantasies, and behavior, intimate relationships, and bodily phenomena.

Each session uses moments of strong feelings as an entry point into the client's inner world. The shifts that occur in working with peak moments of strong experiencing provide the vehicle to help bring about deep-seated change (Mahrer, 1996/2004a). It is from within that the potential for substantive changes is accessed. It is a particularly apt approach for working with powerful impulses, intrusive and menacing images, painful feelings, or bodily phenomena. Precisely the same material that clients typically try to ward off, manage, or control (unsuccessfully) provides the perfect fodder for Experiential sessions. Whether it is the rape victim's flashbacks and nightmares, the intense anxiety of the man reporting erectile dysfunction, the pain of the woman with vaginismus, or the fantasies of the individual with paraphilic fantasies (Kleinplatz, 1998, 2004, 2007, 2012), the distressing symptoms are never to be eliminated without attention to their value, meaning, purpose, and clinical usefulness. Sexual problems, including unusual sexual proclivities and troubling behaviors, are ideal to work with in Experiential Psychotherapy because the initial feelings that accompany them are so strong and close to the surface and therefore easy to reach (Kleinplatz, 2006, 2010; Mahrer, 2012; Mahrer & Boulet, 2001). The therapist and client are to enter into and dilate them. High or low desire or the "wrong" desires, compelling and recurring fantasies and impulses, can each provide the intensity required to begin an Experiential session.

The first step of each session involves finding a moment of strong feeling and using it to find something within that is accessed in the opening scene. In dealing with someone who is referred for treatment of a paraphilia, the content and context for this strong feeling could be a recurring fantasy, a disturbing desire, a fear of being discovered; it could be anything. The important thing is for the therapist to be open to letting whatever feeling is front and center at the outset intensify so as to access the inner experiencing. When that emerges, something shifts: What seemed ominous suddenly becomes less foreboding and instead is to be welcomed. What had been warded off now changes in character and is to be appreciated. New ways of being become possible. In order to make them real and attainable, the therapist is to accompany the client to live in moments from the past, where this new way of being could have, should have, or perhaps actually did surface. By making them increasingly vivid and by having the client live fully in such moments, the likelihood of enduring change increases. In the concluding step, the client, who has now lived as this inner, deeper potential, contemplates and rehearses actually being this new way in the real world. The patient has "a taste of what it is like to be this whole new person, to think, act, feel and experience as this whole new person who is living and being in the world outside the office" (Mahrer, 1996/2004a, p. 337). If therapy has been successful, the person who entered therapy is rather different from the one who has completed the process. He becomes what he might have been all along.

In Experiential Psychotherapy, the therapist is aligned with the client and listens experientially. That is, the therapist is to be disengaged from his or her usual sense of self and allow the client's experiencing to flow through him or her. Given that the therapist is living in the client's phenomenal world, countertransference issues are minimized or eliminated (Mahrer, 2001). Although there are no contraindications as to *clients* undergoing Experiential Psychotherapy, *therapists* who are uncomfortable in entering the client's inner experiencing are advised to refer clients elsewhere when they are beyond their comfort zone (Mahrer, 1996/2004a). Additional training in Experiential methods can be very helpful in growing one's capacity to deal with taboo material.

In using this approach with couples, the same general format is followed. However, the concluding step involves having the client consider and try on for size the possibility of actually living as this new person, the inner experiencing, beyond this session. In this variation, the client also has the opportunity to include the partner and to experiment with or play out this new way of being with him or her, right then and there near the end of the session. Partners are typically receptive to these initiatives and tend to be eager to participate in the other's growth.

CAN THE OUTCOMES IN EXPERIENTIAL PSYCHOTHERAPY BE COMPARED TO THE TRADITIONAL OUTCOME DATA IN TREATMENT OF THE PARAPHILIAS?

The goal in treatment of the paraphilias is reduction in the frequency of the behavioral manifestation of the paraphilia (e.g., voyeurism, exhibitionism, pedophilia). There is little attention to the client's underlying feelings. The criteria for effective outcome in Experiential Psychotherapy involve profound changes, specifically actualization and integration, rather than treatment of sexual disorders or, indeed, any psychopathology (Mahrer, 1994/2006, 2002, 2011). Such a model does not lend itself to producing traditional outcome data because the intended objectives are unrelated to a particular form of psychopathology—let alone sexual disorders—to be remedied (Mahrer, 2010). The two objectives, however, are quite substantial: Successful Experiential sessions do result in (1) eliminating the original source of pain in the initial painful scene and (2) allowing the individual to become whatever is deeper within. Although Experiential Psychotherapy was not designed to treat sexual problems, it brings about changes so fundamental to personality that it eventuates in better intrapsychic and interpersonal relations, increases embodiment, sexual functioning, and the capacity for intimacy (Kleinplatz, 1998, 1999, 2004, 2006, 2007, 2010; Kleinplatz & Krippner, 2005; Mahrer, 1996/2004a, 2011, 2012; Mahrer & Boulet, 2001).

Based on the clinical and psychotherapy-*process* research evidence, I began to use Experiential Psychotherapy with my clients in sex therapy 25 years ago. As indicated previously, psychotherapy *outcome* research is not usually applied to a paradigm aimed at substantive personality change rather than treatment of psychopathology (Mahrer, 2004b). There is no traditional psychotherapy *outcome* research available on Experiential Psychotherapy for the treatment of voyeurism or, indeed, any of the DSM sexual diagnoses.

Nonetheless, it has been very helpful for a broad array of sexual problems (Kleinplatz, 1998, 2004, 2007, 2010; Mahrer & Boulet, 2001), including the paraphilias (see the case history literature on the paraphilias in Kleinplatz, 2006, 2012; Kleinplatz & Krippner, 2005; Mahrer, 2012), and is worthy of consideration and systematic evaluation in the broader world of sex therapy.

CASE ILLUSTRATION AND DISCUSSION

The following case illustration involved a client who was referred for the treatment of voyeurism and was seen in Experiential Psychotherapy. The case is presented with informed consent. Identifying details have been changed to protect confidentiality.

Jeff and Nancy Sinclair contacted me as a last resort. They had first attempted therapy shortly after Mr. Sinclair was caught by his wife with one hand on his penis and another on his binoculars, pointed toward a neighbor's open window. He had secretly been watching women or couples as his primary source of sexual arousal and release since early adolescence. He was deeply ashamed, not only of his clandestine need to see naked women or couples without their consent for sexual excitement but also of being discovered. He had previously spent 4 years with two therapists. He reported that the prior therapy had led to greater feelings of self-understanding and acceptance but that treatment had not affected his preoccupation with watching. He had also tried a 12-step group for several months and found it "depressing . . . those people kept talking about their shame but nothing ever changed." He was afraid that he was beyond help. During times when their relationship was especially sexually exciting, his pull to look at the forbidden was controlled. "But then it flares up. It will happen . . . it's an obsession . . . it tends to be at a higher level of arousal than any other activity that I participate in." He reported having difficulty reaching orgasm without fantasizing to or enacting the voyeuristic theme.

Mrs. Sinclair had long been dissatisfied with their sex life. She complained that he never initiated sex, would sometimes refuse her, saying he was too tired, and would be unable to get an erection. She remarked that he would often fall asleep while stimulating her sexually. "I take a long time to come, and I hate to nag him." She wanted him to be assessed for narcolepsy but was not optimistic that he would be diagnosed as suffering from a neurological disorder. Mr. Sinclair said he was satisfied with their sexual relationship. When Mrs. Sinclair discovered her husband's voyeurism, she was relieved that the problem was "strictly his." She also wanted to deal with her feelings of betrayal given that his habit had long been clandestine. "He doesn't like to confront me. He always said that it would be much easier to protect and lie to me than to deal with upsetting me." His goal was to "get control" over his "sexual urges," but he did not anticipate giving up his fantasy entirely, nor did he wish to do so. I said that I would offer them the opportunity, if they were so inclined, to change as individuals and as a couple such that the context in which his symptoms existed as a painful source of conflict no longer occurred. They agreed, skeptically. I pointed out that I did not think I would be helpful by trying to change a man who found his sexual behaviour pleasurable but that it was not up to me to make that choice.

Therapy consisted of Experiential Psychotherapy with a shifting focus, more or less from session to session, on the husband and then the wife. Both husband and wife are present for each session. In any given session, we focus on either individual but not both. The other observes and may occasionally participate toward the end of the session.

It is our second session and he is describing his family background—how his parents lavished attention on his older sister and ignored him and how he has always felt like an outsider. The words are insightful, but his feelings are muted. It is when he mentions his inability to urinate in public restrooms, that his feeling level increases noticeably: "I've always been too sensitive." He says it started when he was 5 years old and his father would grab at his penis and mock him with the family present. "To him, it was a game, but I felt violated. It was sick and dirty." (As I allow his words to wash over me, listening experientially, I am feeling ashamed and squirming.) I ask him to speak to his father.

He says, "Leave me alone. Have some respect for me." But his father is answering that he was just joking around and that his son is overreacting. His brother, Colin, is approaching, menacingly. He is scared and looks at his brother, saying, "Don't you fuckin' touch me." He is feeling frustrated, misunderstood, and alone. They continue to tease him. He is becoming increasingly distant and alienated. "I'm not being heard. . . . He's denying that I'm feeling what I'm feeling." I say these words to his father directly but Mr. Sinclair responds, "I could never talk to him. He made me call him 'Sir'!" He then turns to his mother. "Look at her. She's pathetic. She just sits there! Each time it happened, I would pray for her to rescue me but she never said a word, and neither did I." I encourage him to speak right to her. He begins, "How can you stay with him? Do your thing! Just leave him and take me with you. I've always been on the outside looking in but maybe . . . together, just the two of us, it could be different." (There is now a sense of reaching out, of closeness, of wanting to be intimate.)

I repeat his words but with more feeling. He continues, "If I let down my guard, he'd accuse me of being a faggot, but with you, I had hope . . . there was a chance." As he focuses in on his mother, what emerges in the midst of violation, shame, frustration, and alienation is a sense of closeness, of reaching out, of connecting with one another. There is a sad wistfulness, an "if only" quality. I ask if this hint of what might have been evokes similar moments of closeness, warmth, reaching out, that were brought to fruition—full-blown, fulfilled moments of this kind. He responds with memories of his maternal grandfather and of the time they spent together. "I love you because you cared . . . now you're gone and I miss you . . . I wish you'd been my father." (He is speaking with fondness and affection and is beginning to cry quietly.) "I want you to know that I remember the way we would laugh together." He is now sobbing intensely. "I'm longing for missed opportunities; there were times and people I'd been drawn towards, feeling a desire to be closer with them, and I'd blown it."

We begin searching aloud for similar moments when he had felt warm, affectionate, and fond toward another, on the verge of reaching out and perhaps even taking the steps, the initiative to connect. He remembered the gym teacher Mr. Carter, who had protected him from the teasing of his peers. "I think back and I feel so good, so alive. I'd love to write him a letter, telling him how much he meant to me."

From there, Mr. Sinclair began to focus more clearly on the present and future, on those in his current life for whom he feels a special fondness but rarely acts upon it. A whole slew of possibilities seemed to pop up, including reaching out to his older sister, Ellen, and a friend in Montreal, Richard, saying, "I miss you. We don't see eye to eye and that's OK. I still care about you and I miss your crazy sense of humor. I feel more like myself around you than I normally do. . . . Yeah, I guess it's pretty important to choose the people you want to be around carefully."

The next session began with Mr. Sinclair saying that he had written a letter to Mr. Carter. He had also presented his father with a letter, confronting him. The feelings of victimization and alienation had now been replaced with a desire to connect, notwithstanding some trepidation. He discovered that others were receptive to his tentatively making contact and that he wanted more. Most notably, Mr. and Mrs. Sinclair seemed warmer, and her stance seemed to have softened, becoming more intrigued and less condemning.

During our fourth session, Mr. and Mrs. Sinclair enter my office in the middle of a disagreement. He seems intimidated. I ask him what's scaring him. He says he cannot stand opposing her; he can barely handle expressing his opinions to her at all. I am getting fleeting images of a little pipsqueak, an ineffectual boy standing up to a big, powerful adult and feeling scared silly. I describe it aloud: "I am trying to imagine the consequences of standing my ground. What will she do?" I ask. "I'm afraid she'll stop loving me," he answers.

"How can you say that?" she asks. "I'm proud of you for confronting me!" I motion to her to hold off as his feelings are growing stronger. As I listen to him, he seems to shrink. I am seeing a little boy again, only now he is terribly alone, wanting desperately to be accepted. I describe this image to him, and he says, "Yeah! That's me. Always alone. As a kid, I was short and skinny with two left feet. I was the last one picked for every team. They'd tease me and I'd go inside, alone. They'd be out in the fields playing and I'd go home, into the basement to read."

His wife interjects, "He told me all about it. He was really smart and he'd get into all these books and make up this whole, rich fantasy world. He'd live in it. . . . " I interrupt her, explaining that I prefer to hear Mr. Sinclair talk about his childhood in his own words so that I can attend to what it felt like to actually be him as a little boy. "How old were you?" I ask. "Describe it, take me along so I can be there with you."

"I was 8 years old and I was so shy. Our house faced on to the fields and I would sit on the edge of the stairs, watching from a distance," he clarifies. "I remember once I was listening to their voices and it sounded like they were having so much fun. Just once, I wanted to belong. So I went over there to say 'Can I play with you?' but they just laughed."

As we continue reliving this memory, my attention shifts from the initial feeling of being hurt, rejected, alone, and inadequate to that moment of leaving the porch and heading toward the other children. I ask him to return to that window of opportunity wherein he attempted to join his peers. What exactly is to be found there? As we delve into that moment, making it more and more vivid, what emerges is a sense of venturing forward, of reaching out and of offering himself, on the verge of connecting. We stop here for a few minutes in freeze frame just to take it all in, to appreciate how special this feeling is. There is a warmth in our bodies, a lightness in our chests, a building excitement and quickening energy. This is distinctly, qualitatively different from the prior feeling of being a loser, destined to be alone forever, watching the fun from a distance. This new feeling is barely familiar to him. He can recall lots of moments of his usual feelings of alienation but few in which he is acting on this inner feeling. I ask him to see if he can recall moments in which the kernel, a hint, of this new feeling was present but in which he refrained from following through and acting on it.

"Yes," he says, "there are a lot of those! Like when the guys from work are going out for drinks at five o'clock. When I first started working there, they used to invite me along, but I told them that I don't like to drink and drive. I'd get all uptight and rigid—awkward—and they'd look pretty uncomfortable, too. Eventually, they stopped asking me all together. What I really wanted to say was, 'Great! I'd love to join you.'" (I am now [virtually] in his office saying, "Me? You want me to go out for drinks with you? I'd love to.")

We go through a series of such moments, occasions when he was on the verge of risking, of venturing forward, of reaching out and extending himself toward others but customarily withdrew. In each instance, we go back and try out this new potential way of being in place of his previous inclination to feel alone and inadequate. As he delves into each of these past moments, he experiences the potential for extending himself that had been untapped. With every attempt to reenter such scenes and to discover how it would have felt to actually be this new person in past moments, the new way of being seems to change a little, becoming more comfortable, fitting, and real; it seems to suit him. Each of these moments seems to draw us into the future, into the possibility of becoming this newly activated potential in his current life.

Mr. Sinclair considers the possibility of actually allowing himself to be this way in a variety of situations that currently exist: going out with the group at work after presentations for drinks; going to baseball games with the office support staff; attending the upcoming annual company picnic (for the first time); and so forth. Furthermore, given that these possibilities seem not only viable but attractive, Mr. Sinclair now creates a slew of entirely new situations in which he could arrange to venture forth and extend himself in his local community. He detests the Conservative government and feels tempted to join the opposition party's riding association (local party organization office) . . . and his eyes twinkle as he looks over at his wife, who is giggling her assent. He has always been shy, but he suggests that he could offer to come to speak to elementary school students on career day.

I point out that he has come up with quite a list of options but we have been playing exuberantly; now, as the session is winding down, I ask if there is anything that he would seriously like to initiate right away, within the next 24 hours, to make these ideas into reality. He answers that he would like to invite the neighbors over for a barbecue. He is tired of making polite, small talk with them from a distance. Second, he has always wanted to play bridge with his sister and brother-in-law, but they would need a fourth. He turns to his wife and asks if he could teach her how to play bridge. She agrees and seems somewhat dumbfounded that these ideas are actually springing from her previously socially recalcitrant and withdrawn husband.

By now Mr. and Mrs. Sinclair have learned that Experiential Psychotherapy is most effective when one allows oneself to be immersed fully in past memories or future imagery. This means focusing for as long as it is one's "turn," uninterrupted by the spouse, who may have questions, reactions, and so forth, but who is to appreciate this work from the sidelines until invited to participate. It is the comfort that the couple have developed with that position that allows Mr. Sinclair to delve within while Mrs. Sinclair is quietly attentive during the following session.

At the beginning of the seventh session, Mr. Sinclair said that in order to move ahead, he wanted to deal with his past and, in particular, his unresolved feelings about his first love, Michelle. He closes his eyes as he describes his relationship with Michelle when they met at summer camp at age 16. He had spent the summer falling more and more deeply in love with her. During their last week they spent every possible moment together. "It was like I'd died and gone to heaven. . . . I felt so close to her . . . we were making out for hours." He had been sure that they would finally engage in intercourse, but she refused. He had been frustrated and frozen at that point, not quite knowing what to do, but saying that he would wait for her. "I respected her." He spent the entire following year turning down opportunities to date other women while holding out for Michelle. But when he arrived at camp the next July, he found out that Michelle had become serious about another man. He would see her occasionally over the years, but they never discussed their feelings for one another. "There are still a lot of what-if's. I would like to let go if it will help me connect with Nancy."

I instruct him to speak directly with Michelle. He begins, "I'm angry. I hung on to my virginity for you." [I am looking at Michelle longingly with frustration and resentment.] He continues, "That last night . . . I'd never felt so close to anyone before. I wanted you so much I thought I'd die. I couldn't wait. But you made me stop. You said, 'No, I want to wait till we're married. . . . ' That we had to get hold of ourselves. That if I loved you, I'd wait. And I did. I can't believe we stayed dressed the whole time! I was such an idiot but I'd have done anything you asked."

As I listen experientially I am attending to that moment just prior to Michelle calling a halt to the sexual contact and exploration. The feelings are of erotic closeness and passion, being sexually driven and intense, on the verge of sexual frenzy and overwhelmed. I name and describe these feelings for him, identifying the mounting sexual passion in my body (the body of a 16-year-old male), the power of my blood surging, the throbbing in the tip of my penis, the intense desire for this woman. He responds that he rarely feels that kind of excitement anymore, that he recognizes that throbbing sensation in his penis but that the explosive passion is a thing of the past. We linger in these feelings for a few moments, savoring them.

I ask Mr. Sinclair to return to that moment just before it was interrupted and to imagine what it would have been like had the feelings that were building at that moment been given free rein. He returns to that basement couch, taking her clothes off and then his own. This time there are no impediments to sexual expression, and he is flooded by sexual passion. He allows himself to experience how it would have felt to make love with Michelle, to let go with her and to explode together. As he revels in his own capacity for overwhelming sexual passion, he begins to imagine calling her, arranging to meet, and describing his fantasy to her of how it might have been between them in glorious detail. "I'd tease her and make her see what she was missing. I'd bring her upstairs and make her beg for it. . . . " But when he contemplates following through on the fantasy, he thinks of Nancy. He was filled with trepidation at the possibility of endangering his marriage; the arousal was diminishing.

"Well, how about Nancy? How would it feel to have this kind of intense, driven, overwhelming sex with her?" I asked. "Can you even imagine what it might be like if you let yourself go wild with Nancy? I don't know . . . are you allowed to do that with a wife?"

"Yeah, I could lift her straight up onto the dining room table while I stand next to her and then really fuck her. And then we could shower together afterward—we haven't done that since we were dating—and be really close. You know what else? We could go back to that bed and breakfast with the whirlpool. The last time we were there we just looked at it, and each other, and never said a word. But this time, I could get a bottle of champagne and we could make love with bubbles everywhere."

"That's very sweet, but there's more, though, more that you and Nancy never do, never try, never talk about, wouldn't even dare think about together . . . not that you should, of course. But I can feel it coming up. . . . "

"You know what I really want? I want her to take control," he says.

"Now that's more like it. Say it to Nancy," I suggest. He turns to his wife, saying, "I want you to be rough with me and command me to go down on you. That's what I'd really like! I want you to entice me and spread your legs and tease me. I don't want to be responsible. I want to be a plasticene doll. I want to burn and have to have you to release me. I want you to be forceful but gentle. I want you to have balls." Mrs. Sinclair is now looking gleefully mischievous and nodding.

As he winds down, I ask, "Okay, that's a pretty good start. Is there more?" Mr. Sinclair comes up with one scene after another, each involving overwhelmingly intense, outrageous sex and/or passionately close sex—with moments of easy closeness.

By the eighth session, Mr. and Mrs. Sinclair had followed up on all the possibilities he'd imagined during the previous session. More important, he said that he had experienced the *feelings* that had permeated the previous session while with his wife. "I saw the creative side of Nancy." He was feeling much freer and no longer worried about her reactions. "It makes a big difference. . . . I'd buried my sexuality but I'm feeling what I felt at 16." She confirmed that they had each dared to share their fantasies together, uncertain of what to expect. Both were thrilled with the outcome. "Nancy was perfect . . . I experienced some sensations while she was teasing me that I'd never experienced before. It was the ultimate! I'm more easily turned on, more present, and I'm able to tell her if I'm not entirely in the mood. It should be like this all the time."

He added that he felt no desire to reach for his binoculars nor to prowl the streets for open windows. "Even my need to gawk at every woman who walks by isn't there anymore."

At the 6-month, 18-month, and 5-year follow-up marks, Mr. Sinclair reports that his voyeurism has been eliminated. Mr. and Mrs. Sinclair report that although there have been daunting moments, the erotic intimacy between them has continued to grow. In addition, his shyness, stuttering, and lifetime low-level depression and fears of losing control are gone.

CONCLUSIONS

This clinical illustration is quite different from what is ordinarily seen as the methods and goals in working with the paraphilias. Unfortunately, there is no empirical support for the treatments of voyeurism in the conventional literature (Mann et al., 2008). What accounts for the outcome in Experiential Psychotherapy? The alternative to behavioral/pharmacological management is to consider transforming the underlying experiencing. In the conventional treatment of the paraphilias, the individual is taught to keep the fantasies at bay and to stay away from whatever stimuli might trigger his or her behaviors. In parallel with the treatment of sexual dysfunctions in general, the predominant approach to the paraphilias targets the symptom while leaving the source of the problem unexplored (Kleinplatz, 2012.). The focus is on reducing the strength, frequency, or impetus to act on unacceptable urges, but there is no talk of changing the person who has the proclivities or his or her desires.

In the sex offender literature, the goals have traditionally been to eliminate dangerous behavior, to contain corresponding desires, and to promote public safety. From the Experiential perspective, these goals duplicate the problem already there for the patient/offender: He or she feels his or her deepest desires are unacceptable and wants to reduce or at least control them. In each instance, the treatment models and methods involve modulating and attenuating the disturbing symptoms, as if they were the problems themselves (Kleinplatz, 2007). By contrast, in Experiential Psychotherapy, it is in entering into whatever is front and center for the client, no matter how menacing or innocuous, that profound change can be effected. The goal is not to remove the symptoms, although, fortunately, those, too, tend to fade away. In this instance, that means not only change in behavior but also in the nature of one's desires (Kleinplatz, 2006, 2007, 2012; Mahrer, 2012).

Mr. Sinclair felt alienated, unlovable, and ashamed. Underlying that was a longing, a reaching out, a capacity for warmth and affection. Similarly, beyond his cool, safe, inhibited sexuality was a long-inaccessible capacity for passionate, intense, almost frenzied erotic intimacy. His capacity to integrate these potentials allowed him to be more authentically fulfilled in his marriage and to relinquish his voyeurism. Whatever might arise in moments of peak feeling can be used as an avenue toward substantive personality change. Similarly, there is discussion of the history of attachment problems in the genesis of the paraphilias in the sex offender literature (e.g., Marshall & Marshall, 2010). We can go further than social skills training by entering directly into the patient's loneliness, if that is what arises, as it did here.

Are these the characteristics that lie deeper in each voyeur? There is no way of knowing what is to be found within any patient a priori except that it is unique. Dealing with sexual fantasies may be a particularly crucial but often overlooked element required for substantive change to come about in dealing with paraphilias in therapy (Vanhoeck, Van Daele, & Gykiere, 2010).

There are myriad advantages that come with the use of Experiential Psychotherapy with paraphiliacs. In conventional treatment, the first step is often to stop sexual behavior; patients generally do not like giving up activities that are so rewarding. This approach is less intrusive. As illustrated here, there are often increases in "conventional" sex, and thus this approach is less prone to problems of compliance. There is no judging or pathologizing of the patient; this frees the therapist from acting as an agent of social control. By merely controlling behavior, we may help to fuel the alienation from within and thereby make forbidden sexual desires, shrouded in secrecy, seem more compelling and menacing (Kleinplatz, 2012). It is only by entering into the heart of it that we may find hope for transformation.

REFERENCES

Ahlers, C. J., Schaefer, G. A., Mundt, I. A., Roll, S., Englert, H., Willich, S. N., et al. (2011). How unusual are the contents of paraphilias?: Paraphilia-associated sexual arousal patterns in a community-based sample of men. *The Journal of Sexual Medicine, 8*(5), 1362–1370.

American Psychiatric Association. (2000). *Diagnostic and statistical manual of mental disorders* (4th ed., text rev.). Washington, DC: Author.

American Psychiatric Association. (2013). *Diagnostic and statistical manual of mental disorders* (5th ed.). Arlington, VA: Author.

Blanchard, R. (2009a, April 3). *Paraphilias vs. paraphilic disorders, pedophilia vs. pedo- and hebephilia, and autogynephilic vs. fetishistic transvestism.* Paper presented at the annual meeting of the Society for Sex Therapy and Research, Arlington, Virginia.

Blanchard, R. (2009b). The DSM diagnostic criteria for pedophilia. *Archives of Sexual Behavior, 39*(2), 304–316.

Blanchard, R., Cantor, J. M., & Robichaud, L. K. (2006). Biological factors in the development of sexual deviance and aggression in males. In H. E. Barbaree & W. L. Marshall (Eds.), *The juvenile sexual offender* (2nd ed., pp. 77–104). New York: Guilford Press.

Blanchard, R., Lykins, A. D., Wherrett, D., Kuban, M. E., Cantor, J. M., Blak, T., et al. (2009). Pedophilia, hebephilia, and the DSM-V. *Archives of Sexual Behavior, 38*, 335–350.

Briken, P., & Kafka, M. P. (2007). Pharmacological treatments for paraphilic patients and sexual offenders. *Current Opinion in Psychiatry, 20*, 609–613.

Cantor, J. M. (2012). Is homosexuality a paraphilia?: The evidence for and against. *Archives of Sexual Behavior, 41*(1), 237–247.

Corabian, C., Dennett, L., & Harstall, C. (2011). Treatment for convicted adult male sex offenders: An overview of systematic reviews. *Sexual Offender Treatment, 6*(1). Retrieved from *www.sexual-offender-treatment.org/93.html.*

Darcangelo, S. (2008). Fetishism: Psychopathology and theory. In D. R. Laws & W. O'Donohue (Eds.), *Sexual deviance: Theory, assessment, and treatment* (pp. 108–118). New York: Guilford Press.

Darcangelo, S., Hollings, A., & Paladino, G. (2008). Fetishism: Assessment and treatment. In D. R. Laws & W. O'Donohue (Eds.), *Sexual deviance: Theory, assessment, and treatment* (pp. 119–130). New York: Guilford Press.

Fedoroff, J. P., & Marshall, W. L. (2010). Paraphilias. Cognitive-behavioral therapy for refractory cases: Turning failure into success. In D. McKay, J. S. Abramowitz, & S. Taylor (Eds.), *Cognitive-behavioral therapy for refractory cases: Turning failure into success* (pp. 369–384). Washington, DC: American Psychological Association.

Freund, K. (1990). Courtship disorder. In W. L. Marshall, D. R. Laws, & H. E. Barbaree (Eds.), *Handbook of sexual assault: Issues, theories, and treatment of the offender* (pp. 341–342). New York: Plenum.

Freund, K., & Blanchard, R. (1993). Erotic target location errors in male gender dysphorics, paedophiles, and fetishists. *British Journal of Psychiatry, 162*, 558–563.

Gijs, L. (2008). Paraphilia and paraphilia-related disorders: An introduction. In D. L. Rowland & L. Incrocci (Eds.), *Handbook of sexual and gender identity disorders* (pp. 491–528). Hoboken, NJ: Wiley.

Greenfield, D. P. (2006). Organic approaches to the treatment of paraphilics and sex offenders. *Journal of Psychiatry and Law, 34*(4), 437–454.

Guay, D. R. P. (2009). Drug treatment of paraphilic and nonparaphilic sexual disorders. *Clinical Therapeutics, 31*, 1–31.

Hanson, R. K., Bourgon, G., Helmus, L., & Hodgson, S. (2009). The principles of effective correctional treatment also apply to sexual offenders: A meta-analysis. *Criminal Justice and Behavior, 36*, 865–891.

Hucker, S. J. (2008). Sexual masochism: Assessment and treatment. In D. R. Laws & W. O'Donohue (Eds.), *Sexual deviance: Theory, assessment, and treatment* (pp. 264–271). New York: Guilford Press.

Kleinplatz, P. J. (1998). Sex therapy for vaginismus: A review, critique and humanistic alternative. *Journal of Humanistic Psychology, 38*(2), 51–81.

Kleinplatz, P. J. (1999). Infertility: "Experientially oriented" couples therapy and subsequent pregnancy. *Journal of Couples Therapy, 8*(2), 17–35.

Kleinplatz, P. J. (2004). Beyond sexual mechanics and hydraulics: Humanizing the discourse surrounding erectile dysfunction. *Journal of Humanistic Psychology, 44*(2), 215–242.

Kleinplatz, P. J. (2006). Learning from extraordinary lovers: Lessons from the edge. *Journal of Homosexuality, 50*(3/4), 325–348.

Kleinplatz, P. J. (2007). Coming out of the sex therapy closet: Using experiential psychotherapy with sexual problems and concerns. *American Journal of Psychotherapy, 61*(3), 333–348.

Kleinplatz, P. J. (2010). Desire disorders or opportunities for optimal erotic intimacy. In S. R. Leiblum (Ed.), *Treating sexual desire disorders: A clinical casebook* (pp. 92–113). New York: Guilford Press.

Kleinplatz, P. J. (2012). Is that all there is?: A critique of and new alternative to the goals of sex therapy. In P. J. Kleinplatz (Ed.), *New directions in sex therapy: Innovations and alternatives* (2nd ed., pp. 101–118). New York: Routledge.

Kleinplatz, P. J., & Krippner, S. (2005). Spirituality and sexuality: Celebrating erotic transcendence and spiritual embodiment. In S. G. Mijares & G. S. Khalsa (Eds.), *The psychospiritual clinician's handbook: Alternative methods for understanding and treating mental disorders* (pp. 301–318). New York: Haworth.

Kleinplatz, P. J., & Moser, C. (2004). Toward clinical guidelines for working with BDSM clients. *Contemporary Sexuality, 38*(6), 1–4.

Kleinplatz, P. J., & Moser, C. (2005). Is SM pathological? *Lesbian and Gay Psychology Review, 6*(3), 255–260.

Krueger, R. B. (2009a). The DSM diagnostic criteria for sexual sadism. *Archives of Sexual Behavior, 32*(1), 325–345.

Krueger, R. B. (2009b). The DSM diagnostic criteria for sexual masochism. *Archives of Sexual Behavior, 32*(1), 346–356.

Krueger, R. B., & Kaplan, M. S. (2008). Frotteurism: Assessment and treatment. In D. R. Laws & W. O'Donohue (Eds.), *Sexual deviance: Theory, assessment, and treatment* (pp. 150–163). New York: Guilford Press.

Langevin, R., Lang, R. A., & Curnoe, S. (1998). The prevalence of sex offenders with deviant fantasies. *Journal of Interpersonal Violence, 13*, 315–327.

Laws, D. R., & O'Donohue, W. T. (2008). Introduction. In D. R. Laws & W. O'Donohue (Eds.), *Sexual deviance: Theory, assessment, and treatment* (pp. 1–20). New York: Guilford Press.

Lussier, P., & Piché, L. (2008). Frotteurism: Psychopathology and theory. In D. R.

Laws & W. O'Donohue (Eds.), *Sexual deviance: Theory, assessment, and treatment* (pp. 131–149). New York: Guilford Press.

Mahrer, A. R. (2001). An experiential alternative to countertransference. *Journal of Clinical Psychology, 57,* 1021–1028.

Mahrer, A. R. (2002). *Becoming the person you can become: The complete guide to self-transformation.* Boulder, CA: Bull Publishing.

Mahrer, A. R. (2004a). *The complete guide to experiential psychotherapy.* Boulder, CO: Bull. (Original work published 1996)

Mahrer, A. R. (2004b). *Why do research in psychotherapy? Introduction to a revolution.* Chichester, UK: Wiley.

Mahrer, A. R. (2010). *What is psychotherapy for? An alternative to the profession of psychotherapy.* Montreal, Quebec, Canada: Howard Gontovnick.

Mahrer, A. R. (2011). *Transformation: A glimpse into the future of how change will come about.* Montreal, Quebec, Canada: Howard Gontovnick.

Mahrer, A. R. (2012). Goodbye sex therapy, hello undergoing my own transformation. In P. J. Kleinplatz (Ed.), *New directions in sex therapy: Innovations and alternatives* (2nd ed., pp. 231– 252). New York: Routledge.

Mahrer, A. R., & Boulet, D. (2001). How can Experiential Psychotherapy help transform the field of sex therapy? In P. J. Kleinplatz (Ed.), *New directions in sex therapy: Innovations and alternatives* (pp. 234–257). Philadelphia: Brunner-Routledge.

Mann, R. E., Ainsworth, F., Al-Attar, Z., & Davies, M. (2008). Voyeurism: Assessment and treatment. In D. R. Laws & W. O'Donohue (Eds.), *Sexual deviance: Theory, assessment, and treatment* (pp. 320–335). New York: Guilford Press.

Marshall, W. L., & Marshall, L. E. (2010). Attachment and intimacy in sexual offenders: An update. *Sexual and Relationship Therapy, 25*(1), 86–90.

Marshall, W. L., Marshall, L. E., Serran, G. A., & O'Brien, M. D. (2011). *Rehabilitating sexual offenders: A strength-based approach.* Washington, DC: APA Books.

Money, J. (1986). *Lovemaps: Clinical concepts of sexual/erotic health and pathology, paraphilia, and gender transposition in childhood, adolescence, and maturity.* New York: Irvington.

Morin, J. W., & Levenson, J. S. (2008). Exhibitionism: Assessment and treatment. In D. R. Laws & W. O'Donohue (Eds.), *Sexual deviance: Theory, assessment, and treatment* (pp. 76–107). New York: Guilford Press.

Moser, C., & Kleinplatz, P. J. (2002). Transvestic fetishism: Psychopathology or iatrogenic artifact? *New Jersey Psychologist, 52*(2) 16–17.

Moser, C., & Kleinplatz, P. J. (2005). DSM-IV-TR and the paraphilias: An argument for removal. *Journal of Psychology and Human Sexuality, 17*(3/4), 91–109.

Newring, K. A. B., Wheeler, J., & Draper, C. (2008). Transvestic fetishism: Assessment and treatment. In D. R. Laws & W. O'Donohue (Eds.), *Sexual deviance: Theory, assessment, and treatment* (pp. 285–304). New York: Guilford Press.

Nichols, M. (2006). Psychotherapeutic issues with "kinky" clients: Clinical problems, yours and theirs. *Journal of Homosexuality, 50*(2/3), 281–300.

Quinsey, V. L. (2009). Coercive paraphilic disorder. *Archives of Sexual Behavior, 39*(2), 405– 410.

Reiersøl, O., & Skeid, S. (2006). The ICD diagnoses of fetishism and sadomasochism. *Journal of Homosexuality, 50,* 243–262.

Rice, M. E. (2010, September). *Treatment for adult sex offenders: May we reject the null hypothesis?* Paper presented at the conference of the International Association for the Treatment of Sexual Offenders, Oslo, Norway.

Seto, M. C., Marques, J. K., Harris, G. T., Chaffin, M., Lalumière, M. L., Miner, M., et al. (2008). Good science and progress in sex offender treatment are intertwined. *Sexual Abuse: A Journal of Research and Treatment, 20*, 247–255.

Vanhoeck, K., Van Daele, E., & Gykiere, K. (2010). Fantasy management in sex offender treatment. *Sexual Offender Treatment, 6*(1). Retrieved from *www.sexual-offender-treatment.org/94.html.*

Wilson, R. J., Cortoni, F., & McWhinnie, A. J. (2009). Circles of Support and Accountability: A Canadian national replication of outcome findings. *Sexual Abuse, 21*, 412–430.

CHAPTER 10

"Gold-Star" Pedophiles in General Sex Therapy Practice

James M. Cantor

Cantor argues that the treatment of men who have a sexual interest in or preference for children is well within the skill set of sex therapists. He makes the important distinction between child molestation (a criminal offense) and pedophilia (a sexual interest). One of the major reasons for the reluctance of many sex therapists to treat clients with pedophilic interests is that their treatment raises ethical and legal questions that are not easily answered: Does the use of erotica increase or decrease the likelihood of sexual offending? Where does confidentiality end and duty to warn begin? Although this chapter does not provide easy answers to such questions, the author does guide us in thinking about these issues.

According to Cantor, most pedophiles commit sexual offenses when they have nothing in their lives worth protecting. And so he advises that "although the focus of one's sex drive cannot be meaningfully addressed by talk therapies, the feelings of hopelessness and isolation often can be." He notes that as sex therapists we have a unique opportunity to help someone before they commit an offense ("gold-star pedophiles"), both aiding the individual and addressing social safety concerns as well.

James M. Cantor, PhD, is Associate Professor of Psychiatry at the University of Toronto Faculty of Medicine. Additionally, he is Senior Scientist of the Campbell Family Mental Health Research Institute at the Centre for Addiction and Mental Health in Toronto, Ontario, Canada. Dr. Cantor is Editor-in-Chief of *Sexual Abuse: A Journal of Research and Treatment.*

Few aspects of human sexual desire remain taboo in the practice of sex therapy. When confronted with the possibility that a client might have a sexual interest in children, however, even very experienced sex therapists find themselves struggling with competing instincts: unconditional positive regard for the client versus sympathy for victims of child molestation; client confidentiality versus ethical and legal obligations to protect children; the recognition of the potential stakes in clinical decision making versus the current limitations of the field's empirical knowledge; and many other concerns. There is a large and growing forensic literature regarding the assessment, treatment, and recidivism risk of sex offenders—people who have already committed sexual offenses against children and are under legal supervision (e.g., Seto, 2007)—but there is scant discussion regarding persons who recognize or fear that they experience sexual fantasies or interests involving children and voluntarily consult a (nonforensic) sex therapist for help.

> Jason was a 34-year-old male presenting to a general sex therapy practice, reporting difficulties during intercourse with his wife of 6 years, Mai. The couple had enjoyable intercourse several times per week for the first 3–3½ years of their relationship, until Jason began experiencing increasingly frequent erectile dysfunction, an inability to achieve orgasm during intercourse, and increasing feelings of depression. Jason reported no erectile or orgasmic difficulties during masturbation, in which he continued to engage approximately weekly. The couple's sexual contact together decreased to less often than monthly.
>
> Jason told Mai he was seeking help for his depression rather than for any sexual concerns, and he attended therapy alone. A previous trial of PDE5 inhibitors had no effect on his sexual function, and he decided against a trial of antidepressants, due to their potential to exacerbate his anorgasmia.

Such initial presentations are well known to sex therapists: Male clients will often emphasize their physiological symptoms, especially at the beginning of therapy, and such symptoms can be an unclear combination of erectile dysfunction, delayed or rapid ejaculation, and decreases in or lack of sexual desire. Generalist clinicians (non-sex therapists) will sometimes focus first on what seems to be a diagnostic issue: Do the symptoms represent erectile dysfunction, anorgasmia, or both? Is one of these symptoms driving the others? To sex therapists, however, such symptoms are commonly conjoined and can reflect any of many etiologies. Marital conflict, lack of sufficient partner novelty, and cultural differences in expectations about sex all have the potential to interfere with sexual function, necessitating a broad assessment. With Jason, a particular question was why he was attending alone.

Jason grew up in a middle-class, suburban neighborhood of a North American city. He was a talented student and athlete, receiving high grades throughout his schooling and graduating from a university with a degree in engineering. He reported no health difficulties. Although attractive and athletic, he was relatively reclusive socially and did not date until his university years. During his 20s, Jason's family of origin settled a wrongful-death lawsuit, which provided him with enough money to support him comfortably without other income. He began to travel widely, with Thailand being a favorite destination. It was there that he met and married Mai. The couple lived there until a family illness required that Jason relocate with her to North America.

Jason professed great affection for Mai but described her as traditional, even subservient, and psychologically unsophisticated. He gave that as the reason for not including her in therapy. He noted that she was not reserved sexually but never complained about Jason's changes in sexual function; nor did she ever make demands of him (sexually or nonsexually).

Jason's description of Mai's lack of psychological sophistication led to exploration of what he does find attractive about her (sexually and nonsexually), as well as his history of sexual and romantic attractions. He indicated that he had a preference for Asian women in general, which he attributed to their having more slight builds on average and a characteristic he hesitatingly referred to as androgyny. Although identifying as heterosexual, he noted that he had wondered during adolescence whether he was gay. He never had any sexual contact with other males, either in adulthood or before, and he did not sexually fantasize about men outside of transient images while masturbating during adolescence. However, he indicated he never felt as sexually obsessed with women as his peers seemed to be.

The fact that it appears in this chapter at all will make the eventual revelation about Jason's sexual interests already obvious, and editing the case to fit this short space places the relevant clues closer together than they would typically appear during therapy. The most salient (and often the most diagnostic) of these include the breadth of the sexual dysfunctions (except during masturbation to covert fantasies), the history of sexual orientation confusion, and the atypical preferences for physical features in sexual partners. These features do not, in and of themselves, indicate a paraphilia, but they do seem to emerge in a substantial proportion of men who are paraphilic, homosexual, or transsexual and suggest that an assessor acquire much greater detail than usual about exactly what features such clients do find to be of greatest sexual interest.

Jason's recollection of thinking he might be gay suggested the possibility that he might still (or again) be struggling with such issues. Because his implied denial of being gay obviated very direct questioning, he was instead asked about his preferences for various physical features in

fantasized sexual partners. In addition to being Asian, he preferred partners who had small breasts and trimmed (or, more preferably, shaved)
pubic hair. As the description of Jason's optimal sexual contacts became
clearer, and as the therapeutic rapport developed, Jason acknowledged
first that he preferred younger women and later that he felt sexually
aroused by girls as young as 12 or 13. Although Jason's explicit goal for
therapy was the resumption of his prior sexual activities with Mai, his
underlying goal was for therapy and his marriage to manage his sexual
interest in children, which he had been doing so far by effortfully redi-
recting his attractions to approximations of his ideal.

COMMENT

Research on pedophiles outside a forensic context consists of only a small
handful of studies, and these are based on self-reports of members of online
or real-world social groups for self-acknowledged pedophiles and hebephiles
(e.g., Bernard, 1975; DeYoung, 1989; Durkin & Bryant, 1999; Wilson & Cox,
1983). These are descriptive surveys of community samples; none pertains to
providing treatment or support in a clinical context. Unlike treatment protocols tested for use with pedophilic offenders, there are no therapy manuals and
no empirically based treatments endorsed as "best practices" by professional
organizations of clinicians. Therapists, both forensic and otherwise, can rely
only on general principles, doing the best we can with what we have. Indeed,
working with clients on these and related situations is one of the remaining
frontiers in the field of sex therapy.

Pedophilia and hebephila refer to the sexual preferences for prepubescent
and early pubescent children (typically < 11 years and 11–14 years, respectively; Cantor, 2012, p. 59). There is often a belief among sex therapists that
such interests, or any other paraphilic interest whose expression might involve
illegal or harmful activities, requires referral to a forensic specialist. It is an
error to confuse pedophilia or hebephilia with actual child molestation, however. Whereas child molestation refers to overt sexual contact with children,
pedophilia and hebephilia refer to the sexual interest or preference for children, regardless of whether the person acts upon it or spends his life actively
and successfully resisting it. Sex columnist Dan Savage referred to these latter individuals as gold-star pedophiles (Savage, 2010), and helping them to
live productive, offense-free lives is very often within the skill set both of sex
therapists and of general mental health providers.

Although few data are available, it is my experience that the pedophilic
and hebephilic men who go on to commit sexual offenses against children
appear to do so when they feel the most desperate—when they have nothing
to lose, nothing in their lives worth protecting. Although the focus of one's
sex drive cannot be meaningfully addressed by talk therapies, the feelings of
hopelessness and isolation often can be. Cognitive-behavioral therapy (CBT)

and other structured techniques have been particularly useful in that regard. In public health care systems (frequently serving individuals less wealthy than those in private clinics), clients can similarly benefit from addressing basic life needs, including regular employment, a stable living environment, and the pursuit of hobbies or other recreational interests.

In general sex therapy, the use of sexual fantasy, visual pornography, and written erotica are mainstays. When working with a person with pedophilia, however, those techniques pose certain ethical and legal questions. That is, with clients unable to express their sexual interests in the real world, one logical strategy is to help them develop enjoyable fantasy lives, and erotica is usually a substantial component of that life. Complicating that strategy, however, is that the content of erotica for pedophiles can constitute child pornography. A legitimate concern exists regarding whether any children were harmed in the production of stimuli that pedophiles would find erotic; however, stimuli involving no actual people (e.g., written-text-only and drawn or cartoon depictions of children) have also been subject to legal challenges. The legal definitions of child pornography continue to evolve; so, should such erotica be considered for therapeutic use, their current legal status should be checked first.

The foregoing embeds another complicated question: Can the use of (or the permission to use) erotica depicting even fictional children increase the probability that a self-acknowledged pedophile would go on to seek sexual contact with a real child? A widely used therapeutic model for actual sex offenders is "relapse prevention," which includes as a tenet that someone who committed a sexual offense must never use erotica (or masturbatory fantasies) involving children. Unfortunately, there are no strong data to reveal whether such erotica can either increase or decrease the probability of committing an offense. Rather, the recommendations to ban versus to employ such erotica are based on the theoretical stances of the therapists.

ETIOLOGY

During initial sessions, clients seek, often desperately, to understand themselves and their interests, and their greatest need is information: Why are they different from everyone else? Why were they born this way? The need for and benefits of psychoeducation are one of the ways in which these cases are no different from typical sex therapy situations. The sexual interest Jason was hoping to escape was the most stigmatized of all paraphilic sexual interests. His initial presentation and incremental revealing of his genuine concern, however, can occur with any paraphilic or stigmatized sexual interest or behavior. Unlike homosexuality, consensual BDSM, autogynephilic transsexuality, and other alternative sexualities, Jason cannot easily enact his sexual interests without risking harm to someone.

The nature–nurture debate over the causes of pedophilia dates back more

then a century. Krafft-Ebing claimed in 1886 that pedophilia was a neurological disorder (Krafft-Ebing, 1886/1965). Most 20th-century authors, however, instead referred to "nurture" arguments, typically citing reports that
the majority of child molesters were themselves victims of molestation during
their own childhoods. Contemporary findings, however, have revealed that
men who sexually prefer children manifest multiple physical, neuropsychological, and neuroanatomical differences from nonpedophiles. They perform
significantly lower on IQ and other neuropsychological tests (Blanchard, Cantor, & Robichaud, 2006; Cantor et al., 2004; Cantor, Blanchard, Robichaud,
& Christensen, 2005) and demonstrate significant differences in the grey and
white matter of the brain, relative to nonpedophilic controls (Cantor, Kabani,
Christensen, Zipursky, Barbaree, et al., 2008; Schiffer et al., 2007; Schlitz et
al., 2007). They have more frequently suffered head injuries causing unconsciousness before but not after age 13 (Blanchard et al., 2002, 2003), and
they have significantly greater probabilities of having failed a grade or having
been assigned to special education classes during their school years (Cantor et
al., 2006), suggesting that any neuroanatomical differences existed before the
commission of any sexual offenses (and before any effects of incarceration or
other sequelae). They are physically shorter in height than controls (Cantor et
al., 2007), indicating suboptimal physical development overall—indeed, the
magnitude of the height deficit (approximately 2.5 cm) is roughly double the
effect found from a mother smoking cigarettes during pregnancy (cf. Fogelman & Manor, 1988). Pedophilic men are also up to three times as likely as
nonpedophiles to be non-right-handed (Blanchard et al., 2007; Bogaert, 2001;
Cantor et al., 2004; Cantor, Klassen, et al., 2005), indicating that the differences in brain development were likely present prenatally. (Fetuses demonstrate on sonograms a hand preference for thumb-sucking; Hepper, Wells, &
Lynch, 2005.) Considered together, this body of findings suggests that pedophilia might be considered a sexual orientation, that is, an innate and likely
immutable characteristic. Indeed, some authors have referred to pedophilia as
an *age* orientation (e.g., Seto, 2012).

   Notwithstanding those findings, there remain claims that having been
a victim of sexual abuse in childhood causes or predisposes one to develop
pedophilia in adulthood. This putative association appears intuitive to several
schools of psychological thought, including conditioning, social learning, and
psychoanalytic formulations (e.g., Araji & Finkelhor, 1985; Burton, Miller,
& Tai Shill, 2002; Laws & Marshall, 1990). Despite the near ubiquity of the
belief of a causal link between being a victim of sexual abuse and developing
pedophilia, it is not clear to what extent the association actually exists. The
claim that pedophiles were themselves victimized comes from the pedophiles
themselves, suggesting the possibility that they generate such claims to evoke
sympathy. In a very interesting report, sex offender clients were asked whether
they were sexually abused in childhood; 67% reported that they were. After
that clinic began informing its clients that they would be undergoing testing with a polygraph ("lie detector"), however, only 29% claimed to have

been abused (Hindman, 1988). More recently, Jesperson, Lalumière, and Seto (2009) meta-analyzed reports of the proportions of sex offenders and sex offender subtypes who reported having been victims. On the one hand, sexual offenders against children reported being childhood victims significantly more frequently than did sexual offenders against adults; however, no significant difference was detected between pedophilic child molesters and nonpedophilic child molesters. Their findings are consistent with the interpretation that suffering childhood sexual abuse (or other adverse developmental circumstances with which it is associated) facilitates inappropriate sexual behavior but does not cause pedophilia or hebephilia themselves. Because the data entered into the Jesperson et al. (2009) meta-analysis were, in turn, from self-reports, it remains unclear to what extent the child molesters might still be providing inflated rates of their own abuse.

Regardless of the magnitude of the association between sexual abuse in childhood and subsequent pedophilia, the aforementioned developmental theories also fail to account for multiple other observations. The majority of victims of child molestation are female (Snyder, 2000), whereas pedophilia appears to be a phenomenon nearly exclusive to males. Thus, if the aforementioned models account for the development of pedophilia, some other factor(s) must also be involved. The intuitiveness of the correlation comes from a "like makes like" perspective; however, the similarity between the stimuli is only superficial. From the point of view of the child victim, the putatively sexual stimulus (the abuser) is an adult, not another child. Were the mechanism one of simple learning, one would expect the sexual interaction to cause a sexual interest in *older* sexual partners, rather than in much younger ones. Similarly, sex play between peers in childhood is common. Were early sexual experiences central to the development of pedophilia, one would expect sexual interactions with other children, not adults, to be associated with a future sexual preference for children.

LIFE IN THE *DUNKELFELD*

It is unsurprising that convicted child molesters show elevated depression scores (e.g., Raymond, Coleman, Ohlerking, Christenson, & Miner, 1999), but the same has been reported among pedophile self-help group members (Wilson & Cox, 1983). The unparalleled stigma and lifelong inability to have sexual contact with the objects of one's attractions would challenge most men—depression in this group would seem unsurprising, too.

One of the hindrances to reliable data about pedophiles and hebephiles who voluntarily seek out treatment are their perceptions (right or wrong) about the reportability of their cases. North American clinicians have noted the calamitous drop in the number of people seeking treatment or support after the enactment of mandatory reporting laws, leaving neither the opportunity to help them stay offense-free nor the scientific opportunity to develop and test new methods of intervention and improve public safety. There is an exception, however. In 2004–2005, Prevention Project Dunkelfeld was launched in Germany, with an extensive media campaign announcing (translated) "You are not guilty because of your sexual desire, but you are responsible for your sexual behavior. There is help! Don't become an offender!" (Beier, Neutze, et al., 2009). A prevention project such as the PPD is possible there, as Germany requires strict confidentiality on the part of therapists should the client disclose any offenses or plans to commit such offenses (unless the plan includes an intent to commit homicide; Beier, Ahlers, et al., 2009). With such a protection, research and prevention efforts can be aimed at situations otherwise unknown to legal authorities, existing only in the "dark field" (*dunkelfeld*). After its initiation, more than 450 men contacted the PPD, and nearly 300 provided data in screening procedures. Of these, 26.3% reported "strong" and 43.3% reported "very strong" distress, 30.0% reported "some/medium" and 20.9% reported "strong/very strong" fear of offending, and 68.4% reported previously seeking psychiatric or psychotherapeutic treatment.

INTERVENTIONS

There are no compelling data to suggest that pedophiles might be converted into *teleiophiles* (persons with a primary sexual interest in adults). Multiple types of interventions have been attempted, including sex-drive-reducing medications and talk therapies informed by any of many theoretical orientations. Although there exist authors who have claimed that their interventions changed their clients' fundamental sexual interests (e.g., Fedoroff, 1988, 1992), such reports do not include comparison groups, long-term follow-up, or any validated, objective measure to verify the claims of successful change. Typically, such reports describe sexual offenders who claim that they have ceased to be pedophilic, but those reports are unable to distinguish such claims from demand characteristics and noncritical evaluation by the treatment provider(s). In the absence of a technique that might alter one's fundamental sexual interests, therapy must instead be aimed at helping clients to manage or suppress those interests or to express them in way that would cause no harm to any other person.

The Internet—and its anonymity—has provided the opportunity for people with even the rarest of sexual interests to gather and form communities for mutual support, education, socializing, and political advocacy. In general, Internet-mediated contact with peers who share an atypical sexual interest can serve as an important component in combating isolation and in developing one's self-identity and sexual identity. Individuals with pedophilia and their online communities are no exception.

I have not yet encountered a client who had contacted such a group before attending therapy. (This is unlike persons attending therapy to help in their coming-out process as homo- or bisexual or as transsexual. In my experience, such individuals very often have already explored online social or support groups.) Clinicians need to apply caution in recommending such groups to individuals with pedophilia seeking peer support, however. Social media groups can be very prosocial in their cultures, with their sexual interests being only an infrequent topic of conversation (Malesky & Ennis, 2004). As is true with other sexuality interest groups, however, groups can and do discuss a range of political ideologies, and some advocate (or have vocal members who advocate) controversial agendas. That is, their views vary from emphasizing responsibility for one's behavior to opposing increases in the age of consent to the complete legalization of adult–child sexual contact (e.g., Durkin & Bryant, 1999). Unfortunately, a printed book chapter cannot easily include an evaluation of the existing online communities. Although such a list would be a handy reference, Internet groups are not without their internal drama, splintering, and rapid revision of agendas as their leadership changes. It can be fruitful for the therapist to explore potential online venues together with the client. This should include discussion of the policy or philosophical statements that such groups typically include on their mainpages, but should also include exploration of their members' actual discussions: It is my experience that mainpages contain only the least controversial and most prosocial philosophies, but that many or most of the members and their comments pursue less productive agendas.

PPD recently released an evaluation of the use of anti-androgenic medications in men seeking treatment, but outside a forensic context (Amelung, Kuhle, Konrad, Pauls, & Beier, 2012). Although it was not possible to assign participants randomly to treatments, those researchers compared the treatment seekers who opted for pharmacological interventions (with cyproterone acetate or gonadatropin-releasing hormone [GnRH] analog) with those selecting nonpharmacological treatment only, both on their pretreatment and posttreatment characteristics. On pretreatment questionnaires, the men opting for medications perceived themselves as less able to control their sexual interests and more aware of potentially dangerous situations. After completion of the trial, they indicated greater ability to control their sexual interests, but, remarkably, *lower* self-esteem. Amelung et al. indicated this to be consistent with their clinical impression that the clients often view their need for medication as having lost the fight with themselves to resist their own impulses.

CONFIDENTIALITY VERSUS DUTY TO WARN/REPORT

Confidentiality has long been a backbone of sex therapy, but in the context of sexual interests in children, it becomes pitted against professionals' duty to report cases or warn potential victims, leaving clinicians in less familiar situations. (In some jurisdictions, not only licensed professionals but even private citizens are legislated to report; "State-by-state look," 2011.) Further complicating the situation is that multiple levels of government and other regulatory bodies have overlapping jurisdiction, each with regulations in place: child protection laws, licensure laws, professional regulatory boards, and each of the (sometimes numerous) professional associations to which a clinician might belong. They contain analogous but differently worded versions of two opposing principles (confidentiality and duty to warn/report), giving little clear guidance to a clinician for navigating them without tripping either a false positive or false negative. More difficult still is the frequent use in such regulations of terms that have no objective referent, such as what might constitute a reasonably foreseeable or substantial risk. Although there now exist multiple, empirically validated instruments for use in quantifying the risk of *re*offending posed by men who have already committed one or more sexual offenses—including the Rapid Risk Assessment of Sexual Offense Recidivism (Hanson, 1997), Sex Offender Risk Appraisal Guide (Quinsey, Harris, Rice, & Cormier, 2006), and Static-99 (Hanson & Thornton, 2000)—there do not exist any such instruments validated for men without such a history. (The field also lacks validated instruments for predicting reoffenses among men convicted of child pornography but no "hands on" offenses.) Alleviating some of the pressure, perhaps, is that regulations that require therapists to break confidentiality often contain a clause such that no action can be taken against a clinician who makes such a report in good faith.

Notwithstanding the laws, in my experience many clinicians are guided (for better or for worse) by their awareness of potential civil litigation and of action by their professional licensure boards, to whom a future hypothetical victim might report them. There is unfortunately little guidance from the civil courts. Although there exist such cases (e.g., Bruni, 1998a, 1998b), they typically arrive at financial settlements outside of court rather than a ruling that might set a precedent and guide clinicians in the future. There is still less guidance regarding the attitudes of licensure boards. The opinions of such boards vary still more widely, according to the cultures of the local professional associations. Indeed, contacting the licensing board to ascertain its opinion (and documenting doing so) can often be an optimal approach to conflicting principles in practice.

Although Jason disclosed his sexual interests later in therapy, there also exist men who disclose their attractions to children to the therapist up front. Very often, such individuals are keenly aware of either the clinical reporting requirements or of client confidentiality and will ask about the limits of confidentiality at the outset. In most situations in general mental health practice, a general indication of limits is sufficient for the client to make an informed decision about whether and what to disclose. In the present context, however, the task can be more complicated, and most therapists will feel the need to check the current requirements in their jurisdictions. The limits of confidentiality can be the deciding factor in what a client decides to disclose, and such disclosures can sometimes result in triggering a mandatory report. Thus it can be useful, or even necessary, to halt conversations to allow the clinician time to verify the status or receive an outside opinion about reportability (such as by the licensing board). With clients in this situation, it can often be helpful to acknowledge the ambiguity of the situation at the outset, to conduct initial information gathering by telephone or e-mail (so that whole sessions do not become forestalled), and to interrupt as necessary.

DIAGNOSTIC ISSUES

A primary issue surrounding diagnostic criteria for pedophilia pertains to its cutoff point: Should the sexual preference for the average 11-year-old be diagnosable? The average 13-year-old? 15? That is, at what point do we cease to classify the "age orientation" as a mental illness? Few authors have argued that the sexual preference for persons with Tanner stage 4 characteristics (ages 15–16, on average; called *ephebophilia*) should be diagnosable, and few that the sexual preference for Tanner stage 1 characteristics (before age 11, on average) should not be diagnosed. Rather, the debates have centered on the status of hebephilia (preference for Tanner stages 2–3; ages 11–14, on average). There is a general consensus that hebephilia exists and is meaningfully distinct from the sexual preference for adults (Tanner Stage 5; *teleiophilia*), but there remains debate regarding whether it ought to be considered a mental illness, with opinions (often strong opinions) offered by expert witnesses paid to testify in court on behalf of accused or convicted child molesters, by victim advocates, and even by alternative sexuality advocates who philosophically reject the idea that any sexual interest (including pedophilia) should ever be deemed a mental illness. Unfortunately, many of the discussions surrounding the issue have been fraught with multiple factual inaccuracies (cf., Franklin, 2010; Cantor, 2012), hampering sober discussion. In the context of clients seeking assistance for their sexual interests in either age group, however, this distinction can be moot: The sexual interest in either age group presents the same issues for the client seeking to manage those interests.

Not all clients who self-refer for sexual interests in children are actually pedophilic—a nontrivial portion of such clients instead suffer from obsessive–compulsive disorder (OCD), manifesting as an obsessive fear that they will molest a child (e.g., O'Neil, Cather, Fishel, & Kafka, 2005). No data from samples of such cases have yet been published in either the forensic, sexological, or OCD literatures. In my own clinical experience, however, such cases differentiate themselves the most strongly from genuine pedophilia when the clients are asked to describe their sexual interests: Whereas individuals with pedophilia express (if hesitatingly) the physical (or, sometimes, emotional) features that arouse them, the "pseudo-pedophiles" instead express disgust. That is, although both those with genuine pedophilia and with OCD pseudo-pedophilia fear that they might molest a child, only those with genuine pedophilia express sexual attraction to children. Whereas those with pedophilia experience a motivation to contact a child sexually, those with pseudo-pedophilia do not.

WHEN TO REFER

Despite the potential instinct to refer out to forensic specialists any case involving pedophilia or hebephilia, such issues can often be addressed by nonforensic sex therapists and by many general practitioners. There do exist situations, however, for which at least consultation with forensic or other professionals can be necessary.

One of the most common potential referral issues is for clients considering sex-drive-reducing medications and their management. As noted by Amelung et al. (2012), this kind of therapy may have a beneficial effect on clients' ability (or perception of their ability) to control their behavior, but a referral to an endocrinologist or other specialist should accompany psychotherapy to assess and address any sense of failure that may accompany the perceived need for pharmacotherapy. Depending on the local availability of a laboratory equipped to conduct it, therapy may also be aided by psychophysiological testing of a client's sexual responses to stimuli depicting males or females ranging in age from adult to prepubescent (e.g., Blanchard, Klassen, Dickey, Kuban, & Blak, 2001). Objective testing such as this (called *phallometry* or *penile plethysmography*) would generally provide little information in cases wherein the client admits to his sexual interests; however, it can be an important tool in differentiating clients who experience genuine pedophilia or hebephilia from those with (for example) an obsessive or irrational fear of having it. Finally are situations wherein a client does commit or reveal a sexual offense. Such situations are not an automatic end to therapy. They can, however, evoke a complicated set of issues, for which consulting clinicians with specific forensic experience can be more than helpful.

It is outside the scope of the present chapter to outline those issues themselves. A resource for identifying colleagues from any of multiple disciplines, however, is the Association for the Treatment of Sexual Abusers (ATSA; *www.atsa.com*). In addition to ATSA, other resources that may aid over the course of treatment are Stop It Now! (*www.stopitnow.org*) and publications from the Safer Society Press (*www.safersociety.org/safer-society-press*).

CONCLUSIONS

Over the course of therapy, Jason came to acknowledge the nature of his sexual interests. He realized that his interest in Mai (and their instances of successful sexual intercourse) were related to his desire to approximate the sexuality he could not actualize. The couple eventually divorced, and Jason found that being divorced rather than never married reduced the social pressure he experienced to be in a romantic relationship. He continued in therapy, however, indicating that it was the only venue in which he could unburden himself without risk.

Mai, interestingly, turned out to be less unsophisticated than Jason first described her. Upon disclosing his full story to her, she indicated both that she was already aware of Jason's status and that he was not the first person to be attracted to her due to her physical resemblance to underage girls. She continued to live in North America with her citizenship via marriage, started a house cleaning business, and helps support her family in Thailand.

The great majority of the treatment literature pertains to treating victims of abuse and to preventing convicted offenders from repeating their crimes. Both of these efforts, however, apply only after an offense has already occurred: That is, the best a therapist could do is to help minimize consequences or prevent a second offense. But when meaningful attention is to paid to persons struggling with their sexual urges—on both the individual level and the social safety policy level—we have the opportunity to help prevent the first offense.

REFERENCES

Amelung, T., Kuhle, L. F., Konrad, A., Pauls, A., & Beier, K. M. (2012). Androgen deprivation therapy of self-identifying, help-seeking pedophiles in the Dunkelfeld. *International Journal of Law and Psychiatry, 35*, 176–184.

Araji, S., & Finkelhor, D. (1985). Explanations of pedophilia: Review of empirical research. *Bulletin of the American Academy of Psychiatry and the Law, 13*, 17–37.

Beier, K. M., Ahlers, C. J., Goecker, D., Neutze, J., Mundt, I. A., Hupp, E., et al. (2009). Can pedophiles be reached for primary prevention of child sexual abuse? First results of the Berlin Prevention Project Dunkelfeld (PPD). *Journal of Forensic Psychiatry and Psychology, 20*, 851–867.

Beier, K. M., Neutze, J., Mundt, I. A., Ahlers, C. J., Goecker, D., Konrad, A., et al. (2009). Encouraging self-identified pedophiles and hebephiles to seek professional help: First results of the Prevention Project Dunkelfeld (PPD). *Child Abuse and Neglect, 33*, 545–549.

Bernard, F. (1975). An enquiry among a group of pedophiles. *Journal of Sex Research, 11*, 242–255.

Blanchard, R., Cantor, J. M., & Robichaud, L. K. (2006). Biological factors in the development of sexual deviance and aggression in males. In H. E. Barbaree & W. L. Marshall (Eds.), *The juvenile sex offender* (2nd ed., pp. 77–104). New York: Guilford Press.

Blanchard, R., Christensen, B. K., Strong, S. M., Cantor, J. M., Kuban, M. E., Klassen, P., et al. (2002). Retrospective self-reports of childhood accidents causing unconsciousness in phallometrically diagnosed pedophiles. *Archives of Sexual Behavior, 31*, 511–526.

Blanchard, R., Klassen, P., Dickey, R., Kuban, M. E., & Blak, T. (2001). Sensitivity and specificity of the phallometric test for pedophilia in nonadmitting sex offenders. *Psychological Assessment, 13,* 118–126.

Blanchard, R., Kolla, N. J., Cantor, J. M., Klassen, P. E., Dickey, R., Kuban, M. E., et al. (2007). IQ, handedness, and pedophilia in adult male patients stratified by referral source. *Sexual Abuse: A Journal of Research and Treatment, 19,* 285–309.

Blanchard, R., Kuban, M. E., Klassen, P., Dickey, R., Christensen, B. K., Cantor, J. M., et al. (2003). Self-reported injuries before and after age 13 in pedophilic and non-pedophilic men referred for clinical assessment. *Archives of Sexual Behavior, 32,* 573–581.

Bogaert, A. F. (2001). Handedness, criminality, and sexual offending. *Neuropsychologia, 39,* 465–469.

Bruni, F. (1998a, April 19). A child psychiatrist and pedophile; his therapist knew but didn't tell; a victim is suing. *The New York Times.* Retrieved from *www.nytimes.com/1998/04/19/nyregion/child-psychiatrist-pedophile-his-therapist-knew-but-didn-t-tell-victim-suing.html?pagewanted=all&src=pm.*

Bruni, F. (1998b, October 9). Jury finds psychiatrist was negligent in pedophile case. *The New York Times.* Retrieved from *www.nytimes.com/1998/10/09/nyregion/jury-finds-psychiatrist-was-negligent-in-pedophile-case.html.*

Burton, D. L., Miller, D. L., & Tai Shill, C. (2002). A social learning theory comparison of the sexual victimization of adolescent sexual offenders and nonsexual offending male delinquents. *Child Abuse and Neglect, 26,* 893–907.

Cantor, J. M. (2012). The errors of Karen Franklin's *Pretextuality* [Commentary]. *International Journal of Forensic Mental Health, 11,* 59–62.

Cantor, J. M., Blanchard, R., Christensen, B. K., Dickey, R., Klassen, P. E., Beckstead, A. L., et al. (2004). Intelligence, memory, and handedness in pedophilia. *Neuropsychology, 18,* 3–14.

Cantor, J. M., Blanchard, R., Robichaud, L. K., & Christensen, B. K. (2005). Quantitative reanalysis of aggregate data on IQ in sexual offenders. *Psychological Bulletin, 131,* 555–568.

Cantor, J. M., Kabani, N., Christensen, B. K., Zipursky, R. B., Barbaree, H. E., Dickey, R., et al. (2008). Cerebral white matter deficiencies in pedophilic men. *Journal of Psychiatric Research, 42,* 167–183.

Cantor, J. M., Klassen, P. E., Dickey, R., Christensen, B. K., Kuban, M. E., Blak, T., et al. (2005). Handedness in pedophilia and hebephilia. *Archives of Sexual Behavior, 34,* 447–459.

Cantor, J. M., Kuban, M. E., Blak, T., Klassen, P. E., Dickey, R., & Blanchard, R. (2006). Grade failure and special education placement in sexual offenders' educational histories. *Archives of Sexual Behavior, 35,* 743–751.

Cantor, J. M., Kuban, M. E., Blak, T., Klassen, P. E., Dickey, R., & Blanchard, R. (2007). Physical height in pedophilia and hebephilia. *Sexual Abuse: A Journal of Research and Treatment, 19,* 395–407.

DeYoung, M. (1989). The world according to NAMBLA: Accounting for deviance. *Journal of Sociology and Social Welfare, 16*(1), 111–126.

Durkin, K. F., & Bryant, C. D. (1999). Propagandizing pederasty: A thematic analysis of the on-line exculpatory accounts of unrepentant pedophiles. *Deviant Behavior: An Interdisciplinary Journal, 20,* 103–107.

Fedoroff, J. P. (1988). Buspirone hydrochloride in the treatment of transvestic fetishism. *Journal of Clinical Psychiatry, 49*, 408–409.

Fedoroff, J. P. (1992). Buspirone hydrochloride in the treatment of an atypical paraphilia. *Archives of Sexual Behavior, 21*, 401–406.

Fogelman, K. R., & Manor, O. (1988). Smoking in pregnancy and development in early adulthood. *British Medical Journal, 297*, 1233–1236.

Franklin, K. (2010). Hebephilia: Quintessence of diagnostic pretextuality. *Behavioral Sciences and the Law, 28*, 751–768.

Hanson, R. K. (1997). *The development of a brief actuarial scale for sexual offense recidivism* (Research Report No. 1997-04). Ottawa, Ontario, Canada: Public Safety Canada.

Hanson, R. K., & Thornton, D. (2000). Improving risk assessments for sex offenders: A comparison of three actuarial scales. *Law and Human Behavior, 24*, 119–136.

Hepper, P. G., Wells, D. L., & Lynch, C. (2005). Prenatal thumb sucking is related to postnatal handedness. *Neuropsychologia, 43*, 313–315.

Hindman, J. (1988). Research disputes assumptions about child molesters. *NDAA Bulletin, 7*, 1–3.

Jespersen, A. F., Lalumière, M. L., & Seto, M. C. (2009). Sexual abuse history among adult sex offenders and non-sex offenders: A meta-analysis. *Child Abuse and Neglect, 33*, 179–192.

Krafft-Ebing, R. von (1965). *Psychopathia sexualis: A medico–forensic study* (H. E. Wedeck, Trans.). New York: Putnam. (Original work published 1886)

Laws, D. R., & Marshall, W. L. (1990). A conditioning theory of the etiology and maintenance of deviant sexual preference and behavior. In W. L. Marshall, D. R. Laws, & H. E. Barbaree (Eds.), *Handbook of sexual assault: Issues, theories, and treatment of the offender* (pp. 209–230). New York: Plenum.

Malesky, L. A., & Ennis, L. (2004). Supportive distortions: An analysis of posts on a pedophile Internet message board. *Journal of Addictions and Offender Counseling, 24*, 92–100.

O'Neil, S. E., Cather, C., Fishel, A. K., & Kafka, M. (2005). "Not knowing if I was a pedophile . . . ": Diagnostic questions and treatment strategies in a case of OCD. *Harvard Review of Psychiatry, 13*, 186–196.

Quinsey, V. L., Harris, G. T., Rice, M. E., & Cormier, C. A. (2006). *Violent offenders: Appraising and managing risk* (2nd ed.). Washington, DC: American Psychological Association.

Raymond, N. C., Coleman, E., Ohlerking, F., Christenson, G. A., & Miner, M. (1999). Psychiatric comorbidity in pedophilic sex offenders. *American Journal of Psychiatry, 156*, 786–788.

Savage, D. (2010, February 4). Gold star pedophiles. *The Stranger.* Retrieved from *www.thestranger.com/seattle/savagelove?oid=3347526.*

Schiffer, B., Peschel, T., Paul, T., Gizewski, E., Forsting, M., Leygraf, N., et al. (2007). Structural brain abnormalities in the frontostriatal system and cerebellum in pedophilia. *Journal of Psychiatric Research, 41*, 753–762.

Schiltz, K., Witzel, J., Northoff, G., Zierhut, K., Gubka, U., Fellman, H., et al. (2007). Brain pathology in pedophilic offenders: Evidence of volume reduction in the right amygdala and related diencephalic structures. *Archives of General Psychiatry, 64*, 737–746.

Seto, M. C. (2007). *Pedophilia and sexual offenses against children: Theory, assessment, and intervention.* Washington, DC: American Psychological Association.

Seto, M. C. (2012). Is pedophilia a sexual orientation? *Archives of Sexual Behavior, 41,* 231–236.

Snyder, H. N. (2000). *Sexual assault of young children as reported to law enforcement: Victim, incident, and offender characteristics.* (Report No. NCJ 182990.) U.S. Department of Justice, Office of Justice Programs, Bureau of Justice Statistics. Retrieved from *http://bjs.ojp.usdoj.gov/content/pub/pdf/saycrle.pdf.*

State-by-state look at abuse-reporting laws. (2012, January 2). *USA Today.* Retrieved from *www.usatoday.com/news/nation/story/2012-01-02/unreported-abuse-state-laws/51982310/1.*

Wilson, G. D., & Cox, D. N. (1983). Personality of paedophile club members. *Personality and Individual Differences, 4,* 323–329.

CHAPTER 11

Gender Dysphoria

Kenneth J. Zucker and Nicola Brown

A profound disconnection between one's felt or experienced gender (most often the gender assigned at birth) and one's biological sex is the basis for the diagnosis of gender dysphoria (GD). Although there is some controversy about whether GD is a psychiatric disorder or nonpsychiatric medical condition, it is clear that GD is not a sexual dysfunction. However, Brown and Zucker note that an important therapeutic task is helping individuals suffering from GD to have clarity with regard to their sexuality and their gender identity. "The kind of sexual activity, the way it is enacted, and how one relates and is related to in the interaction, the sexual language used, and the degree to which sex can be embodied are all factors that contribute to our experience of the quality and enjoyment of sex, and also can powerfully affirm or undercut our sense of gender." Sex therapists may be uniquely suited to discuss these issues with transgender patients. Brown and Zucker provide a critical review of the relevant literature, including recent changes to the DSM-5 diagnosis of GD. They also adopt a lifespan developmental approach, discussing the important theoretical and clinical differences between GD in childhood, adolescence, and adulthood.

Kenneth J. Zucker, PhD, is a certified psychologist with the College of Psychologists of Ontario. He is the Psychologist-in-Chief at the Centre for Addiction and Mental Health (CAMH) and the Head of the Gender Identity Service for children and adolescents in the Child, Youth, and Family Program at CAMH. He is a Professor in the Department of Psychiatry, University of Toronto. Since 2002, he has been Editor of the *Archives of Sexual Behavior.* Dr. Zucker was the chair of DSM-5 Sexual and Gender Identity Disorders Work Group.

Nicola Brown, PhD, is a certified psychologist with the College of Psychologists of Ontario. Dr. Brown completed a Postdoctoral Fellowship at Harvard University in the

Victims of Violence Program. She is a staff psychologist in the Gender Identity Clinic for adults at the Centre for Addiction and Mental Health (CAMH) and also has a private practice.

In this chapter, we review therapeutic approaches and clinical management strategies for children, adolescents, and adults with gender dysphoria (GD). Although GD is not a sexual dysfunction, interpersonal sexual relationships (whether functional or dysfunctional) for adolescents and adults are an important part of the clinical picture, and thus the practicing sex therapist should be cognizant of this diagnostic class. Moreover, as there is evidence that an increasing number of people identify along the transgender spectrum, it is likely that more clients with GD or its variants will be seen in the clinical practice of sex therapists who work with adults. It is also quite likely that sex therapists will encounter some couples who have a child or adolescent with GD, and thus they should have some familiarity with clinical management approaches for the pediatric population.

PHENOMENOLOGY

In DSM-IV-TR (American Psychiatric Association, 2000), the diagnosis of gender identity disorder (GID) can be given to children, adolescents, or adults. There are separate criteria sets for children versus adolescents/adults. "Gender dysphoria" was a term coined by Fisk (1973) that can be used to characterize individuals who, at one time or another, experience sufficient discomfort with their biological sex to form the wish for sex reassignment. GD refers to a sense of awkwardness or discomfort in the anatomically congruent gender role and the desire to possess the body of the opposite sex (or at least "parts" of that body), together with the negative affect associated with the marked incongruence between the gender they have been assigned to (usually at birth, referred to as natal gender) and their experienced or expressed gender. This discrepancy is the core component of the diagnosis. There must also be evidence of distress or impairment about this incongruence. As we note in more detail later, DSM-5 (American Psychiatric Association, 2013) has renamed the diagnosis of GID as GD. Hence, we predominately use the GD diagnostic term in this chapter.

EPIDEMIOLOGY

There have been no formal epidemiological studies of GD in children, adolescents, or adults (Zucker & Lawrence, 2009). Accordingly, estimates of prevalence have relied on less sophisticated approaches.

Children and Adolescents

The Child Behavior Checklist (CBCL; Achenbach & Edelbrock, 1983), a parent-report behavior problem questionnaire, and the Youth Self-Report Form (YSR; Achenbach & Edelbrock, 1986) are two widely used assessment measures that include items related to cross-gender identification.

On both the CBCL and the YSR, *behaving* like the opposite sex was reported to be more common than *wishing* to be of the opposite sex and was more common in girls than in boys. In the nonreferred standardization sample for children ages 4–11 years, only 1.0% of mothers of boys indicated that their sons wished to be of the opposite sex "sometimes," and 0% indicated that this was "very true." The comparable percentages among nonreferred girls were 2.5% and 1.0%, respectively (Zucker, Bradley, & Sanikhani, 1997). On the YSR, for youth ages 11–18 years, the percentages of nonreferred boys who indicated a desire to be of the other gender were 2.5% and < 1%, respectively. For nonreferred girls, the corresponding percentages were 11% and 2%, respectively.

A limitation of such data is that they do not adequately identify patterns of cross-gender behavior that would determine "caseness," that is, the presence or absence of a disorder using DSM diagnostic criteria. Therefore, such data can be best viewed as screening information for more intensive evaluation.

Sex Differences in Referral Rates

For the clinician, a more practical matter concerns information about sex differences in referral rates of children and adolescents to specialized gender identity clinics (Wood et al., 2013). Three facts are noted here: First, among children (12 years of age and younger), the sex ratio favors boys. In our clinic for children and youth, for the years 1975–2011, the sex ratio among referred children was 4.49:1 of boys to girls (N = 577), which was significantly larger than the 2.02:1 sex ratio of boys to girls (N = 468) from the Amsterdam clinic in the Netherlands. Second, for our adolescent cases, the sex ratio was near parity, at 1:04:1 of boys to girls (N = 253), quite comparable to the Dutch sex ratio of 1.01:1 (N = 393). Third, the number of referred adolescent cases has increased dramatically over the past 8 years, with an almost fivefold increase in annual referrals from prior years.

Adults

Given the absence of epidemiological studies, estimates of GD have been attempted using other methods. This process has been aided by the fact that adults are eligible for treatments, such as hormone therapy and sex reassignment surgery (SRS), which theoretically equate with "caseness." These methods have included surveys of primary care or surgical care providers, analysis of case series from specialty hospitals and clinics that serve as principal gateways for sex reassignment, and examination of central medical and legal registries in countries in which these are available. Limitations in these methods likely result in underestimates of prevalence. In particular, the increase in community-based or alternative care settings for transgender people may lead to many adults with GD escaping notice, simply because care providers in these settings are less likely to publish information on the number of clients served.

Regarding prevalence rates inferred from the number of individuals who present at specialized gender identity clinics at university- or hospital-based centers, DSM-IV used data from several European studies to suggest a rate of 1 out of 30,000 for natal males and 1 out of 100,000 for natal females. In Zucker and Lawrence's (2009) review of data from 25 adult clinics, it was concluded that there was evidence for an increase in prevalence rates from the earlier DSM-IV estimate—at least a threefold increase (and perhaps as high as an eightfold increase).

Asking about GD in population-based surveys has been advocated in order to more accurately estimate prevalence rates. Recent efforts using probability samples and using the term "transgender" yield much higher rates: 1 out of 300 (Gates, 2011) and 1 out of 215 (Conron, Scott, Stowell, & Landers, 2012). However, it is quite likely that these numbers would include many individuals subthreshold for a clinical diagnosis of GD. The range provided, however, suggests how complex a task it is to establish solid prevalence rates among hidden and stigmatized populations.

DIAGNOSIS

In early 2008, the American Psychiatric Association announced the formation of the DSM-5 Task Force that was responsible for recommending changes to the DSM-IV. The launching of the Task Force opened the door for a long-simmering debate on whether GID should remain in the DSM as a psychiatric diagnosis (Drescher, 2010; Meyer-Bahlburg, 2010; see also the special issue of the *International Journal of Transgenderism*, guest edited by Knudson, De Cuypere, & Bockting, 2010). Some argued for various kinds of improvements in the conceptualization of GID, along with modifications to the diagnostic criteria; others argued that it should be deleted and reconceptualized as some kind of nongeneral medical condition or even as a central nervous system (CNS) limited form of a physical intersex condition (see Meyer-Bahlburg, 2011). However, in the absence of data to support a reclassification as a nonpsychiatric medical condition, others argued that it should remain in the DSM so that people could access medical treatment through public health care systems or private insurers (Drescher, 2010).

It was the decision of the Board of Trustees of the American Psychiatric Association to retain the GID diagnosis in DSM-5 (American Psychiatric

Association, 2013). There are 9 substantive changes from DSM-IV: (1) change in name of the diagnosis from gender identity disorder to gender dysphoria; (2) decoupling of the GD diagnosis from the sexual dysfunctions and paraphilias and placement in a separate chapter; (3) change in the introductory descriptor to the Point A criterion, including the specification of a 6-month duration criterion; (4) merging of what were the Point A and Point B criteria in DSM-IV-TR; (5) for children, the desire to be of the other gender as a necessary indicator for the GD diagnosis; (6) for adolescents and adults, much more detailed diagnostic criteria than in DSM-IV-TR and, like the criteria for children, polythetic in form; (7) elimination of the sexual attraction specifier for adolescents/adults; (8) inclusion of a subtype pertaining to the presence (or absence) of a disorder of sex development; and (9) inclusion of a "posttransition" specifier (for adolescents/adults).

From GID to GD

The diagnostic name change was based on several considerations. First, it represented a conceptual shift in focus to the incongruence between a person's experienced/expressed gender and his or her natal (biological) sex, not a person's gender identity per se (De Cuypere et al., 2010). Second, it captures the essence ("dysphoria") of the distress/impairment criterion. Third, it was a term that has a long history in clinical sexology, as noted before. Fourth, removal of the "disorder" label was considered to be helpful in destigmatizing the diagnosis (Vance et al., 2010). The diagnostic name change is already reflected in the seventh version of the *Standards of Care for the Health of Transsexual, Transgender, and Gender-Nonconforming People* (SOC) issued by the World Professional Association for Transgender Health (WPATH; Coleman et al., 2011).

Elimination of the Sexual Attraction Specifier

In DSM-IV-TR, for sexually mature individuals, there is a sexual attraction (sexual orientation) specifier to measure whether an individual is sexually attracted to males, sexually attracted to females, sexually attracted to both, or sexually attracted to neither.

There is considerable evidence that the sexual attraction specifier (perhaps better characterized as a subtype) is associated with meaningful differences among adolescent and adult patients with GD (for a review, see Lawrence, 2010), such as age-of-onset of symptoms, degree of expression of cross-gender behavior in childhood, age at presentation for clinical evaluation, marital status, co-occurrence with transvestic disorder, and so forth. These findings likely reflect underlying differences in causal mechanisms among subgroups of patients with GD. This has been particularly so for natal males with GD, who show much more variability in their sexual attraction patterns than do natal females with GD.

In the early years of sex reassignment surgeries, it was posited that male-to-female transsexuals with late-onset histories (typically attracted sexually to women or bisexual) had poorer outcomes. Nonetheless, the absolute percentage of regrets of carefully assessed clients is rather low (Gijs & Brewaeys, 2007). Moreover, more recent research has shown that the levels of presurgery distress, as well as improvement on numerous postsurgery outcome measures among male-to-female (MTF) transsexuals with early and late-onset GD, are comparable, regardless of sexual orientation (Lawrence, 2003). There is also a growing body of literature among large community-based samples suggesting that sexual attractions and practices are quite diverse. In contemporary clinical practice, therefore, it has been argued that sexual attraction (sexual orientation) per se plays only a minor role in treatment protocols or decisions. Because sexual attraction (sexual orientation) subtyping is of interest to researchers, this associated feature of GD is discussed in the DSM-5 text. Clinicians also need to be mindful of the variation in sexual attraction among patients with GD, as it will help understand relational issues that are important for the therapeutic context.

Posttransition Specifier

For adolescents and adults, the GD diagnosis contains a "posttransition" specifier colloquially referred to as the "out" clause. The addition of this specifier was prompted by the observation that many individuals, after transition, no longer meet the criteria for GD but that they require ongoing hormone treatment, further gender-confirming surgery, or intermittent psychotherapy or counseling to facilitate the adaptation to life in the desired gender and the social consequences of the transition. Although the concept of "posttransition" is modeled on the concept "in [partial or full] remission" as used for mood disorders, "remission" has implications in terms of symptom reduction that do not apply directly to GD. Cross-sex hormone treatment of gonadectomized individuals could, of course, be coded as treatment of hypogonadism, but this would not apply to individuals who have not undergone gonadectomy but receive hormone treatments. In the DSM-5 text, there is mention that the course specifier of "full remission" in its original meaning does apply to many children with the diagnosis of GD and perhaps to a small number of adolescents and adults.

ASSESSMENT

Apart from a clinical interview to ascertain the presence of the GD diagnosis, the practicing clinician can also utilize a variety of quantitative assessment measures that are available in the published literature. For children, a summary of measures can be found elsewhere (Zucker, 2005; Zucker & Bradley, 1995; Zucker & Wood, 2011). For adolescents and adults, options include the gender-related scales of the Minnesota Multiphasic Personality Inventory–2 (*Mf*, *GM*, and *GF*; Martin & Finn, 2010), which provide objective measures of clients' gender-typical or atypical attitudes and interests. The Utrecht Gender Dysphoria Scale is now available in English (Steensma et al., in press). The Gender Identity/Gender Dysphoria Questionnaire for Adolescents and Adults (Deogracias et al., 2007) is a recently developed, published instrument with good sensitivity and specificity and has been cross-validated (Singh et al., 2010). Some advantages of this last measure are that the items were developed, in part, based on DSM indicators; it is relatively brief (27 items); and it appears well suited to identifying caseness.

ETIOLOGICAL MODELS

The causal mechanisms that might account for the development of GD include a range of conceptual models: an emphasis on biological mechanisms, an emphasis on psychosocial mechanisms, or an emphasis on some type of biopsychosocial framework that attempts to integrate both biological and psychosocial factors. For the contemporary clinician who studies this literature, it will become apparent that there is much that we still do not know and that one has to tolerate this ambiguity.

Biological Factors

Several lines of evidence provide some support for biological mechanisms in the genesis of GD. These include genetic factors, as judged by a higher rate of concordance for GD in identical twins than in nonidentical same-sex twins (Heylens et al., 2012). Candidate gene studies, however, have yielded mixed results in adult males and females with GD, including high rates of "false positives" in control groups and failures to replicate (Ngun, Ghahramani, Sánchez, Bocklandt, & Vilain, 2011).

It has long been noted that classic prenatal hormone theory does not easily account for GD, as the vast majority have a grossly normal somatic phenotype. Thus, there is little reason to believe that the prenatal hormonal milieu was grossly atypical. However, it is conceivable that more subtle variations in patterns of prenatal sex hormone secretion play a predisposing role. A relevant rhesus monkey animal model demonstrates the dissociation between sex-dimorphic behavioral differentiation and genital differentiation that is related to prenatal hormonal exposure and has the most direct relevance for explaining the marked cross-gender behavior of individuals with GD (Goy, Bercovitch, & McBrair, 1988). Another example potentially related to prenatal hormone exposure is 2D:4D digit ratios that demonstrate normative sex differences (Grimbos, Dawood, Burris, Zucker, & Puts, 2010). Whether these differences are related to GD is not clear (Wallien, Zucker, Steensma, & Cohen-Kettenis, 2008).

More recently, several studies have assessed, via structural magnetic resonance imaging, whether or not there are neuroanatomical regions in the brain that are altered in adults with GD when compared with unaffected males and females (Luders et al., 2009; Zubiaurre-Elorza et al., 2012).These studies suggest that the brains of individuals with GD are shifted, although not completely, in the direction of the opposite sex. This conclusion is somewhat qualified by sexual orientation differences. Homosexual MTF transsexual brains are shifted toward a more female-typical structural pattern (Zubiaurre-Elorza et al., 2012). Conversely, nonhomosexual transsexual brains are similar to those of control males, not control females, and instead differ from controls for aspects of brain morphology that are not sexually dimorphic among controls (Savic & Arver, 2011).

Psychosocial Factors

To merit truly causal status, psychosocial factors should be able to account for the emergence of GD in the first few years of life, when its behavioral expressions are first manifested (at least for those patients who have the early-onset form of GD). Otherwise, psychosocial factors would be better conceptualized as having a perpetuating role.

Parental tolerance or encouragement of the early cross-gender behavior of children with GD has been reported on by clinicians of diverse theoretical persuasions and has also marshaled some degree of empirical support (Green, 1987; Zucker & Bradley, 1995).

The reasons that parents might tolerate, if not encourage, early cross-gender behaviors appear to be quite diverse, suggesting that the antecedents to this "end state" are multiple in origin. For example, if one listens to the reports by contemporary parents of children who have made an early gender social transition (later discussion), a common narrative is that the parents are simply "supporting" what they view as their child's essential "nature." Such parents would argue that the direction of effect is from child to parent, not the other way around, or even some kind of interactive, iterative transactional process. In an earlier generation, parents of children with GD have reported being influenced by ideas regarding nonsexist child rearing and thus were as likely to encourage cross-gender behavior as same-gender behavior. In other parents, the antecedents seem to be rooted in pervasive conflict that revolves around gender issues (Zucker & Bradley, 1995, pp. 213–215).

In the normative-development literature, the role of parental reinforcement efforts in inducing sex-typed behavioral sex differences was studied extensively between the 1970s and the early 1990s. Lytton and Romney's (1991) meta-analysis concluded that, with one exception, there was "little differential socialization for social behavior or abilities" (p. 267). The exception was in the domain of "encouragement of sex-typed activities and perceptions of sex-stereotyped characteristics" (p. 283), for which the mean effect sizes for mothers, fathers, and parents combined were 0.34, 0.49, and 0.43, respectively. Although Lytton and Romney's overall conclusion minimized the influence of parental socialization on sex-dimorphic behavior, the domain for which clear parental gender socialization effects were found is precisely the domain that encompasses many of the initial behavioral features of GD (see also Zucker & Bradley, 1995, pp. 222–226).

Over the past couple of decades, cognitive-developmental models have come to play a much more central role in the normative-development literature regarding gender development (Martin, Ruble, & Szkrybalo, 2002), building on the seminal theoretical work from the 1960s through the 1980s and its emphasis on "self-socialization."

Studies of children with GD have shown that they are more likely than control children to mislabel themselves as of the other gender and to also show a "developmental lag" in cognitive gender constancy (Zucker et al., 1999). Perhaps this early cognitive mislabeling of gender contributes to their cross-gender identification, although the reasons why such mislabeling occur is unclear. It could, for example, be argued that there is some kind of interactive effect between gender cognitions and the strong interest in cross-gendered behavior.

A second aspect of the cognitive-developmental literature pertains to the observation that young children have rather rigid, if not obsessional, interests in engaging in sex-typed behavior: for girls, Halim et al. (2013) dubbed this the "pink frilly dress" phenomenon. Halim et al. argued that this gender rigidity was part of the young child's effort to master gender categories and to securely (affectively) place him- or herself in the "right" category. Parents of such children do not particularly encourage the rigidity, but they also do not discourage it, and there is the assumption that such rigidity will wane over developmental time and that there will be a concomitant increase in gender flexibility.

Halim et al.'s (2013) observations jibe rather nicely with empirical data suggesting that many children with GD show very focused and intense cross-gendered interests (VanderLaan et al., in press). If these early cross-gendered intense interests are reinforced rather than ignored or compensated for by efforts to increase gender-flexible thinking and behavior, perhaps this contributes to their continuation and an increase in the likelihood that a cross-gender identity will persist.

A multifactorial model of gender development can take into account biological predisposing factors, precipitating factors, and perpetuating (maintenance) factors. Because so much is still not even known about normative gender development (Fausto-Sterling, Garcia Coll, & Lamarre, 2012), clinicians, patients, and their families vary in how much weight (or variance) each of these factors is given. At one extreme, some would argue that biological factors account for the bulk of the variance; at the other extreme, some would argue that psychosocial factors are most influential (see Zucker & Bradley, 1995, Chs. 6–7). As noted by Nieder and Richter-Appelt (2011), the propensity for practicing clinicians (and clients) to utilize dichotomous "either/or" paradigms in conceptualization is a common problem that should be avoided.

APPROACHES TO TREATMENT

Children

If one studies the follow-up literature on children with GD, current data show that:

1. The majority of children, when followed up in adolescence or adulthood, no longer have GD and are relatively content with a gender identity that matches their birth sex (for boys, 97.8%, n = 44, Green, 1987); 79.7%, n = 59, Wallien & Cohen-Kettenis, 2008; 87.8%, n = 139, Singh, 2012; for girls, 88%, n = 25, Drummond, Bradley, Peterson-Badali, & Zucker, 2008; 50%, n = 18, Wallien & Cohen-Kettenis, 2008). For children who show a persistence of their GD, almost all are sexually attracted to members of their natal sex; however, because these youth identify as members of the other gender, their *subjective* sexual identity is heterosexual or "straight."
2. The majority of children with GD, especially boys, in whom the GD has desisted are sexually attracted to members of their natal sex and identify as gay.
3. A minority of children with GD for whom it has desisted are sexually attracted to the opposite sex and identify as heterosexual or "straight." Thus, to date, the most common long-term outcome for children with GD, especially boys, is a homosexual/gay sexual identity with no continued occurrence of GD.

In the treatment literature for children with GD, three broad approaches appear: (1) psychosocial treatments designed to reduce the GD in order to increase the likelihood that a long-term gender identity will be more congruent with the natal sex; (2) a neutral or "watchful waiting" approach in which the clinician suggests that the child be given time to sort out his or her gender identity, in one way or another, but without active interventions; and (3) psychosocial support for an "early" gender social transition, in which the child is given the opportunity to live in the social role of the "desired" gender (e.g., via a name change, presenting socially via hairstyle and clothing style in the desired gender, etc.).

These three treatment approaches need to be understood in relation to underlying theoretical, philosophical, and social-value perspectives (for a broad overview of these approaches, see the guest-edited volume by Drescher & Byne, 2012, in the *Journal of Homosexuality*).

The first approach, which Dreger (2009) has characterized as the "therapeutic model," has the longest history. It has also taken many forms: behavior therapy, psychodynamic therapy, peer group therapy, family therapy, parent counseling, and interventions in the naturalistic environment carried out by parents with input from the clinician. From a theoretical perspective, psychosocial treatments have likely assumed that the child's GD is not yet fixed and thus amenable to change (Zucker, Wood, Singh, & Bradley, 2012). From philosophical and social-values perspectives, clinicians probably assume that a child's life would be easier and less complicated if a gender identity that matches his or her birth sex could be achieved. For example, it would reduce the social ostracism that many of these children experience because of their cross-gender or gender-variant behaviors (Meyer-Bahlburg, 2002), and it would avoid the complex medical treatments required to achieve a gender transition. As noted by Cohen-Kettenis and Pfäfflin (2003), "Relatively little dispute exists regarding the prevention of transsexualism" (p. 120). Although much less apparent in the contemporary treatment literature, some clinicians have also advocated treatment with the expressed goal of preventing homo-sexuality (see Zucker, 1990). Although it has been noted for years that there is little evidence that treatment of children with GD alters their eventual sexual orientation (see Green, 1987), the contemporary clinician must be mind-ful that parents vary tremendously in the degree to which they would be able to accept and support their child if he or she later developed and expressed a gay or lesbian sexual identity: for some parents, it is not an issue; for other parents, it is an outcome that they eventually are able to embrace; but for other parents, it is an outcome that causes intense anxiety (for a whole host of reasons—personal, cultural, religious, etc.). Thus, there is considerable room for psychoeducational discussion with parents about what one might expect from a psychosocial treatment designed to reduce GD.

Although there is a reasonably large literature using psychosocial treat-ments, a perusal of it yields the sobering fact that there is not even one ran-domized controlled treatment trial for children with GD (Byne et al., 2012). Although there have been some treatment effectiveness studies, which might qualify as Level II standards (e.g., "evidence obtained from well-designed cohort or case-control analytic studies"), much is lacking in these investiga-tions (Zucker, 2008). To put it plainly: There is a large empirical black hole in the treatment literature for children with GD. As a result, the therapist must rely largely on the "clinical wisdom" that has accumulated in the case report literature and the conceptual underpinnings that inform the various approaches to intervention.

In contrast to the psychosocial treatment approaches designed to reduce GD in children, the recent emergence of a therapeutic approach that supports an early gender social transition, which Dreger (2009) has termed the "accom-modation model," provides the contemporary clinician (and parents) with a very different conceptual perspective (e.g., Vanderburgh, 2009; see also the essays in the edited volume by Drescher & Byne, 2012). In this approach, there appears to be an underlying theoretical assumption that the child's gen-der identity is fixed and unalterable, likely rooted in some type of biological cause. Thus, any attempt to try to change the child's gender identity is viewed with great skepticism. Interestingly, this therapeutic approach nowadays is the one that receives the most media attention (Padawer, 2012; Rosin, 2008), and it certainly dominates Internet discourse.

An interesting and important empirical question is whether or not these three approaches will result in different long-term psychosexual outcomes for children with GD. Steensma, McGuire, Kreukels, Beekman, and Cohen-Kettenis (2013) have now shown that children with GD who had socially transitioned prior to puberty were more likely to persist in their GD by mid-adolescence than children who had not and that early social transition as a predictor variable accounted for unique variance in predicting outcome. In itself, this is an important finding. What is less clear at present is whether or not these different treatment approaches are predictive of variation in more general psychosocial and psychiatric adjustment.

Adolescents

Since the mid-1990s, one model of therapeutic care, developed by Dutch clinicians and researchers, has been to initiate the biomedical aspects of sex reassignment in early to mid-adolescence, rather than waiting for the legal age of adulthood (18 years in many countries) or even later. After careful psychological evaluation, adolescents deemed appropriate for such treatment are prescribed hormonal medication to delay or suppress somatic puberty (prior to the age of 16 years). If the GD persists, then cross-sex hormonal therapy is offered at the age of 16 years, and, if the adolescent so desires, surgical sex change procedures are then offered at a lower-bound age of 18 years (Cohen-Kettenis, Steensma, & de Vries, 2011; Zucker et al., 2011).

The rationale for this treatment protocol includes the following assumptions: (1) for some adolescents with GD (and perhaps even the majority), there is little systematic empirical evidence that psychological interventions can resolve it, even if the adolescent desires this; (2) the use of hormonal blockers can be helpful to the adolescent because it reduces the incongruence between the development of natal-sex secondary physical characteristics (e.g., in males, facial hair growth, hair growth on other parts of the body, deepening of the voice; in females, breast development, menstruation) and the felt psychological gender, thereby reducing stress; (3) reduction of the incongruence makes it easier for adolescents to present socially in the cross-gender identity/role (when they so desire), which is also helpful in reducing stress during the gender transition process. Because the suspension of the patient's biological puberty reduces the preoccupation with it, it has also been argued that this affords the adolescent greater opportunity to explore his or her longer term gender identity options in psychosocial counseling or psychotherapy in a more reflective and less pressured manner.

The sequence of this biomedical treatment is progressively irreversible. On the one hand, the use of hormonal medication to suppress or delay puberty is a reversible procedure; on the other hand, surgical interventions (e.g., in males, vaginoplasty; in females, chest surgery) are irreversible. Accordingly, if clinicians are going to support adolescents with GD in moving down a pathway that, in the end, results in a completely irreversible intervention, it is important to have a relatively high degree of confidence that the likelihood of regret will be low.

In the Dutch model, several factors have been identified as important in deeming an adolescent eligible for early biomedical treatment. According to Cohen-Kettenis, Delemarre-van de Waal, and Gooren (2008), these include the following: (1) the presence of GD from early childhood on; (2) an increase in the GD after the first signs of puberty; (3) the absence of psychiatric comorbidity that would interfere with a diagnostic evaluation or treatment; (4) adequate psychological and social support during treatment; and (5) a demonstration of knowledge of the sex-reassignment process.

The use of hormonal blockers to treat adolescents with GD has been well received in the professional literature (Hembree et al., 2009). There are, however, a number of uncertainties that require further explication. Perhaps the most acute issue is how to best identify adolescents deemed eligible for early biomedical treatment from those who are not. As noted earlier, one criterion used by the Dutch group is a history of GD from early childhood on. Yet, in clinics such as our own, we see some adolescents with GD who showed very little or absolutely no evidence of GD in early childhood (Zucker, Bradley, et al., 2012). In many respects, the presentations of these adolescents resemble the "late-onset" form of GD that has been described in the literature on adults (Lawrence, 2010). The GD appears to emerge, at least in the eyes of significant others (e.g., parents, therapists who have known the patient since childhood), only after the onset of puberty. It is not clear whether this late-onset group should be deemed ineligible for early hormonal therapy. Other adolescents have a history of pervasive cross-gender behavior during childhood but without apparent GD until adolescence. It is unclear whether a childhood history of pervasive cross-gender behavior without the explicit wish to be of the other gender would count as an example of "early onset" in the Dutch model.

Another issue that deserves consideration concerns the Dutch group's view on the role of psychiatric comorbidity in making treatment decisions about early biomedical interventions. It is, for example, unclear what is meant when it is stated that the presence of such comorbidity interferes with a diagnostic evaluation or in what ways the presence of such comorbidity interferes with treatment.

There are several ways to conceptualize such comorbidity. In some instances, it may be that the GD has emerged as secondary to another, more "primary" psychiatric disorder, such as autism spectrum disorder or borderline personality disorder, or as a result of a severe trauma (e.g., sexual abuse). In such situations, it could be argued that the GD would dissipate if the more primary condition was treated. In other instances, it could be that the presence of other psychopathology (e.g., substance abuse) would interfere with the adolescent's ability to adhere to a biomedical treatment and that there would be risks in trying to institute a regimen of hormonal therapy until stabilization was achieved. Last, there is the thorny issue regarding the extent to which the presence of other psychopathology (e.g., depression, suicidality) is due to the stress of having GD or is secondary to the social ostracism and rejection that results from it. On this point, one could argue that institution of treatment of the GD may reduce the secondary psychopathology.

Given that that there are likely multiple reasons as to why adolescents with GD also present with other kinds of psychiatric issues, the clinician needs to formulate the extent to which these other difficulties are merely secondary to the GD, may actually be fueling it, or are related to other factors (e.g., a biological predisposition, family psychopathology). This kind of case formulation can help the clinician decide whether biomedical treatments should be instituted after the diagnostic assessment or delayed until the other issues can be worked through.

Case 1

Katie was a 15-year-old natal female with a childhood history of cross-gender behavior but without an expressed desire to be a boy. Her childhood was chaotic: Katie's biological mother left the family without notice when she was 4. She was raised primarily by her biological father, who was preoccupied with his own physical health and mental health (substance abuse, depression, etc.). At the age of 12, Katie was sexually abused by a male neighbor. Three years later, Katie could still not talk about it. During the assessment, her father fell asleep while the issue was being explored. Shortly after the abuse, Katie began to masculinize her phenotypic appearance and informed her father that she was thinking about a sex-change operation. In addition to her emerging GD, Katie began to manifest other behavioral and emotional issues: She would run away from home after arguing with her father, was often truant from school, and engaged in a lot of self-harming behavior (e.g., cutting). At the time of the assessment, Katie indicated that she was attracted sexually to girls and was trying to sort out if she was "just a lesbian" or was "really" transsexual. Katie commented: "I know why I want to be a guy. It's to protect myself. . . . I know it's related to the abuse." In Katie's case, we did not recommend hormonal treatment but recommended more psychosocial treatment to stabilize her from a psychiatric and psychological point of view and to provide her with a therapeutic space to work through the trauma that resulted from the sexual abuse and to explore further her gender identity and sexual orientation.

Case 2

Mark was a 16-year-old natal male with no history of cross-gender behavior in childhood. He began to express a desire to be female at the age of 15. His sexual orientation was, if anything, for females, but Mark described himself as "asexual." He did not report any behaviors associated with fetishistic cross-dressing, and there was no history of taking his mother's undergarments or the clothing of other females. His parents noted that in childhood he had had a lot of social difficulties. Although a gifted youth, with a superior-range IQ, Mark had a lot of trouble with social cues and was very rule bound. He preferred to stay at home with his mother (who was a homemaker) and play with his older sister. He never had a best friend in childhood. During childhood, he was seen by several psychiatrists, who questioned whether he might have Asperger's disorder. At the time of assessment, Mark had developed sufficient social skills so that he could interact with other gifted, "nerdy" youth. Much of their interactions revolved around online computer games. Mark had never actively cross-dressed in women's clothing or attempted to pass in the female gender role. At assessment, he wore his hair long, which often concealed his eyes, but this was as much to "hide" himself from others when he was anxious as it was to have a hairstyle similar to some teenage girls. He was unable to verbalize why he wanted to become a woman other than "I just don't fit in as a male." His father commented that he was puzzled as to how Mark could say that he "felt" like a woman because he did not seem to understand the feelings of other people. The clinical impression was that Mark met criteria for an autism spectrum disorder. Hormonal treatment was not recommended. Mark agreed to a trial of psychosocial therapy in which his gender-dysphoric feelings could be explored further.

Adults

Therapeutic guidelines for adults have long adhered to the WPATH SOC (Coleman et al., 2011). Here we summarize some of the significant changes in Version 7. The guidelines no longer require a diagnosis for medical interventions, only that the GD be "persistent and well documented." This reflects a significant shift from seeing somatic treatments as only for those with severe GD and opens the way for individuals who may identify as more "genderqueer" (i.e., as not strongly either gender or as psychologically between genders) to receive interventions. Practically speaking, this may mean more expression of gender variation through the use of hormone therapy; however, many public health care models and insurers require a diagnosis for surgical interventions.

The previous SOC had the real-life experience (RLE) eligibility criterion, which necessitated individuals to be involved in full-time work, school, or volunteer activities in their chosen gender. The idea was driven by the importance of people having a "lived informed consent," that they adjusted socially and understood the consequences of transition before beginning a medical intervention with irreversible aspects. The wording grated on many community members ("This is my real life!"), and some felt the attitude behind it paternalistic and representing an undue hardship on trans women, who had a more difficult time integrating socially without physical intervention. The criterion also de facto required people to be functional. This, too, was criticized as holding trans people to an unfairly high standard (i.e., "If cisgender people [i.e., those whose gender identities align with their natal sex] can stay at home on social assistance, why can't trans people?"). The spirit of the RLE is carried forward into the new language of a continuous gender-role experience for genital surgery only, opening up alternatives for people to document their lives and understanding of the social consequences of transition, offering time to adjust and adapt to the challenges inherent within. Readiness for hormones and surgery is captured in the stipulation that mental health issues be "well controlled."

The SOC represent minimum standards and leave significant room for providers or sites as to how they will be interpreted. Because this will unavoidably lead to some amount of discrepancy in philosophy and practice, it has led to discussions in communities with multiple providers. Some providers are working on an informed consent model for hormones in the most liberal sense (i.e., "Is the person mentally capable of consenting to treatment?"), with less attention to readiness per se, which is what others consider holistically (e.g., Has a person reasonably anticipated, and is he or she mentally prepared for, the potential consequences of this decision? Is he or she sufficiently psychiatrically stable, and is social support adequate to help him or her with the ways in which his or her life might become unraveled?). These discrepancies have resulted in some psychiatrically vulnerable patients pursuing a surgery track who do not meet the higher standard for surgery and are left in physical limbo. Another tension in this work is differences in what might be considered to be medically necessary and what government health policies consider to be medically necessary and, therefore, insured services. One example of this seen in Canada is considering the mastectomy portion of a female-to-male chest surgery medically necessary, while the chest contouring is seen as cosmetic in nature. Surgeons make no distinction; they are considered part of the same surgery, and they will not provide one without the other because it would lead to poor results, such as the possibility for concave depressions in the chest. Our gender identity clinic team thinks a certain amount of cosmesis is medically necessary to relieve the dysphoria, but these are larger policy issues.

Subtypes and Gender Differences

There has been a significant amount of controversy in the literature and at the community level regarding the existence of "subtypes" of those with significant GD and their meaning. In brief, researchers have identified a taxonomy largely organized by natal sex (male, female) and sexual orientation (most often seen as "homosexual" vs. "nonhomosexual" in the literature). These have also gone by other names in the literature: primary versus secondary and early versus late onset.

MALE-TO-FEMALE TRANSSEXUALS

Trans women (MTF) are considered more variable in presentation than trans men (female-to-male [FTM] transsexuals). Among these, the most controversial concept may be that of autogynephilia, based largely on the work of Blanchard (1989) and subsequently Lawrence (2009, 2013). Autogynephilia is specific to male-to-females and is characterized by sexual arousal to the idea of being a woman—an "erotic target location error" in which a male himself becomes the object of his (heterosexual) desire (Lawrence, 2009). It casts the motivation for transition in these cases as largely an erotic, and indeed paraphilic, one. Further to this, autogynephilia is proposed as a sexual orientation. Features considered typical of autogynephilia include more male gender-typed childhoods, a primary attraction to women, and a history of erotic cross-dressing that evolves into a sustained cross-gender identity.

This concept has been incredibly politically laden and has also emerged within trans community circles as a divisive issue. Some high-profile women of trans experience have supported the concept as an accurate representation of their experience, whereas others have felt that the concept was "insulting to their senses of self" (see Dreger, 2008) and highly pathologizing, delegitimizing their identities. There is less debate that, for many who transition later in life, sexuality has played a developmental or mediating role in coming into their gender identities. But what this means, or what can reasonably be thought of as causal, continues to be strongly contested. Some women of trans experience describe this sexual element as a kind of phase that passes or as one that plays an important role in the exploration or clarification of their identity. Some have likened the initial practice of embodiment as having a transcendental or charged quality without being reducible to sexual desire per se (Dreger, 2008).

There has been significant narrative and clinical evidence for varied presentations, with significantly more attention paid to variations among MTFs. In clinical practice, although we may describe cases as early or late onset for the purpose of communicating someone's gender identity trajectory, it serves little functional value in terms of the evaluation itself from an eligibility perspective regarding somatic treatments, such as hormone therapy and surgery. It is useful insofar as anticipating the differing life circumstances.

Early- and late-onset trans women tend to have different vulnerabilities and strengths. Early-onset trans women often recount significant histories of social exclusion and harassment over long periods of time. They tend to have high degrees of social anxiety and may be less socially skilled on account of having lesser practice within peer networks. Some of this may be resolved through transition, but there is typically quite a bit of residual work regarding grieving the experiences they have missed out on, low self-esteem, and the anxiety of being discovered as trans, as early transitioners often choose to live "stealth" (i.e., not disclose their transition history to most others). If their families are not supportive, this group is much more vulnerable to homelessness, to using substances to cope, and/or to survival sex work. Late-onset trans women have mostly grown up with fairly traditional masculine childhoods and the psychological steadiness and resilience that acceptance and "fitting in" (at least from the outside) can bring. Contemplating transition is often frightening, as the stripping of privilege and potential losses in relationship and employment can be sudden and staggering. If they lose core parts of their lives, which many do, there may also not be an easy transition into new communities or employment opportunities. Many could be helped with grief work and/or by finding new supports or activities.

FEMALE-TO-MALE TRANSSEXUALS

Most trans men are heterosexual in their sexual orientation, that is, desiring of women. Although some of them partner with heterosexual women, others partner with queer-identified women. The reason may be that queer-identified women are less invested in gender and bodies per se in considerations of partnering. It may also be that a significant percentage of trans men have histories in the lesbian community. Their initial identity trajectories are in many ways similar to those who later identify as lesbians (Rowniak & Chesla, 2012). Because there is a fair amount of acceptable gender variance in queer women's communities (and, indeed, sometimes an overvaluing of masculine-type gender expression and presentation), some FTMs initially believe that they belong in the lesbian community. Some will figure out, based on the degree of their body dysphoria and/or discomfort with how they are responded to culturally or sexually, that they are not similar to lesbians. The exploration of this conflict may be difficult to untangle from internalized homophobia in some cases by client and clinician alike. Some FTMs already know they are not lesbian but may take on "lesbian" as a transitory identity to "test the waters" in terms of social acceptance and/or bide some time for themselves as they strengthen their internal and external resources necessary for the often overwhelming task of coming out to others as transgender. Still, precisely because many have been involved in communities of difference and marginality, there is typically more open-mindedness in their social circles, and many can retain core aspects of their existing communities if they wish.

A significant minority of trans men identify as gay, that is, desiring of men (and an even lesser percentage as bisexual or pansexual). In our experience, this group has had less success integrating socially within gay men's communities and finding sexual partners among cisgender men whose cultures tend to be more body focused (and phallocentric, in particular). We more typically see gay trans men partnering with each other.

Trans men as a group tend to fare better psychiatrically than trans women. This may be because they have been, relatively speaking, subject to less relational trauma than trans women. Tomboyish girls enjoy a certain normativity that effeminate boys do not. When FTMs decide to transition, they can sometimes pass for young men with changes to their appearance alone, and testosterone often creates significant masculinization over a relatively short period of time. Although this minimizes the time that they are visibly transitioning, gay trans men and trans men of color will be adapting to a new social identity role in which they may be subject to more overt discrimination than before. Because of this, they may need help navigating social spaces or responding to harassment, but their histories may have both instilled a decent sense of worth from which to work and already taught them about how discrimination operates (through previous experiences of sexism, homophobia, or racism).

Specific Therapeutic Issues

Clarifying sexuality from gender identity may be one of the important thera-peutic tasks in working with GD, particularly in cases with young adults. Despite the fact that they are separate constructs, in practical terms the edges of their boundaries are sometimes not. For example, some younger trans women interested in men have talked about a period of community and sexual exploration to better understand whether they might be a very feminine gay man or a woman. Similarly, some younger trans men interested in women have done similar exploration to better understand the shadings between being a very masculine lesbian woman and a man, especially when some amount of body dysphoria may be common among some sexual-minority subgroupings. Desire is often relational, and issues of admiration and wanting to "be like" can sometimes get confused with sexual desire. Some of our FTM clients talk about being curious and interested in men pretransition and that only in retro-spect did they see their sexual involvement with them as being more an oppor-tunity to explore men's bodies and to learn, more in a kind of role modeling or mirroring process. In getting up close to see what they wanted for themselves, it allowed them to more easily imagine how they might proceed, appear, and behave. This is not to say this is always or even mostly the case, just that it is another developmental phase for some clients in which distinctions between sexuality and gender identity may feel less clear.

Case 3

Edward was a 22-year-old natal female who presented for approval for hor-mone therapy and chest surgery. He had already undergone a legal name change and was presenting male insofar as possible. He remembered early fan-tasies of being a boy and being closer to his male cousins and enjoying sports that he could not play with his sisters. He was said to be quite "beautiful," received a lot of praise, and knew his parents were happy to see him presenting as more feminine. He joined the Reserves when he was old enough, resenting being in the female divisions and taking secret pleasure when people took him for a boy. Puberty was uncomfortable, but he began to realize that his discom-fort was not the same as that of his peers—many of them seemed to want the changes and faster, but he did not want them at all. He felt alone in realizing that, despite the complaints they had, girls did not "hate" being girls as he did. He did not like the uneven look of his growing chest and was revolted by the idea that this was understood to be sexually desirable. He wanted, even expected, a deeper voice and was disappointed that this did not come to be and jealous of his male peers. He did not feel likeable and went through a phase of presenting as more feminine to try to attract male attention. In fic-tion and fantasy, male couplings were the most exciting, and he would place himself in one of the characters. He dreamed about his body being different and would be angry to wake up and find it was not so. It struck him as impor-tant that he felt normal and happy in these dreams. He did some reading on the Internet and found information about FTMs/trans men, which was not as easy to find as it was on MTFs/trans women, but for some time he did not want to think he was "like this." He understood that the surgeries would not be perfect, and this reality was also difficult for him to accept. His first true introduction was a drag performance, which included someone who identified as transgender, and he spoke about his feelings openly for the first time. He bought his first binder and packer, things that brought him much more comfort, confidence, and joy. After some failed attempts at dating mostly men but some women, he began a relationship with a male who was aware of how he felt, was reportedly supportive, and addressed him using male pronouns. He wished to pursue chest surgery before hormones.

Trans people with sexual-minority identities have more identity work to do and are sometimes less understood by others (hearing iterations of "If you want to attract men, why go through the trouble of transition?"). Indeed, in this vignette, there was a small period of time that this client feminized his gender presentation to be able to enact aspects of his sexuality (albeit likely unknown to the former partners, who may have themselves experienced it as a heterosexual encounter). This tends not to be satisfying in the long term, for a holistic understanding of attractions and sexual activity involves the interaction of both gender and sexuality. The kind of sexual activity, the way it is enacted, and how one relates and is related to in the interaction, the sexual language used, and the degree to which sex can be embodied are all factors that contribute to our experience of the quality and enjoyment of sex and also can powerfully affirm or undercut our sense of gender.

Shame and loss often feature prominently in early stages of help seeking, sometimes especially so for trans women who present or transition later in life. This difficult affective combination increases the sense of internal conflict regarding a decision to live in a manner congruent with one's identity. It can also increase the risk for suicide, because the patient may feel trapped between two seemingly felt impossibilities: living what feels like a lie and keeping one's life intact, albeit fairly miserably, or living congruently and likely facing rejection by family, as well as significant losses in social status and networks. When women's gender identities have evolved from a history of what they previously felt was cross-dressing, many come to us with a sense of failure of control and/ or questions about how to stop their behaviors or desires. A number of them have gone through cycles of acquiring and purging clothes and makeup and report feeling quite guilt-ridden.

Case 4

Fatima, a natal male in her 30s, presented as female at the assessment. It was the first time she had presented to others as female, despite many years of practice in secret, and she had told no one other than her doctor, who referred her. Growing up, she was more effeminate (and has worked to keep a petite frame), and she wished to be doing what girls of her age were doing. Her family caught her once as a teen in makeup and women's clothing and threatened to have her institutionalized. There was taunting about the incident, but the family also considered it a phase. Having immigrated from a South Asian country years ago, Fatima was now married to a woman and had two young children. She felt more comfortable being feminine and wanted to be female, but she felt transitioning would go against her Muslim faith, and she also worried about losing custody of her children. As time went on, she had felt increasingly desperate and depressed, particularly because her marriage had meant that she had had less opportunity (she kept female clothes in her car), and she found thoughts of transitioning fairly preoccupying in her day-to-day life. She and her wife do not have an emotionally intimate life. Fatima tried to bring up her dysphoria indirectly: She shaved her legs and once tried on her wife's undergarments in her presence to see if she would ask her about it (she didn't). She and her wife had a sexual life, despite Fatima's discomfort having sex that involved her penis. As sexual attractions often remain stable through transition, she worried about another religious conflict if she transitioned: reconciling her attraction to women, which as a woman would be same sex, also inconsistent with her current beliefs.

We felt clear in a diagnosis of GD—her feelings had been consistent and persistent, despite her concerns over them. She had significant dysphoria both for social role and her body, her genitals in particular, which she used somewhat reluctantly and with great discomfort. Living incongruently was negatively affecting her happiness and productivity at work. In initial therapy sessions, she alternated between wishing "to be cured" and hoping that we could help her be happy as a man and wanting to start hormones before she told her wife. Part of our initial work is psychoeducational, in sharing more about what the diagnosis means and that it is not something to be cured; that our role is not to rid her of these feelings but to help her come to terms with them. This is different from having any investment in what clients then do with this diagnosis. Some of our clients decide living congruently is the most important thing; to many, it no longer feels like a decision at some point. Some of our clients continue to live with these feelings without acting on them publicly because they decide that their marriages or relationships with their children are too important to risk (the latter of which we mean only in emotional terms—there is legal precedence whereby gender identity is not a determinant of child custody). As with working with any issue involving ambivalence, we do clients a disservice in becoming "cheerleaders"; taking up one side often only results in their taking up the other side. It is important that they come to their own resolution.

Patients may present in treatment at any one of a number of stages, but as with therapy in general, many individuals or couples are typically motivated by an urgent matter or crisis. Some may present when there has been a disclosure or discovery (e.g., if the dressing has been secret, a wife finds the clothes and believes her spouse is having an affair). Sometimes, gender variance has been an open feature of a relationship, but one or both parties have assumed it to be "just that"; having a partner consider transition puts a very different frame on the future of their lives together. In some of these cases, one or both parties knew of transgender feelings but believed they could live without transition and/or that marriage would rid them of the feelings. There may also have been a genuine evolution, from being satisfied with less gender expression to feeling that it is not enough. Lev's (2004) volume reviews a number of helpful case illustrations of working with couples in which one partner has gender questions or concerns. Brown (2010) has reviewed the literature on partners' experiences, both in cases of MTFs and FTMs, which may also be helpful to providers.

Many relationships break up under these circumstances, but a good minority do not. It is more common for FTMs in relationships with cisgender women to stay together. We have also seen a number of MTFs in relationships with cisgender women stay together through transition, albeit infrequently. Of these couples we've seen many have had ongoing quality communication and have taken transition slowly. Some people continue on as life partners without a sexual component to the relationship. Some maintain sexual intimacy and adapt to a new life being seen as a lesbian couple. Our use of "being seen as" is not meant to demean the legitimacy of this, only to draw attention to the fact that the cisgender spouses may not identify this way and may continue to think of themselves as being part of a "mixed orientation" dyad. In other cases, they do truly renegotiate their sexual orientations.

There may also be negotiations regarding the gender expression of the trans-identified spouse and mutual compromises to come to regarding when or how much the relationship context can manage. We hear about people's decisions to not transition or to delay transition until their children reach a certain age. An interesting case study is presented in Levine and Davis (2002), in which a trans woman made a series of returns to the male role for her wife's career events as what she could conceptualize as a "gift of love." Similarly, one of our clients dresses more plainly at home as part of honoring her partner, motivated by her interpretation of fairness in which she feels her wife deserves the right to see and connect with more of the person she agreed to marry.

If a relationship breaks up, one may also see people struggling both with their grief and with the worry of there being a smaller dating pool in the future. Our experience is that this is based in some reality; some people have partnered successfully (more so with women), whereas others have been single for years and describe significant loneliness.

A number of trans women partner with men. A number of these men appear to have a heterosexual orientation, particularly those partnered with early transitioners, and are able to incorporate a trans body into their sexuality. Men partnered with trans women who transition later in life may have paired with them *because* of their preoperative status. This may be an explicit aspect of their connection, having met, for example, on a trans-specific dating website. This may also be a covert aspect of a relationship, which emerges we suspect when women approaching surgery reveal that their partners are concerned and may be couching their resistance in loving terms—"I love you just the way you are. The surgery is so risky. Are you sure you want to go through with this?" We try to prepare people for the possibility that their relationship may end as part of undergoing sex reassignment surgery. Certainly, women who date preoperatively have mixed experiences, the majority sharing relatively disappointing stories of men who appear to be interested primarily for sexual encounters rather than relationships; they may say that there is a strong fantasy or fetishistic aspect to the interaction in which the men are quite interested in the anatomy that the woman wishes to be rid of. Some see it as a concession of types—a price to pay in more of an exchange framework of intimacy. As one of our clients said, "It's bittersweet."

Regretters

In carefully evaluated patients, narrative literature reviews have estimated the regret rate for sex reassignment to be quite low—about 2%—and "dissatisfaction" with surgical treatment to be also quite low—about 4% (Gijs & Brewaeys, 2007). Gijs and Brewaeys noted, however, that these are likely lower-bound estimates of dissatisfaction and regrets, because a substantial percentage of postsurgical patients are lost to follow-up. Dhejne et al. (2011) used a population-based registry in Sweden and found that the overall mortality for sex-reassigned patients was higher during follow-up than for controls of the same sex, with an adjusted hazard ratio of 2.8, and with death from suicide particularly high, with an adjusted hazard ratio of 19.1.

Lawrence (2003) reviewed the follow-up literature and some of the methodological problems associated with these studies. Research has identified several factors relating to an increased likelihood of postsurgical dissatisfaction or regret. Of preoperative factors relating to developmental trajectory, these included older age, late-onset desire for SRS, and a history of fetishistic cross-dressing. Of preoperative factors relating to compliance with established treatment, the evidence is more limited, but it includes a lack of social experience in the desired gender role and noncontinuous hormone use. Preoperative factors relating to the psychosocial environment included coexisting psychopathology and poor social support. Of postoperative factors, the most significant factor associated with dissatisfaction or regret relates to poor surgical outcome.

In our clinic, we try to elicit and assess the expectations of all candidates as part of our work. Where necessary, our approach is to be clear and factual. For the FTM who believes he can secure a heterosexual woman who would not know of his transsexual history, he must come to terms with the fact that he will have a scarred body that will invite questions and require explanation and that phalloplasty does not offer a phallus that looks or operates like a biological one. People who regret their transition or surgery are typically distressed and may seek counseling as part of coming to terms with their regret and deciding how to proceed with their lives. Others do not regret transitioning but have had difficult surgeries with significant complications and must come to terms with continuing dysphoria related to functional or cosmetic limitations.

As the SOC have become less stringent for approval of hormonal treatment and SRS, it will be important to continue to monitor rates of regret and satisfaction with these biomedical therapies.

CONCLUSIONS

In the past decade, there has been a genuine increase in the number of patients (and their families) seeking out mental health care for GD and, in the majority of adolescents and adults, biomedical treatment. Thus, for the practicing clinician who wishes to work with this population, it is critical to gain some familiarity with the extant treatment approaches, including SOC guidelines (see Byne et al., 2012; Coleman et al., 2011).

In this chapter, we have summarized the literature on therapeutics, taking into account what is known about developmental trajectories. Whereas biomedical treatment for adolescents and adults is probably the most common method to ameliorate GD, it should be recognized that not all clients wish to pursue SRS and, for them, a supportive psychosocial therapeutic approach can be provided as a first-step alternative. For children, the field is currently in a great state of flux regarding best-practice principles, with a tremendous range of clinical opinion. It is important, therefore, for the practicing clinician to gain some familiarity with the different therapeutic approaches in designing a plan of care for individual children and their families.

REFERENCES

Achenbach, T. M., & Edelbrock, C. (1983). *Manual for the Child Behavior Checklist and Revised Child Behavior Profile*. Burlington: University of Vermont, Department of Psychiatry.

Achenbach, T. M., & Edelbrock, C. (1986). *Manual for the Youth Self-Report and Profile*. Burlington: University of Vermont, Department of Psychiatry.

American Psychiatric Association. (2000). *Diagnostic and statistical manual of mental disorders* (4th ed., text rev.). Washington, DC: Author.

American Psychiatric Association. (2013). *Diagnostic and statistical manual of mental disorders* (5th ed.). Arlington, VA: Author.

Blanchard, R. (1989). The concept of autogynephilia and the typology of male gender dysphoria. *Journal of Nervous and Mental Disease, 177*, 616–623.

Brown, N. R. (2010). The sexual relationships of sexual-minority women partnered with trans men: A qualitative study. *Archives of Sexual Behavior, 39*, 561–572.

Byne, W., Bradley, S. J., Coleman, E., Eyler, A. E., Green, R., Menvielle, E. J., et al.

(2012). Report of the American Psychiatric Association Task Force on Treatment of Gender Identity Disorder. *Archives of Sexual Behavior, 41*, 759–796.

Cohen-Kettenis, P. T., Delemarre-van de Waal, H. A., & Gooren, L. J. G. (2008). The treatment of adolescent transsexuals: Changing insights. *Journal of Sexual Medicine, 5*, 1892–1897.

Cohen-Kettenis, P. T., & Pfäfflin, F. (2003). *Transgenderism and intersexuality in childhood and adolescence: Making choices.* Thousand Oaks, CA: Sage.

Cohen-Kettenis, P. T., Steensma, T. D., & de Vries, A. L. C. (2011). Treatment of adolescents with gender dysphoria in the Netherlands. *Child and Adolescent Psychiatric Clinics of North America, 20*, 689–700.

Coleman, E., Bockting, W., Botzer, M., Cohen-Kettenis, P., DeCuypere, G., Feldman, J., et al. (2011). Standards of care for the health of transsexual, transgender, and gender-nonconforming people, Version 7. *International Journal of Transgenderism, 13*, 165–232.

Conron, K. J., Scott, G., Stowell, G. S., & Landers, S. J. (2012). Transgender health in Massachusetts: Results from a household probability sample of adults. *American Journal of Public Health, 102*, 118–122.

De Cuypere, G., Knudson, G., & Bockting, W. (2010). Response of the World Professional Association for Transgender Health to the proposed DSM-5 criteria for gender incongruence. *International Journal of Transgenderism, 12*, 119–123.

Deogracias, J. J., Johnson, L. L., Meyer-Bahlburg, H. F. L., Kessler, S. J., Schober, J. M., & Zucker, K. J. (2007). The Gender Identity/Gender Dysphoria Questionnaire for Adolescents and Adults. *Journal of Sex Research, 44*, 370–379.

Dhejne, C., Lichtenstein, P., Boman, M., Johansson, A. L., Langstrom, N., & Landen, M. (2011). Long-term follow-up of transsexual persons undergoing sex reassignment surgery: Cohort study in Sweden. *PLoS One, 6*(2), e16885.

Dreger, A. D. (2008). The controversy surrounding "The Man Who Would Be Queen": A case history of the politics of science, identity, and sex in the Internet age. *Archives of Sexual Behavior, 37*, 366–421.

Dreger, A. (2009). Gender identity disorder of childhood: Inconclusive advice to parents. *Hastings Center Report, 39*, 26–29.

Drescher, J. (2010). Queer diagnoses: Parallels and contrasts in the history of homosexuality, gender variance, and the *Diagnostic and Statistical Manual. Archives of Sexual Behavior, 39*, 427–460.

Drescher, J., & Byne, W. (2012). Introduction to the special issue on "The Treatment of Gender Dysphoric/Gender Variant Children and Adolescents." *Journal of Homosexuality, 59*, 295–300.

Drummond, K. D., Bradley, S. J., Peterson-Badali, M., & Zucker, K. J. (2008). A follow-up study of girls with gender identity disorder. *Developmental Psychology, 44*, 34–45.

Fausto-Sterling, A., Garcia Coll, C., & Lamarre, M. (2012). Sexing the baby: Part 1. What do we really know about sex differentiation in the first three years of life? *Social Science and Medicine, 74*, 1684–1692.

Fisk, N. (1973). Gender dysphoria syndrome (the how, what, and why of a disease). In D. Laub & P. Gandy (Eds.), *Proceedings of the second interdisciplinary symposium on gender dysphoria syndrome* (pp. 7–14). Palo Alto, CA: Stanford University Press.

Gates, G. J. (2011). *How many people are lesbian, gay, bisexual, and transgender?* Los Angeles: University of California School of Law, Williams Institute.

Retrieved from *http://williamsinstitute.law.ucla.edu/wp-content/uploads/gates-how-many-people-lgbt-apr-2011.pdf*.

Gijs, L., & Brewaeys, A. (2007). Surgical treatment of gender dysphoria in adults and adolescents: Recent developments, effectiveness, and challenges. *Annual Review of Sex Research, 18,* 178–224.

Goy, R. W., Bercovitch, F. B., & McBrair, M. C. (1988). Behavioral masculinization is independent of genital masculinization in prenatally androgenized female rhesus macaques. *Hormones and Behavior, 22,* 552–571.

Green, R. (1987). *The "sissy boy syndrome" and the development of homosexuality.* New Haven, CT: Yale University Press.

Grimbos, T., Dawood, K., Burris, R., Zucker, K. J., & Puts, D. A. (2010). Sexual orientation and the second to fourth finger length ratio: A meta-analysis in men and women. *Behavioral Neuroscience, 124,* 278–287.

Halim, N. L., Ruble, D. N., Tamis-Lemonda, C. S., Zosuls, K. M., Greulich, F. K., & Lurye, L. E. (2013). The pink frilly dress and the avoidance of all things "girly": Children's appearance rigidity and cognitive theories of gender development. *Developmental Psychology*.

Hembree, W. C., Cohen-Kettenis, P., Delemarre-van de Waal, H. A., Gooren, L. J., Meyer, W. J., Spack, N. P., et al. (2009). Endocrine treatment of transsexual persons: An Endocrine Society Clinical Practice Guideline. *Journal of Clinical Endocrinology and Metabolism, 94,* 3132–3154.

Heylens, G., De Cuypere, G., Zucker, K. J., Schelfaut, C., Elaut, E., Vanden Bossche, H., et al. (2012). Gender identity disorder in twins: A review of the literature. *Journal of Sexual Medicine, 9,* 751–757.

Knudson, G., De Cuypere, G., & Bockting, W. (2010). Process toward consensus on recommendations for revision DSM diagnoses of gender identity disorders by the World Professional Association for Transgender Health. *International Journal of Transgenderism, 12,* 54–59.

Lawrence, A. A. (2003). Factors associated with satisfaction or regret following male-to-female sex reassignment surgery. *Archives of Sexual Behavior, 32,* 299–315.

Lawrence, A. A. (2009). Erotic target location errors: An underappreciated paraphilic dimension. *Journal of Sex Research, 46,* 194–215.

Lawrence, A. A. (2010). Sexual orientation versus age of onset as bases for typologies (subtypes) of gender identity disorder in adolescents and adults. *Archives of Sexual Behavior, 39,* 514–545.

Lawrence, A. A. (2013). *Men trapped in men's bodies: Narratives of autogynephilic transsexualism.* New York: Springer.

Lev, A. I. (2004). *Transgender emergence: Therapeutic guidelines for working with gender-variant people and their families.* New York: Haworth Press.

Levine, S. B., & Davis, L. (2002). What I did for love: Temporary returns to the male gender role. *International Journal of Transgenderism, 6.* Retrieved from *www.symposiom.com/ijt/ijtvo6no4_04.htm*.

Luders, E., Sanchez, F. J., Gaser, C., Toga, A. W., Narr, K. L., Hamilton, L. S., et al. (2009). Regional gray matter variation in male-to-female transsexualism. *NeuroImage, 46,* 904–907.

Lytton, H., & Romney, D. M. (1991). Parents' differential socialization of boys and girls: A meta-analysis. *Psychological Bulletin, 109,* 267–296.

Martin, C. L., Ruble, D. N., & Szkrybalo, J. (2002). Cognitive theories of early gender development. *Psychological Bulletin, 128,* 903–933.

Martin, H., & Finn, S. E. (2010). *Masculinity and femininity in the MMPI-2 and MMPI-A*. Minneapolis: University of Minnesota Press.

Meyer-Bahlburg, H. F. L. (2002). Gender identity disorder in young boys: A parent- and peer-based treatment protocol. *Clinical Child Psychology and Psychiatry, 7*, 360–377.

Meyer-Bahlburg, H. F. L. (2010). From mental disorder to iatrogenic hypogonadism: Dilemmas in conceptualizing gender identity variants as psychiatric conditions. *Archives of Sexual Behavior, 39*, 461–476.

Meyer-Bahlburg, H. F. L. (2011). Transsexualism ("gender identity disorder"): A CNS-limited form of intersexuality? *Advances in Experimental Medicine and Biology, 707*, 75–79.

Ngun, T. C., Ghahramani, N., Sánchez, F. J., Bocklandt, S., & Vilain, E. (2011). The genetics of sex differences in brain and behavior. *Frontiers in Neuroendocrinology, 32*, 227–246.

Nieder, T. O., & Richter-Appelt, H. (2011). *Tertium non datur*: Either/or reactions to transsexualism amongst health care professionals: The situation past and present, and its relevance to the future. *Psychology and Sexuality, 2*, 224–243.

Padawer, R. (2012, August 12). Boygirl. *New York Times Magazine*, pp. 18–23, 36, 46.

Rosin, H. (2008, November). A boy's life. *Atlantic*, pp. 56–71.

Rowniak, S., & Chesla, C. (2012). Coming out for a third time: Transmen, sexual orientation, and identity. *Archives of Sexual Behavior, 42*, 449–461.

Savic, I., & Arver, S. (2011). Sex dimorphism of the brain in male-to-female transsexuals. *Cerebral Cortex, 21*, 2525–2533.

Singh, D. (2012). *A follow-up study of boys with gender identity disorder*. Unpublished doctoral dissertation, University of Toronto.

Singh, D., Deogracias, J. J., Johnson, L. L., Bradley, S. J., Kibblewhite, S. J., Owen-Anderson, A., et al. (2010). The Gender Identity/Gender Dysphoria Questionnaire for Adolescents and Adults: Further validity evidence. *Journal of Sex Research, 47*, 49–58.

Steensma, T. D., Kreukels, B., Jürgensen, M., Thyen, U., de Vries, A., & Cohen-Kettenis, P. T. (in press). The Utrecht Gender Dysphoria Scale: A validation study. *Archives of Sexual Behavior.*

Steensma, T. D., McGuire, J. K., Kreukels, B. P. C., Beekman, A. J., & Cohen-Kettenis, P. T. (2013). Factors associated with desistence and persistence of childhood gender dysphoria: A quantitative follow-up study. *Journal of the American Academy of Child and Adolescent Psychiatry, 52*, 582–590.

Vance, S. R., Cohen-Kettenis, P. T., Drescher, J., Meyer-Bahlburg, H. F. L., Pfäfflin, F., & Zucker, K. J. (2010). Opinions about the DSM gender identity disorder diagnosis: Results from an international survey administered to organizations concerned with the welfare of transgender people. *International Journal of Transgenderism, 12*, 1–14.

Vanderburgh, R. (2009). Appropriate therapeutic care for families with pre-pubescent transgender/gender-dissonant children. *Child and Adolescent Social Work Journal, 26*, 135–154.

VanderLaan, D. P., Postema, L., Wood, H., Singh, D., Fantus, S., Hyun, J., et al. (in press). Do children with gender dysphoria have intense/obsessional interests? *Journal of Sex Research.*

Wallien, M. S. C., & Cohen-Kettenis, P. T. (2008). Psychosexual outcome of gender dysphoric children. *Journal of the American Academy of Child and Adolescent Psychiatry, 47,* 1413–1423.

Wallien, M. S. C., Zucker, K. J., Steensma, T. D., & Cohen-Kettenis, P. T. (2008). 2D:4D finger- length ratios in children and adults with gender identity disorder. *Hormones and Behavior, 54,* 450–454.

Wood, H., Postema, L., VanderLaan, D. P., Singh, D., Fantus, S., Leef, J., et al. (2012). *Do children with gender identity disorder have intense/obsessional interests?* Manuscript submitted for publication.

Wood, H., Sasaki, S., Bradley, S. J., Singh, D., Fantus, S., Owen-Anderson, A., et al. (2013). Patterns of referral to a gender identity service for children and adolescents (1976–2011): Age, sex ratio, and sexual orientation [Letter to the editor]. *Journal of Sex and Marital Therapy, 39,* 1–6.

Zubiaurre-Elorza, L., Junque, C., Gómez-Gil, E., Segovia, S., Carrillo, B., Rametti, G., et al. (2012). Cortical thickness in untreated transsexuals. *Cerebral Cortex.*

Zucker, K. J. (1990). Treatment of gender identity disorders in children. In R. Blanchard & B. W. Steiner (Eds.), *Clinical management of gender identity disorders in children and adults* (pp. 25–47). Washington, DC: American Psychiatric Press.

Zucker, K. J. (2005). Measurement of psychosexual differentiation. *Archives of Sexual Behavior, 34,* 375–388.

Zucker, K. J. (2008). Children with gender identity disorder: Is there a best practice? *Neuropsychiatrie de l'Enfance et de l'Adolescence, 56,* 358–364.

Zucker, K. J., & Bradley, S. J. (1995). *Gender identity disorder and psychosexual problems in children and adolescents.* New York: Guilford Press.

Zucker, K. J., Bradley, S. J., Kuksis, M., Pecore, K., Birkenfeld-Adams, A., Doering, R. W., et al. (1999). Gender constancy judgments in children with gender identity disorder: Evidence for a developmental lag. *Archives of Sexual Behavior, 28,* 475–502.

Zucker, K. J., Bradley, S. J., Owen-Anderson, A., Kibblewhite, S. J., Wood, H., Singh, D., et al. (2012). Demographics, behavior problems, and psychosexual characteristics of adolescents with gender identity disorder or transvestic fetishism. *Journal of Sex and Marital Therapy, 38,* 151–189.

Zucker, K. J., Bradley, S. J., Owen-Anderson, A., Singh, D., Blanchard, R., & Bain, J. (2011). Puberty-blocking hormonal therapy for adolescents with gender identity disorder: A descriptive clinical study. *Journal of Gay and Lesbian Mental Health, 15,* 58–82.

Zucker, K. J., Bradley, S. J., & Sanikhani, M. (1997). Sex differences in referral rates of children with gender identity disorder: Some hypotheses. *Journal of Abnormal Child Psychology, 25,* 217–227.

Zucker, K. J., & Lawrence, A. A. (2009). Epidemiology of gender identity disorder: Recommendations for the standards of care of the World Professional Association for Transgender Health. *International Journal of Transgenderism, 11,* 8–18.

Zucker, K. J., & Wood, H. (2011). Assessment of gender variance in children. *Child and Adolescent Psychiatric Clinics of North America, 20,* 665–680.

Zucker, K. J., Wood, H., Singh, D., & Bradley, S. J. (2012). A developmental, biopsychosocial model for the treatment of children with gender identity disorder. *Journal of Homosexuality, 59,* 369–397.

CHAPTER 12

Persistent Genital Arousal Disorder

David Goldmeier, Hossein Sadeghi-Nejad, and Thomas M. Facelle

Persistent genital arousal disorder (PGAD) is a relatively "new" disorder that was originally termed persistent sexual arousal syndrome. The change in name is important as it reflects the fact that the genital arousal is not necessarily indicative of sexual arousal or pleasure. According to Goldmeier, Sadeghi-Nejad, and Facelle, women who suffer from PGAD experience relatively long periods of heightened genital sensation that are unbidden, unwanted, and highly distressing. The genital symptoms do not subside easily even after prolonged masturbation resulting in multiple orgasms. Partnered sexual activity may even worsen the symptoms. Although not a sexual disorder per se, PGAD is included in this volume because it has significantly deleterious effects on sexuality. In addition, PGAD and hypersexuality sufferers may appear similar because repeated masturbation is a symptom of both problems. This superficial resemblance, however, ignores the underlying motivations, which are very different. Goldmeier and his colleagues describe the different potential physiological (e.g., neurological) and psychological (e.g., anxiety-related) pathways that may be responsible for PGAD. The authors propose a treatment approach that involves a combination of physical and psychological remedies, including medication, pelvic floor physical therapy, and mindfulness-based CBT.

David Goldmeier, MD, is clinical lead for the multidisciplinary Jane Wadsworth Sexual Function Clinic at Imperial College and Imperial College NHS Healthcare in London, England. He has written 115 peer-reviewed academic papers and is chair of the sexual dysfunction special interest group of the British Association of Sexual Health and HIV. In his practice, he combines organic with psychological treatments (particularly mindfulness).

263

Hossein Sadeghi-Nejad, MD, graduated Magna Cum Laude from Bowdoin College in Brunswick, Maine, where he was the recipient of the Goodwin Commencement Prize. He received his MD from the McGill University School of Medicine in Montreal, Quebec, Canada, and served as an Intern and Resident in General Surgery at the University of California in San Francisco. Dr. Sadeghi-Nejad completed his urological residency and fellowship training in Male Reproductive Medicine (infertility and erectile dysfunction) and microsurgery at the Boston University Medical Center under the auspices of Drs. Robert Krane, Irwin Goldstein, and Robert Oates.

Thomas M. Facelle, MD, is a resident in Urology at Rutgers University Medical School, University Hospital, in Newark, New Jersey. He received his undergraduate degree from Wesleyan University in Middletown, Connecticut, and his medical degree from New York University School of Medicine. Additionally, he is a candidate member of the American Urologic Association.

Persistent genital arousal disorder (PGAD) is a newly recognized condition, in which the woman (or rarely man) complains of long periods of subjective genital arousal that come on unbidden (i.e., are not associated with sexual desire) and are highly distressing. PGAD may be associated with a feeling described by some patients as "restlessness," and many women with PGAD masturbate and orgasm repeatedly in order to rid themselves of these symptoms—usually unsuccessfully. It is possible that Soranus of Ephesus (trans. 1991) alluded to the condition in his text "Midwifery and Diseases of Women" in the second century A.D., but it was first accurately described and defined by Sandra Leiblum and Sharon Nathan in 2001. They presented five cases of women suffering from what they called persistent sexual arousal syndrome (PSAS; Leiblum & Nathan, 2001). This was more accurately renamed persistent genital arousal disorder (PGAD) in light of the fact that most women did not see it as a sexually related condition (Goldmeier & Leiblum, 2006).

Fewer than 500 cases of PGAD have been described in the literature. However, some evidence suggests that it may not be such a rare condition (Garvey, West, Latch, Leiblum, & Goldmeier, 2009), and many sex therapists and psychologists anecdotally report to us at conferences that they are now seeing and managing such cases.

WHAT PRECISELY IS PGAD AND WHAT IS IT NOT?

Following are six features of PGAD that we believe are relevant for its diagnosis (Leiblum & Nathan, 2001; Goldmeier & Leiblum, 2006; Waldinger & Schweitzer, 2009):

1. Genital symptoms characteristic of sexual arousal (genital fullness/ swelling and sensitivity with or without nipple fullness/swelling) or

unpleasant genital sensations (dysesthesia), that persist for an extended period of time (hours or days) and do not subside completely on their own.

2. Genital symptoms characteristic of sexual arousal or genital dysesthesia that do not resolve with ordinary orgasmic experience and may require multiple orgasms over hours or days to remit.

3. Genital symptoms characteristic of sexual arousal or genital dysesthesia that are usually experienced as unrelated to any subjective sense of sexual excitement or desire.

4. Genital symptoms that may be triggered not only by a sexual activity but also by nonsexual stimuli or by no apparent stimulus at all.

5. Genital symptoms that are experienced as unbidden, intrusive, and unwanted.

6. Genital symptoms that cause the woman a significant degree of distress.

PGAD needs to be differentiated from hypersexuality (Kafka, 2010), which can be defined as frequently repetitive sexual urges, fantasies or behaviors. Urges and fantasies are subjective mental events that have a desire quality—something patients with PGAD do not report in relation to their symptoms. Repetitive sexual behavior such as masturbation may be a clinical feature of both PGAD and hypersexuality. However, only in PGAD is this undertaken because of unbidden genital arousal or dysesthesia.

Other women report spontaneous and persistent genital arousal but are not distressed by these sensations. They may feel neutral about them (Leiblum & Chivers, 2007) or may even welcome and enjoy these genital feelings, which they can either act on by engaging in sexual activity or dismiss (Leiblum, Seehuus, & Brown, 2007). Such women should not be diagnosed with PGAD. To complicate matters, some women with frequent genital arousal can be distressed about their condition some of the time but welcome it at other times.

SPECTRUM OF SYMPTOMATOLOGY

The most common locations of symptoms of PGAD are the clitoris, vagina, labia, or a combination of all three. Less commonly it is felt in the pubic bone or around the anal area. Symptoms may be continuous or intermittent. Common symptoms include feelings of congestion, tingling, and wetness. Genital contractions and/or a feeling of imminent orgasm are commonly reported. Spontaneous vaginal and clitoral pain (28.6%) and pain with vaginal penetration (45.7%) have also been reported (Leiblum, Brown, Wan, & Rawlinson, 2005). The pain is of a throbbing quality. Original and current triggers for the onset of PGAD include physical stimulation, such as intercourse or masturbation, and psychological stress or anxiety. Seemingly innocuous stimuli such as sitting, wearing tight clothes, genital pressure, or vibrations from a motor vehicle are likely to exacerbate symptoms in most women. Erotic visual stimulation exacerbated symptoms in about 60% of women. The most frequently reported relieving factors include masturbation, orgasm, distraction, intercourse, exercise, and cold compresses. Many of the women reported fatigue or a severe loss of energy (Leiblum et al., 2005; Waldinger, Venema, van Gils, & Schweitzer, 2009).

CONCEPTUALIZING PGAD

Atypical Pudendal Nerve Neuropathy

It has been suggested that PGAD is a neuropathy involving the pudendal and the dorsal clitoral nerves. The pudendal nerve derives from the second to fourth sacral levels of the spinal cord and sends sensory information from the perineum, anal area, and labia. A terminal branch of this nerve, the dorsal clitoral nerve, innervates the clitoris. These nerves under normal circumstances (e.g. digital stimulation) send sensory information to more central sites. It is postulated that in the pathological state they may spontaneously (i.e., without stimulation) produce pain (pudendal neuralgia) or, in the case of PGAD, a sensation of local sexual arousal and sometimes pain.

In the case of classical pudendal neuralgia, the symptoms may alter depending on posture. Similarly, many women with PGAD demonstrate exacerbation of genital symptoms with tight underwear and/or prolonged sitting (Waldinger, Venema, van Gils, & Schweitzer, 2009). Investigators have mapped mechanical "trigger points" based on hypersensitivity to static pressure in 23 volunteers with symptoms of PGAD. All women demonstrated preorgasmic or orgasmic sensations upon cotton swab examination along various points within the pudendal and dorsal clitoral nerve sensory areas. Eight women received local anesthetic blocks at one or more trigger points, and 5 reported resolution of all symptoms of PGAD for the duration of the block. It is suggested that C (small and unmyelinated) and A delta (myelinated) pudendal and/or dorsal clitoral nerve dysfunction, possibly caused by compression or irritation, underlies PGAD (Waldinger, Venema, et al., 2009). Further evidence of a pudendal neuropathic etiology comes from a recent paper by Rosenbaum (2010), who reported the case of a 27-year-old pregnant women with PGAD and hypertonic obturator internus muscles (part of the pelvic floor group) on physical exam. Two men with PGAD have recently been described who likely had a small fiber sensory neuropathy (Waldinger, Venema, van Gils, deLint, & Schweitzer, 2011).

Cognitive Disorder

Leiblum and Chivers (2007) have proposed a psychological model for PGAD. This model suggests that PGAD develops when anxious individuals become overly focused on their spontaneous genital arousal. This hypervigilance results in a vicious cycle of increased anxiety, elevated sympathetic tone, and more genital arousal. In addition, anxiety itself may decrease sensory thresholds, thus increasing the perception of genital arousal. Leiblum and Chivers (2007) have speculated that a history of abuse could further contribute to anxiety and negative association with genital arousal. This theory was motivated, in part, by an online survey of PGAD sufferers (Leiblum et al., 2007) which showed a high rate of psychological symptomatology, including panic attacks (31.6%), obsessive–compulsive illnesses (24%), and major depression (57.9%). Nearly two-thirds of these women reported that their anxiety and/ or depression predated their PGAD symptoms by at least 1 year. Fifty-three percent of women with PGAD in this survey reported suffering sexual abuse as children; however, only 16.7% thought that their current symptoms could be attributed to their prior abuse.

In clinical practice women with PGAD may have features suggestive of both of the preceding conceptualizations, that is, genital symptoms that are altered by posture as well as a background history of anxiety and unwanted sex. They may also complain of pain as well as unbidden arousal.

OTHER MEDICAL CONDITIONS ASSOCIATED WITH PGAD

Pharmacologically Induced

Several authors have noted a potential association between the initiation and withdrawal of selective serotonin and serotonin–norepinephrine reuptake inhibitors (SSRIs or SNRIs) and the onset of PGAD (Leiblum et al., 2007). Proposed mechanisms include rebound anxiety (on withdrawal of medication), C-nerve fiber pathology at the spinal level (Waldinger, de Lint, Venema, van Gils, & Schweitzer, 2009), genital vasodilatation following antidepressant withdrawal (Goldmeier & Leiblum, 2006), as well as a return to baseline libido and newfound awareness of genital sensations previously suppressed by the medication (Goldmeier & Leiblum, 2008).

Restless Legs and Bladder Symptoms

Waldinger and Schweitzer (2009) investigated 18 women with PGAD and found that two-thirds of these women also complained of overactive bladder symptoms (OAB; i.e., increased urgency for micturition) and restless leg syndrome (RLS). The authors suggest that PGAD may share an underlying neuropathic pathological state with OAB and RLS. As such, they propose that the new term "restless genital syndrome" (RGS) be adopted when PGAD is coincident with RLS.

Miscellaneous

There are a variety of other medical conditions that have been described in association with PGAD including epileptic foci, brain arteriovenous fistulas, and poststroke states (Anzellotti et al. 2010; Goldstein, De Elise, & Johnson, 2006); enlarged labial or pelvic veins (varices; Rosenbaum, 2010; Waldinger, van Gils, et al., 2009; Thorne & Stuckey, 2008); high soy intake (Amsterdam, Abu-Rustum, Carter, & Krychman, 2005); and sleep onset (Wylie, Levin, Hallam-Jones, & Goddard, 2005). These potentially important associations are not as yet well established, as they are based on case reports or small uncontrolled studies.

SEXUAL DYFUNCTIONS IN PGAD

Our clinical experience is that some women with PGAD have normal spontaneous or responsive sexual desire and enjoy genital stimulation and arousal and intercourse with their partners. They report, however, that the context of the genital stimulation is of major importance—that is, genital arousal with a partner is a positive and pleasant event, whereas unbidden genital arousal is distressing and unpleasant. Others, particularly those whose symptoms are controlled on pharmacotherapy, may have low desire and be subjectively nonresponsive but may agree to engage in sex to please their partners or because they derive emotional pleasure from such activity. Many such patients with PGAD would prefer not to have genital stimulation or vaginal intercourse, as it exacerbates or induces unpleasant genital arousal. A recent study of sexual functioning in women with a PGAD diagnosis used the Female Sexual Function Index (FSFI) questionnaire and compared their scores with those of women with female sexual arousal disorder (FSAD) and with controls (Leiblum & Seehuus, 2008). Women with PGAD showed a mean level of desire that was only slightly higher than control women, supporting the idea that PGAD is not a hypersexual state. Sexual satisfaction and pain were similar in the FSAD and PGAD groups. In all other respects the scores of women with PGAD fell between those of controls and the women with FSAD. The authors conclude that frequent unprovoked sexual arousal "is not necessarily indicative of either especially good or especially poor sexual function, at least as assessed by the FSFI."

DIAGNOSIS

Making a Clinical Assessment of PGAD

Full assessment of a woman with potential PGAD may require input from more than one health care professional. The initial clinical interview should be undertaken by a health care professional with sufficient time and expertise to get a full psychosocial, psychosexual, and medical history while making the woman feel comfortable. Figure 12.1 illustrates the crucial assessment areas that need to be covered. A psychologist or sex therapist may often be an ideal health professional to undertake this initial assessment, as he or she will be familiar with the relevant psychosocial and psychosexual issues and methods of assessment. A psychologist or sex therapist, however, would have to familiarize him- or herself with the relevant medical domains and, if appropriate, get help from a suitable professional. The important medical areas to be assessed are also listed in Figure 12.1. An appropriately trained physician or nurse can also carry out such an assessment. Time and comfort are essential, because many women suffering from PGAD have previously felt rejected or not listened to by clinicians or, worse still, may have been diagnosed with a primary delusional illness. The assessor needs to carefully yet compassionately obtain a full description of the PGAD symptom profile, including site, quality, duration, exacerbating and relieving factors, whether the genital arousal is preceded by desire, whether there is concomitant pain, and how long the women spends masturbating in an attempt to relieve the symptoms. Exacerbating factors include pressure on the genitals, vibrations (e.g., car driving), visual sexual stimuli, genital stimulation or intercourse, and anxiety. Relieving factors include medications, masturbation, orgasm, distraction, and physical exercise. For a clinician to make a working diagnosis of PGAD, patients should complain of unbidden sexual arousal/dysesthesia that (1) persists for an extended period of time (i.e., at least several hours); (2) does not subside spontaneously or with ordinary orgasmic experience (i.e., may require

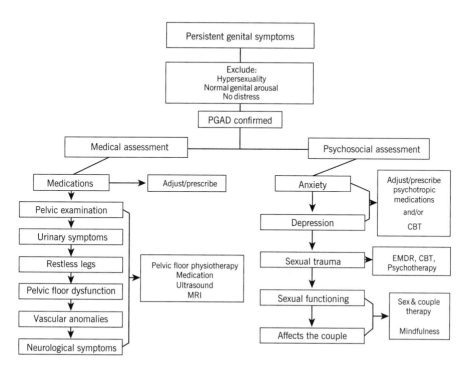

FIGURE 12.1. Treatment algorithm for PGAD.

multiple orgasms over hours or days in order to gain some relief); (3) causes a clinically significant degree of distress.

Working with the Physician/Gynecologist

Once PGAD is suspected, the nonmedical clinician should work with a physician or gynecologist to carry out the necessary medical assessment. At a minimum, this should involve a lower genital examination (to look for sensory changes and genital varices) and a pelvic examination. Where pelvic varices or pudendal nerve entrapment is suspected, working with an experienced radiologist using MRI scanning will yield the most meaningful data. Current and past medications should be reviewed, as well as possible comorbid conditions, including voiding symptoms, urinary tract infections, restless leg symptoms, and a history suggestive of seizures, epilepsy, or temporal lobe events. Pelvic floor dysfunction is best assessed by a pelvic floor physical therapist.

THE TREATMENT PROCESS

The algorithm in Figure 12.1 illustrating the potential process of assessment and associated treatments is based on our clinical experience. As far as we are aware, there are no empirically validated diagnostic criteria or treatment algorithms for PGAD. Thus we cannot as yet define how long genital symptoms must last or the degree of distress necessary; this must be left to clinician judgment. It is not yet known in which order treatments should be tried or whether they should be tried simultaneously. It is logical that if PGAD symptoms started with the initiation of a particular medication or life event, then this should be carefully investigated. Because of this lack of knowledge, it seems crucial for one clinician to monitor and coordinate the assessment and treatment process.

Unless there is a simple remediable medical cause, mindfulness-based cognitive-behavior therapy (CBT) is recommended as a treatment for most patients. As a result, we highlight the role of the psychologist/sex therapist.

TREATMENT BY A SEX THERAPIST/PSYCHOLOGIST

Mindfulness-Based CBT

For the majority of women with PGAD, the role of the clinical psychologist/sex therapist is to help the patient manage and cope with symptoms of PGAD rather than finding a cure. CBT is a useful tool for women with genital pain and therefore likely to be useful for PGAD (Lofrisco, 2011). PGAD can easily rule over all other aspects of the patient's life so that the woman's thinking becomes very negative. Explaining to the woman that she likely has a subtle derangement of her pudendal nerve that won't cause damage but can be exacerbated by anxiety is very important. Reassuring her that she is neither a sex maniac nor insane is also crucial. Women suffering from PGAD often think catastrophically (e.g., "this problem rules my whole life," "my genitals must be grossly abnormal," or " this must be due to masturbating too much as a teenager"). Such thinking should be challenged point by point.

There is often an understandable urge to masturbate to orgasm to relieve symptoms. This can take on features of a compulsion. Many women find that refraining from masturbation leads to an overall lessening of their symptoms, as well as to freeing up the women from spending a lot of her time trying to relieve their symptoms. Other women find that their PGAD builds up to a crescendo over days and that a session of repeated masturbation and orgasm over hours can bring some degree of relief. Working with the patient to explore extending periods of masturbation abstinence may guide therapist and patient. So, for instance, an exacerbation of physical symptoms with little anxiety might suggest that masturbation at intervals would be useful. However, if the major theme is an increase in anxiety at abstinence, then exploring and managing this may be more beneficial than repeated masturbation.

Mindfulness is now seen by many psychologists as an important additional therapy to be used in conjunction with CBT (Kabat-Zinn, 2005). There is reasonable evidence that its regular use decreases anxiety, depression, and the suffering aspect of pain, as well as altering brain structure, function, and immune responses (Goldmeier & Mears, 2010). The practice of mindfulness requires that the patient focus on the breath and also observe distractions such as thoughts or physical discomforts. One way that mindfulness may work is by increasing focus on any event or situation, with distractions becoming increasingly peripheral. Thus one can learn to observe the sensations of PGAD rather than experiencing them with negative thoughts ("Will this ever stop?" "I can take this no longer," "When will I have to masturbate next?"). Focusing on the "naked" PGAD symptoms, that is, observing the exact site and quality of the PGAD sensations for 10–20 minutes a day, alongside mindfully observing the mind's reaction to it, has had very useful outcomes in some of our patients. After some weeks of mindfulness training, which might include 20 minutes of focusing on the breath and 20 minutes focusing on the PGAD itself, patients may feel they can more easily live alongside the PGAD symptoms and can learn to recognize thoughts and emotions secondary to these and gently put those on one side. In effect, the patient comes to be more accepting of her PGAD symptoms. Such acceptance has been shown to help pain and therefore likely to help PGAD symptoms (Vowles, McCracken, & O'Brien, 2011). Our own patients who are motivated to do regular mindfulness exercises anecdotally report significant improvement in their quality of life. In light of the associated psychological aspects of PGAD described before, it should not be surprising that management of anxiety and depression has yielded good results in some of our patients. Those who have been sexually assaulted may derive great benefit from specific therapies such as revisiting and reconstructing these events under carefully controlled conditions (Littrell, 1998).

Enhancing Sexual Functioning in the Patient with PGAD

Most women with PGAD are highly focused on alleviating their symptoms rather than being sexual. They find that genital touching or sexual arousal precipitates or exacerbates their symptoms, at least in certain trigger areas (Leiblum et al., 2005; Waldinger, Venema, et al., 2009). Our experience is that being sexual and being sexually stimulated are very far from their minds. The prescribed pharmacotherapy may also cause problems with desire, subjective and genital arousal, and orgasm. It is only a minority of women with PGAD who are able to respond to sexual desire in relation to a partner and then proceed to arousal that is pleasurable. Many women may find pleasure in nongenital stimulation, but find that once sexual arousal is present, so is the PGAD. Women who have intermittent symptoms are often sexual between exacerbations, and women whose symptoms are controlled want to return to intercourse in order to keep their relationships going. Most women with PGAD find that connecting emotionally rather than sexually is what they want to achieve.

The clinician should broach the topic of sexual functioning in all women suffering from PGAD. We feel we are on a learning curve in regard to addressing this issue, so we stress the importance of a thorough assessment. We suggest asking the patient for details of how her PGAD affects sex with her partner, including the following:

1. Does sexual arousal with her partner always trigger PGAD? If not, when does the PGAD get triggered and when does it not?
2. Are there certain places on her body where she can enjoy sexual stimulation or sexual/sensual touch that does not trigger PGAD? Similarly, are there certain sexual activities that do or do not become triggers?
3. If all sexual arousal causes an exacerbation of the PGAD, does stimulating her partner also result in an increase in symptomatology? Is the idea or thought of sex problematic?

Input from the partner is important. However, we recommend interviewing the patient privately, as in a conjoint session she may hide the extent of her symptoms in order not to hurt or upset her partner. A later interview with the couple will allow for the partner's perceptions to be included in the assessment and may also help the patient understand how the PGAD affects him or her. Many partners are perplexed regarding the fact that sexual activity is avoided, even though it reliably results in orgasm. The partner's need or desire for sex, as well as the patient's own sexual problems or dysfunctions, should be part of the assessment, as these issues will inform treatment decisions.

Treatment directed toward the couple's sexual relationship focuses on the same issues that individual treatment does: managing and coping with the symptoms of PGAD, rather than "curing" them. Reassurance is also important. Sharing the diagnosis and the results of the assessment with the couple can alleviate tensions built on misconceptions regarding the nature and origin of the problem. It is important to distinguish PGAD from hypersexuality or sexual aversion and also to dispel the notion that somehow the partner is responsible for the problem. Treatment options for patient and partner will depend on their interest in having sex, as well as the way that PGAD manifests in the sexual relationship. These options range from no sexual activity to sexual stimulation only for the partner (or limited sexual or sensual stimulation for the PGAD sufferer) to sex between exacerbations of PGAD to sexual activity knowing that the symptoms of PGAD will likely worsen. In the latter scenario, the patient should be encouraged to engage in mindfulness during sex, noticing the genital sensations but focusing on the emotional connection. After sex, masturbation, mindfulness, yoga, or cold compresses may help to control the symptoms.

CONTEMPORANEOUS TREATMENT BY A PHYSICIAN

Based on the findings of the medical assessment, the physician's major role may be to prescribe or adjust medication (see Facelle, Sadeghi-Nejad, & Goldmeier, 2012, for a review). SSRIs, SNRIs, and tricyclic antidepressants have been reported to have useful effects as anxiolytics, antidepressants, analgesics, and in some cases antiobsessionals. Other drugs with which success has been reported are antipsychotics (e.g., quetiapine), dopaminergic agents (e.g., varenicline), benzodiazepines (e.g., clonazepam; however, continuous use may lead to dependence), and atypical opiates (e.g., tramadol). The composite clinical picture and its spectrum of symptoms should help dictate the medication choice. The final decision should be taken after consultation with all the health care workers involved plus the patient. For example, if the major symptomatology is PGAD in the absence of psychiatric features, then gabapentin might be the initial drug of choice; if it is PGAD associated with anxiety, then a low-dose antipsychotic might be appropriate; if it is PGAD associated with depression, then tricyclics or SSRI antidepressants might be most appropriate.

CONTEMPORANEOUS TREATMENT
WITH PELVIC FLOOR PHYSICAL THERAPY

The pudendal nerve can become "entrapped" or compressed, usually causing vulval/clitoral pain that is worse on sitting and relieved on standing. Rosenbaum (2010) has described a case of a pregnant woman in whom the PGAD symptoms were immediately relieved on massaging and manipulating one of the pelvic floor muscles (the obturator internus), which in this woman's case was overcontracted. The patient reported "that something had been released." Rosenbaum (2010) theorizes that the pelvic floor tonicity may have compressed the pudendal nerve in Alcock's canal, leading to her symptoms, and that the soft tissue mobilization released this tension

TENS (transcutaneous electrical nerve stimulation) produces its effects by activation of opioid receptors in the central nervous system. Some of our patients have found it very helpful. Similar anecdotal successes have been described in the literature (Waldinger, de Lint, et al., 2010).

In principle, pelvic floor physical therapy should be very useful when there is sensory disruption of the pelvic floor musculature. There has been little systematic work reported to date, and it is not clear whether biofeedback or the full range of manual techniques used by pelvic floor physical therapists will be useful. In our clinical experience, physical therapy has been helpful in only a very few cases.

CASE DISCUSSION

Development of Symptoms

Belinda was a 52-year-old primary school teacher. Two years ago she became depressed after her father died of lung cancer. The grief reaction of the first 6 months after his passing seemed to exacerbate after the onset of her menopause at that time. Her family practitioner diagnosed a mixed affective disorder in that she displayed quite high levels of anxiety as well as depression. She suffered morbid thoughts but no active suicidal ideation. Along with the depression, she began to develop disturbing sensations in her genital area. These included a sensation as if she were sexually aroused. She found these feelings highly distressing inasmuch as she had had no sexual interest since her father died. Belinda was at this stage too ashamed to reveal or discuss this issue with anyone. The sensations "rippled" up and down her genital area all day long and kept her awake much of the night. Although she found it difficult to precisely describe the sensations, they included a "tingling" and almost "pain-like congestion" quality. At times, she felt she was very close to orgasm, so she tried clitoral stimulation to see if that would help. Orgasm relieved the uncomfortable sensations for 1–2 minutes but seemed to initiate muscle "twitching" just inside the outer genital area that was equally distressing. Two to 3 minutes after orgasm, Belinda found herself back with both the distressing genital sensations and the muscle twitchings. Many days she masturbated up to 30 times in a row.

Belinda felt that these sensations "hounded " her and that her genitals were about to explode. She felt that they had taken over her thoughts and her life and often thought of nothing else. The more tense she got, the worse they became.

Her general practitioner prescribed sertraline at this point. Her depression gradually improved over 8–10 weeks. However, her genital sensations continued with the same frequency and intensity. She eventually discussed her symptoms with one of the doctors in her general practice, who was sympathetic but confessed she did not know what the cause of her problem might be. At this point she came to see one of us, having looked up what her condition might be on the Internet.

Belinda's Background

Belinda was born and brought up in northern England. Her parents were Catholic but had very broadminded and liberal views on most matters, including sex and sex education. She had no significant physical illness in childhood but suffered from enuresis till age 9. Looking back over her adolescent and teenage years, she felt she was very shy and thought she might have had panic attacks in her early 20s. She went to a Catholic school where she was very happy and achieved high marks, studying art at a university and then going on to teacher's training college, where she met her first husband, Tom, also a teacher. She describes him as very attractive and very sexually needy, from the outset having to have sex every night when possible. In the first 2 years of their relationship, she mostly enjoyed this, but once the children came along and she "had two jobs—one at work and the other at home," she began to dread sex. In many other respects, he was a caring father and husband but seemed to "thoughtlessly and selfishly demand sex"—although when he did so it was not rough but rather an emotionless event for Belinda. This went on for 20 years, at which time she was 43 and felt she could no longer live with him. Her three children had by this time all grown up and left home.

At age 45 she met Joe, her second husband, who was a year younger than she. She said she was emotionally very close to him and that their sexual life was consensual, although for Belinda intercourse was more of an emotional than a sexual event. However, at times when she made love with Joe she found herself thinking about sex with Tom and "froze up." She told Joe about this, and he reacted in a "very understanding way."

Assessment

On direct questioning Belinda still reported high anxiety levels with occasional panic attacks. She had a somewhat perfectionistic personality (e.g., she liked the house very tidy) but no overt obsessional–compulsive illness and had no features of depression.

Her genital symptoms were continuously present in the background but became worse at night, preventing and interrupting sleep. Once every week or so the symptoms reached a peak, when she had to clitorally stimulate herself to orgasm repeatedly over a period that lasted up to 5 hours (her "sorting out"), after which she was exhausted but symptomatically much improved. Because of her genital symptoms, she had to take a long-term sick leave from schoolteaching.

Belinda did not have restless legs or urinary symptoms, had no other illnesses, and had sustained no pelvic or head trauma. External genital examination appeared normal apart from a small patch of psoriasis on the left labium majus. There was no allodynia in the vulvar vestibule but definite hypersensitivity on cotton bud testing of the periclitoral and suprapubic area. Digital palpation of the left pubococcygeus muscle showed it to be hypertonic and tender.

Pelvic ultrasound was normal, as was a gadolinium-enhanced MRI scan of the pelvis—no incompetent veins, pelvic masses, or visible pathology along the path of the pudendal nerve. An MRI of the brain and spinal cord, as well as an EEG, were normal. A full blood count, thyroid, renal, and liver function tests were normal. Hormonally she presented a postmenopausal picture.

Therapy

The patient's dose of sertraline was increased to 40 mg per day. This and adding, in sequence, amitriptyline, nortriptyline, and quetiapine did not help and caused major side effects, so none of these medications were continued. Varenicline was not given because of her history of depression. Gabapentin (300 mg at night) was well tolerated but caused somnolence, which was a therapeutic advantage. TENS also proved unhelpful. Hormone replacement therapy given for 6 months was also unhelpful. She had sessions with a pelvic floor physiotherapist but did not find these helpful.

Belinda also undertook sessions in CBT. The likely pathology of PGAD was explained insomuch as it might be seen as a pudendal/clitoral nerve neuralgia that was exacerbated by stress and fear of the condition itself. The sensations coming from the genital area, it was explained, could be modified by a positive emotional and affective outlook on the issue. Pleasant imagery was taught for her to use when the PGAD symptoms became very severe. Cognitive restructuring was also initiated, so that negative cognitions (e.g., "PGAD is taking over my life") were replaced with more positive ones (i.e., "I can have a productive and enjoyable life in spite of having PGAD"). During therapy she was taught to use this type of thinking over increasingly large parts of the day.

She was also taught mindfulness meditation in the clinic, as well as by book and CD (Williams, Teasdale, Segal, & Kabat-Zinn, 2007), and practiced it for 30 minutes a day. This was done by learning to focus on both her breath and other parts of her body. Distracting thoughts and feelings were to be seen as important in that they were to be observed, followed by a gentle return to the focus of the meditation. Belinda also spent 15 minutes a day mindfully looking at the PGAD itself—examining its exact site, texture, and radiation. Once again, she was taught to observe the thought that came with the PGAD (e.g., "PGAD is so awful—can I cope?") and to observe these cognitions for 1–2 minutes and then compassionately and gently return to the focus of the meditation.

In terms of the unwanted sex with her first husband, she did 10 sessions of revisiting, reexperiencing, and reprocessing these events with an expert in psychological trauma therapy (Littrell, 1998). Six months later Belinda was back at work teaching and was, on the whole, enjoying life. She was much better at coping with the PGAD during the day and slept well by night. She reported being much less anxious and had not had a panic attack. However, she still had to spend up to 5 hours about once a week "sorting out." Intercourse continued as an emotional but not a sexual event for her. However, there were no longer psychological "freeze ups."

This case history reflects many of the typical features of the cases of PGAD that we have treated. The range of comorbid problems and reactions to different therapies is, however, very wide. Some women suffering with PGAD do not have antecedent or current psychiatric problems or past unwanted sex. Others are similar to Belinda. Some respond remarkably well to simple mindfulness-based CBT; others refuse all psychological therapies and demand medication. A few of our patients have done so well that they no longer require our care. However, the majority continue to see us, albeit with some degree of improvement in the quality of their lives.

CONCLUSIONS

Without the groundbreaking work of Sandra Leiblum and Sharon Nathan (2001), we probably would not have a label for the problem of PGAD, and this chapter would not exist. Although it is still not clear whether PGAD is a unitary syndrome, we are now in a position to investigate this issue and some of the explanatory mechanisms that have been proposed. It is hoped that the chapter on PGAD in the next edition of *Principles and Practice of Sex Therapy* will report significant therapeutic advances.

REFERENCES

Amsterdam, A., Abu-Rustum, N., Carter, J., & Krychman, M. (2005). Persistent sexual arousal syndrome associated with increased soy intake. *Journal of Sexual Medicine*, 2(3), 338–340.

Anzellotti, F., Franciotti, R., Bonanni, L., Tamburro, G., Perrucci, M. G., Thomas, A., et al. (2010). Persistent genital arousal disorder associated with functional hyperconnectivity of an epileptic focus. *Neuroscience*, 167(1), 88–96.

Facelle, T. M., Sadeghi-Nejad, H., & Goldmeier, D. (2013). Persistent genital arousal disorder: Characterization, etiology, and management. *Journal of Sexual Medicine*, 10(2), 439–450.

Garvey, L. J., West, C., Latch, N., Leiblum, S., & Goldmeier, D. (2009). Report of spontaneous and persistent genital arousal in women attending a sexual health clinic. *International Journal of STD and AIDS*, 20(8), 519–521.

Goldmeier, D., & Leiblum, S. R. (2006). Persistent genital arousal in women: A new syndrome entity. *International Journal of STD and AIDS*, 17(4), 215–216.

Goldmeier, D., & Leiblum, S. (2008). Interaction of organic and psychological factors in persistent genital arousal disorder in women: A report of six cases. *International Journal of STD and AIDS*, 19(7), 488–490.

Goldmeier, D., & Mears, A. J. (2010). Meditation: A review of its use in western medicine and, in particular, its role in the management of sexual dysfunction. *Current Psychiatry Reviews, 6*(1), 11–14.

Goldstein, I., De Elise, J. B., & Johnson, J. A. (2006). Persistent sexual arousal syndrome and clitoral priapism. In I. Goldstein, C. M. Meston, S. Davis, & A. Traish (Eds.), *Women's sexual function and dysfunction: Study, diagnosis and treatment* (pp. 674–685). London: Taylor & Francis.

Kabat-Zinn, J. (1990). *Full catastrophe living: Using the wisdom of your body and mind to face stress, pain, and illness.* New York: Bantam Doubleday Dell.

Kafka, M. P. (2010). Hypersexual disorder: A proposed diagnosis for DSM-V. *Archives of Sexual Behavior, 39*(2), 377–400.

Leiblum, S., Brown, C., Wan, J., & Rawlinson, L. (2005). Persistent sexual arousal syndrome: A descriptive study. *Journal of Sexual Medicine, 2*(3), 331–337.

Leiblum, S., Seehuus, M., & Brown, C. (2007). Persistent genital arousal: Disordered or normative aspect of female sexual response? *Journal of Sexual Medicine, 4*(3), 680–689.

Leiblum, S. R., & Chivers, M. L. (2007). Normal and persistent genital arousal in women: New perspectives. *Journal of Sex and Marital Therapy, 33*(4), 357–373.

Leiblum, S. R., & Nathan, S. G. (2001). Persistent sexual arousal syndrome: A newly discovered pattern of female sexuality. *Journal of Sex and Marital Therapy, 27*(4), 365–380.

Leiblum, S. R., & Seehuus, M. (2008). FSFI scores of women with persistent genital arousal disorder compared with published scores of women with female sexual arousal disorder and healthy controls. *Journal of Sexual Medicine, 6*(2), 469–473.

Littrell, J. (1998). Is the reexperience of painful emotion therapeutic? *Clinical Psychology Review, 18*(1), 71–102.

Lofrisco, B. M. (2011). Female sexual pain disorders and cognitive-behavioral therapy. *Journal of Sex Research, 48*(6), 573–579.

Rosenbaum, T. Y. (2010). Physical therapy treatment of persistent genital arousal disorder during pregnancy: A case report. *Journal of Sexual Medicine, 7*(3), 1306–1310.

Soranus of Ephesus. (1991). *Soranus' gynecology* (Owsei Temkin, Trans.) [electronic resource]. Baltimore: Johns Hopkins University Press.

Thorne, C., & Stuckey, B. (2008). Pelvic congestion syndrome presenting as persistent genital arousal: A case report. *Journal of Sexual Medicine, 5*(2), 504–508.

Vowles, K. E., McCracken, L. M., & O'Brien, J. Z. (2011). Acceptance and values-based action in chronic pain: A three-year follow-up analysis of treatment effectiveness and process. *Behaviour Research and Therapy, 49*(11), 748–755.

Waldinger, M. D., de Lint, G. J., Venema, P. L., van Gils, A. P., & Schweitzer, D. H. (2009). Successful transcutaneous electrical nerve stimulation in two women with restless genital syndrome: The role of A delta and C-nerve fibers. *Journal of Sexual Medicine, 7*(3), 1190–1199.

Waldinger, M. D., & Schweitzer, D. H. (2009). Persistent genital arousal disorder in 18 Dutch women: Part II. A syndrome clustered with restless legs and overactive bladder. *Journal of Sexual Medicine, 6*(2), 482–497.

Waldinger, M. D., van Gils, A. P., Ottervanger, H. P., Vandenbroucke, W. V., & Tavy, D. L. (2009). Persistent genital arousal disorder in 18 Dutch women: Part I. MRI,

EEG, and transvaginal ultrasonography investigations. *Journal of Sexual Medicine*, 6(2), 474–481.

Waldinger, M. D., Venema, P. L., van Gils, A. P., de Lint, G. J., & Schweitzer, D. H. (2011). Stronger evidence for small fiber sensory neuropathy in restless genital syndrome: Two case reports in males. *Journal of Sexual Medicine*, 8(1), 325–330.

Waldinger, M. D., Venema, P. L., van Gils, A. P., & Schweitzer, D. H. (2009). New insights into restless genital syndrome: Static mechanical hyperesthesia and neuropathy of the nervus dorsalis clitoridis. *Journal of Sexual Medicine*, 6(10), 2778–2787.

Williams, J. M. G., Teasdale, J. D., Segal, Z. V., & Kabat-Zinn, J. (2007). *The mindful way through depression: Freeing yourself from chronic unhappiness*. New York: Guilford Press.

Wylie, K., Levin, R., Hallam-Jones, R., & Goddard, A. (2005). Sleep exacerbation of persistent sexual arousal syndrome in a postmenopausal woman. *Journal of Sexual Medicine*, 3(2), 296–302.

CHAPTER 13

Nonparaphilic Hypersexuality Disorders

Martin P. Kafka

In recent years, there has been a veritable explosion in therapeutic approaches, self-help books, and groups aimed at the treatment of "sexual addiction." In this chapter, Kafka uses the term "nonparaphilic hypersexuality disorder" to describe this phenomenon, while leaving aside the issue of cause. Hypersexual disorders (HDs) feature "disinhibited or exaggerated expressions of human sexual arousal and appetites. . . . involving sexual behaviors that are culturally considered within the range of normal or conventional." According to Kafka, HDs and paraphilias are "arguably the most shame- and guilt-inducing contemporary psychiatric conditions." HDs are often kept secret from the person's partner and friends, and its clinical presentation is often masked, appearing paradoxically as low desire. Kafka describes how the symptom constellation of HDs is actually quite complex and that these problems are often accompanied by paraphilias, severe relationship distress, and comorbid psychiatric conditions, such as bipolar disorder, depression, anxiety, and attention-deficit/hyperactivity disorder (ADHD). Given this complexity, treatment cannot be a prepackaged in a one-size-fits-all approach. Sex therapy will often be the point of entry for an individual or couple struggling with HD, but medication, self-help support groups, behavior therapy techniques, couple therapy, and individual psychotherapy will often be part of the treatment armamentarium.

Martin P. Kafka, MD, is a Clinical Associate Professor of Psychiatry at Harvard Medical School in Boston, Massachusetts, a Senior Clinical Associate at McLean Hospital, Belmont, Massachusetts, and a Distinguished Life Fellow of the American Psychiatric Association. He was a member of the DSM-5 Sexual and Gender Disorders Work Group. In 2010, Dr. Kafka was awarded the Carnes Award for achievement by the Society for Sexual Health.

HISTORICAL OVERVIEW

Nonparaphilic hypersexuality disorders are disinhibited or exaggerated expressions of human sexual arousal and appetites. In contrast to paraphilic disorders, a group characterized by unconventional or even "deviant" sexual arousal, nonparaphilic hypersexuality disorders are "normophilic," that is, involving sexual behaviors that are culturally considered within the range of normal or conventional. The modern clinical view of these disorders dates from the late 19th century, with the pioneering work in Europe of Richard von Krafft-Ebing (1886/1965), Havelock Ellis (1905), and Magnus Hirschfeld (1948). These investigators observed a spectrum of persistent, socially deviant sexual behaviors that we now call paraphilias (PAs). They further noted clinical examples of males and females whose nonparaphilic sexual appetites, including compulsive masturbation, appeared insatiable. Their clinical characterizations were amplified in the 20th century with other disorders, such as protracted promiscuity, identified as "Don Juanism" or satyriasis in men and nymphomania in women.

CONTEMPORARY CLINICAL CONCEPTUALIZATIONS OF NONPARAPHILIC HYPERSEXUALITY

In 1978, Orford suggested that excessive sexual appetites and activities, including promiscuity, could be understood as a syndrome with many resemblances to addiction, even in the absence of an actual substance being abused (Orford, 1978, 1985). The clinical concept of "sexual addiction" was further popularized by the publication of Carnes's descriptive book *Out of the Shadows: Understanding Sexual Addiction* (Carnes, 1983) and other publications (Carnes, 1989, 1990, 1991). The clinical term has been enthusiastically embraced by the popular press. It has particularly struck a chord with people who feel themselves subject to either repetitive paraphilic or nonparaphilic hypersexual behaviors that they find difficult to control and that lead to undesirable and significant psychosocial consequences.

The term "sexual compulsivity" was introduced by Quadland (1985) around the time of Carnes's first publication. He suggested this term to describe volitional impairment associated with nonparaphilic hypersexual behavior. His term has subsequently been taken up as a descriptor for both paraphilic and nonparaphilic sexual behavior disorders by a number of investigators (Coleman, 1986, 1987; Anthony & Hollander, 1993; Black, 1998; Black, Kehrberg, Flumerfelt, & Schlosser, 1997). The applicability to both paraphilic and nonparaphilic disorders has been the subject of some debate (Coleman, 1986), with the upshot that a hybrid term, "sexual compulsivity/addiction" (or the reverse), is now used to cover both cases (Shaffer, 1994).

Kinsey Institute researchers have outlined a theoretical model for sexual appetite and have illustrated its applicability to nonparaphilic "out-of-control" sexual behaviors (Bancroft & Vukadinovic, 2004). Bancroft and associates put forward a dual-control model of sexual arousal (Bancroft & Janssen, 2000) that postulates a centrally mediated homeostasis between sexual excitation and sexual inhibition in males and females. They have developed a validated scale of proneness to excitation and inhibition to assess how social or clinical groups might differ in these regards. In this view, "sexual risk takers" would show low inhibition or high excitation or both and would thus tend in particular toward promiscuous behavior. They concur with other investigators (Carnes, 1989; Coleman, 1987; Kafka, 1991) that "negative" mood states, especially anxiety and depression, can be associated with both sexual promiscuity and increased masturbation (Bancroft, Janssen, Strong, Carnes, et al., 2003; Bancroft, Janssen, Strong, & Vukadinovic, 2003). They have applied their model and rating instruments to a small group of "sexual addicts" and found that those self-identified persons had low sexual inhibition and high sexual excitation and that these characteristics were associated with anxious/depressive mood states (Bancroft & Vukadinovic, 2004).

I have suggested the term "paraphilia-related disorder" (PRD; Kafka & Hennen, 1999; Kafka & Prentky, 1994, 1998) for specific nonparaphilic hypersexual conditions. Unlike "impulsivity," "compulsivity," or "addiction," this term is not bound to explanatory models for these specific actions and behaviors. Nevertheless, it acknowledges that such behaviors, although not socially deviant, may share many of the same clinical characteristics as the family of paraphilic disorders.

Following the DSM nosology (American Psychiatric Association, 2000), PRDs like PAs, persist for at least 6 months, are manifested by intense and arousing sexual fantasies, urges, and activities, and produce personal distress or significant psychosocial impairment (Kafka, 2007).

In organized American psychiatry, sexual deviations were recognized as personality disorders in the second edition of the *Diagnostic and Statistical Manual of Mental Disorders* (DSM-II; American Psychiatric Association, 1968), but that document made no mention of nonparaphilic hypersexuality disorders. By 1980, however, DSM-III (American Psychiatric Association, 1980) had subclassified paraphilic disorders as distinct pathologies, that is, as sexual disorders. Don Juanism and nymphomania were included as psychosexual disorders not otherwise specified. In DSM-IV (American Psychiatric Association, 1994) and DSM-IV-TR (American Psychiatric Association, 2000), there were no specific designations describing paraphilia-related disorders, although sexual disorders not otherwise specified (302.9) includes a condition described as "distress about a pattern of repeated sexual relationships involving a succession of lovers who are experienced by the individual only as things to be used" (American Psychiatric Association, 2000, p. 582)

Over the past 30 years, sufficient empirical data have been published from these aforementioned clinical perspectives to allow the formulation of a composite diagnostic entity, hypersexual disorder (HD) (Kafka, 2010), which was proposed for but not included in the fifth edition of the *Diagnostic and Statistical Manual of Mental Disorders* (DSM-5; American Psychiatric Association, 2013). The most current formulation for HD is presented in Table 13.1.

The diagnosis of HD was constructed from the in-common core factors derived from the most rigorously validated and reliable rating scales published in refereed Journals. Rating scales included the Sexual Compulsivity Scale (Kalichman & Rompa, 1995), the Sexual Addiction Screening Test (Carnes, 1991), the Kinsey Institute's rating scales (Janssen, Vorst, Finn, & Bancroft, 2002a, 2002b), the Compulsive Sexual Behavior Inventory (Coleman, Miner,

---

TABLE 13.1. Proposed Diagnostic Criteria for Hypersexual Disorder

A. Over a period of at least 6 months, recurrent and intense sexual fantasies, sexual urges, and sexual behavior in association with four or more of the following five criteria:
   1. Excessive time is consumed by sexual fantasies and urges, and by planning for and engaging in sexual behavior.
   2. Repetitively engaging in these sexual fantasies, urges, and behavior in response to dysphoric mood states (e.g., anxiety, depression, boredom, irritability).
   3. Repetitively engaging in sexual fantasies, urges, and behavior in response to stressful life events.
   4. Repetitive but unsuccessful efforts to control or significantly reduce these sexual fantasies, urges, and behavior.
   5. Repetitively engaging in sexual behavior while disregarding the risk for physical or emotional harm to self or others.

B. There is clinically significant personal distress or impairment in social, occupational, or other important areas of functioning associated with the frequency and intensity of these sexual fantasies, urges, and behavior.

C. These sexual fantasies, urges, and behavior are not due to direct physiological effects of exogenous substances (e.g., drugs of abuse or medications), a co-occurring medical condition, or to manic episodes.

D. The person is at least 18 years of age.

Specify if:
   Masturbation
   Pornography
   Sexual behavior with consenting adults
   Cybersex
   Telephone Sex
   Adult entertainment venues/clubs
   Other:

Specify if:
   In remission (no distress, impairment, or recurring behavior for 5 years and in an uncontrolled environment)
   In a controlled environment

Note. Copyright 2013 by the American Psychiatric Association. Reprinted by permission.

Ohlerking, & Raymond, 2001), and, most recently, the Hypersexual Behavior Inventory (Reid, Ganes, & Carpenter, 2011). In an independent multicenter field trial testing how well these proposed criteria "fit" persons seeking treatment for "sexual addiction" or "hypersexual behavior," Rory Reid and associates reported robust reliability and discriminative validity administering a rating scale devised directly from the specific HD criteria and administered to men seeking such treatment ($N = 152$) in comparison with those with nonsexual psychiatric disorders ($N = 35$), as well as substance abuse disorders ($N = 20$; Reid et al., 2012). The diagnostic criteria for HD also were significantly associated with theoretically related measures of hypersexuality, impulsivity, emotional dysregulation, and stress proneness. Patients assessed for HD also reported a vast array of consequences for hypersexual behavior that were significantly greater than for those diagnosed with a general psychiatric condition or substance-related disorder. The behavioral specifiers that would accompany the diagnosis of HD are also behaviors described in the sexual addiction, sexual compulsivity, paraphilia-related disorders, and other hypersexual behavior empirical literatures.

There has been recent controversy as to whether HD is really just "sexual addiction" but with a new appellation. DSM-5 is intended as an "atheoretical" text, listing disorders in broad categories until the etiology of a specific disorder has been clearly elaborated. At present, the etiologies of paraphilias or HD are unknown. It should be noted, however, that the five proposed "A criteria" for HD (see Table 13.1) are all compatible with the definition of a dependence syndrome or a behavioral addiction (e.g., as in psychoactive substance dependence in DSM-IV). The rating instruments reviewed to synthesize HD, however, do not sufficiently measure important domains associated with addictions, such as behavioral tolerance (e.g., escalation of behaviors or increased risk taking) and withdrawal phenomenology. This does not mean that these phenomena do not clinically exist; we need carefully constructed rating scales to look at these phenomena to see how frequently they can accompany HD behaviors and how to best operationalize these phenomena. There are both similarities and differences between pathological gambling and HD and whether HD behavioral addiction requires further research (Kor, Fogel, Reid, & Potenza, 2013).

Although HD was considered for placement in the section of DSM-5 saved for newly proposed psychiatric disorders that require more empirical research, it was ultimately rejected for such placement. Researchers and clinicians should further explore the clinical utility of the proposed diagnostic criteria, as well as investigate aspects such as family history, specific developmental vicissitudes, and neurobiological components. It would also be important to obtain larger epidemiological studies to assess whether the proposed criteria for HD adequately discriminate prospective patients from those who do not have a nonparaphilic sexual impulsivity disorder. For example, would there be a high false-positive diagnosis of HD among adolescents in a large nonpatient community sample? As has been stated so commonly in published journal articles, "more research is needed" to establish the diagnostic reliability and validity of HD. This adage is particularly true when constructing a psychiatric disorder characterizing sexual behavior in general and normophilic sexual behaviors specifically.

The failure of HD to achieve any designated placement in DSM-5 leaves clinicians in a quandary of how to adequately diagnose or categorize persons who would otherwise have been designated by sexual disorder not otherwise specified, a residual diagnostic category, in Prior DSM editions. While HD is not a sexual dysfunction nor a paraphilia, it can be considered an impulsivity disorder and thus can be diagnosed as "Other Specified Disruptive, Impulse-Control, and Conduct Disorder: hypersexual disorder" (ICD 312.89) (American Psychiatric Association, 2013, p. 479). For physicians who favor other designations for nonparaphilic sexual behavior disorders requiring clinical assessment and treatment or who have patients who do not meet criteria for HD, the ICD 312.89 code can be followed by other clinical descriptors, such as, but not limited to, sexual addiction/compulsivity, or nonparaphilic hypersexual behavior.

In the following sections of this chapter, I use the term HD when its use would appear consistent with the rejected DSM-5 proposal.

In men (and presumably in women), HD shares some clinical characteristics that are also associated with paraphilic disorders. First, although the male–female prevalence ratio of HD, estimated at 5:1 (Black et al., 1997; Carnes & Delmonico, 1996), is not as high as the estimated ratio for paraphilias (20:1; American Psychiatric Association, 1987, 1994), HD and PAs are still predominantly male disorders. Second, PAs and HD both show themselves during adolescence (Abel, Mittleman, & Becker, 1985; Black et al., 1997; Kafka, 1997). Third, several empirical studies have reported that people presenting for treatment of sexual impulsivity disorders (Abel, Becker, Cunningham-Rathner, Mittelman, & Rouleau, 1988; Freund, Sher, & Hucker, 1983; Carnes, 1983, 1989, 1991) commonly report having multiple rather than single hypersexual outlets over their lifetimes. These studies reveal a general diathesis or vulnerability to PAs and/or HD. Fourth, although many studies of paraphilic sex offenders do not systematically assess HD, nevertheless HD may be common among males with PA (Anthony & Hollander, 1993; Black et al., 1997; Kafka & Hennen, 2003; Kafka & Prentky, 1998; Levine, Risen, & Althof, 1990). Fifth, men and women with HD, as well as those with PAs, describe their sexual behavior as obligatory, repetitive, and stereotyped at times. In addition, sexually arousing fantasies, urges, and behaviors can be time-consuming, often occupying several hours per day (Black et al., 1997; Carnes, 1983; Kafka, 1997). Sixth, like paraphilic arousal (American Psychiatric Association, 2000), HD can wax and wane, be either ego-syntonic or ego-dystonic, and is more likely to occur or intensify during periods of "stress" (Black et al., 1997; Reid, Carpenter, Spackmen, & Willes, 2008). Seventh, men with PAs or PRDs (HD) are equally likely to report periods of persistently heightened sexual behaviors leading to orgasm, compared with the general population (Kafka, 1997; Kafka & Hennen, 2003). Last, as with PAs, people with HD may come to prefer unconventional sexual activities to sex with a partner. This may lead to extramarital activity, reliance on mastur-bation, and /or severe relationship problems.

The frequency distribution of HD in females is less thoroughly stud-ied, although compulsive masturbation, protracted promiscuity (including prostitution), and the paraphilia of sexual masochism have been reported. Carnes, Coleman, and others describe pathological "crushes," "obsessional fixations," or "love addictions" (Carnes, 1991; Kasl, 1989; Schaef, 1989) as predominant female expressions of sexual compulsivity/addiction. Currently, however, there is a substantial lack of empirical data on these conditions. For example, it is not evident whether these are primarily genital/sexual behavior disorders or, perhaps, attachment disorders or obsessional symptoms not pri-marily mediated by sexual appetitive behavior.

CLINICAL AND DIAGNOSTIC ASSESSMENT OF HD

General Principles

Several principles are of particular relevance in the evaluation and treat-ment of HD. First, PA and HD behaviors are secretive because they engen-der considerably more shame, guilt, and blame than other sexual disor-ders. Indeed, these sexuality disorders are arguably the most shame- and guilt-inducing contemporary psychiatric conditions. Sometimes it may take years before a person with these conditions acknowledges them to a pro-fessional or is "caught" by a spouse or significant other engaging in an unconventional sexual behavior. Thus the first principle for the evaluation of HD (or paraphilias) is to ask specific clinically relevant questions and to inquire without a spouse or significant other present. In this regard, I always inform patients that when I ask them personal questions about sexual behavior, it is because sexual disorders are highly misunderstood by the lay public and are, in fact, readily treatable conditions. I suggest that the failure to address and diagnose these conditions during the early part of evaluation and treatment can lead to misdiagnosis, costly and unproductive psychotherapy, and an incomplete understanding of the causes of a person's suffering. This helps to establish a rationale for self-disclosure early in the process of evaluation or treatment of both PAs and HD. A clinician can inquire about problematic sexual behavior by referring to the proposed cri-teria for HD in a safe, clinical context. For a full assessment and treatment algorithm, see Figure 13.1.

The Importance of Assessing Comorbidity

In the few studies that systematically evaluated psychopathology-related diagnoses in "sexually compulsive" males and females (Black et al., 1997,

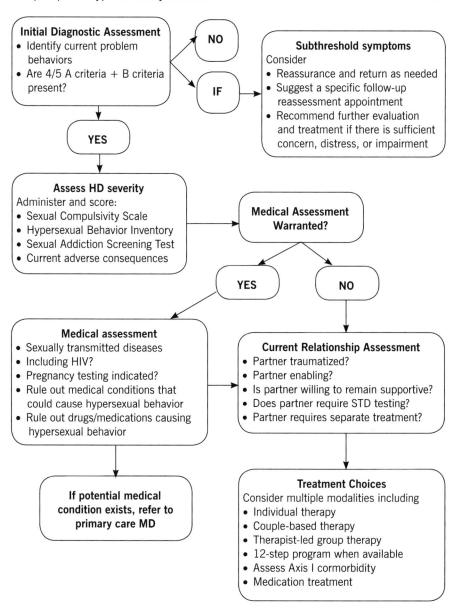

FIGURE 13.1. Assessment–treatment algorithm for hypersexuality disorder.

Morgenstern et al., 2011), paraphilia-related disorders (Kafka & Hennen, 2002; Kafka & Prentky, 1994, 1998), or nonparaphilic HD (Reid, Carpenter, et al., 2011), one of the major findings is that most individuals with these disorders have multiple lifetime comorbid disorders, especially mood, anxiety, and psychoactive substance abuse disorders and ADHD. Anxious and depressive affect (as opposed to specific clinical disorders) can be associated with sexual risk-taking behaviors and "out-of-control" sexual behaviors in both heterosexual and homosexual men (Bancroft, Janssen, Strong, Carnes, et al., 2003; Bancroft, Janssen, Strong, & Vukadinovic, 2003; Bancroft & Vukadinovic, 2004).

The clinical implications of these reports are significant for several reasons. First, these findings strongly suggest that all persons, male or female, who seek evaluation for a sexual behavior disorder should be systematically questioned about symptoms consistent with dysthymic disorder, bipolar spectrum disorders such as cyclothymia and bipolar disorder—not otherwise specified, and social anxiety disorder, as well as ADHD. The appropriate assessment of these conditions requires retrospective as well as current symptom ascertainment. In addition, many persons with current psychoactive substance abuse may deny the severity of their use of these substances. Thus the concurrent presence of these clinically significant and common comorbid psychiatric conditions may be undetected and thus untreated. Comorbid psychiatric conditions may be risk factors that substantially contribute to the onset, severity, escalation, and social deviance of hypersexual behaviors (Kafka & Prentky, 1998).

Comorbidity with Other Sexual Disorders

The coassociation of PAs with HD has already been mentioned. In addition, both males and females with HD commonly report reduced sexual arousal to "conventional" partnered sex, especially when the initial infatuation phase of a relationship has passed. In these circumstances, patients with HD may present to psychotherapists and sex therapists with apparent hypoactive sexual desire disorder, acquired and situational subtypes. In addition, diminished sexual arousal in a current relational context could present as female arousal disorder, male erectile disorder, and, perhaps, sexual aversion. Thus it is imperative to take a full sexual history of patients who present with these sexual dysfunctions as a primary complaint to rule out the presence of paraphilic or nonparaphilic hypersexuality disorders.

HD, General Medical Conditions, and Drugs/Medications

When it can be clearly established that hypersexual behaviors or HD are temporally associated with another concurrent medical or neurological condition, the diagnosis of HD should not be made independently of the medical condition or medication. Medical conditions that may be associated with hypersexual behavior can include, but are not limited to, brain injury, dementias, Huntington's disease, and Kleine–Levin syndrome. Medications or drugs that increase dopamine in the brain can be associated with hypersexual behavior. For example, amphetamine stimulants, cocaine, and medications associated with the treatment of Parkinson's disease can be associated with sexual disinhibition.

The Pair Bond

Although there are no compelling data showing that contemporary relationship dysfunction is a primary etiological factor for HD, the presence of a meaningful pair bond can have profound effects on the clinical course and outcome of treatment. Both PAs (Marshall, 1989) and HD have been described as intimacy dysfunctions by many clinicians (Carnes, 1991; Coleman, 1995; Schneider & Schneider, 1991). At least some significant others, characterized as "codependents," suffer from low self-esteem, depression, overly dependent behavior, "enabling behaviors" (e.g., protecting the identified patient from the brunt of the consequences of his or her behavior), and comorbid impulse-control disorders (Schneider & Schneider, 1991) prior to the disclosure or discovery of a PRD in their partners.

Certainly, the sudden personal disclosure or unexpected discovery of a nonparaphilic (or paraphilic) disorder in a partner during a stable pair-bonded relationship can have devastating consequences because mutual trust has been severely breached. It is clinically helpful, whenever possible, to include the significant other during the assessment process and/or early treatment phases to assess the impact of disclosure on the pair bond and to attempt to contain the relationship crisis that invariably follows disclosure. It may be helpful to send the affected partner for individual or group therapy if conjoint treatment is not feasible. In particular, when protracted sexual promiscuity (sexual behavior with consenting adults) is an identified HD, assessment for sexually transmitted diseases should be prescribed for the identified patient and, if indicated, for the significant other, especially if identified problematic behaviors included unprotected sex. There may be certain clinical situations, however, in which the identified patient is unwilling to include the significant other. For example, he or she may still be unaware of the sexual disorder or too emotionally unstable to tolerate disclosure, or imminent disclosure would almost certainly be followed by divorce or its equivalent.

The extent and timing of disclosure of nonparaphilic hypersexual behaviors in an intimate partnership should be subject to joint negotiation. Both Schneider (Schneider & Schneider, 1991) and Corley (Corley & Schneider, 2002) reported that the honesty that follows full disclosure is most likely to lead to the best marital outcome but that the reestablishment of trust might take years.

TREATMENT MODALITIES FOR HD

Some general principles associated with the evaluation and treatment of HD are enumerated in Table 13.2.

Psychodynamic Psychotherapy

At present, there is no compelling empirically derived evidence to suggest that individual psychodynamic therapy as the solitary treatment modality

TABLE 13.2. Selected Pertinent Psychological or Behavioral Domains to Be Addressed during the Evaluation and Treatment of HD

A. Gaining control over hypersexual symptomatology:
- Psychoeducation about what we know and what we don't know about these conditions and their psychiatric and developmental comorbidities
- Discussion of the range of available therapeutic strategies and selective referral to cognitive and behavior therapies, support groups, marital therapy, and/or pharmacotherapy
- Collaborative limit setting to establish a "bottom line" to hypersexual behavior that the patient can work toward
- Negotiating the use of phone blocks; discarding paraphernalia such as pornography; canceling subscriptions for pornography;installing password protection pornography blocking software; holding or discontinuing credit cards; using an Internet censor with password controlled by partner, family member, or therapist; moving a computer out of a private setting; consider eliminating Internet access completely
- Facilitating decisions about self-disclosure/trust in revealing the details of hypersexual activities to a significant other, involvement of partner if indicated
- Psychotherapeutic interventions that specifically target current sexual symptoms in preference to early developmental conflicts
- Encouraging involvement in 12-step recovery programs

B. Here-and-now issues
- Destigmatization: discussing the paradigm shift from "badness" to "illness" to diminish blame, shame, and guilt
- Clarification of thoughts, affects, behaviors, and common precipitating stressors that might precede hypersexual behaviors
- Developing alternative response strategies for managing dysphoric affects that precede both covert and overt problematic sexual behaviors
- Maintenance of interpersonal boundaries to reduce stressors: assertiveness training, social skills training, relaxation/meditation, recognition and modulation of stressful affects
- If involved in a 12-step group program: establishing a sponsor, monitoring attendance and a bottom line, encouraging and reviewing progress with the 12-step methodology
- Consideration of 6 months of celibacy as a personal growth experience
- Psychoeducation regarding a "healthy" sexual relationship: how to develop and maintain intimacy, how to remain single but not be depressed or lonely, what healthy sexuality is
- Mourning a lifestyle of hypersexual behaviors: the role of suffering, pleasure, and escape from painful affects
- If referred for pharmacotherapy: monitor changes in sexual arousal and impulse control, assess concurrent depressive and anxious symptoms, collaboration with other treaters

C. Developmental factors (issues preferably managed after symptom stabilization)
- Coming to terms with family dysfunction; identification of the role of psychiatric illness in family members
- Events that may have shaped early sexual behaviors, including emotional, physical or sexual abuse or neglect, premature sexualization in relationships
- The development and elaboration of the "false self" or "double life" to compartmentalize nonparaphilic hypersexuality and manage painful affects
- Possible psychodynamic or behavioral contexts for the meaning and perpetuation of sexual symptom formation
- Assessing the developmental effects of concurrent psychiatric diagnoses

is effective for either PAs or HD. Psychodynamic psychotherapy, however, may help to synthesize the role of developmental antecedents; reduce current anxiety, depression, guilt, and shame; and improve social adjustment. As is commonly the case for the treatment of PAs, multimodal treatment approaches utilizing behavioral, psychodynamic, group, psychoeducational, and pharmacological treatments are commonly prescribed and tailored to the specific needs of the patient or couple. The informed individual psychotherapist, regardless of theoretical persuasion, may function as the person to select and integrate different therapeutic interventions, akin to the model of "primary-care therapist" advocated by Khantzian (1986) for the recovering substance abuser. In the sexual addiction literature, the most commonly prescribed combination of therapies associated with successful outcome are 12-step group therapy (see the following section) and individual psychotherapy with a clinician familiar with sexual addiction as a conceptual framework (Carnes, 2004).

Group Psychotherapies

Men with HD have been treated with therapist-led group psychotherapy. Quadland (1985) reported favorable outcome in 30 gay or bisexual men enrolled in a semistructured 20-week group therapy program with a goal of controlling protracted promiscuity. Earle and Crow (1989) and Turner (1990) report the use of outpatient group psychotherapy with "sexual addicts," but no outcome was included. A model for outpatient group therapy combining psychodynamic and cognitive-behavioral techniques has been reported as well (Line & Cooper, 2002).

Case 1: Sam

Sam was a 33-year-old married man who was referred by an experienced psychotherapist after many years of sexual addiction treatment, including active participation in 12-step programs. Although Sam was "better" and "understood some of my triggers," he episodically continued to engage in promiscuous behaviors with women. His wife was aware of his problem and history of treatment and stayed married because "I am a good father." Their relationship, although still affectionate, no longer included sexual relations.

Sam grew up in a household in which there was significant interpersonal turmoil. His mother was likely depressed, and his father had unpredictable moods, punctuated by bouts of alcohol intoxication. At times, his father unleashed harsh and undeserved criticism, especially at Sam, such that Sam withdrew from his dad but also felt little support from his mother. The father eventually sobered up but was characterized as a "dry drunk" by Sam and his younger sister.

Sam's escape from his dysfunctional family was his ability to do well in school and have active friendships. Known for his creativity and general high energy, Sam graduated from a distinguished business school, joined a start-up technology group, and was financially successful. At business meetings he was described as a natural leader, although he could be narcissistic and argumentative when he perceived that his peers were "not as bright."

Sam's promiscuous behavior started in college and had included one-night stands with peer females, progressing to escort services once he was in business. Typically he planned and looked forward to having sex with women, sometimes staying up the night before checking out ads on the Internet for sexual services. When he traveled for business, he almost always looked to hook up with either women he met through business or escort services. His addiction could cost over $2,000 some months, but he used a separate credit card until his wife discovered some of his receipts. He rarely sought out pornography and was not an enthusiast for masturbation, either.

A careful psychiatric evaluation of Sam's developmental and behavioral symptoms revealed that he had had two past episodes of major depression. His promiscuous behavior appeared associated with either an anxious/depressive mood state or bursts of increased energy, increased talkativeness, and "racing thoughts" lasting 1–2 days. It was hard to sort out whether these "energy bursts" were caused by his anticipated sexual trysts, but he also recalled other such periods when he was working on business plans and could get by with less sleep for up to 3 days in a row.

Sam's DSM-5 Diagnoses

- Other specified bipolar and related disorders: short-duration hypomanic episodes and major depressive episodes
- Other specified disruptive, impulse-control, and conduct disorder: hypersexual disorder, sexual behavior with consenting adults

TREATMENT

Sam's treatment with me was limited to pharmacological management of a bipolar mood disorder associated with the bipolar spectrum. He was prescribed lamotrigine, a limbic anticonvulsant mood stabilizer. He began to notice a calming effect on lamotrigine 100 mg/day but the optimal effect when a daily dose of 200 mg/day was reached. He described improved emotional resilience and greatly improved ability to think before he made plans, whether it was at business meetings or fantasizing about having a sexual liaison. Unexpectedly, with the help of his individual psychotherapist, he was better able to emotionally process how much damage he had perpetrated on his wife over the years through his persistent philandering. He was ready to join a therapist-led group with other men who had similar sexual impulsivity disorders. Both psychotherapies contributed to his ability to address issues associated with narcissism, self-esteem, and the compartmentalization of his emotional life. In 1 year at follow-up he reported only one slip—while away on a business trip.

After 6 months of abstinence from sexual impulsivity, Sam wanted to taper lamotrigine. He did so slowly with check-ins to my office. He noticed increased emotional lability, and he self-monitored his emotional states, made sure he had regular and sound sleep, and learned to moderate his mood swings with mindfulness techniques. After an additional year of follow-up, he had not had a recurrence of promiscuous sexual behavior, and his marriage was substantially mended. He continued in both individual and group therapy.

Self-Help Groups

Since the formation of Alcoholics Anonymous and the articulation of the 12-step recovery program, self-help groups based on 12-step methodology have been formed for many forms of impulsive/addictive behaviors, including behavior involving drugs, sex, and food, as well as gambling, kleptomania, and others. These programs can have a profound effect on the process of recovery, especially if the program is zealously adhered to. For example, 12-step recovery programs commonly require daily attendance at a 12-step meeting for the first 3 months of recovery from alcoholism (Galanter, Talbott, & Gallegos, 1990), and recovery from bulimia nervosa (Malenbaum, Herzog, & Eisenthal, 1988) was associated with five or more 12-step meetings per week for at least 3 years.

Although HD does not meet the criteria necessary to qualify as a behavioral addiction, the primary resources available for the treatment of this condition are based in the addiction model. There are now several different 12-step programs for recovering "sex addicts," some of which are distinguished by geographic location or differing philosophies as to what constitutes "recovery," "abstinence," and "bottom line" in the context of normalizing sexual behaviors (Salmon, 1995). Naditch and Barton (1990) and Carnes (1991) noted a positive long-term outcome associated with 12-step sexual addiction programs in conjunction with individual psychotherapy in a retrospective survey of men and women recovering from both nonviolent PAs and HD. Resources for locating such groups are available via the Internet (e.g., Sexaholics Anonymous, *www.sa.org*; Sex Addicts Anonymous, *http://saa-recovery.org*; Sex and Love Addicts Anonymous, *www.slaafws.org*).

The self-help fellowships for treatment of HD can offer several important advantages. First, these groups have become increasingly prevalent in many parts of the country, so they are generally readily accessible, especially in metropolitan areas. Second, there is no financial burden associated with this form of treatment. Third, these groups are very helpful in lessening the shame, secrecy, stigmatization, and blame that accompanies nonparaphilic hypersexuality. Fourth, there can be a sense of "healing community" that includes fellowship, spiritual values, association with other persons in recovery, self-help support groups for the "coaddict," and the provision of a sponsor relationship that can include daily check-in phone calls and crisis management. Fifth, in many respects, the program offered by zealous adherence to the

12-step recovery model for sexual addiction or HD bears some resemblance to a relapse prevention program based on cognitive-behavioral therapy (CBT), a model of psychological treatment prevalent for the treatment of sex offenders with PAs (Carnes, 1991; Laws, 1989).

On the other hand, 12-step programs such as Sex and Love Addicts Anonymous (SLAA), Sexaholics Anonymous, and Sexual Compulsives Anonymous require an intensive evening-and-weekend time commitment, a sponsor, the regional availability of appropriate groups, and, most important, a person who is willing to work in an intensive recovery program over a period of several years.

Note that self-help resources are also available for partners of individuals with HD (e.g., COSA, *www.cosa-recovery.org*; Recovering Couples Anonymous, *www.recovering-couples.org*; S-Anon International Family Groups, *www.sanon.org*). For additional resources for clinicians and patients with HD, please consult the books and websites included in this chapter's reference list (e.g., Society for the Advancement of Sexual Health, 2012; Edwards, Delmonico, & Griffin, 2011; Delmonico, Griffin, & Moriarity, 2001; Carnes, Delmonico, Griffin, & Moriarity, 2007; Maltz & Maltz, 2008).

Case 2: Alan

Alan was a 33-year-old single male who was self-referred after he received a threatening e-mail from a man he had encountered online. They had engaged in cybersex repetitively using web cameras, and the e-mailer threatened to "out" him in his work setting using recordings he surreptitiously kept of Alan masturbating. He demanded $1,000.

Alan was an avid user of cybersex chatrooms and cybertechnology (most typically webcams). He had engaged in these behaviors several times per week for about 5 years. He stated that he had a high sexual drive but was typically too anxious to meet men in person if his intent was to develop an intimate relationship. Cybersex allowed him to maintain anonymity and reduce his social anxiety but, at least with some men he encountered online, fantasize that he could meet them eventually and have already "gotten through the preliminaries" of a romantic relationship.

Alan had discovered the world of online sex through lifestyle websites that encouraged him to develop an alternative personality with an avatar. He could build a lifestyle, acquire a home, money, and friends, and engage in sex. Although he was gainfully employed, outside of the work setting he had very few friendships, had only a single former romantic partner, and described feeling anxious and depressed when he "stepped outside my safety zone." Alan had unsuccessfully tried to meet men at bars and in gay cruising areas, but he was too reticent to come out to his family or work colleagues.

When Alan was unable to meet someone for cybersex chat, he would view gay pornography and masturbate. These were his primary evening activities, sometimes extending into the late-night hours. He was also increasingly concerned because he noted that the pornography that turned him on the most seemed to involve younger males, some perhaps under age 18.

Alan already had an individual psychotherapist, who had counseled him to retain an attorney but to have no contact whatsoever with the man who had threatened him. After beginning to psychologically process the blackmail threat that had been made against him, it dawned on Alan that he had never revealed where he was employed to this particular male and had no Facebook page or other simple means by which his workplace could be readily identified. His DSM-5 psychiatric diagnoses were as follows: persistent depressive disorder: late onset, with pure dysthymic syndrome; mild social anxiety disorder; and other specified, disruptive, impulse-control, and conduct disorder: hypersexual disorder; cybersex, pornography, and masturbation.

TREATMENT

Alan needed "connection" as a primary modality for his treatment. He felt safely connected to his therapist, who had specialized skills with gay men who had sexual addiction. Both his therapist and I made a strong case for his attending local 12-step groups, as he lived in an urban environment and these were readily available. Alan balked at first, but when I asked whether he would begin attending if he were accompanied by another patient in my practice, he agreed. This turned out to be a crucial turning point for Alan, as he was able to attend multiple 12-step groups with many gay males and, especially because this was to be deliberately "unromantic," he began to establish a broader network of platonic friendships. He established his "bottom line" behaviors and was able to abstain from cybersex. One year later he was able to abstain from pornography, except for occasional use.

Eventually the 12 steps and the strong fellowship that the groups fostered became central to his lifestyle. Over a 2- to 3-year period, Alan matured socially and eventually came out to his family and then to some work colleagues. As his social anxiety decreased, so did his low self-esteem and other depressive symptoms. He did not return to cybersex.

Cognitive–Behavioral Therapies

Relapse prevention is an integrated cognitive-behavioral and group therapy treatment approach that originally evolved from a theoretical understanding of and treatment for addictive disorders such as alcohol abuse, nicotine dependence, and compulsive overeating (Marlatt & Gordon, 1980). Several different techniques are used: (1) identifying and modifying cognitive distortions and beliefs that rationalize hypersexual behavior, (2) helping the patient to recognize and then anticipate high-risk situations, (3) identifying specific behavioral-affective-cognitive precursors to relapse, and (4) extensive behavior rehearsal of new comprehensive problem-solving techniques, as well as social and sexual skills training.

The relapse prevention model and accompanying cognitive-behavioral and social learning techniques are now becoming commonly employed in specialized sex offender treatment programs in the United States and Canada. To my knowledge, there are no published data on this comprehensive approach to the treatment of HD.

Behavioral Therapy Techniques

Behavioral therapy techniques are used frequently in treatment centers specializing in the assessment and treatment of sexually aggressive persons with PAs. These techniques appear to be applicable to nonviolent PAs and HD as well. Aversive techniques, for example, can be applied to a wide range of human behaviors, including sexual behaviors, when accompanied by the voluntary consent and understanding of the patient.

McConaghy and Armstrong (1985) reported that imaginal desensitization was as effective as covert sensitization in reducing compulsive sexual behaviors in a group of 20 men with PAs and HD (promiscuity) at both 1-month and 1-year follow-up.

Olfactory aversion was designed to reduce unconventional sexual arousal with aversive smells, such as ammonia (Colson, 1972). The advantage of olfactory aversion is the immediacy of a powerful noxious odor that can be rapidly introduced during the repetition of specific sexually arousing fantasies. Ammonia aversion utilizes encapsulated ammonia ampoules that are portable and can be broken and inhaled in conjunction with both behavioral homework and *in vivo* practice in situations that trigger sexual urges. As is the case for any conditioning therapy, aversion therapy requires persistent and repetitive practice involving specific self-identified precursor situations that are sexually arousing.

Psychopharmacology

As is the case for the previously mentioned psychological treatment modalities, published data supporting a pharmacological approach for the amelioration of nonparaphilic hypersexuality disorders are scant but encouraging. A persuasive rationale for the use of psychopharmacological agents for these conditions can be based on the clinical evidence of psychiatric comorbidity. There are pharmacological treatments that target specific disorders, such as chronic mood and anxiety disorders and ADHD and nonparaphilic hypersexuality disorders (see the section on comorbidity earlier in this chapter).

In my clinical experience with the pharmacological treatment of more than 500 males with HD who have failed a panoply of psychological treatments, the use of mood stabilizers, antidepressants, atypical neuroleptics, psychostimulants, opiate antagonists, and an orally administered anti-androgen, medroxyprogesterone, alone or in various combinations, can have profound effects in ameliorating nonparaphilic as well as paraphilic hypersexuality disorders (Kafka, 2008) . We do not currently have sufficient outcome data to determine whether these agents need to be prescribed for the short term (e.g., 1 year) while other psychological therapies are ongoing or whether pharmacological therapy requires longer term prescription for the successful continued management of nonparaphilic hypersexuality disorders.

Psychopharmacological treatment for HD should not be reserved only for situations in which other therapeutic endeavors have either failed or been only partially successful. If an individual is still struggling with strong urges or acting out repetitively despite involvement in therapies to help him stop his destructive sexual behaviors, a psychopharmacological consultation should be considered. The careful diagnosis of chronic psychiatric disorders that have been empirically demonstrated to have a genetic/biological component should be followed by a discussion of all available treatment modalities, both psychological and biological. Since the last edition of this text, my clinical practice has been shaped significantly by referrals of individuals with HD or sexual addiction who have "spectrum" manifestations of bipolar mood disorders in particular. The thorough assessment of such patients requires a clinician to understand that hypomania, the pathognomonic mood state distinguishing bipolar from unipolar mood disorders, is not always easy to detect and has its own spectrum. Recurrent hypomania can be of brief duration (1–3 days) and is not necessarily associated with elevated mood or euphoria (e.g., it can include irritability and anxiety instead); hypomanic symptoms can co-occur even while a person is dysthymic or having a major depressive episode. Recent research suggests that the hallmark of hypomania is increased energy and activity accompanied by racing or "crowded" thoughts, rather than a specific "elevated" mood state (Judd & Akiskal, 2003; Judd et al., 2003; Benazzi, 2001).

I have noticed several clinical situations in which the apparent mitigating effect of medication is less robust for HD. This outcome can be noted in psychological treatments as well. On closer inspection of patients whose outcomes are less robust, I have repeatedly observed several common clinical concomitants. First, such patients no longer feel as intense an urgency to their sexual desire after pharmacotherapy in combination with psychological treatments. For example, many are able to willfully control themselves when requested to do so for a period of several weeks. Second, many patients with HD may continue to maintain a reduced frequency of a nonparaphilic sexual behavior when they have no current or regular sexual partners, when the financial cost of the specific outlet is modest, when a sexual dysfunction in a partner precludes sexual intimacy, or when pair-bond intimacy dysfunction that affects sexual relations is apparent. In these situations, the sexual behavior no longer is described as ego-dystonic and therefore may not meet criteria for a "disorder." I see this most commonly with continued pornography use.

Case 3: Ted

Ted was a 37-year-old married male whose Internet pornography viewing while at work was discovered when the company's computer operating system was upgraded. He had planned to delete his Internet browser's viewing history, but he had not done so. There was sufficient evidence, along with his general work underperformance, that led to his being asked to take a "medical leave" or be fired. Choosing the former option, Ted was panicked when he called for an appointment. A married man with two young children, he was the family breadwinner and desperately wanted help. He had noted that even after a few weeks of his taking leave, he could not help himself to resist urges at home to view pornography and masturbate while smelling and stroking his wife's underpants.

Ted started masturbating (without ejaculation) while smelling or stroking his older sister's undergarments when he was about age 8. He had viewed his sister scantily clad on only a few occasions but felt an intense urge to steal her underpants. During adolescence and into adulthood, Ted had collected women's panties from girlfriends or by sneaking into the bedrooms of adults when he visited them as an adolescent with his family and he had amassed a small collection. He had intermittently tried to discard them but then would collect others. He was highly aroused by smelling or stroking these underpants, not by wearing them.

During his courtship, Ted had mentioned to his fiancée that he enjoyed viewing pornography and had done so starting in early adolescence. He did not tell her, however, about his fetishistic attraction to female lingerie. Although the majority of his pornography viewing was of adult heterosexuals engaging in diverse sexual activities, he enjoyed looking at and masturbating while viewing female underwear sites online. He denied promiscuous behavior or persistent visits to strip clubs.

Ted was criticized by his father during childhood and adolescence because he underperformed at schoolwork, procrastinated with his homework, and seemed more at ease with action games than interacting with family members. There was no overt abuse or neglect in his family, but an older brother had similar school underachievement problems and barely graduated high school. He had some close male friends and dated girls during high school but "always loved my pornography," at times masturbating at least one to three times a day and sometimes spending 3–5 hours viewing pornography, especially as he had Internet access.

Ted tried college but found the workload too demanding, handed in his assignments and papers at the last moment, and never finished college. His school underperformance was further compromised by smoking marijuana, eventually on a daily basis "to help me concentrate better." Even while married, Ted enjoyed getting stoned on weekends, even though it upset his wife.

Ted's marriage had been troubled because, from his wife's perspective, he was self-centered and a poor communicator. She had noted his distractibility and procrastination but attributed those characteristics to his marijuana smoking. She also described increasing social withdrawal, pessimism, irritability, and passivity during the past 3 years. As well, he took to overeating when stressed, so she felt he was less and less physically attractive.

Ted's primary DSM-5 psychiatric diagnoses included: attention-deficit/hyperactivity disorder (ADHD), predominantly inattentive type; cannabis use disorder; persistent depressive disorder: late onset, with pure dysthymic syndrome, moderate; fetishistic disorder, nonliving object; other specified disruptive, impulse control, and conduct disorderL hypersexual disorder; pornography and masturbation.

TREATMENT

Ted agreed to attend 12-step support groups (SLAA) but was unable to maintain the bottom line of abstinence from viewing pornography or masturbating while stroking stolen women's undergarments. He stopped using marijuana, to the relief of his wife. He was encouraged to purchase pornography-blocking software, and his wife placed a password on his home laptop computer. He confided with me that he was using his smartphone to access pornography, however, and just couldn't stop himself. He started psychotherapy with an experienced sexual addiction–trained therapist, but he never agreed to give up his smartphone for one without Internet access. He was referred back to me to "treat my ADD." Prescription of a long-acting psychostimulant and a serotonergic antidepressant, sertraline, had substantial effects on improving his emotional resilience and his executive functions. He experienced sufficient relief that he was able to agree to give up a smartphone and redouble his efforts in psychotherapy and 12-step group participation. He called his sponsor to check in regularly. After an additional year of treatment, he was able to use a smartphone without accessing pornography except during unusual stress points in his life. He told me that he had discarded almost all of the underpants he had stashed, although he kept "a few pairs." He returned to work in another company.

CONCLUSIONS

When persons afflicted with HD are effectively relieved of their target symptoms by medications, self-help groups, and/or psychotherapies, it is rare that they miss their sexually impulsive behaviors. They are most often relieved to be more productive, feel less sexually preoccupied, and have more emotional resilience. There is generally no "symptom substitution" but, rather, a sense of feeling unburdened, perhaps for the first time in many, many years.

In contrast to other disturbances of human sexuality, the status of HD remains controversial because we lack sufficient empirical studies of these behaviors and their treatment outcomes. As a result, these serious conditions are only cursorily addressed in most textbooks and academic courses teaching about human sexuality disorders. Despite the lack of empirical information regarding nonparaphilic hypersexuality disorders, there is certainly clinical lore evidencing that they are prevalent conditions that may remain hidden from spouses and family members.

It is imperative to form a trusting and collaborative therapeutic alliance and to offer hope and effective treatment modalities to persons impaired by these conditions. As demonstrated by the case examples in this chapter, the successful treatment of these conditions commonly requires more than one type of mental health intervention. As clinicians, then, it behooves us to sustain collegial relationships with a collaborative network of resources and specialized clinicians who may share differing competencies but can work collaboratively.

The healing and recovery period that is necessary when HD has disrupted the pair bond should be measured in years, not months. Marriages and other intimate partnerships need time to heal and reestablish a trusting bond, even if problematic sexual behavior ceases early in treatment. In most cases, especially during the first few years of treatment, we need to speak about "effective treatment" or "control" rather than "cure" as an outcome measure. In kind, we can analogously think of the successful amelioration of other chronic medical conditions, such as psychoactive substance abuse, obsessive–compulsive disorder, diabetes mellitus, atherosclerotic vascular disease, and hypertension in similar terms.

REFERENCES

Abel, G. G., Becker, J. V., Cunningham-Rathner, J., Mittelman, M., & Rouleau, J. L. (1988). Multiple paraphilic diagnoses among sex offenders. *Bulletin of the American Academy of Psychiatry and Law, 16*, 153–168.

Abel, G. G., Mittleman, M., & Becker, J. V. (1985). Sex offenders: Results of assessment and recommendations for treatment. In H. H. Ben-Aron, S. Hucker, & C. D. Webster (Eds.), *Clinical criminology: Assessment and treatment of criminal behavior* (pp. 191–205). Toronto, Ontario, Canada: M&M Graphics.

American Psychiatric Association. (1968). *Diagnostic and statistical manual of mental disorders* (2nd ed.). Washington, DC: Author.

American Psychiatric Association. (1980). *Diagnostic and statistical manual of mental disorders* (3rd ed.). Washington, DC: Author.

American Psychiatric Association. (1987). *Diagnostic and statistical manual of mental disorders* (3rd ed., rev.). Washington, DC: Author.

American Psychiatric Association. (1994). *Diagnostic and statistical manual of mental disorders* (4th ed.). Washington, DC: Author.

American Psychiatric Association. (2000). *Diagnostic and statistical manual of mental disorders* (4th ed., text rev.). Washington, DC: Author.

American Psychiatric Association. (2013). *Diagnostic and statistical manual of mental disorders* (5th ed.). Arlington, VA: Author.

Anthony, D. T., & Hollander, E. (1993). Sexual compulsions. In E. Hollander (Ed.), *Obsessive–compulsive-related disorders* (pp. 139–150). Washington, DC: American Psychiatric Press.

Bancroft, J., & Janssen, E. (2000). The dual control of male sexual response: A theoretical approach to centrally mediated erectile dysfunction. *Neuroscience and Biobehavioral Review, 24,* 571–579.

Bancroft, J., Janssen, E., Strong, D., Carnes, L., Vukadinovic, Z., & Long, S. L. (2003). The relation between mood and sexuality in heterosexual men. *Archives of Sexual Behavior, 32,* 217–230.

Bancroft, J., Janssen, E., Strong, D., & Vukadinovic, Z. (2003). The relation between mood and sexuality in gay men. *Archives of Sexual Behavior, 32,* 231–242.

Bancroft, J., & Vukadinovic, Z. (2004). Sexual addiction, sexual compulsivity, sexual impulsivity or what? Toward a theoretical model. *Journal of Sex Research, 41,* 225–234.

Benazzi, F. (2001). Is 4 days the minimum duration of hypomania in bipolar II disorder? *European Journal of Psychiatry and Clinical Neuroscience, 251,* 32–34.

Black, D. W. (1998). Compulsive sexual behavior: A review. *Journal of Practical Psychiatry and Behavioral Health, 4,* 217–229.

Black, D. W., Kehrberg, L. L. D., Flumerfelt, D. L., & Schlosser, S. S. (1997). Characteristics of 36 subjects reporting compulsive sexual behavior. *American Journal of Psychiatry, 154,* 243–249.

Blankenship, R., & Laaser, M. (2004). Sexual addiction and ADHD: Is there a connection? *Sexual Addiction and Compulsivity, 11,* 7–20.

Carnes, P. (1983). *Out of the shadows: Understanding sexual addiction.* Minneapolis, MN: CompCare.

Carnes, P. (1989). *Contrary to love: Helping the sexual addict.* Minneapolis, MN: CompCare.

Carnes, P. (1990). Sexual addiction. In A. Horton, B. L. Johnson, & L. M. Roundy (Eds.), *The incest perpetrator: A family member no one wants to treat* (pp. 126–143). Newbury Park, CA: Sage.

Carnes, P. (2004). Sexual addiction. In B. J. Sadock & V. A. Sadock (Eds.), *Comprehensive textbook of psychiatry* (Vol. 1, pp. 1991–2001). Philadelphia: Lippincott Williams & Wilkins.

Carnes, P. (1991). *Don't call it love: Recovery from sexual addiction.* New York: Bantam Books.

Carnes, P., & Delmonico, D. (1996). Childhood abuse and multiple addictions: Research findings in a sample of self-identified sexual addicts. *Sexual Addiction and Compulsivity, 3,* 258–268.

Carnes, P. J., Delmonico, D. L., Griffin, E., & Moriarity, J. (2007). *In the shadows of the net: Breaking free of compulsive online sexual behavior.* Center City, MN: Hazelden.

Coleman, E. (1986, July). Sexual compulsion vs. sexual addiction: The debate continues. *SIECUS Report,* pp. 7–11.

Coleman, E. (1987). Sexual compulsivity: Definition, etiology, and treatment considerations. *Journal of Chemical Dependency Treatment, 1,* 189–204.

Coleman, E. (1995). Treatment of compulsive sexual behavior. In R. C. Rosen & S. R. Lieblum (Eds.), *Case studies in sex therapy* (pp. 333–349). New York: Guilford Press.

Coleman, E., Miner, M., Ohlerking, F., Raymond, N. (2001). Compulsive sexual behavior inventory: A preliminary study of reliability and validity. *Journal of Sex and Marital Therapy, 27,* 325–332.

Colson, C. E. (1972). Olfactory aversion for homosexual behavior. *Journal of Behavior Therapy and Experimental Psychiatry, 3,* 185–187.

Corley, M. D., & Schneider, J. P. (2002). Disclosing secrets: Guidelines for therapists working with sex addicts and co-addicts. *Sexual Addiction and Compulsivity, 9,* 43–67.

Delmonico, D. L., Griffin, E., & Moriarity, J. (2001). *Cybersex unhooked: A workbook for breaking free of compulsive online sexual behavior.* Wickenburg, AZ: Gentle Path Press. Available at *www.internetbehavior.com/services/cyber_unhooked.htm.*

Earle, R., & Crow, G. (1989). *Lonely all the time: Understanding and overcoming sexual addiction.* New York: Pocket Books.

Edwards, W., Delmonico, D. L., & Griffin, E. (2011). *Cybersex unplugged: Finding sexual health in an electronic world.* Seattle, WA: CreateSpace.

Ellis, H. (1905). *Studies in the psychology of sex* (Vols. 1 and 2). New York: Random House.

Freund, K., Sher, H., & Hucker, S. (1983). The courtship disorders. *Archives of Sexual Behavior, 12,* 369–379.

Galanter, M., Talbott, D., & Gallegos, K. (1990). Combined Alcoholics Anonymous and professional care for addicted physicians. *American Journal of Psychiatry, 147,* 64–68.

Hirschfeld, M. (1948). *Hypereroticism in sexual anomalies: The origins, nature and treatment of sexual disorders* (pp. 86–100). New York: Emerson Books.

Janssen, E., Vorst, H., Finn, P., & Bancroft, J. (2002a). The Sexual Inhibition (SIS) and Sexual Excitation (SES) Scales: I. Measuring sexual inhibition and excitation proneness in men. *Journal of Sex Research, 39,* 114–126.

Janssen, E., Vorst, H., Finn, P., & Bancroft, J. (2002b). The Sexual Inhibition (SIS) and Sexual Excitation (SES) Scales: II. Predicting psychophysiological response patterns. *Journal of Sex Research, 39,* 127–132.

Judd, L. L., & Akiskal, H. S. (2003). The prevalence and disability of bipolar spectrum disorders in the U.S. population: A re-analysis of the ECA database taking into account subthreshold cases. *Journal of Affective Disorders, 73,* 123–131.

Judd, L. L., Akiskal, H. S., Schettler, P. J., Coryell, W., Endicott, J., Maser, J. D., et al. (2003). A prospective investigation of the natural history of the long-term weekly symptomatic status of bipolar II disorder. *Archives of General Psychiatry, 60,* 261–269.

Kafka, M. P. (1991). Successful antidepressant treatment of nonparaphilic sexual addictions and paraphilias in men. *Journal of Clinical Psychiatry, 52,* 60–65.

Kafka, M. P. (1997). Hypersexual desire in males: An operational definition and clinical implications for men with paraphilias and paraphilia-related disorders. *Archives of Sexual Behavior, 28,* 505–526.

Kafka, M. P. (2007). Paraphilia-related disorders: The evaluation and treatment of nonparaphilic hypersexuality. In S. R. Leiblum (Ed.), *Principles and practice of sex therapy* (4th ed., pp. 442–476). New York: Guilford Press.

Kafka, M. P. (2008). Neurobiological processes and comorbidity in sexual deviance. In D. R. Laws & W. O'Donohue (Eds.), *Sexual deviance: Theory, assessment and treatment* (2nd ed., pp. 571–593). New York: Guilford Press.

Kafka, M. P. (2010). Hypersexual disorder: A proposed diagnosis for DSM-5. *Archives of Sexual Behavior, 39*, 377–400

Kafka, M. P., & Hennen, J. (1991). The paraphilia-related disorders: An empirical investigation of nonparaphilic hypersexuality disorders in 206 outpatient males. *Journal of Sex and Marital Therapy, 25*, 305–319.

Kafka, M. P., & Hennen, J. (2002). A DSM-IV Axis I comorbidity study of males (*n* = 120) with paraphilias and paraphilia-related disorders. *Sexual Abuse, 14*, 349–366.

Kafka, M. P., & Hennen, J. (2003). Hypersexual desire in males: Are males with paraphilias different from males with paraphilia-related disorders? *Sexual Abuse, 15*, 307–321.

Kafka, M. P., & Prentky, R. A. (1994). Preliminary observations of DSM-III-R Axis I comorbidity in men with paraphilias and paraphilia-related disorders. *Journal of Clinical Psychiatry, 55*, 481–487.

Kafka, M. P., & Prentky, R. A. (1998). Attention-deficit/hyperactivity disorder in males with paraphilias and paraphilia-related disorders: A comorbidity study. *Journal of Clinical Psychiatry, 59*, 388–396.

Kalichman, S. C., & Rompa, D. (1995). Sexual sensation seeking and sexual compulsivity scales: Reliability, validity and HIV risk behavior. *Journal of Personality Assessment, 65*, 586–601.

Kasl, C. (1989). *Women, sex and addiction*. New York: Harper & Row.

Khantzian, E. J. (1986). A contemporary psychodynamic approach to drug abuse treatment. *American Journal of Drug and Alcohol Abuse, 12*, 213–222.

Kor, A., Fogel, Y. A., Reid, R. C., & Potenza, M. N. (2013). Should hypersexual disorder be classified as an addiction? *Sex Addiction and Compulsivity, 20*, 27–47.

Krafft-Ebing, R. (1965). *Psychopathia sexualis*. New York: Putnam. (Original work published 1886)

Laws, D. R. (1989). *Relapse prevention with sex offenders*. New York: Guilford Press.

Levine, S. B., Risen, C. B., & Althof, S. E. (1990). Essay on the diagnosis and nature of paraphilia. *Journal of Sex and Marital Therapy, 16*, 89–102.

Line, B. Y., & Cooper, A. (2002). Group therapy: Essential component for success with sexually acting out problems among men. *Sex Addiction and Compulsivity, 9*, 15–32.

Malenbaum, R., Herzog, D., & Eisenthal, S. (1988). Overeaters Anonymous: Impact on bulimia. *International Journal of Eating Disorders, 7*, 139–143.

Maltz, W., & Maltz, L. (2008). *The porn trap: The essential guide to overcoming problems caused by pornography*. New York: HarperCollins.

Marlatt, G. A., & Gordon, J. R. (1980). Determinants of relapse: Implications for the maintenance of behavior change. In P. O. Davidson & S. M. Davidson (Eds.), *Behavioral medicine: Changing health lifestyles* (pp. 410–452). New York: Brunner/Mazel.

Marshall, W. L. (1989). Intimacy, loneliness, and sexual offenders. *Behaviour Research and Therapy, 27*, 491–503.

McConaghy, N., & Armstrong, M. S. (1985). Expectancy, covert sensitization and imaginal desensitization in compulsive sexuality. *Acta Psychiatrica Scandinavica, 72*, 176–187.

Morgenstern, J., Muench, F., O' Leary, A., Wainberg, M., Parsons, J. T., Hollander, E., et al. (2011). Non-paraphilic compulsive sexual behavior and psychiatric co-morbidities in gay and bisexual men. *Sex Addiction and Compulsivity, 18*, 114–134.

Naditch, M. P., & Barton, S. N. (1990). Outcome study of an inpatient sexual dependence progam, *American Journal of Preventive Psychiatry and Neurology, 2*, 27–32.

Orford, J. (1978). Hypersexuality: Implications for a theory of dependence. *British Journal of Addiction, 73*, 299–310.

Orford, J. (1985). Excessive sexuality. In *Excessive appetites: A psychological view of the addictions* (pp. 91–106). Chichester, UK: Wiley.

Quadland, M. C. (1985). Compulsive sexual behavior: Definition of a problem and an approach to treatment. *Journal of Sex and Marital Therapy, 11*, 121–132.

Reid, R. C., Carpenter, B. N., Gilliland, R., & Karim, R. (2011). Problems of self-concept in a patient sample of hypersexual men with attention-deficit disorder. *Journal of Addiction Medicine, 5*, 134–140.

Reid, R. C., Carpenter, B. N., Hook, J. N., Garos, S., Manning, J. C., Gilliland, R., et al. (2012). Report of findings in a DSM-5 field trial for hypersexual disorder. *Journal of Sexual Medicine, 9*, 2868–2877.

Reid, R. C., Carpenter, B. N., Spackman, M., & Willes, D. L. (2008). Alexithymia, emotional instability, and vulnerability to stress proneness in patients seeking help for hypersexual behavior. *Journal of Sex and Marital Therapy, 34*, 133–149.

Reid, R. C., Garos, S., & Carpenter, B. N. (2011). Reliability, validity, and psychometric development of the Hypersexual Behavior Inventory in an outpatient sample of men. *Sexual Addiction and Compulsivity, 18*, 1–22.

Salmon, R. F. (1995). Therapist's guide to 12-step meetings for sexual dependencies. *Sexual compulsivity and Addiction, 2*, 193–213.

Schaef, A. W. (1989). *Escape from intimacy.* San Francisco: Harper & Row.

Schneider, J. P., & Schneider, B. (1991). *Sex, lies and forgiveness: Couples speak out on the healing from sexual addiction.* Center City, MN: Hazelden Educational Materials.

Shaffer, H. (1994). Considering two models of excessive sexual behavior: Addiction and obsessive–compulsive disorder. *Journal of Sex Addiction and Compulsivity, 1*, 6–18.

Society for the Advancement of Sexual Health. (2012). *Bookstore.* Retrieved from *www.sash.net/en/bookstore.html.*

Turner, M. (1990). Long-term outpatient group therapy as a modality for treating sexual addiction. *American Journal of Preventive Psychiatry and Neurology, 2*, 23–26.

PART III

THERAPEUTIC CHALLENGES FOR SEX THERAPY

Specific Groups

CHAPTER 14

Therapy with LGBTQ[1] Clients

Working with Sex and Gender Variance from a Queer Theory Model

Margaret Nichols

> We do not even in the least know the final cause of sexuality.
> The whole subject is hidden in darkness.
> —CHARLES DARWIN

> I argued that psychiatric diagnosis was the child of morality and
> that Judeo-Christian values controlled psychiatric practice.
> —GAY PSYCHOLOGIST CHARLES SILVERSTEIN (2009),
> referring to the 1973 removal of homosexuality
> from the DSM

Deviant or different? Sex therapy has moved beyond this question for individuals who identify as members of a sexual minority, defined in this chapter as lesbian, gay, bisexual, transgender, or queer (LGBTQ). Members of sexual minorities now seek sex therapy not for help in changing or accepting their orientation but for help improving their sexual satisfaction. Although many of the sexual problems may be the same

---

[1]LGBTQ: lesbian, gay, bisexual, transgender, queer. "Queer" includes other sex/gender variations, such as BDSM and polyamory, or is used by some to indicate membership in more than one sex/gender minority.

(e.g., low desire, anorgasmia), Nichols cautions us not to apply heterosexual standards of normal, ideal, or healthy sexuality to our treatment of sexual minority clients; in other words, "All forms of sex and gender variance are innocent until found guilty." Nichols places sex therapy for sexual minorities in historical and cultural context and raises basic questions about the nature of sexuality, such as: What constitutes a sexual orientation? Is sexual orientation static? Why is monogamy privileged over other sexual arrangements? Above all, Nichols encourages clinicians working with sexual minority clients to keep an open mind and to be flexible in both the method and goals of treatment.

Margaret Nichols, PhD, is a Licensed Clinical Psychologist, an AASECT-Certified Sex Therapist and a Sex Therapy Supervisor. She is the founder and Executive Director of the Institute for Personal Growth, a psychotherapy center in New Jersey, and has been working with the LGBTQ community since 1983. She received her PhD from Columbia University in 1981 and her postgraduate training in sex therapy at the University of Medicine and Dentistry of New Jersey in 1983. Dr. Nichols is an author, activist, and an advocate for LGBTQ mental health issues.

The first edition of *Principles and Practice of Sex Therapy,* published in 1980, contained a chapter on gay male sexuality written by David McWhirter, MD, and Drew Mattison, PhD. It was provocative for its time because even though homosexuality had been officially removed from the *Diagnostic and Statistical Manual of Mental Disorders* (DSM) in 1973, many sexologists and sex therapists were not fully on board with this idea. Masters and Johnson (1979) had just published a book purporting to "cure" homosexuals, and Helen Singer Kaplan (1979) had claimed that same-sex orientation was a form of desire disorder. Yet Leiblum and Pervin (1980) chose two openly gay men for a chapter showcasing solid, long-lasting—and nonmonogamous—gay male relationships.

Starting in 1989 with the second edition of *Principles and Practice of Sex Therapy,* I have written the "queer chapter" as an openly queer sex therapist running a therapy agency specializing in work with the LGBTQ community.[2] Over the years the queer subculture has grown more inclusive: In 2013 "the community," virtual and in the flesh, contains not only people who identify as LGBTQ but also those interested in BDSM, fetishes, and nonmonogamy. Because of this, in this chapter I address LGBTQ issues as well as polyamory/nonmonogamy, leaving BDSM to Kleinplatz (Chapter 9). I define "sex therapy" as not only the treatment of sexual dysfunction but also what it has been historically, treatment of those with atypical sexuality or gender expression, and I cover both types of issues here.

---

[2]The chapter in the fourth edition is coauthored with my dear late friend and colleague Michael Shernoff.

THE PATHOLOGY MODEL
AND ITS SOCIAL CONSEQUENCES

From the birth of sexology, marked by the publication of Kraft-Ebbing's *Psychopathia Sexualis* in 1886, sex researchers and their psychiatric colleagues have been concerned, one might even say obsessed, with atypical sexual behavior and gender presentation. And since that time, there have been two competing views of nonstandard sexual behaviors: the belief that these behaviors and attractions are deviant and the view that they are simply variant. Kraft-Ebbing favored deviance, whereas Havelock Ellis and Magnus Hirschfeld saw variance; Freud framed deviant sexuality as developmental immaturity, whereas Kinsey imagined the natural variation found in his original field, entomology (Drescher, 2010).

The American Psychiatric Association's *Diagnostic and Statistical Manual of Mental Disorders* codified our understanding of sex and gender variance with its first edition in 1952 (Grob, 1991). Dominated by psychoanalytic thought, grounded in psychiatric opinion rather than, for example, the scientific work of Kinsey, the diagnosis of OOQ-x63, Sexual Deviation, included descriptors and subtypes ranging from homosexuality and transvestitism to nymphomania and syphilophobia (fear of syphilis). We now see some of these diagnoses as ridiculous, but at the time psychiatrists saw them as true mental disorders.

Biological theories now rival or overshadow psychoanalytic ones in psychiatry and sexology, but both models are rooted in the assumption that procreation is the sole or primary function of sex. This belief in turn issues from a narrow interpretation of Darwin's theory of sexual selection, for example, "survival of the fittest," the idea that the transmission of desirable genetic traits is accomplished when the fittest male and fittest female mate and produce offspring. This model makes heterosexual intercourse a biological imperative, whereas sex or gender presentations that do not lead directly to reproduction are "evolutionarily maladaptive" (Bailey, 2003, p. 115) or a "developmental error" (Bailey, 1999, p. 884).[3] In the deviance model, statistically unusual forms of sex and gender are mistakes, whether diseases caused by birth defects (biology based) or immature development (psychoanalytically based). And if they are mistakes, if possible these atypical forms should be treated and cured. Just as the medical model upon which psychiatry rests views deviations from the norm as disease indicators, so by extension sex and gender outliers are abnormal as well.

The deviance model became incorporated into the new field of sex therapy, the clinical application of sexology science. The leaders in the field,

---

[3]In fact, there is a virtual cottage industry of evolutionary psychological theories just to explain homosexuality, because according to a strict Darwinian model, genes for homosexual behavior should have vanished eons ago.

Masters and Johnson and Helen Singer Kaplan, clearly saw homosexuality as less desirable than heterosexuality; besides their books, these pioneers played deplorable roles in the AIDS era of the late 1980s, exaggerating the risks of transmission, spreading misinformation about gay men, and amplifying the heightened homophobia of the nation (Irvine, 2005).

Although sexologists and psychiatrists assume that their work is neutral and above the fray of social norms and customs, history shows us that the opinions of these experts have enormous social consequences, intended or not. The pathologization of homosexuality by sexologists in the 1800s is widely credited with bringing about increased social oppression of same-sex people, including the criminalization of sodomy (D'Emilio & Freedman, 1988). In the first part of the 20th century, homophile activists, ironically, turned to psychiatry in the hope that being classified as "mentally ill" rather than criminals would soften public opinion, only to find that their psychiatric status became the justification for other forms of discrimination, particularly employment (Hirshman, 2012). As the Silverstein quote that starts this chapter suggests, so clearly was psychiatry seen as the enemy that the Gay Activist Alliance demonstrated at the American Psychiatric Association (APA) meeting within 6 months of the "Stonewall Revolution" that started modern gay activism. And the removal of the diagnosis in 1973 was instrumental in changing the public image of homosexuality (Bayer, 1981; Drescher, 2010). Although the APA, pushed by the activists, did not see the change as an endorsement that homosexuality was "normal," it was widely interpreted that way, and this helped efforts to overturn the criminal and civil laws founded on the view that gays were mentally ill. The practice of therapy changed: Involuntary hospitalization and aversive conditioning techniques, formerly routine, were abolished and attempts at "cure" mostly discredited. The declassification reinforced "gay pride" and helped diminish shame and self-hatred (Bayer, 1981). In part because of the APA decision, lesbians and gay men in the United States have achieved a remarkable degree of acceptance in a few decades.

Although the removal of the diagnosis in 1973 was a victory, Silverstein (2009), who was one of the activists involved, acknowledges that it fell far short of their goal of removing all "sexual deviancies" from the DSM. It by no means signaled the fall of the pathology paradigm: Even psychiatrists who favored removal believed that homosexuality was inferior to heterosexuality (Bayer, 1981), and as recently as 2012 sexologists could wonder whether homosexuality was a "paraphilia" (Cantor, 2012).

Thus debates about "cures" for homosexuality continue to rise up periodically. Although "conversion therapy" became scientifically discredited and homosexuality largely seen as "inborn," Christian Right groups in the United States still consider homosexuality a (sinful) "choice." Some have continued to try to change sexual orientation via what is called "reparative" or "ex-gay" therapy. In 2003, prominent psychiatrist Robert Spitzer, a leading proponent of the 1973 DSM decision, published an article reporting the success of ex-gay treatment (Spitzer, 2003), which was published in the prestigious *Archives of Sexual Behavior* without peer review. Spitzer's study was widely used by Christian ex-gay groups to justify their treatment methods.

The reparative therapy issue made headlines once again in the spring of 2012, when journalist Gabriel Arana published an account of his own ex-gay therapy. During an interview Arana obtained for the story, Spitzer admitted that "he had been wrong" in his conclusions in the 2003 study (Arana, 2012). Later, Spitzer made public a letter to the *Archives* retracting his 2003 views and a video apology to the gay community (Besen, 2012). But Spitzer's rationale for his apology was simply the ineffectiveness of conversion therapy. Despite his 1973 advocacy of removal of the diagnosis, Spitzer never saw gayness as normal. Says Hirshman (2012): "To this day, Spitzer thinks there's something not optimal about homosexuality, a behavior that does not lead to survival in a simple Darwinian world" (p. 140).

A QUEER THEORY OF SEX AND GENDER VARIANCE

I write as an openly queer therapist, the director of an LGBTQ psychotherapy center since 1983. But the model I describe here reflects the views of many of my LGBTQ-oriented peers and increasing numbers of leaders in sexology and mental health. The American Psychological Association Practice Guidelines for LGBTQ clients state that "same-sex attractions, feelings and behavior are normal variants of human sexuality" (2012, p. 14). The World Association for Transgender Health (WPATH) endorses a "normal variance" model, and the *International Classification of Diseases* (ICD) codes of many European countries already reflect the WPATH guidelines. Some European countries have also eliminated consensual paraphilias from the ICD. The following paradigm is mine, but it is not unique.

An important subtext of the queer model I describe is a postmodern view of science. Queer theorists assume that science is never unbiased, that it is always distorted by the often unarticulated beliefs that the entire culture takes for granted to be true, even when it seems to be completely "objective." Consider this *Scientific American* report on song sparrows, birds that form long-lasting pair bonds to rear offspring but are sexually nonmonogamous (Fecht, 2012). Biologists describe the birds as "cheating" and "promiscuous" and label their behavior "infidelity." If a "hard" science such as biology is so clearly biased by cultural beliefs, queer theorists reason, the "softer" social sciences are hopelessly skewed. Queer theory considers history, sociology, direct observation, and clinical experience as data sources equal in significance to experimentally designed research.

Here are some fundamental assumptions of the queer theory paradigm:

- *Sex and gender variance is part of evolution's plan.* The traditional interpretation of Darwin is being challenged more and more in biology (Bagemihl, 1999), evolutionary science (Bailey & Zuck, 2009; Roughgarden,

2004) and psychology (Ryan & Jetha, 2010). Noting the lack of evidence to support the traditional mate-competition hypothesis and the observed fact that most sexual acts engaged in by animals are nonprocreative, dissenters suggest that sexual behavior is multipurposed and for many animals functions as an affiliative tool more often than a mechanism of reproduction. Thus, "recognized as a way to build and maintain a network of mutually beneficial relationships, nonreproductive sex no longer requires special explanations" (Ryan & Jetha, 2010, p. 103). Because "normal" sex does not have to be procreative, heterosexual intercourse and a rigid binary system of gender are not privileged.

- *All forms of sex and gender variance are innocent until found guilty.* If sex and gender variance are part of natural design, then they are presumed useful, even necessary, unless proven otherwise. This concept is in direct opposition to the psychiatric model that considers outliers problematic, and the clash of these beliefs has produced the ongoing hostile relationship between psychiatry/sexology and the LGBTQ community. What psychiatry sees as suboptimal adjustment, LGBTQ people consider normal and benign. Diagnosis, cure, and treatment is not only unnecessary, it is oppressive to sex and gender atypical people, who consider themselves in need of civil rights, not mental health intervention. A graphic on *GIDreform.org* is labeled "Let Us Out" and shows three trans people "escaping" from the DSM.

- *Our current knowledge of sex and gender variance is primitive; we don't yet know what dimensions are relevant.* For example, our current Western model assumes that sexual orientation and gender identity are completely separate dimensions, but many other cultures, including our own less than 100 years ago, see them as blended or even identical. The very way we "slice up the pie" may be wrong, and contemporary research on sex and gender may largely turn out to be irrelevant, like the old Greek medical concept of "vapors."

For example, there is current dialogue within the LGBTQ community—and confusion among professionals—about what constitutes an "orientation." Some nonmonogamous people, many kinky people and some self-identified asexuals experience their respective sexual desires as outside of conscious control, compelling, and organic, that is, something that has "always" been part of them. We have no tangible definition of "orientation," which traditionally has referred only to same- or opposite-sex attraction. Do sex- and gender-variant people share common underlying traits that might represent dimensions of sexuality we have yet to consider? And think of our different measurements: Does "orientation" reference desire, fantasy, behavior, or self-identification? To queer theorists, our current category constructs must be thought of as working models, not "reality."

- *Variant forms of sex and gender expression have existed in all cultures since the beginning of human existence.* Exhibit 1: the "gay caveman" (Gast & Aarthun, 2011). Interestingly, these are actually the remains of a gender-variant but not necessarily same-sex-attracted individual.

• *Biology may predispose toward sex and/or gender variance, but culture determines the extent to which it will get expressed and the ways it may manifest.* The interdisciplinary approach favored by queer sexologists makes us appreciate the vitally important role of culture. We understand that different cultures determine whether sex and gender variance will be permitted any open expression at all and, if permitted, what forms are sanctioned (Eliason & Schope, 2007; Nichols, 2012). Iran exemplifies extreme cultural shaping: The country ranks second worldwide in its rate of gender reassignment surgery (GRS) (Drescher, 2010) with little (open) expression of homosexual behavior, because in Iran homosexuality is a crime punishable by death, and GRS is sanctioned and funded by the state.

Even in cultures in which same-sex attraction has been allowed, its expression has taken many forms. Our 21st-century Western model of homosexuality is far from universal. We define orientation by the gender of one's partners, but in many cultures the particular sexual acts engaged in, and the role one plays during sex, are more important. For example, Brazilian "travesti" have a feminine gender presentation but keep their penises and are sexually involved with other men (Phua, 2010), and in Mexico a homosexual is defined as being the person who is the "insertee" in sex and bisexual behavior is accepted in heterosexually identified "inserter" males (Jeffries, 2009). In Western First World countries, egalitarian relationships between self-identified gay people are the norm, but age-structured relationships between older men or women and young boys or girls are most common historically and still exist in some non-Western cultures. Culture affects whether sex and gender variance is expressed openly, how much it is stigmatized, and what lifestyles and identities are available to variant people.

• *In Western culture, sex and gender expression are also determined by the LGBTQ subculture.* Unlike other minorities, LGBTQ people usually have sex- and gender-normative parents who may not support their children, and often this spurs the formation of communities that take the place of family. The LGBTQ subculture provides a "tribe" that validates, protects, and nurtures its members against a hostile mainstream, and like all tribes it has its own norms, philosophies, and beliefs that determine available identities—how one can self-label—and permitted behaviors. Most important, the LGBTQ subculture continuously evolves. In North America and Western Europe it has evolved and morphed at warp speed in the past 40 years. I discuss current trends in the LGBTQ community later in the chapter.

• *It's not "dysphoria," it's "minority stress."* Consistently higher rates of depression, suicidality, and substance abuse have been solidly documented among LGBTQ people for at least three decades (Mustanski, Garofalo, & Emerson, 2010). LGBTQ teens are twice as likely to use alcohol or drugs as their heterosexual peers and half as likely to report that they are happy, and they are more likely to report eating disorders, self-harm, depression, or suicide (Human Rights Campaign, 2012). Proponents of a deviance model have suggested that elevated rates of mental disorders are genetically linked to sexual orientation or gender atypicality (Bailey, 1999). In contrast, queer theory sees an LGBTQ person's dysphoria as the result of "minority stress." Borrowed from research on racial and ethnic minorities, the concept of "minority stress" refers to the physical violence, legal sanctions, discriminatory practices, and social disapproval that members of stigmatized groups routinely encounter in their lives. There is a substantial body of research linking minority stress and LGBTQ mental and sexual health (Herek & Garnets, 2007). LGBTQ people who live in states that have banned gay marriage exhibit elevated rates of psychiatric disorders after passage of the laws (Hatzenbuehler, Rosario, Corliss, Koenen, & Austin, 2012), and among transgender people depression is directly linked to the extent to which they have suffered abuse because of their atypical gender presentation (Roberts et al, 2012). School victimization fully mediates the relationship between LGBTQ youth and depression (Toomey, Ryan, & Diaz, 2010).

Minority stress affects different LGBTQ subgroups differentially, with the most stigmatized subgroups suffering the most. Gender-variant people and bisexuals appear to have the highest rates of depression, suicidality, sexual assault history, and sexual health problems (Mustanski et al., 2010). Black LGBTQ people suffer more than whites; black gay and transgender youth are more likely to end up homeless, for example (Yu, 2010). The queer model asserts that LGBTQ people do not suffer psychological distress because they are variant but rather because society can't handle their variance.

- *Families do not create sex and gender variance, but their reaction to their variant children greatly influences the young person's mental health.* Supportive families and schools can reduce minority stress. The top reasons depressed and suicidal LGBTQ teens give for their distress are family rejection and LGBTQ-related victimization by peers and others (Diamond et al., 2011). Family acceptance seems to be a "buffer" against extrafamilial stressors (LaSala, 2010; Kuper, Nussbaum, & Mustanski, 2012).

DSM-5: A CLASH OF PARADIGMS

The revisions to DSM-5 (American Psychiatric Association, 2013) include two areas of great concern to the LGBTQ community: diagnoses about gender atypicality and the paraphilias. I address only the first here.

When the diagnosis of gender identity disorder (GID) was added to DSM in 1980, transgender people hoped it would lead to increased access to medical care, but over the years most transgender activists came to view GID as the equivalent of the psychiatric diagnosis of homosexuality, a tool of social control (Lev, 2005). Since the publication of the first Harry Benjamin Society Standards of Care (SOC) in 1979, mental health practitioners have been gatekeepers for hormone treatment and surgery, and as such they have sometimes denied or blocked access to medical treatment based on their interpretations of the SOC. Certain theories, such as the theory of autogynephilia, have caused concern among the transgender community that people who fit this definition will not be seen as "true" transsexuals, and thus they will be denied access to medical treatment. As transgender people feel more empowered, they are becoming more vocal: At the 2009 American Psychiatric Association meeting, transactivists protested the composition of the DSM-5 Work Group on Gender Identity Disorders (Peggy Cohen-Kettenis, chair, Heino F. L. Meyer-Bahlburg, Jack Drescher, Friedemann Pfafflin), complaining in particular about the lack of transgender representation and Kenneth Zucker's leadership, as Zucker's therapy methods with gender-variant children have been a target of such activists (Wingerson, 2009). Transactivists continue to protest the GID, gender identity disorder in children (GIDC), and TD (transvestic disorder) diagnoses. Many providers of transgender care have joined them, and as a consequence, the renamed Harry Benjamin Society—the World Professional Association for Transgender Health (WPATH)—version of the Standards of Care released in 2011 radically depart from past editions, changing the role of the mental health professional from gatekeeper to advisor/advocate (Knudson, Cuypere, & Bockting, 2010) and asserting that "gender variance is not in and of itself reflective of pathology and having a cross- or transgender identity is not a psychiatric disorder" (Knudson et al., 2010, p. 116). WPATH has recommended that the World Health Organization change the name of GID and GIDC and move them out of the psychiatric disorder classification and into one of medical disorder; many European countries have already done so. Meanwhile, many LGBTQ counseling centers and health clinics have already rejected the "gatekeeper" model and offer hormones to those who can give informed consent without the recommended letter from a mental health practitioner (Drescher, 2010).

GIDC has been a controversial diagnosis as well. The primary issue has been the recommended treatment for these children, which, until recently, consisted of getting them to become more behaviorally gender conforming. The WPATH SOC now considers this treatment unethical. Instead, WPATH endorses support for younger children and a protocol of medical treatment beginning in early puberty that has been in place in the Netherlands for 20 years (Cohen-Kettenis, Delemarre-van de Waal, & Gooren, 2008). Increasingly, queer-theory-based practitioners and parents of gender-variant children, allied with LGBTQ groups, are demanding this medical treatment and/or social transition for gender-variant children and teens (Ehrensaft, 2011). Mental health professionals practicing within the traditional paradigm are resistant, urging "caution" (Levine, Zucker, & Meyer-Bahlburg, 2012), and in the United States it has primarily been nonpsychiatric M.D.s who have replicated this treatment modality, with apparent success (Spack et al., 2012).

EMERGING TRENDS IN THE LGBTQ COMMUNITY TODAY

In 2013, there are breaking trends in behavior and self-identification in the LGBTQ urban communities that will eventually affect all queer communities in North America. Professionals working with this community need to stay abreast of changes; here are some that have relevance to sex therapists and sexologists:

• *Gender lines are blurring.* Transgender people have increasingly become incorporated into the LGBTQ subculture. Transwomen who are attracted to other women identify as lesbians; transmen attracted to women often partner with bisexual women and remain within the LGBTQ community. This integration of trans people into the queer subculture has produced a new way of viewing gender: rejection of the gender binary in favor of a continuum. This in turn has resulted in a proliferation of new gender identities, especially among women. In truth, there has always been an overlap between gender identity/expression and sexual orientation, for example, "butch" lesbians and "sissy" gay men, despite the politically correct trope that they are separate. Lesbians, who historically have eroticized "butchness," have ultimately embraced transmen, and the younger ones have enthusiastically adopted newly emerging identities. Dykes and butches have been joined by those who identify as bois, AG's, genderqueer, gender fluid, or just plain queer. It is probable that the acceptance of "butchness" within the lesbian community has helped drive the explosion of female-to-male (FtM) transmen. Once thought to be uncommon, FtMs now equal male-to-female (MtF) transgender people in number (Beemyn & Rankin, 2011), and two-thirds of FtMs first identified as "butch" lesbians. Gender identity and sexual orientation are blending in new and unexpected ways: There are FtMs who are only attracted to other FtMs, bisexual women just attracted to transmen or transwomen, and FtMs who pretransition were only attracted to women but afterward are attracted to gay men and self-identify as gay male (Bockting, Benner, & Coleman, 2009).

Transgender people themselves are choosing more "blended" identities, eschewing the former labels of "transsexual" and "cross-dresser." In fact, among those under 40, "genderqueer" is the single most commonly chosen identity label (Beemyn & Rankin, 2011). As the binary has broken down, so has the traditional trajectory of hormones, full transition to the "other" gender, and GRS. Providers used to the psychiatric model become confused when, for example, a young FtM wants chest reconstruction surgery but eschews the use of testosterone, and yet this is becoming increasingly common.

• *The overlap increases.* As transgender people become incorporated into the LGBTQ community, so have others whose sexual expression is variant from the mainstream. Alliances between BDSM and polyamory[4] activists

---

[4]Polyamory is a specific form of "open" relationship, espousing multiple sexual and romantic partners, unlike "swinging" and typical gay male open relationships, both of which emphasize sex and not intimate connection. In practice, the boundaries between these types of open relationships can get blurred.

and LGBTQ groups are growing, and there is increasing overlap between all groups. Gay men, lesbians, and especially bisexuals are overrepresented among those who are interested in nonstandard sexual practices and open relationships (Richters, de Visser, Rissel, Grulich, & Smith, 2008; Barker & Langdridge, 2010). The professional used to working with one group will increasingly need to be aware of all types of sex and gender atypicality.

• *The notion of fixed identity and orientation is changing.* Sex- and gender-variant identity is more fluid than we have imagined, perhaps more for women than men (Diamond, 2008). Moreover, the very meaning of identity may be changing. Most sexologists regard identity as a fixed, essential quality of the individual. But Lisa Diamond, who followed a cohort of self-identified bisexual and lesbian college women over nearly 12 years, found that her participants changed identities two or more times, using the labels more as descriptions of their current lives than unchangeable attributes. Increasingly, many younger sex- and gender-variant people feel that *no* identity label captures their experience (Savin-Williams, 2005). One such person's self-description is "first as a guy, then as a gay man, then as an FtM, then perhaps. . . . as a queer FtM who still has sex with women (usually butch women or MtFs) once in a while" (Bockting et al., 2009, p. 693).

CLINICAL ISSUES

Assessing with Whom You Are Working and What the Sexual Problem Is

Not all nonheterosexual clients will self-identify as gay, lesbian, bisexual, or transgender, so it is important for the clinician to recognize the relationship between self-proclaimed identity and other measures of sex and gender variance, such as attractions, fantasy, or behavior. In any society that stigmatizes homosexuality, many more people will *experience* same-sex attractions than will *act* upon them, and fewer still will *identify* as gay, lesbian, or bisexual (Chandra, Mosher, & Copen, 2011). Also, when gender nonconformity is vilified, people attempt to hide their atypicality. Therefore, heterosexually identified people may have same-sex desires and behavior (Reback & Larkins, 2010), and some clients who appear to be cisgendered[5] have internal feelings of gender incongruence. Because gay people have historically had difficulty with bisexuals, self-identified lesbians and gay men may have extensive heterosexual experience that they hide. And the label "bisexual" is itself complex—it is a residual category that includes people who have little in common besides an attraction to both sexes. There are bisexuals who are monogamous, those who consider bisexuality and polyamory intrinsically linked, individuals with

---

[5] "Cisgender" = the opposite of transgender. Cisgender people experience their gender as congruent with their body, presentation, traits, and behaviors and with others' experience of them.

equal attraction to both genders, those with a primary attraction to one gender, and some who feel their desires transcend gender.

To capture this complex information and to avoid offending LGBTQ clients, who usually notice language based on the "heterosexual assumption," initial assessment tools need to be gender and sexual orientation neutral. Include the option of "other" when asking about gender, ask for information about the client's partner instead of "husband" or "wife," talk about vaginal penetration, not intercourse. Information about multiple dimensions—attractions, fantasy, behavior, and self-identification—should be ascertained separately and examined for incongruencies. When present, incongruencies should be explored gently: A client's identity may seem at odds with his or her behavior or attraction, but it symbolizes an important, deeply held belief the person holds about him- or herself. As a clinician, you may suspect that the man sitting across from you, who regularly has sex with other men but identifies as heterosexual, is fooling himself, but it may take years before the client can come to terms with that—or it may never happen at all.

There are no widely used instruments measuring sexuality and sexual dysfunction that are geared to LGBTQ clients. Most existing tools focus on heterosexual intercourse as a measure of sexual function, so clinicians working with LGBTQ clients will need to design their own instruments.[6] The sexual questionnaire we give clients at the Institute for Personal Growth (IPG) includes questions about more than two dozen sex acts, including some "kinky" and "fetish" acts, questions about male and female sex partners, and questions about open, consensual outside sexual activity, as well as about "infidelity." Therapists should be aware that despite such TV shows as *Modern Family,* LGBTQ people do not all model their sex and relationship lives according to heterosexual norms. As previously noted, BDSM and open relationships are quite common in LGBTQ populations, especially among younger people in urban areas.

For LGBTQ clients in need of sex therapy, DSM-5 (American Psychiatric Association, 2013) diagnostic categories can be used without issue, as they are notably free of heterosexual bias in their wording. There are some specific sexual problems that LGBTQ clients may bring that are uncommon among heterosexuals and related to differences in sexual behavior—for example, an aversion to oral or anal sex. These may need to be classified as "not otherwise specified" (NOS) disorders in DSM-5.

Lesbian Sexual Issues

The sparse research on lesbian sexuality, mostly survey data, suggests that woman-to-woman sex is different from heterosexual sex in some important ways (Matthews, Hughes, & Tartaro, 2006; Nichols, 2006; van

[6]I will send electronic versions of my questionnaires upon request.

Rosmalen-Nooijens, Vergeer, & Largo-Janssen, 2008). Lesbians seem to spend more time on sex, incorporate a larger sexual repertoire (particularly those acts commonly considered "foreplay"), are more frequently orgasmic when they do have sex, are less likely to have sex just because their partners want it, and report fewer pain disorders, lower overall rates of sexual dysfunction, and lower rates of STDs. Like their heterosexual female counterparts, the most common lesbian sexual complaint is lack of desire, although, unlike heterosexual women, lesbians are as likely to complain of lack of desire in their partners as lack of desire in themselves.

"Lesbian bed death" is a phrase that describes lesbian relationships that over time become devoid of genital sex, if not nongenital affection. The term emerged in the 1980 from within the lesbian community, and it has been discussed and debated ever since. Some critics (Rothblum & Brehony, 1993; Cole, 1993) challenge the belief that sex is needed for healthy relationship functioning, arguing that genital sex may be redundant in egalitarian, intimately connected relationships: "sex therapy currently assumes that the goal is to be sexual, whereas in some situations it is better simply to validate a 'Boston marriage'"(Cole, 1993, p. 192). Others argue that lesbian bed death is a myth. The data on frequency is mixed, with some surveys showing lesbians having somewhat lower frequency than heterosexual couples (Nichols, 2006) and others no difference (Matthews et al., 2006) In any case, lesbian bed death appears to occur less often than the urban legend would have it. But the focus on sexual frequency may reflect a heteronormative bias. Frequency aside, it appears that when two women do have sex, it seems to be at least as pleasurable as heterosexual sex is for straight women, it lasts longer, contains more of the sexual behaviors many women desire, and is more likely to be consensual.

Whatever the truth about lesbian bed death, existing data indicate that low frequency or desire is the main, indeed virtually the only, sexual problem gay women report. Many, though not all, lesbian couples present in a distinct way: They often have high-functioning, physically affectionate relationships with minor nonsexual relationship problems. Therapists who are familiar with the ideas of David Schnarch and Esther Perel may posit that the intense togetherness of these relationships contributes to the loss of sex passion, and in these cases individuation of each partner may be a therapeutic goal.

When a lesbian couple presents with problems of low sexual frequency, before initiating treatment the clinician should probe the reasons for the complaint and explore motivation before agreeing to attempt to resurrect sex for the couple. Coles's admonition is worth remembering: Some couples just need to have their lack of a genital sexual relationship validated.

Case 1: "Lesbian Bed Death"

Elle and Cara, together 12 years, came to sex therapy complaining that sex had dwindled to once or twice a year. Cara had been the first to lose interest, several years into the relationship, whereas Elle's diminished desire appeared to be a reaction to repeated rejection. Recently, Elle had experienced a strong attraction to another woman. Although she did not act on these feelings, the experience made her realize how much she missed sex, and she insisted that the couple seek sex therapy. Cara agreed. The couple reported good intimacy in nonsexual aspects of their relationship, and though Cara was not experiencing active sexual desire, her love for Elle motivated her to try to regain libido. The therapist's first intervention was to teach Elle and Cara about Rosemary Basson's (Basson, 2000) alternative model of the female sexual response cycle, which conceptualizes female desire as typically moving from "active" to "receptive" in long-term relationships. The women were told that they could not rely on physical lust to propel them to sexual behavior. Lesbian relationships sometimes suffer from what might be termed the "Basson squared" effect: If both women lose active desire, then no one initiates sex at all. Educating the couple about the Basson model validated Cara's experience and helped Elle depersonalize Cara's rejection of her sexual advances.

Once they accepted that "sexual willingness" would need to replace "lust," the couple was disabused of their belief that sex should be spontaneous and convinced to make "dates." They were also encouraged to dress and behave seductively and flirtatiously. Both women were trained to foster "simmering": They were taught to make themselves ready for sex by consciously thinking and fantasizing about sex hours or days before "date night," thus facilitating arousal over time.

The couple needed to shed other romantic but unrealistic myths. For example, they believed that all sexual encounters had to end in orgasm for both partners and that orgasm had to result from partner stimulation. But Elle had a higher sex drive and easier arousal and orgasm than Cara. Cara recognized her own willingness to pleasure Elle if she herself did not feel the pressure to have an orgasm that made sex into work. Cara and Elle redefined sex as sensual and/or genital contact that might (but did not have to) result in orgasm for one or both partners and in which the orgasms might or might not be partner facilitated. This freed the couple to have more sexual encounters, and the overall frequency of their sex life increased in a way that gave pleasure to them both.

This couple had a sexual repertoire that included lots of touching, oral and manual genital sex, and occasional digital–vaginal penetration. Although varied, it had become routine, and therapy shifted to encouraging exploration of new territory. They spent a session with the IPG toy box—a collection of sex toys ranging from vibrators, dildos, and butt plugs, to feathers, bondage cuffs, and lube samples. The therapist explained the use of these toys in an enthusiastic and matter-of-fact way in order to dispel the women's anxiety and encourage a playful stance toward sex, and afterward the women accepted a "homework" assignment to purchase some sex toys together. Because the therapist believed that "kinky sex," far from being pathological, could be an enhancer of sex, the women were asked to "interview" each other using copies of sexual negotiation questionnaires developed by BDSM groups, documents promoting open, specific communication about sexual likes and dislikes. The use of a BDSM questionnaire might have been a risky intervention with a heterosexual couple, but given the acceptance of kink in the lesbian community, these women found it unremarkable. The exercise was successful and led the women to experiment with dominant–submissive role play. Thus BDSM introduced a power and role differential in this couple's sexual dynamic that did not exist in the rest of their relationship, and this individuation may have fueled erotic desire. The couple increased their sexual encounters to a frequency of about once every 6 weeks, and they were both satisfied with this result.

Gay Men, Gay Male Sexuality, and HIV

Since the beginning of the AIDS epidemic, research on gay male sexuality has focused almost exclusively upon HIV transmission and prevention, with less attention paid to gay male sexual dysfunction. Sandfort and de Keizer (2001), in a comprehensive review of research on gay sexuality, found that reports of erectile dysfunction (ED) were higher for gay men than for heterosexual men but that complaints about rapid ejaculation (RE) or delayed ejaculation (DE) were uncommon, as were reports of low sexual desire, except among HIV positive men.[7] Bancroft, Carnes, Janssen, Goodrich, and Long (2005) found similar results, and Hart, Wolitsky, and Purcell (2003) also report high ED rates in gay men. These differences may reflect the specific common sexual behaviors of gay men. Gay men do not experience the pressure felt by heterosexual men to ejaculate during intercourse while "lasting" long enough to pleasure their partners, but they do feel pressure to "perform," which may account for the high rates of reported ED.

Gay men are more sexual than women or heterosexual men, with all studies comparing them showing more frequent sex, more casual sex, and greater numbers of partners (Martin, 2006; Sandfort & de Keizer, 2001). Despite AIDS, sex is still a dominant force in the lives of gay men, providing social networks, affirmation of identity, and access to transcendent, spiritual experience (Martin, 2006). Therapists should expect that sex will be very important to most of their gay male clients and that clients will engage in a wide range of sexual encounters and behaviors. Moreover, nearly half of all male couples are nonmonogamous (LaSala, 2004; Parsons, Starks, DuBois, Grov, & Golub, 2011). The most common form of sexual openness, sometimes called "monogamish" relationships, are couples who regularly bring a third man into their sexual encounter, and often the couples who have this kind of sexual arrangement report the highest levels of relationship satisfaction (LaSala, 2004). BDSM, often called "leather sex," has been an integral part of gay male sexuality for decades, with the terms "top" and "bottom,"

---

[7]HIV appears to lower testosterone, as do some of the medications used to treat it.

borrowed from BDSM, used by gay men to designate inserter versus insertee in oral and anal sex (Hart et al., 2003). Clinicians working with gay couples should expect many of them to be sexually nonmonogamous and be prepared to help the couple with problems that arise from this openness without judging the arrangement. It may be even be appropriate to question why a couple does *not* have an open relationship in cases of very discrepant interests or desire.

HIV remains a huge problem in the gay male community. Gay and bisexual men remain most affected in the United States, with 61% of all new seroconversions in 2009 (Centers for Disease Control and Prevention, 2011). "Barebacking"—anal sex without a condom—remains common, especially among younger men. Because prevention techniques developed in the 1980s appear to have reached the limit of their effectiveness, many now advocate a harm-reduction approach through techniques such as "serosorting," or encouraging men to bareback only with men of similar HIV status (Philip, Yu, Donnell, Vittinghoff, & Buchbinder, 2010).

Case 2: Using Harm Reduction with a Sexual Risk Taker

Toby, a 30-year-old HIV-negative man, entered therapy with concerns about his practice of barebacking with partners found on the Internet. Toby had never known anyone who died of AIDS, and although a friend of his had recently become HIV positive, the friend was on combination antiretroviral therapy with no apparent adverse side effects, and this probably muted Toby's concern about becoming infected. Toby did not want to be HIV positive, but he felt unwilling or unable to give up barebacking. He believed that barebacking increased his sexual currency, that it enabled him to have sex with men he deemed more attractive than himself, who he feared would not be interested in him if he insisted on safe sex. Because of the riskiness of Toby's behavior, the gay male therapist treating Toby decided on an initial harm-reduction approach rather than a deeper exploration of the self-esteem and body image issues that probably drove Toby's somewhat compulsive sexuality.

Toby was not confident that he would use condoms regularly. Although he readily agreed that he should, he was unsure of his ability to do so in the heat of a sexual encounter. The therapist suggested he try serosorting as an alternative. Toby felt more capable of using serosorting, but he needed to develop skills to accomplish this method of prevention. Toby felt unable to raise the topic of HIV status with men he encountered online for fear that he would be rejected. His therapist suggested that in order to develop the skill of asking about serostatus, Toby begin by asking about HIV status only with men to whom he was *not* attracted. Toby learned that although some men were offended by this, others responded well, and some were even relieved. After learning to ask the HIV status of men he did not desire, he was coached to do this with men to whom he was moderately attracted. After about 3 months he was able to ask all the men he flirted with online their HIV status, and he had sex only with men who identified as being HIV negative. Although the serosorting method is clearly not foolproof and relies upon the honesty of partners, for Toby it was a step toward reducing the possibility of seroconverting.

The clinician in this case, the late Michael Shernoff, incorporated a "queer" perspective in his acceptance of frequent, casual sexual encounters with multiple partners and barebacking and in his practical, objective view of risky behavior. This allowed him to enthusiastically endorse a harm-reduction approach instead of labeling this man a "sex addict," which many pathology-paradigm clinicians would have done.

Bisexuality

Within the LGBTQ community, as well as without, bisexuals have historically been either invisible, labeled "straight" or "gay" according to the gender of their current partners, or feared, mistrusted, and despised, although younger people are more accepting and more likely themselves to identify as bi- or pansexual. When homosexuality was more highly stigmatized, the use of the label became associated with gay people who couldn't accept their homosexuality and were prone to desert their same-sex lovers for socially acceptable heterosexual relationships. In addition, lesbians have mistrusted bisexual women because they are seen as bringing sexually transmitted infections (STIs) into the women's community (Nichols, 2006; van Rosmalen-Nooijens et al., 2008). Among heterosexuals, a study rating attitudes toward a multitude of stigmatized racial, social, religious, and sexual groups revealed that bisexual men and women were rated lower than all other groups except injecting drug users (Herek, 2002). The negative attitudes about bisexuality are probably related to widespread ignorance and misunderstanding. Many people simply do not believe bisexuality exists, including, in the recent past, some sex researchers.

There are substantial data that suggest that bisexual attraction, behavior, and identity are more common among women than men, including studies of physiological arousal (Chivers, Seto, & Blanchard, 2007; Cerny & Janssen, 2011) and survey data (Chandra et al., 2011). Three times more women identify as bisexual than lesbian, whereas among men slightly more identify as gay than bisexual, and same-sex sexual behavior appears to be increasing among young women but not young men (Gartrell, Bos, & Goldberg, 2012), although it is not known how these young women will eventually identify themselves. Many self-identified bisexuals are also transgender, "kinky," or polyamorous. The clinician needs to pay close attention to what each client means by self-identifying as bisexual and to be mindful of the double stigma attached to the label that may leave the person feeling isolated and alone even within the LGBTQ community.

Special Problems of Gender-Variant Youth

It is beyond the scope of this chapter to fully discuss the highly controversial issues of transgender clients, but it is important to touch on the problems faced by gender-variant youth, as they are becoming the fastest growing and most visible members of the LGBTQ community. LGBTQ teens have higher rates of abuse and distress than other adolescents, and, within this group, distress is highest among gender-variant youth (Skidmore, Linsenmeier, & Bailey, 2006), because they are more visible than their gender-conforming peers. They get less support from parents (LaSala, 2010), and they are often the targets of bullying in school.

Because they suffer such distress, gender-variant young people are more likely than other queer youths to come for treatment. With treatment aimed at getting these young people to conform to traditional gender roles discredited, queer clinicians are developing alternative models of treatment that involve affirming and validating the child's nonconformity, encouraging parental support, and finding ways to protect children from peer abuse.

Like gay, lesbian, and bisexual youth, transgender people are "coming out" at earlier ages, and clinicians will increasingly see younger teens and even preteens who identify this way or who identify as "genderqueer" or "gender fluid." Some young people will need help sorting out their identity, and clinicians will increasingly be asked by parents to assess whether their children are "really" transgender, an assessment that is by definition imprecise because so little is known of the developmental trajectories of gender-variant children. Many clinicians will not be comfortable assuming this responsibility, and they should be able to refer to colleagues who will. When the adolescent already is certain of his or her gender identity, different issues come into play. The treatment protocols for young gender-variant people approved by WPATH and the U.S. Endocrine Society (Hembree et al., 2009) call for administering "puberty blocking" hormones early in the process, for social transition in the early teens, for cross-gender hormone treatment as young as 16, and for GRS as early as 18. Outcome research on these young people has shown that they do not regret their early transition and that they are as psychologically well adjusted as their nontransgender peers (Cohen-Kettenis et al., 2008). Because puberty blockers prevent the emergence of body changes associated with biological gender, young people given growth-blocking hormones at early stages of puberty never develop the physical characteristics that might "give them away" in their affirmed gender. Administered appropriately, growth-blocking hormones, followed 2 or more years later by cross-gender hormones, can make the difference between a transgender person who can "pass" and one who will not. Because the blockers are reversible, their use provides a "time-out" for the teen to explore gender issues and clarify identity. From a queer perspective, "the suspension of puberty is not only not unethical: if it is likely to improve the child's quality of life or even save his or her life, then it is indeed unethical to defer treatment" (Giordano, 2008, p. 580). Norman Spack and his colleagues, who released data on nearly 100 gender-variant youth using the preceding protocol in 2012, obtained the same result as Cohen-Kettenis and colleagues. Spack et al. (2012) noted that their sample contained a large percentage of young people with emotional disturbances such as depression, suicidality, and self-injurious behavior and that treatment with puberty-blocking and cross-gender hormones caused most of the disturbance to abate. Our experience at IPG parallels these findings. Many of us are used to treating older transgender people who transition after decades of hiding and whose lives are often shattered by transition. By contrast, it is notable that many gender-variant young people are free of mental illness or emotional disturbance once they are affirmed and supported and receive proper treatment.

Supported by parents and advocacy organizations such as TransYouthFamilyAllies (TYFA), some gender-variant children are socially transitioning as early as 5 or 6 (Ehrensaft, 2011), although the WPATH Standards of Care recommend caution with such early transition because longitudinal studies show that less than 50% of gender-variant children persist in a transgender identity into adulthood (Wallien & Cohen-Kettenis, 2008). How does a therapist respond to a 5-year-old natal boy who has insisted since his first words that he is a girl and whose parents want a social transition? Although we know that not all such children persist in their gender dysphoria, we are currently unable to predict which of them will. At IPG we are more cautious about prepubescent gender-variant children. When possible, we help parents structure an environment in which the child's nonconforming expression is permitted, validated, and supported, and where the child is not stigmatized in his or her school and community. Young natal boys have been more common in our practice than very young girls, possibly because gender-role norms for young males are so rigid and they are so viciously punished when violated. With these young boys we have advocated and educated the school system, guided the parents to activities in which nonconformity is permitted, for example, dance, and referred to groups for young gender-nonconforming children to decrease the child's isolation. But as of this writing we have had one young client, a 6-year-old natal boy, who was so severely dysphoric about his assigned gender that we supported the parents in a full social transition. At this juncture, 2 years after transition, the child seems to be doing well living as a girl in her school and community. However, parents and therapist give frequent reminders to the child that her identity can be fluid if she chooses.

Polyamory: The New Critique of Monogamy

Space does not permit more than a passing mention of polyamory and other forms of open relationships. As noted, open relationships are common among gay men and polyamorous ones increasingly common among lesbian and bisexual women (Munson & Stelbourn, 1999). Consensual nonmonogamy (as distinct from "cheating") is not new, even among heterosexuals. In the United States, nonmonogamy movements have been popular at several different points over the last century or two, with "swinging" the most prominent in recent decades. Polyamory, the practice of having multiple sexual and romantic relationships concurrently, is a newer iteration. In recent years, nonmonogamy as a valid lifestyle has received public visibility and curiosity, if not full acceptance. A number of books aimed at sophisticated general audiences have increased awareness of open relationships (Taormino, 2008; Ryan & Jetha, 2010), including a best-selling memoir by a polyamorous suburban wife and mother (Block, 2009). Therapists working with polyamorous people become accustomed to doing relationship counseling with three or more people in the room, and accepting therapists might even occasionally suggest some form of open relationship to a receptive monogamous couple searching to revive a boring sex life.

Case 3: Two "Lifestyle" Couples Attempt Polyamory

Roy and Connie entered treatment together as a late-middle-aged couple with a fundamentally sound 30-year marriage, the last 20 of which had been spent as "lifestylers"—swingers. Swinging as it is practiced today often goes beyond purely casual encounters; both Roy and Connie had occasionally had ongoing outside partners with whom they developed somewhat intimate, as well as sexual, relationships. Recently, Roy had ended such a liaison and, as often happens in open relationships, the balance shifted in the marriage and problems emerged that needed tending, problems not directly related to sex or swinging. The couple saw me regularly for a few months, and we "fine-tuned" the relationship, helping Connie become more assertive, Roy more attentive, and so on. In addition, I helped them "come out" to their grown children, as they had grown tired of secrecy. Although the couple feared a negative reaction, after some initial shock the children decided their parents' lifestyle was "cool." Then the couple became involved in their first clearly polyamorous network. They became intensely intimate, sexually and in other ways, with another swinging couple, Adelle and Jason. When some problems of insecurity and jealousy emerged, they sought my help. Both couples had had previous experience with more traditional therapists who saw their nonmonogamy as an escape from intimacy, and so they were grateful when I assured them that I would work toward their collective goal of remaining together as a foursome. Over a period of 6 months I saw them in various combinations and permutations in what has been challenging but fascinating work. Much of my work involved guiding them to make their expectations explicit, helping them set boundaries, rules, and guidelines for interactions, and avoiding triangulation or hidden alliances. We established ways for the marital relationships to stay primary, such as reserving certain times, places, and activities as "special," not to be shared with the other couple. At this writing the two couples remain a happy foursome. Although I cannot predict how long the polyamorous relationship will last, I have seen relationships like this last for many years. Far from using outside partners to replace sex in the primary relationship, many open couples maintain exceptionally good sex with each other even after decades together. Roy and Connie and Adelle and Jason, married two and three decades respectively, reported frequent and hot sex in their marriages throughout treatment, and both couples asserted that the "heat" had never left their marriages. My queer perspective with this case is obvious: I am enthusiastic about nonmonogamy as an option and knowledgeable about many of the common issues encountered when negotiating such alternative relationships.

CONCLUSIONS

Good clinical work with LGBTQ minorities involves more than acceptance of homosexuality. To be effective, the therapist must discard the traditional view that variations in sexual attractions and behavior and gender expression are symptoms of psychiatric disorder, suboptimal adjustment, or biological mistakes. This must be replaced by the perspective that variance is normal and adaptive and that "all sex and gender variance is innocent until proven guilty." The sex therapist adopting a "normal variance" paradigm will work more skillfully with their LGBTQ clients and understand their special needs. Beyond this, therapists can learn from their LGBTQ clients: about alternative forms of relationships and family, about the range of gender expression, about issues that are universal to all couples versus those related to gender. The queer theory paradigm promotes good practice and the genuine celebration of diversity.

REFERENCES

American Psychiatric Association. (1968). *Diagnostic and statistical manual of mental disorders* (2nd ed.). Washington, DC: American Psychiatric Association.

American Psychiatric Association. (2013). *Diagnostic and statistical manual of mental disorders* (5th ed.). Arlington, VA: Author.

American Psychological Association. (2012). Guidelines for psychological practice with lesbian, gay, and bisexual clients. *Journal of the American Psychological Association, 67*(1), 10–42.

Arana, G. (2012, April 11). *My so-called ex-gay life.* Retrieved June 7, 2012, from *http://prospect.org/article/my-so-called-ex-gay-life.*

Bagemihl, B. (1999). *Biological exuberance: Animal homosexuality and natural diversity.* New York: St. Martin's Press.

Bailey, J. M. (1999). Commentary: Homosexuality and mental illness. *Archives of General Psychology, 56,* 876–880.

Bailey, J. M. (2003). *The man who would be queen: The science of gender-bending and transsexualism.* Washington, DC: Joseph Henry Press.

Bailey, N. W., & Zuk, M. (2009). Same-sex sexual behavior and evolution. *Trends in Ecology and Evolution, 24*(8), 439–446.

Bancroft, J., Carnes, L., Janssen, E., Goodrich, D., & Long, J. S. (2005). Erectile and ejaculatory problems in gay and heterosexual men. *Archives of Sexual Behavior, 34*(3), 285–297.

Barker, M., & Langdridge, D. (2010). Whatever happened to non-monogamies? Critical reflections on recent research and theory. *Sexualities, 13*(6), 748–772.

Basson, R. (2000). The female sexual response: A different model. *Journal of Sex and Marital Therapy, 26,* 51–65.

Bayer, R. (1981). *Homosexuality and American psychiatry.* New York: Basic Books.

Beemyn, G., & Rankin, S. (2011). *The lives of transgender people.* New York: Columbia University Press.

Besen, W. (2012, May 30). *Interview with Dr. Robert Spitzer who discusses retracting his infamous "ex-gay" study.* Retrieved June 7, 2012, from *www.truthwinsout.org/blog/2012/05/25725.*

Block, J. (2009). *Open: Love, sex, and life in an open marriage.* Berkeley, CA: Seal Press.

Bockting, W., Benner, A., & Coleman, E. (2009). Gay and bisexual identity development among female-to-male transsexuals in North America: Emergence of transgender sexuality. *Archives of Sexual Behavior, 38*(5), 688–701.

Cantor, J. (2012). Is homosexuality a paraphilia? The evidence for and against. *Archives of Sexual Behavior, 41*(1), 237–347.

Centers for Disease Control and Prevention. (2011, August). *HIV incidence.* Retrieved December 15, 2011, from *www.cdc.gov/hiv/topics/surveillance/incidence.htm.*

Cerny, J. A., & Janssen, E. (2011). Patterns of sexual arousal in homosexual, bisexual, and heterosexual men. *Archives of Sexual Behavior, 40*(4), 687–697.

Chandra, A., Mosher, W. D., & Copen, C. (2011, March). *Sexual behavior, sexual attraction, and sexual identity in the United States: Data from the 2006–2008 National Survey of Family Growth* (National Health Statistics Reports No. 36). Retrieved December 15, 2011, from *www.cdc.gov/nchs/data/nhsr/nhsr036.pdf.*

Chivers, M. L., Seto, M. C., & Blanchard, R. (2007). Gender and sexual orientation differences in sexual response to sexual activities versus gender of actors in sexual films. *Journal of Personality and Social Psychology, 93*(6), 1108–1121.

Cohen-Kettenis, P. T., Delemarre-van de Waal, H. A., & Gooren, L. J. G. (2008). The treatment of adolescent transsexuals: Changing insights. *Journal of Sexual Medicine, 5,* 1892–1897.

Cole, E. (1993). Is sex a natural function?: Implications for sex therapy. In E. Rothblum & K. Brehony (Eds.), *Boston marriages: Romantic but asexual relationships among contemporary lesbians* (pp. 188–193). Amherst: University of Massachusetts Press.

Coleman, E., Bockting, W., Botzer, M., Cohen-Kettenis, P., DeCuypere, G., Feldman, J., et al. (2011). Standards of care for the health of transsexual, transgender, and gender-confirming people: Version 7. *International Journal of Transgenderism, 13,* 165–232.

D'Emilio, J. D., & Freedman, E. B. (1988). *Intimate matters: A history of sexuality in America.* New York: Harper & Row.

Diamond, G. M., Shilo, G., Jurgensen, E., D'Augelli, A., Samarova, V., & White, K. (2011). How depressed and suicidal sexual minority adolescents understand the causes of their distress. *Journal of Gay and Lesbian Mental Health, 15*(2), 130–151.

Diamond, L. (2008). *Sexual fluidity: Understanding women's love and desire.* Cambridge, MA: Harvard University Press.

Drescher, J. (2010). Queer diagnoses: Parallels and contrasts in the history of homosexuality, gender variance, and the *Diagnostic and Statistical Manual. Archives of Sexual Behavior, 39*(2), 427–460.

Ehrensaft, D. (2011). *Gender born, gender made: Raising healthy gender-nonconforming children*. New York: The Experiment Publishing.

Eliason, M. J., & Schope, R. (2007). *The health of sexual minorities: Shifting sands or solid foundation* (1st ed., Part 1, 3–26). New York: Springer-Verlag.

Fecht, S. (2012, June 6). *Lady liaisons: Does cheating give females an evolutionary advantage?* Retrieved June 2, 2012, from *www.scientificamerican.com/article. cfm?id=why-do-females-cheat*.

Gartrell, N. K., Bos, H. M. W., & Goldberg, N. G. (2012). New trends in same-sex sexual contact for American adolescents? [Letter to the editor]. *Archives of Sexual Behavior, 41*(1), 5–7.

Gast, P., & Aarthun, S. (2011, April 10). *Scientists speak out to discredit "gay caveman" media reports*. Retrieved June 7, 2012, from *http://articles.cnn. com/2011–04–10/world/czech.republic.unusual.burial_1_archaeologists-caveman-sexual-orientation?_s=pm:world*.

Giordano, S. (2008). Lives in a chiaroscuro: Should we suspend the puberty of children with gender identity disorder? *Journal of Medical Ethics, 34*, 580–584.

Grob, G. N. (1991). Origins of DSM-I: A study in appearance and reality. *American Journal of Psychiatry, 148*(4), 421–431.

Hart, T. A., Wolitski, R. J., & Purcell, D. W. (2003). Sexual behavior among HIV-positive men who have sex with men: What's in a label? *Journal of Sex Research, 40*(2), 179–188.

Hatzenbuehler, M. L., O'Cleirigh, C., Grasso, C., Mayer, K., Safren, S., & Bradford, J. (2012). Effect of same-sex marriage laws on health care use and expenditures in sexual minority men: A quasi-natural experiment. *American Journal of Public Health, 102*, 285–291.

Hembree, W. C., Cohen-Kettenis, P., Delemarre-van de Waal, H. A., Gooren, L. J., Meyer, W. J., III, Spack, N. P., et al. (2009). Endocrine treatment of transsexual persons: An endocrine society clinical practice guideline. *Journal of Clinical Endocrinology and Metabolism, 94*(9), 3132–3154.

Herek, G. M. (2002). Heterosexuals' attitudes towards bisexual men and women in the United States. *Journal of Sex Research, 39*(4), 264–274.

Herek, G. M., & Garnets, L.D. (2007). Sexual orientation and mental health. *Annual Review of Clinical Psychology, 3*, 353–375.

Hirshman, L. (2012). *Victory: The triumphant gay revolution*. New York: HarperCollins.

Human Rights Campaign. (2012). *Growing up LGBT in America: Key findings*. Retrieved from *www.hrc.org/youth#.t9-c3ilzeso*.

Irvine, J. M. (2005). *Disorders of desire: Sexuality and gender in modern American sexology*. Philadelphia: Temple University Press.

Jeffries, W., IV. (2009). A comparative analysis of homosexual behaviors, sex role preferences, and anal sex proclivities in Latino and non-Latino men. *Archives of Sexual Behavior, 38*(5), 756–778.

Kaplan, H. S. (1979). *Disorders of sexual desire and other new concepts and techniques in sex therapy* (Vol. 2). New York: Brunner/Mazel.

Knudson, G., Cuypere, G., & Bockting, W. (2010). Recommendations for revision of the DSM diagnoses of gender identity disorders: Consensus statement of the World Professional Association for Transgender Health. *International Journal of Transgenderism, 12*(2), 115–118.

Kuper, L. E., Nussbaum, R., & Mustanski, B. (2012). Exploring the diversity of gender and sexual orientation identities in an online sample of transgender individuals. *Journal of Sex Research, 49*(2–3), 244–254.

LaSala, M. (2004). Monogamy of the heart: Extradyadic sex and gay male couples. *Journal of Gay and Lesbian Social Services, 17*(3), 1–24.

LaSala, M. (2010). *Coming out, coming home.* New York: Columbia Press.

Leiblum, S., & Pervin, L. (Eds.). (1980). *Principles and practice of sex therapy.* New York: Guilford Press.

Lev, A. I. (2005). Disordering gender identity: Gender identity disorder in the DSM-IV-TR. In D. Karasic & J. Dresher (Eds.), *Sexual and gender diagnoses of the diagnostic and statistical manual (DSM): A reevaluation* (pp. 35–69). Binghamton, NY: Hawthorn Press.

Levine, S. B., Zucker, K. J., & Meyer-Bahlberg, H. F. L. (2012, March). *Social and medical gender transitioning on demand: The case for caution.* Paper presented at the 37th annual meeting of the Society for Sex Therapy and Research, Chicago.

Martin, J. I. (2006). Transcendence among gay men: Implications for HIV prevention. *Sexualities, 9*(2), 214–235.

Masters, W. H., & Johnson, V. E. (1979). *Homosexuality in perspective.* New York: Bantam Books.

Matthews, A. K., Hughes, T. L., & Tartaro, J. (2006). Sexual behavior and sexual dysfunction in a community sample of lesbian and heterosexual women. In A. M. Omoto & H. S. Kurtzman (Eds.), *Sexual orientation and mental health: Examining identity and development in lesbian, gay, and bisexual people* (pp. 185–206). Washington, DC: American Psychological Association.

Munson, M., & Stelbourn, J. (Eds.). (1999). *The lesbian polyamory reader.* New York: Harrington Park Press.

Mustanski, B. S., Garofalo, R., & Emerson, E. M. (2010). Mental health disorders, psychological distress, and suicidality in a diverse sample of lesbian, gay, bisexual, and transgender youths. *American Journal of Public Health, 100*(12), 2426–2432.

Nichols, M. (2006). Sexual function in women with women: Lesbians and lesbian relationships. In I. Goldstein, C. M. Meston, S. R. Davis, & A. M. Traish (Eds.), *Women's sexual function and dysfunction* (pp. 307–313). New York: Taylor & Francis Group.

Nichols, M. (2012). Same sex sexuality from a global perspective. In K. Hall & C. Graham (Eds.), *The cultural context of sexual pleasure and problems: Psychotherapy with diverse clients* (pp. 22–46). New York: Routledge.

Parsons, J. T., Starks, T. J., DuBois, S., Grov, C., & Golub, S. A. (2011). Alternatives to monogamy among gay male couples in a community survey: Implications for mental health and sexual risk. *Archives of Sexual Behavior, 42*(2), 303–312.

Philip, S. S., Yu, X., Donnell, D., Vittinghoff, E., & Buchbinder, S. (2010). Serosorting is associated with a decreased risk of HIV seroconversion in the EXPLORE study cohort. *PLOS One, 5,* 1–7.

Phua, V. C. (2010). Negotiating sex and sexualities: The use of sexual tags in the Brazilian sex trade workplace. *Archives of Sexual Behavior, 39,* 831–842.

Reback, C. J., & Larkins, S. (2010). Maintaining a heterosexual identity: Sexual meanings among a sample of heterosexually identified men who have sex with men. *Archives of Sexual Behavior, 39*(3), 766–773.

Richters, J., de Visser, R., Rissel, C., Grulich, A., & Smith, A. (2008). Demographic and psychosocial features of participants in bondage and discipline, "sadomasochism" or dominance and submission (BDSM): Data from a national survey. *Journal of Sexual Medicine, 5*(7), 1660–1668.

Roberts, A. L., Rosario, M., Corliss, H. L., Koenen, K. C., & Austin, S. B. (2012). Childhood gender nonconformity: A risk factor for childhood abuse and posttraumatic stress in youth. *Pediatrics, 129*(3), 411–417.

Rothblum, E., & Brehony, K. (Eds.). (1993). *Boston marriages: Romantic but asexual relationships among contemporary lesbians.* Amherst: University of Massachusetts Press.

Roughgarden, J. (2004). *Evolution's rainbow.* Berkeley: University of California Press.

Ryan, C., & Jetha, C. (2010). *Sex at dawn: The prehistoric origins of modern sexuality.* New York: HarperCollins.

Sandfort, T. G. M., & de Keizer, M. (2001). Sexual problems in gay men: An overview of empirical research. *Annual Review of Sex Research, 12*, 93–120.

Savin-Williams, R. C. (2005). *The new gay teenager.* Cambridge, MA: Harvard University Press.

Silverstein, C. (2009). The implications of removing homosexuality from the DSM as a mental disorder [Letter to the editor]. *Archives of Sexual Behavior, 38*(2), 161–163.

Skidmore, W. C., Linsenmeier, J. A. W., & Bailey, J. M. (2006). Gender nonconformity and psychological distress in lesbians and gay men. *Archives of Sexual Behavior, 35*(6), 685–697.

Spack, N. P., Edwards-Leeper, L., Feldman, H. A., Leibowitz, S., Mandel, F., Diamond, D. A., et al. (2012). Children and adolescents with gender identity disorder referred to a pediatric medical center. *Pediatrics, 129*(3), 418–425.

Spitzer, R. L. (2003). Can some gay men and lesbians change their sexual orientation? 200 participants reporting a change from homosexual to heterosexual orientation. *Archives of Sexual Behavior, 32*(5), 403–417.

Taormino, T. (2008). *Opening up: A guide to creating and sustaining open relationships.* San Francisco: Cleis Press.

Toomey, R., Ryan, C., & Diaz, R. M. (2010). Gender-nonconforming lesbian, gay, bisexual, and transgender youth: School victimization and young psychosocial adjustment. *Developmental Psychology, 46*(6), 1580–1589.

van Rosmalen-Nooijens, K. A. W. L., Vergeer, C. M., & Largo-Janssen, A. L. M. (2008). Bed death and other lesbian sexual problems unraveled: A qualitative study of the sexual health of lesbian women involved in a relationship. *Women and Health, 48*(3), 339–362.

Wallien, M. S. C., & Cohen-Kettenis, P. T. (2008). Psychosexual outcome of gender-dysphoric children. *Journal of American Academy of Child and Adolescent Psychiatry, 47*(12), 1413–1423.

Wingerson, L. (2009, May 19). Gender identity disorder: Has accepted practice caused harm? *Psychiatric Times.* Available at *www.psychiatrictimes.com/gender-identity-disorder-has-accepted-practice-caused-harm.*

Yu, V. (2010). Shelter and traditional housing for transgender youth. *Journal of Gay and Lesbian Mental Health, 14*, 340–345.

CHAPTER 15

Culturally Sensitive Sex Therapy

The Need for Shared Meanings
in the Treatment of Sexual Problems

Kathryn S. K. Hall and Cynthia A. Graham

Hall and Graham challenge both clinicians and researchers to view culture as central to understanding sexuality. They begin with the following premise: "Sexual problems are experienced by people worldwide, but we contend that the sexual concerns of diverse cultures do not necessarily mirror those of Western populations." Reviewing the literature on immigrant populations, as well as survey data and research from various parts of the world, the authors find that although Western-defined sexual dysfunction may be found in other cultures, the rates of occurrence, the significance of the problems, and the distress experienced vary greatly. In addition, the sexual concerns of other cultures sometimes differ significantly from those identified in the DSM.

Ethnic and cultural minorities seek out therapy less often, but when they do, they often drop out of treatment early. To more adequately address the treatment needs of culturally diverse clients, Hall and Graham describe a model for culturally sensitive sex therapy (CSST) that stresses the value of understanding sexual problems in a cultural context such that there is a shared understanding of the meaning and significance of the sexual problem between client and therapist. Recognizing that culture is not the problem but part of the solution, CSST necessarily requires adaptation, innovation, and flexibility in the treatment process.

Kathryn S. K. Hall, PhD, is a clinical psychologist in private practice in Princeton, New Jersey. She is the author of *Reclaiming Your Sexual Self,* a popular book on female sexual desire and is the co-editor (with Cynthia A. Graham) of *The Cultural Context of Sexual Pleasure and Problems: Psychotherapy with Diverse Clients.* Dr. Hall is the book review editor for the *Journal of Sex and Marital Therapy.*

Cynthia A. Graham, PhD, is currently a Senior Lecturer in the Department of Psychology at the University of Southampton in the United Kingdom, a Research Fellow at the Kinsey Institute for Research in Sex, Gender, and Reproduction, and a visiting Research Fellow at the Rural Center for AIDS/STD Prevention, Indiana University. She is Editor-in-Chief of *The Journal of Sex Research* and is an editorial board member for the *Journal of Sex and Marital Therapy* and the *International Journal of Sexual Health.* She is a Chartered Psychologist, an Associate Fellow of the British Psychological Society, a Fellow of the Society for the Scientific Study of Sexuality, and a member of the Sexual and Gender Identity Disorders Workgroup for the DSM-5. She was elected President of the International Academy of Sex Research in 2009.

Mr. Li looked at me blankly. He had been referred by an infertility clinic for repeatedly failing (refusing?) to give a semen sample. Now he sat expectantly in my office, wondering what I was going to do to help him. I was wondering the same thing.

Feeling incompetent in the role of sex therapist is an uncomfortable feeling. It is especially uncomfortable when you encounter this feeling midway through your career, when you have long ceased to feel the anxiety of a newly minted therapist. Whatever our level of experience, when we encounter clients, situations, or problems that are alien to us, anxiety is a natural response. So it is for many ethnic minority clients who walk into a therapy office with little shared understanding of the process of sex therapy. Many of these clients, like Mr. Li, never return for a second appointment and remain an underserved population (Barrett et al., 2008; Moreira et al., 2005).

This chapter focuses on the need for cultural sensitivity in the practice of sex therapy. We begin with the premise that sexual problems are experienced by people worldwide, but we contend that the sexual concerns of diverse cultures do not necessarily mirror those of Western populations. Culturally sensitive sex therapy is required to meet the needs of people in other countries and cultures and also to address the needs of cultural minorities and immigrant populations in the Western world.

SEXUALITY IN A GLOBAL PERSPECTIVE

Sexuality is best understood as a biopsychosocial phenomenon (Bancroft, 2009). Although the biological, psychological, and social aspects of sexuality are clearly interrelated, the unique contribution of culture has been much neglected in the understanding of human sexuality and its problems and treatment.

Culture is defined as the shared meanings and values of a group that are passed on from one generation to the next or, as defined by Williams (1983), "the way of life for an entire society." What constitutes ideal, acceptable, and offensive sexual behavior is culturally defined. To illustrate, we can examine the cultural variations in what is considered appropriate for marital sex. Although most, if not all, cultures sanction sexuality within some form of marital union, there is a great deal of variation in cultural dictates regarding how that sexuality should be expressed. In the West, marriage is presumably based on mutual love between two adults. There is a growing acceptance of same-sex marriage, with such marriages being legally recognized in Canada, Argentina, and some parts of the United States and Europe (Wright, 2006). Marital sex is expected to be pleasurable, intimate, and consensual. In Western cultures, the standard is that sex should be desired by both parties rather than merely consented to, a fact that has likely contributed to hypoactive sexual desire disorder becoming the most common female complaint seen in sex therapy clinics in the Western world (Robinson, Munns, Weber-Main, Lowe, & Raymond, 2011). In many other parts of the world, however, marriage is the union of two families and is therefore often arranged by the families (Uberoi & Palriwala, 2008). It is always heterosexual, although there is a great deal of variation in what is considered a marriageable age for females. Sometimes the couple has met and consented to the union, but sometimes consent of the individuals is not seen as necessary given that the family has consented to the union. There is usually the expectation that the marriage be consummated quickly, often on the first night following the wedding. This presumes that what is required sexually in a marriage is a potent male and a willing and submissive (and chaste) woman. In many cultures the ability to consummate a marriage signifies not only the likelihood of offspring but also that the union has been blessed by spirits or ancestors (Savage, 2012). Many anxious brides and grooms have taken to cutting themselves in order to show a bloodstained cloth to relatives who are often waiting just outside the door for proof of virility and chastity (Sungur, 2012). So whether marital sex is expected to involve love, good communication, sexual desire, and the ability to give and receive sexual pleasure or whether it requires male potency, female submissiveness, ancestral or spiritual blessing, and ultimately offspring depends on the culture. Because culture defines ideals and norms, it will also then define what is problematic and what treatments are likely to be effective (e.g., medical, spiritual, relational, or psychological). A good resource for the clinician interested in learning about sexuality in different cultures is the *Continuum Complete International Encyclopedia of Sexuality* (Francoeur & Noonan, 2004), available online at *www.kinseyinstitute.org/ccies/index.php*.

SEXUAL DYSFUNCTION IN A GLOBAL CONTEXT

Most epidemiological studies on the prevalence of sexual problems come from the West (North America and Europe). With few exceptions (Laumann et al.,

2005), most of what is known about sexual problems in other parts of the world is based on small numbers, clinical samples or case studies. Furthermore, what little research there is on ethnic minorities has often focused on issues of sexual health and risk for sexually transmitted infections (STIs) or unintended pregnancy rather than on issues related to sexual pleasure (Hall & Graham, 2012; Lewis, 2004)

The first report of a large multinational comparison of sexual dysfunction was the Pfizer-funded Global Study of Sexual Attitudes and Behaviors (GSSAB; Laumann et al., 2005). More than 13,000 men and a similar number of women ages 40–80 years across 29 countries were surveyed. The most common sexual problems reported by women were lack of interest in sex (26–43%), inability to reach orgasm (18–41%), and lubrication difficulties (16–38%). Early ejaculation was the most common complaint made by men (12–31%), closely followed by erectile difficulties (12–28%). The incidence of all reported sexual problems was higher in East Asia and Southeast Asia than in other regions of the world. The authors of the study concluded that "sexual difficulties are relatively common among mature adults throughout the world." (p. 39).

It is difficult to estimate the true prevalence of sexual dysfunction from surveys (Graham & Bancroft, 2006; Mercer et al., 2003). Epidemiological surveys have often resulted in inflated reports of sexual difficulties because both transient, short-term sexual problems (which are very common) and more persistent problems (which are less frequent) have been assessed (Hayes, Dennerstein, Bennett, & Fairley, 2008; Mercer et al., 2003). Although the criterion of "distress" is required for a clinical diagnosis of any sexual disorder (American Psychiatric Association, 2013), the cross-cultural GSSAB did not assess distress about sexual functioning, but only the presence of symptoms. More recent surveys that have assessed distress (Bancroft, Loftus, & Long, 2003; Oberg, Fugl-Meyer, & Fugl-Meyer, 2004; Shifren, Monz, Russo, Segreti, & Johannes, 2008; Witting et al., 2008) show that prevalence estimates drop, usually by at least half, when distress is included in the determination of sexual problems (Brotto, Bitzer, Loan, Leiblum, & Luria, 2010; Hayes et al, 2008).

To further illustrate this point, we can look at the international prevalence data on premature ejaculation (PE). In two multinational studies of intravaginal ejaculation latency times (IELTs), Turkish men had significantly shorter IELTs when compared with their counterparts in The Netherlands, United Kingdom, Spain, and the United States (Waldinger, McIntosh, & Schweitzer, 2009; Waldinger et al., 2005). However, whether these Turkish men were distressed by their relatively short IELTs was not determined in these studies. Yasan and Gurgen (2009) found that Turkish men referred to a sex therapy clinic (usually for fertility-related concerns) who met the DSM-IV criteria for PE were not distressed about their condition. This could be attributed to the fact that these men were more concerned about fertility-related issues, but it could also have reflected a genuine lack of concern about the duration of intercourse. Zargooshi, Rahmanian, Motaee, Kohzadi, & Nourizad (2012) reported that PE was the primary presenting sexual complaint seen at their clinic in rural Iran.

Unlike their Turkish counterparts, men in rural Iran are distressed about the duration of intercourse, even when their IELTs far exceed the standard cutoff of 2 minutes. Zargooshi and his colleagues noted that with the high unemployment rate in rural Iran, sex was one of the few pleasures accorded to married men, and they wanted it to last as long as possible. The opinion of Iranian wives was not solicited, and therefore it is unclear whether they shared a desire for longer lasting vaginal intercourse. Furthermore, whereas the Iranian men were distressed about the brevity of intercourse, Western men are often more concerned about the fact that they lack control over the timing of ejaculation, regardless of how quickly it occurs (Kempeneers et al., 2012). One might predict, therefore, that treatments that focus on extending the length of time before ejaculation (e.g., medications) may be more effective and welcomed in Iran, whereas cognitive-behavioral strategies to help men gain control over the timing of ejaculation will be the treatment modality of choice in the West.

Cross-cultural research invariably raises concerns about the adequacy of translating language and concepts for use with populations other than the originally designated group. This issue was directly addressed by the investigators of the SWAN survey, a study of multiethnic midlife women living in the United States (Cain et al., 2003). Addressing the finding that Chinese and Japanese women were the least likely to report a desire to engage in sex, the authors note, "Despite careful translation, we cannot rule out the possibility that terms such as desire and arousal may have different meanings across cultures or that women will respond to them differently" (p. 275). Furthermore, as Ahrold and Meston (2010) pointed out, the more different a culture is from the mainstream or comparison culture, the more likely it will be that differences will appear in assessment. Therefore, another conclusion regarding the GSSAB and the SWAN study dataset is that Asian sexuality differs significantly from Western sexuality and as such, when measured against Western standards will appear lacking.

The tendency to compare other countries to the standards of the West plagues cross-cultural research (Meston & Ahrold, 2008). The GSSAB asked specific "Western-defined" questions about sexual difficulties. Different sexual concerns may be elicited when the question is broadened to ask "What problems bring men and women to treatment?" For example, in a study of 1,000 consecutive patients attending a sex therapy clinic in India, apart from PE (the most frequent complaint, reported by 77.6% of men), nocturnal emission (71%), masturbatory guilt (33%), and concern about penis size (30%) were all more frequently reported than were complaints of erectile dysfunction (24%; Verma, Khaitan, & Singh, 1998).

Other evidence that the sexual problems of diverse cultures do not mirror those of North America or Western Europe comes from what are typically called culture-bound syndromes (CBS). Examples of CBS include *Dhat syndrome* (excessive worry about penis shrinkage due to masturbation), found on the Indian subcontinent and *koro* or *koro*-like syndromes in West Africa in which men (predominantly) believe that their genitals have either been stolen or have shrunk inside their bodies and will cause their deaths. This syndrome of shrinking genitals is also known as *Suo-yang* (Mandarin) or *Shook-yang* (Cantonese) in China. Unconsummated marriage not due to any specific sexual dysfunction (Zargooshi et al., 2012), "handkerchief stress" (a term coined to reflect the anxiety of having to produce a blood stained cloth on the wedding night to prove virility; Sungur, 2012), and concerns regarding having luck (good and bad) transmitted through sexual behavior (Savage, 2012) may represent real challenges to Western-based notions of what constitutes a sexual problem. Hughes (1998) argued that instead of viewing CBS as a collection of bizarre or exotic sexual problems, they are best seen as examples of the way that culture influences the manifestation of psychopathology.

Western definitions of sexual dysfunction highlight the performance aspect of sexuality, our linear view of sexual response (first desire, arousal, and then orgasm), and the individualism inherent in our culture (the individual nature of the diagnosis and the criterion that the person him- or herself must be distressed about the problem; American Psychiatric Association, 2013). The prevalence of Western-defined sexual dysfunctions in other areas of the world may indicate the extent to which values diverge or are shared. For example, whereas low sexual desire is the most frequent complaint of women in the West, in more male-centric cultures, vaginismus is the primary sexual complaint for which women seek help (Yasan & Gurgen, 2009). The prevalence of vaginismus in these cultures has been attributed to the high premium placed on virginity and the fact that vaginismus interferes with intercourse (and therefore with male pleasure) and can significantly hinder reproduction (Sungur, 2012). Furthermore, as Yasan and Gurgen (2009) have pointed out, "It is understandable that women who have been forced to marry without consent and who know that they have to stay married for the rest of their lives, will have difficulties while experiencing sex unwillingly in their marriage" (p. 73). We agree with these authors that although this is clearly a problem, it is not one best viewed as the problem of an individual woman but a reflection of a culture in which there is little or no autonomy for women.

In summary, we find a paucity of good data regarding the experience of sexual problems in different cultures. Although Western-defined sexual dysfunction may be found in other cultures, the rates of occurrence and the distress experienced vary across different countries (Laumann et al., 2005). The sexual problems that are significant for other cultures may be quite different from those found in the West. A good resource for the interested clinician regarding sexual problems and treatment options may be found in *The Cultural Context of Sexual Pleasure and Problems: Psychotherapy with Diverse Clients* (Hall & Graham, 2012).

ACCULTURATION

Given that sexuality is, at least in part, culturally determined, it follows that when the culture changes, so should sexuality. One of the most striking examples of this phenomenon involved a study of the interaction of two very different cultures: Iran and Sweden (Darvishpour, 1999). Iranian migrants to Sweden were found to have significantly revised their views about sexuality to more closely approximate the values of the host country. They went from a traditional, authoritarian, and patriarchal orientation to a more individual-istic and egalitarian approach to sexuality. People who immigrate to another country will often retain their values and traditions but will also, to a greater or lesser extent, acculturate (adopt the values and traditions of the host coun-try; Ryder, Alden, & Paulhus, 2000). It has been assumed that acculturation proceeds in a linear fashion, with immigrants increasingly assimilating the cultural values and mores of the mainstream culture. However, studies exam-ining the effects of acculturation on the sexual attitudes and behaviors of immigrants have found conflicting results, with some finding that accultura-tion predicts sexual behavior and others reporting no effect (Meston & Ahr-old, 2008). Although this may be due to the different measures of accultura-tion that have been used across studies (questionnaires, length of residency), it is likely that a linear assimilation model does not adequately capture the experience by which people adopt some or all of the tenets of the mainstream culture (Ahrold & Meston, 2010; Brotto, Chik, Ryder, Gorzalka, & Seal, 2005). Brotto and her colleagues found that the degree to which Asian women maintained aspects of their heritage culture influenced the effects of Western-ization on sexual attitudes. Women who relinquished heritage ties adopted the more liberal sexual attitudes of the Western culture, whereas women who maintained strong heritage ties did not. Ahrold and Meston (2010) described two models of acculturation: In one the heritage and mainstream culture blend together and become a third entity—much like tea, "with one element blend-ing into, and changing the original nature of the other" (p. 199). The other model is one in which the two cultures retain their original elements while coexisting, like oil and water when combined. Mutual engagement in both the heritage and the mainstream culture has been found to be the most widely used practice of Hispanic youth who blend their two cultures into a unique cultural identity, whereas Asians tend to retain aspects of their heritage cul-ture while adopting some elements of the mainstream (Ahrold & Meston, 2010). It is not yet known what the impact of age, gender, and other personal-ity variables is on the process of acculturation. Clinicians need to be sensitive to the dual allegiance to heritage and mainstream culture and to be aware that despite assimilation of some aspects of mainstream culture (clothing, occupa-tion, language), clients may retain heritage values with respect to family and sexuality. The same may be true for first-generation clients, who were raised with traditional values of the heritage culture but have greater exposure to mainstream culture.

> Nina, a first-generation Italian woman, came to therapy depressed after having sex with a male friend in college, an occurrence that she deeply regretted. Nina explained, "I was taught that sex is very important,

something sacred for marriage. But for me, it's only right if I'm in a relationship that I could see leading to marriage. I feel pressure with American men. Most of my friends think sex is fun, and it is of course, but I just feel so pressured, I want to say 'No, I don't love you! I would never marry you' but then they would think I was some kind of freak, so I said okay when I meant no."

Cultural sensitivity needs to extend to an awareness and appreciation of various patterns of adherence to the old culture and adoption of the new culture.

CULTURE AND RELIGION

Religion is one way in which values and attitudes and rules regarding sexual behavior are transmitted within a culture. The degree to which a culture embraces religious prohibitions and sexual proscriptions varies. Religion is an important factor in determining sexual behavior in the Arab and Persian countries of the Middle East (Zargooshi et al., 2012) but is a less significant factor in many Western countries and Russia (Hall & Graham, 2012; Temkina, Rotkirch, & Haavio-Mannila, 2012). Gender may moderate the impact of religion and culture on sexuality. In Croatia, inconsistent and weak associations were found between religiosity and sexual behavior among women, whereas no relationship existed for men (Puzek, Stulhofer, & Bozicevic, 2012). Sex guilt, defined as "a generalized expectancy for self-mediated punishment for violating or for anticipating violating standards of proper sexual conduct" (Mosher & Cross, 1971, p. 27), was found to mediate the relationship between religion and culture with sexual desire in women. Woo, Morshedian, Brotto, and Gorzalka (2012) found that the activation of sex guilt reduced sexual desire in Asian Canadian women but not in European Canadians. Simply put, a strong identification with one's heritage culture or religion will mitigate the liberalizing impact of Western acculturation on sexual attitudes and behavior. Strength of religious identification may explain within-ethnic-group differences in sexual attitudes and is therefore an important issue to be addressed during assessment and treatment of sexual problems.

HOW DOES CULTURE INFLUENCE
SEXUAL DYSFUNCTION?

Hughes (1998) outlined three ways in which culture influences psychopathology that we believe have relevance for sexual disorders. The first is the phenomenology of symptoms; for example, culture influences the way distress is experienced. The second is in the syndromization of symptoms into patterns, and the third is in the diagnostic process itself—for example, when the clinician does not understand or is unfamiliar with the culture of the patient, diagnostic errors may result (usually but not always in the direction of over-pathologizing).

We believe that the diagnosis of low sexual desire in women illustrates the three ways that culture influences sexual disorders. Although there is sometimes a biological basis for low desire, the prevalence of this disorder in North America indicates that there are multiple pathways for the diagnosis. The reduction in sexual desire for a loved partner is perhaps a very important way in which Western women manifest the stress, the unfair burden of housework, or other relationship unhappiness. Because refusing sex is a possibility accorded to Western women, a basic right not shared by women worldwide,[1] low sexual desire may be accompanied by avoidance of sex. Nevertheless, sex, when it does occur, may still be enjoyable. Because desire is deemed important and is often equated with love, North American and Western European women often feel distress about their lack of desire. In North America and Western Europe, relationship distress may manifest in low sexual desire (a culturally influenced expression of unhappiness), which will be experienced as a distressing lack of interest in sex, a high rate of refusing sex initiated by a partner, and a somewhat paradoxical enjoyment of the infrequent sex that does occur (the syndromization of symptoms into patterns). This clinical picture will be familiar to Western-trained sex therapists, and a diagnosis of low sexual desire is likely to result. Because female consent, and certainly sexual desire, is not deemed necessary in some other cultures (e.g., traditional Korean culture), unhappy or stressed women may engage in frequent but unwanted sex, may experience disgust regarding sex, and may come to manifest hostility toward their spouses and disdain for men in general (Youn, 2012). This symptom constellation may be unfamiliar to a Western-trained therapist, who, upon encountering one Korean woman with this clinical presentation, may attribute her severe anger and hostility to underlying pathology (e.g., a mood or personality disorder).

CULTURE AND ISSUES RELATED TO DIAGNOSIS OF SEXUAL DYSFUNCTIONS

The assumption that there is a universal model of sexual response leads to the belief in a universal set of sexual dysfunctions. Although there were efforts to enhance the cross-cultural applicability of diagnoses in DSM-IV-TR, critics argued that these efforts fell short and that "the DSM's underlying thesis of universality based on Western-delineated mental disorders is problematic and has limited cross-cultural applicability" (Thakker & Ward, 1998, p. 501). Although the sexual problems of individuals from other cultures may fit into

---

[1]Interestingly there is evidence from a study in sub-Saharan Africa that women who have greater autonomy in general household decision making also have greater ability to choose the timing and frequency of sex (Hindin & Muntifering, 2011).

some of the current *Diagnostic and Statistical Manual of Mental Disorders* (DSM-5) diagnoses for sexual dysfunction, they may more often need to fall into the category of sexual dysfunction not otherwise specified (NOS; American Psychiatric Association, 2013). In DSM-IV-TR, culture-bound syndromes were placed in the Appendix, where few clinicians would access them.

In recent years there has been a growing awareness of the importance of culture in diagnosis and this has been reflected in the development work for DSM-5 published in May 2013 (American Psychiatric Association, 2013). The research agenda for DSM-5 included publications related to cultural issues in diagnosis (Alarcón et al., 2002) and experts on cultural issues were appointed to some of the work groups, including the Sexual and Gender Identity Disorders Work Group (Jack Drescher, MD). There was a study group on gender and cross-cultural issues, convened to "address gender, racial, and ethnic issues in mental disorders, including differences in symptoms, symptom severity, and course of illness" (American Psychiatric Association, 2012). As a result the descriptive text accompanying the DSM-5 diagnostic criteria for sexual dysfunctions highlights the importance of considering cultural factors, such as inhibitions related to prohibitions against sexual activity, attitudes toward sexuality, and so forth.

ASSESSMENT

Culturally sensitive assessment evaluates individuals and couples in the context of culture. Culture is viewed as essential to understanding sexual problems, not as something ancillary or exotic. Cultural values and ties may also be seen as strengths that can guide the treatment process, not solely as part of the pathology (Ahmed & Bhugra, 2004; Hall & Graham, 2012; Kelly & Shelton, 2012).

When encountering an individual or couple from another culture, the clinician must try to understand the unique meaning of the sexual symptoms, rather than diagnosing them using his or her own cultural lens. For example, Ramanathan and Weerakoon (2012) described their treatment of a young Indian man who presented with fears that he had damaged himself by masturbating. The man was concerned because he felt weak, and he worried that his eyesight had been affected and that his acne was a manifestation of the damage caused by his masturbation. These concerns had not stopped the young man from masturbating, and now he worried that he could not control himself and that he would not be able to have sexual intercourse with his wife when he got married. If this young man had encountered a Western therapist, his symptoms might have seemed rather quaint, and the impulse might have been to paternalistically explain that masturbation is not harmful and can indeed help a man prepare for marriage by boosting his confidence in his ability to get and maintain an erection and also to identify what arouses him. Instead, the therapist in this case inquired about the meaning of the fears. The young man was indeed reaching the age where his parents would arrange a match for him. He was anxiously looking forward to marriage, but there was tremendous pressure on him to represent his family well, to please his new wife, and to be found attractive and desirable by her and her family. Indeed, the process that young Indian men and women go through in being evaluated by their potential in-laws is rather daunting and is brilliantly described in the novel *A Suitable Boy* (Seth, 1993). Ramanathan and Weerakoon (2012) did not try to dissuade the young man from his beliefs. Instead they addressed the meaning of the man's distress—his concern about his suitability for marriage. The young man was sent for tests to determine the basis for the weakness, prescribed good nutrition to add strength, had his eyesight tested, and was given a medication for the acne. He was also asked to refrain from masturbating for several days prior to each of the several medical tests. This helped him realize that he could have control over his masturbatory behavior. The therapist also provided information about sex to alleviate anxiety about what to do in order to consummate the marriage.

As in the case just described, we advocate for an approach to assessment in which the clinician tries to understand the presentation of symptoms from the client's perspective, recognizing that this perspective is strongly influenced by the culture in which that client was raised. At present, the best way to do a culturally sensitive assessment is to carry out a thorough diagnostic interview.

ASSESSMENT INSTRUMENTS: TESTS AND QUESTIONNAIRES

Many researchers have noted the limitations in regard to cross-cultural assessment instruments. As Rellini et al. (2005) pointed out, the majority of questionnaires used to assess sexual functioning in women were developed for, and standardized on, a Western, typically U.S., population. The lack of importance accorded to validation of measures in different cultures is grounded in the assumption that the constructs of sexuality that underlie the original questionnaire are unaffected by culture. Rellini et al. (2005) translated the McCoy Female Sexuality Questionnaire into Italian and attempted to validate it on an Italian sample. They found that of the 5 factors that were apparent on the original questionnaire, only 2 had relevance for the Italian sample: sexuality and partnership. These two factors differentiated women with sexual dysfunctions from those who did not have such issues, but the separate constructs underlying the phases of the sexual response cycle (i.e. desire, arousal, and orgasm) were not meaningfully related to sexual problems in the Italian sample. Although these findings may have reflected translation difficulties, they may also reflect differences between Italian and American women in how they experience their sexuality. The Iranian validation of the Female Sexual Function Questionnaire (Quirk et al., 2002) also found a factor structure different from the original test (Khademi et al., 2006). Interestingly, the married women who responded to the questionnaire found a question on "enjoyment of nonpenetrative sex" confusing and rarely responded to it. Other researchers have questioned whether the methods of assessing sexual desire and sexual enjoyment used in North American–European contexts are appropriate in different cultural settings (Graham, Ramos, Bancroft, Maglaya, & Farley, 1995). For example, in a study of the effects of oral contraceptive use on mood and sexuality carried out in women living in Edinburgh, Scotland and Manila, Philippines, there were striking differences between the two samples at baselines. The Manila women, although reporting a somewhat higher frequency of intercourse than the Scottish women, were less likely to initiate sex, had less sexual interest, less sexual enjoyment, and were less likely to feel "close and comfortable" with their partners during sexual activity (Graham et al., 1995). Although the interview and questionnaire measures had been translated and back-translated and the Manila interviewers were trained, the authors questioned whether the method of assessment was appropriate for the Manila women. Personal pleasure for women and the individual (vs. relationship) orientation of many interview formats and questionnaires may be seen as less relevant in collectivist and/or male-centric cultures (Hall & Graham, 2012)

Similar issues affect the assessment of male sexual dysfunction. The International Index of Erectile Function (IIEF; Rosen, Riley, Wagner, Osterloh, Kirkpatrick, et al., 1997) is the most popular measure of erectile dysfunction (ED) and it has been successfully translated into a variety of European languages and validated for use in many European countries (Rosen, Cappelleri, & Gendrano, 2002). The applicability of the IIEF to non-Western cultures has not been established. It was difficult to translate the IIEF into Malaysian because the language often referred to sex obliquely (e.g., intercourse is translated as "joining together in one body") or with moral undertones (sex organs are literally translated as "shame"; Lim et al., 2003).

Although there may be measures that are developed and validated for use with other cultures, it is difficult to find them, if they do exist. When seeing clients from non-Western cultures, we suggest using assessment measures developed in the West with caution—checking to see that the measure in question has been validated for use with a specific population and carefully looking at the answers to specific items, including following up with the client to ensure that the meaning of the question was clear. As Kelly and Shelton (2012) have observed, it is also important to keep in mind that an overreliance on paper-and-pencil tests may be off-putting to certain cultural groups. A diagnostic interview may be the best way at present to gather a sexual history and to diagnose sexual problems.

The most important aspect of the diagnostic interview is the attitude of the interviewer. It is important to be flexible in our style and our openness to understanding problems from other perspectives. For example, an American patient of East Indian background was referred to one of us (Hall) for a court-ordered evaluation regarding homicidal threats she made to her husband. Her husband had succeeded in having her removed from the home and had a restraining order against her. She wanted to reconcile with her husband, but he feared for his life, and the judge was concerned that the woman was mentally ill. In the evaluation the woman readily admitted that she had told her husband (East Indian by birth and ethnicity) that she had put rat poison in some of his food and that she would tell him which food was poisoned if he asked. The background of the story was complex. The wife had recently undergone a hysterectomy for medical reasons, and her in-laws came to visit shortly thereafter. She was required to cook and clean for her in-laws, despite medical advice to rest after the surgery. She also worried (correctly) that her in-laws were there to persuade her husband to divorce her since she could no longer have children. For weeks she cooked and cleaned and listened to her in-laws complain about her to her husband, who never stood up for her. He refused to listen to her worries or her complaints and refused to lift a finger to help her. He felt that the answer to the problem was to show his parents what a good wife she was so that his parents would leave and stop pestering him to divorce her. Instead, his wife was doing the opposite and proving to them that she was not a fit wife for their son. The husband felt caught in the middle and did not know what to do. Ultimately he stopped speaking to his wife altogether. In desperation, she bought rat poison and displayed it prominently in the kitchen (she denied using it, and no food was ever discovered to be poisoned). We believe this was not a case of individual pathology on the part of the wife, or the husband either, but rather an example of the tremendous stress and pressure that couples face and the apparently bizarre ways in which their distress is manifested. The judge and lawyers wondered, "Why didn't she leave him? Why didn't they go to therapy?" Her physicians told her, "You cannot keep doing this housework, you are making yourself sick, you have to stand up to your in-laws. Tell your husband that you cannot cook and clean for 6 weeks. Can't you hire a cleaning lady?" All these are reasonable questions for Western-born and -raised couples, but they fail to understand the context of the distress of this couple.

FROM CULTURALLY COMPETENT TO CULTURALLY SENSITIVE SEX THERAPY

Cultural competence "denotes the capacity to perform and obtain positive clinical outcomes in cross-cultural encounters" (Lo & Fung, 2003, p. 162). Successful treatment of sexual problems will require tailoring treatment to the unique cultural requirements of the individual or couple. In some cases traditional psychotherapy or sex therapy approaches can be modified (Ahmed & Bhugra, 2004; So & Cheung, 2005). Culture-specific modifications to the method of treatment may be most successful when the sexual problems are similar to those for which sex therapy was designed—problems of sexual function, such as erectile dysfunction, ejaculatory problems, and orgasm difficulties—and when the clinician is familiar enough with the culture to make the necessary modifications. For example, So and Cheung (2005) outlined ways in which sex therapy could be modified for Chinese couples, including the admonition that sex therapists be directive and authoritarian. However, tailoring therapy in this way requires the therapist to be a chameleon, may modify the therapeutic relationship to the extent that it is no longer therapeutic, and requires that treatment approaches be adapted in ways that may alter the success of therapy (Sue & Zane, 2009). It also requires a breadth of cultural knowledge that most clinicians simply do not possess, and, as the vignette at the beginning of the chapter illustrates, clients will often not return for the second appointment (when you have done your homework and understood a *little* about the culture). It is simply not workable to have a model of cultural competence that requires that treatments be modified for each culture. This approach also promotes overgeneralizing (Sue & Zane, 2009) or stereotyping, as clearly it is not feasible to understand the diversity and nuances of all cultures.

We believe that a culturally sensitive approach to sex therapy is one that recognizes the centrality of culture in shaping sexuality. Moreover, we argue that the importance of the therapist and client sharing meanings is central to the success of therapy and that, with sensitivity, a shared meaning can be developed between therapists and clients of different cultural backgrounds. Therefore, we prefer the term "culturally sensitive sex therapy," which stresses a flexible attitude, rather than the term "competent," which emphasizes knowledge and behavior.

CASE DISCUSSION

Suleman and Nasreen were a married couple in their early 30s. Both were of Pakistani origin; Suleman was raised in the United Kingdom, while Nasreen was primarily raised in Pakistan and spent only 2 years in London prior to moving to the United States. At the time they came to therapy they had been living in the United States for 2 years. Nasreen made the initial request for therapy, stating on the phone that she had found me (Hall) through an Internet search. She explained that her marriage was in trouble and that she wanted help to fix it. She confirmed that the problem had to do with sex.

When the couple presented together, they seemed to be a bit of a mismatch. Suleman was tall, light-skinned, athletically built, and very attractive. He wore jeans and a t-shirt. Nasreen was short, plump, and rather plain, with a dark complexion. She was dressed in a designer dress and high heels with a scarf loosely draped around her head and neck. (Her appearance bespoke her dual cultural allegiance, as well as the fact that in all things she was trying very [too?] hard). Nasreen explained her worry that her husband had "problems" because he did not seem to want to have sex very often. The frequency of sex was once every 3 weeks or so, but it had been steadily declining since their move to the United States. When asked why this distressed her, Nasreen began to talk about all the hurts, slights, and insults she perceived coming from Suleman's family. Of Suleman, she reported that he was a kind husband and a loving father to their 3-year-old daughter. Suleman sat quietly and never interjected. He answered politely when asked questions. He said that the frequency of sex was not a concern to him. He explained that he was tired during the week from his long commute and that he often brought work home on the weekend because he wanted to be successful in his new job and get a promotion, which would allow them to move into a house and have more children. Suleman agreed to come to therapy to make his wife happy. He was unsure as to whether there really was a sexual problem.

Suleman was the second of three sons born to a Muslim Pakistani family in East London, England. He had been married previously in a match arranged by his parents. Unfortunately, his first wife had been bullied by her family into the marriage and refused to have sex with Suleman in order to annul the marriage. The families got involved, with the bride's family claiming that if Suleman could not have sex with his wife, he must be impotent. Ultimately Suleman's family agreed to a divorce with a monetary settlement in order to avoid further scandal. Suleman felt extraordinarily shamed by the failure of his marriage and betrayed by his parents, who were supposed to vet the bride for him. He isolated himself from friends and family and spent his free time working out at a gym and watching pornography. He began to drink. As Suleman became increasingly estranged from his Islamic faith and his community, he became depressed. In his isolation, Suleman went online to a chat room for Muslims, which is where he met Nasreen.

Nasreen was the only child born to her Pakistani parents. Her father had a business, which had been lucrative at one time, but her father's health began to fail soon after she was born, and after a series of failed financial transactions, the family moved in with her father's eldest and more successful brother. Nasreen reported that although she was treated well, she was aware that her cousins had better clothes and more opportunities than she did. When Nasreen was in her late teens her father's fortunes changed, and the parents moved into their own flat and sent Nasreen to London to go to university. Nasreen was depressed and lonely in London and dropped out of the university after her first term. She tried waitressing at an Indian restaurant for a short period of time, and she did not tell her parents that she had left school. Nasreen felt socially awkward and spent much of her free time on the Internet.

After Nasreen and Suleman met in an online chat room for young Muslims, they began talking on the phone and then meeting for coffee. Both described a feeling of comfort and belonging with each other that they had not felt before. Suleman stopped drinking and going to clubs and was welcomed back into his family. They ultimately accepted his decision to marry Nasreen, as his divorce had negatively affected his chances for a "good" match. Nasreen was Pakistani and Muslim, but she had several points against her, according to Suleman's family: She was not educated, her skin was too dark, her father was not educated nor a professional, and she had worked as a waitress.

Soon after their marriage, Suleman was offered a good position at a financial services company on Wall Street. The couple settled in New Jersey in a Muslim Pakistani community and lived close to Suleman's older brother and his wife. Suleman began to drink again, although only in the privacy of his home, and also returned to watching pornography and masturbating for his sexual pleasure. Nasreen also masturbated to orgasm, although she had never had an orgasm with partnered sex. The couple's sex life had never been very satisfactory for either partner and had consisted of brief kissing and caressing followed by intercourse.

When asked in individual sessions about the reason for their infrequent sex, the couple had two very different interpretations. Suleman said that he loved Nasreen and that she was a good mother and a good wife. However, he did not find her very sexually appealing, and it was easier for him to get his sexual needs met by masturbating to pornography, which he enjoyed a great deal. Suleman had been taught to masturbate by his older cousin when he was 12 years old. His cousin had masturbated him to orgasm and instructed Suleman how he could do this to himself. Suleman did not view this as sexual abuse despite the fact that his cousin was 7 years older than him at the time. Suleman felt pleased to have received the information and instruction, and he remained on good terms with his cousin. Suleman said that he wished someone had taught him how to have sex with a woman, and he still felt very ashamed of the failure of his first marriage. To Suleman it was a good thing that he was not strongly attracted to his wife, as he felt that he needed to be more successful professionally in order to be happy and that the only thing lacking in his family life was a son. He was concerned about his wife's unhappiness, however.

When asked for her belief about the reason for her unhappiness, Nasreen could not stay on topic for any length of time. Instead of talking about her relationship with Suleman, she digressed to discussing slights she perceived coming from his brother, or more particularly her sister-in-law: "She doesn't invite me over, she didn't talk to me at this party or on that occasion, she did not thank me for the gift, she did not put out the food I brought over. . . . " Nasreen expressed the wish for Suleman to talk to his brother so that her sister-in-law would be better behaved toward Nasreen.

An Attempt at Sex/Couples Therapy in the Western Style

At first it appeared that Nasreen's unhappiness about the frequency of sex was due to her unhappiness regarding the relationship. She wanted to have a closer relationship with her husband, who worked a lot and was somewhat withdrawn. Because she was relying on her sister-in-law to help her integrate into the community, she felt lonely and isolated. Also, it appeared that this situation mirrored the situation she was raised in, relying on an older and more successful brother for status in the community. Goals for therapy were to help Nasreen make more connections in the community (without having to rely on her sister in-law) and to increase the connection within the couple using their sexual relationship, which might increase in frequency, but which certainly could improve in the level of pleasure and connection experienced by both.

Suleman became very engaged in treatment and agreed with the goal of improving their sexual relationship. Nasreen also expressed interest in doing "homework" to improve their sexual relationship. Sensate focus I (touching and caressing the body without touching breast and genitals) was assigned with the goal of improving comfort and communication.

Failure

The next several sessions followed a similar path. Suleman made efforts to get home early to be able to spend time with Nasreen and to do the exercises. But there was always a reason Nasreen gave for why the exercise could not happen; she was too tired, their daughter was still awake, she had a stomachache, she had to Skype with her parents in Pakistan. In session it was again hard to keep Nasreen on topic; she continued to obsess and ruminate about slights from her sister-in-law. She did not make any efforts to reach out and make other connections in the community, even when it involved doing things she had expressed an interest in (play groups for her daughter, asking other mothers to come over, going to the library for children's programs). Was Nasreen a help-rejecting complainer? Was she depressed and stuck in obsessive thinking about being slighted? Were her family-of-origin issues significantly interfering with progress? Or was the problem that the therapist had not yet understood what Nasreen was desperately trying to tell her?

Becoming Culturally Sensitive

Amazingly, Suleman and Nasreen continued to come to sessions despite the lack of progress. I determined that I had not sufficiently understood the problem and needed to listen to Nasreen more closely (as she was the one presenting the obstacles). This time I listened to the meaning inherent in her story. Her meaning seemed clear: The problem was that Suleman's family had never really accepted her or the marriage. She felt that this was holding Suleman back from truly loving her. The solution, she felt, was that the marriage needed to be sanctioned by Suleman's family.

I agreed with Nasreen that it was important for the two of them to have family approval for their marriage. When Suleman protested that his family had consented to the marriage, I stated: "Now Nasreen knows it is important that they *accept* the marriage." Both agreed that they could do the sensate focus exercises to strengthen their intimate connection while they also worked on ways to increase familial acceptance. Increasing their intimate connection would help others to see them as a happily married couple and would help Suleman's family see that the marriage was a good one. Nasreen was enthusiastic, but Suleman was pessimistic.

The next week the couple returned and had done the first sensate focus assignment three times. It was very pleasurable for both and new in that Nasreen had been able to communicate her likes and dislikes to Suleman. Suleman felt very pleased with the exercise as well and found it enjoyable to touch and be touched without the pressure to have intercourse. He could tolerate what he would otherwise perceive as criticism, as Nasreen was now the "teacher" he had wanted. Suleman reported that he felt sexually attracted to his wife. The two had also discussed ways in which they could address the family issue. They had decided to have a small gathering, as the youngest brother and his wife were coming to New Jersey from East London for their annual visit. Last year they had not come to Nasreen and Suleman's home—a slight Nasreen felt intensely. As they planned and discussed the party, they reported feeling close to each other. Nasreen felt optimistic about the marriage, and both readily agreed to proceed to sensate focus II—caressing, including breasts and genitals. This exercise again went well. Nasreen worked on communicating her pleasure more overtly and guiding Suleman in constructive and positive ways. Suleman reported feeling more comfortable and confident and basked in his wife's praise during the session. He also reported that he liked the way the Nasreen touched him and that he had an erection during times he was touched and also when he was touching Nasreen. This pleased Nasreen greatly, and she reported feeling desired by Suleman for the first time in their marriage. Nasreen also felt certain that the party would be a success and that the oldest brother, who was the de facto head of the family in the United States, would surely send his parents positive reports about Suleman's wife.

Disaster struck, however, and the next meeting was difficult. The couple did not discuss sex at all. Instead they reported on family events. The sister-in-law had taken exception to Suleman and Nasreen planning a party for the younger brother. She insisted that the party be held at her home, which was a larger and more appropriate venue, as the eldest brother should host. Suleman accepted the situation and shrugged it off, saying that there was nothing to do. Nasreen felt deeply depressed and hurt. She expressed suicidal ideation. Nasreen did not see her reaction as too intense. Rather she felt it was an appropriate reaction to not being treated like a wife and sister-in-law.

Consulting Experts

It was difficult in the session to help Nasreen gain a perspective on the situation that would help her feel less depressed. Suleman offered several options: he would talk to his brother, they would boycott the sister-in-law's party, they would still host their own party; all to no avail. Nasreen continued to be despondent, and Suleman was losing patience. I was unsure of how to proceed. It was time for the experts. My cultural sensitivity was failing me. I knew that Nasreen "Skyped" with her family and felt supported by them, so I encouraged both Nasreen and Suleman to talk to their parents about the situation and ask for guidance. Suleman's parents ultimately supported the older brother, but Suleman's discussion with his parents became known to the younger brother and his wife. While in New Jersey, this sister-in-law reached out to Nasreen, and the two found that they both had difficulties with the superior airs of their eldest sister-in-law. Finally Nasreen had found an ally in the family. Nasreen's parents had been alarmed at the situation and alarmed by Nasreen's depression. After speaking with her, they decided that they needed to come to visit—for 3 months.

For most Americans, a 3-month visit from family, in a small one-bedroom apartment, would be a disaster for sex therapy. In this case it was a bonus. Sex therapy, which had come to a standstill during this time, was restarted anew. Nasreen's parents knew that the couple were having sexual problems and knew that they had exercises to do. So they did what they could to make the exercises easier for the couple. They readily babysat their granddaughter, making dates possible. They cooked and cleaned, alleviating the household burdens for Nasreen. While they slept in the one bedroom in the apartment, the 3-year-old daughter slept in their room, and they agreed not to walk into the hallway during certain hours (necessary to use the bathroom) so that these hours would be available to the couple for working on sex. While his in-laws praised him and extolled Suleman's virtues at every turn, Nasreen felt that their visit really showed their love for her and gave her a sense of family. It was Nasreen's mother who provided the key to success. She told Nasreen, "You are the second wife of a very good man, who is the second son from a very good family. This family accepts you. It is you who does not accept your place in the family. If you don't like it, you don't have to stay here. This is America; you have choices here." In session Suleman and Nasreen agreed that they did not like the option of staying in a second-class place. They began looking for a community to move to, each weekend going to a different town within commuting distance from New York to check it out. These were pleasant family outings (complete with daughter and parents).

Sex therapy proceeded with renewed energy and at a faster pace. With his in-laws staying with them, Suleman had no opportunity to drink or watch pornography. Without his usual diversions, Suleman was more interested in having sex with Nasreen. Pleasing his wife sexually was culturally valued and also valued by Suleman, who genuinely cared for her. With the support of her parents and the knowledge that *she* did not accept the marital family, not the other way around, Nasreen felt that she needed to attend to being a better wife. She made an effort to stay up at night and talk with Suleman about his work, and she began to plan meals and fun outings for the family. It also meant doing the sex homework, which she came to enjoy very much. Nasreen had an orgasm for the first time with Suleman, which thrilled the two of them equally. At the end of 3 months the couple was nervous about the departure of Nasreen's parents, but they were moving to an ethnically diverse town several hours away where they felt a sense of community was possible. Nasreen had already signed up for a "Mommy and me" class with her daughter, and

Suleman's commute was considerably shorter, so he anticipated being home earlier in the evening.

The couple asked for a referral to continue therapy, which they felt was very helpful to them. However, they reported back after several months that they were doing well and were continuing to have regular and enjoyable sex. They declined a referral.

Summary

The important elements to the ultimate success in this case highlight some of the important elements for successful culturally sensitive treatment. It is imperative that therapy begin with a shared understanding of the problem. The way in which the individual or couple discuss their sexual problems provides important information about the meaning of the sexual problem. This will guide treatment. Embracing the culture, which means seeing the culture as a potential source of strength rather than solely a source of problems, allows the clinician access to factors that may further treatment progress. In this case it was extended family. As this case demonstrates, the sex therapy techniques themselves did not radically change, nor did the therapist radically change her therapeutic style, although the context was culturally unique.

FUTURE DIRECTIONS

Sex research, sexual medicine, and sex therapy are either nonexistent or marginalized professions in many parts of the world. As Stulhofer and Arbanas (2009) stated, " The absence of tradition and lack of professional training programs, as well as financial and status-related disincentives for young aspirants, makes sexual problems and dysfunctions nobody's business" (p. 1044). We believe that bringing sex therapy to many parts of the world can raise awareness of sexual problems and can inform the public and related professions that treatment options are available.

It is important to note that although we advocate cultural sensitivity, we are not condoning cultural values and practices that we believe are intrinsically harmful. Gender inequality, which is often culturally entrenched and which affects sexuality, is a case in point. Sexual well-being, as measured by emotional and physical satisfaction with one's sexual relationship, satisfaction with sexual function and stated importance of sex, was higher for men than for women in all the countries surveyed in the GSSAB (Laumann et al., 2006). In many parts of the world, female sexual pleasure is not considered important, or it is considered dangerous. Female genital cutting, forced marriages of girls and women, and the sex trafficking of women and children are dangerous practices. There is a high rate of intimate and partner sexual violence, perpetrated primarily by men against girls and women (World Health Organization, 2005). Sex therapy promotes the equal right to sexual pleasure and safety for men, women, and transgender individuals of all sexual orientations. The ubiquitous presence of sexual medicine, which at present has little to offer women in terms of enhancing sexual pleasure (Hall & Graham, 2012), may further this imbalance if it is also not practiced with sensitivity and augmented with at least some education and counseling. Sex therapy might not save the world, but it can do its part to improve the lives of the people in it.

Improving the lives and the sexual health and pleasure of women and men cannot wait for psychotherapy to be culturally accepted and practiced in communities in which it is not yet established. As Alain Giami (2012) asked, "Who in the culture is authorized or privileged to hear about the sexual problems and offer help?" Often it is the traditional healers. The explanations traditional healers give regarding sexual dysfunction often match the patient's own understanding. They use a common language, and their treatments are based on this mutual understanding, making for better treatment compliance. Perhaps even more important, in cultures in which there is no formal psychotherapy, traditional healers take the time to listen, and this "therapeutic relationship" may be at the core of their effectiveness as healers (Ahmed & Bhugra, 2004). If psychotherapy is to be relevant to the treatment of sexual problems in an ever-changing and varied cultural landscape, adaptation, innovation, and flexibility will be necessary (Hall & Graham, 2012).

REFERENCES

Ahmed, K., & Bhugra, D. (2004). The role of culture in sexual dysfunction. *Psychiatry, 3,* 23–25.

Ahrold, T. K., & Meston, C.M. (2010). Ethnic differences in sexual attitudes of U.S. college students: Gender, acculturation, and religiosity factors. *Archives of Sexual Behavior, 39,* 190–202.

Alarcón, R. D., Alegria, M., Bell, C. C., Boyce, C., Kirmayer, L. J., Lopez, S., et al. (2002). Beyond the funhouse mirrors. In D. J. Kupfer, M. B. First, & D. A. Regier (Eds.), *A research agenda for DSM-V* (pp. 219–307). Washington, DC: American Psychiatric Publishing.

American Psychiatric Association. (2000). *Diagnostic and statistical manual of mental disorders* (4th ed., text rev.). Washington, DC: Author.

American Psychiatric Association. (2013). *Diagnostic and statistical manual of mental disorders* (5th ed.). Arlington, VA: Author.

American Psychological Association. (2012). *Gender and cross-cultural issues.* Available at *www.dsm5.org/meetus/pages/genderandcross-culturalissues.aspx.*

Bancroft, J. (2009). *Human sexuality and its problems* (3rd ed.). London: Elsevier.

Bancroft, J., Loftus, J., & Long, J. S. (2003). Distress about sex: A national survey of women in heterosexual relationships. *Archives of Sexual Behavior, 32,* 193–208.

Barrett, M. S., Chua, W.-J., Crits-Christoph, P., Gibbons, M. B., Casiano, D., & Thompson, D. (2008). Early withdrawal from mental health treatment: Implications for psychotherapy practice. *Psychotherapy: Theory, Research, Practice, Training, 45,* 247–267.

Brotto, L. A., Bitzer, J., Laan, E., Leiblum, S., & Luria, M. (2010). Women's sexual desire and arousal disorders. *Journal of Sexual Medicine, 7,* 586–614.

Brotto, L. A., Chik, H. M., Ryder, A. G., Gorzalka, B. B., & Seal, B. N. (2005). Acculturation and sexual function in Asian women. *Archives of Sexual Behavior, 34,* 613–626.

Cain, V. S., Johannes, C. B., Avis, N. E., Mohr, B., Schocken, M., Skurnick, J., et al. (2003). Sexual functioning and practices in a multi-ethnic study of midlife women: Baseline results from SWAN. *Journal of Sex Research, 40,* 266–276.

Darvishpour, M. (1999). Immigrant women challenge the role of men: Conflict intensification within Iranian families in Sweden. *Nordic Journal of Women's Studies, 7,* 20–33.

Francoeur, R. T., & Noonan, R. J. (Eds.). (2004). *The continuum complete international encyclopedia of sexuality.* Retrieved from *www.kinseyinstitute.org/ccies/index.php.*

Giami, A. (2012). The social and professional diversity of sexology and sex therapy in Europe. In K. S. K. Hall & C. A. Graham (Eds.), *The cultural context of sexual pleasure and problems: Psychotherapy with diverse clients* (pp. 373–393). New York: Routledge.

Graham, C. A., & Bancroft, J. (2006). Assessing the prevalence of female sexual dysfunction with surveys: What is feasible? In I. Goldstein, C. Meston, S. Davis, & A. Traish (Eds.), *Women's sexual function and dysfunction: Study, diagnosis and treatment* (pp. 52–60). London: Taylor & Francis.

Graham, C. A., Ramos, R., Bancroft, J., Maglaya, C., & Farley, T. M. M. (1995). The effects of steroidal contraceptives on the well-being and sexuality of women: A double-blind, placebo-controlled, two-centre study of combined and progestogen-only methods. *Contraception, 52,* 363–369.

Hall, K. S. K., & Graham, C. A. (2012). Introduction. In K. S. K. Hall & C. A. Graham (Eds.), *The cultural context of sexual pleasure and problems: Psychotherapy with diverse clients* (pp. 1–20). New York: Routledge.

Hayes, R. D., Dennerstein, L., Bennett, C. M., & Fairley, C. K. (2008). What is the "true" prevalence of female sexual dysfunctions and does the way we assess these conditions have an impact? *Journal of Sexual Medicine, 5,* 777–787.

Hindin, M. J., & Muntifering, C. J. (2011). Women's autonomy and timing of most recent sexual intercourse in sub-Saharan Africa: A multi-country analysis. *Journal of Sex Research, 48,* 511–519.

Hughes, C. C. (1998). The glossary of culture-bound syndromes in DSM-IV: A critique. *Transcultural Psychiatry, 35,* 413–421.

Khademi, A., Alleyassim, A., Agha-hosseini, M., Dadras, N., Asghari Roodsari, A., Tabatabaeefar, L., et al. (2006). Psychometric properties of Sexual Function Questionnaire: Evaluation of an Iranian sample. *Iranian Journal of Reproductive Medicine, 4,* 23–28.

Kelly, S., & Shelton, J. (2012). African American couples and sex. In K. S. K. Hall & C. A. Graham (Eds.), *The cultural context of sexual pleasure and problems: Psychotherapy with diverse clients* (pp. 48–83). New York: Routledge.

Kempeneers, P., Andrianne, R., Bauwens, S., Georis, I., Pairoux, J.-F., & Blairy, S. (2013). Functional and psychological characteristics of Belgian men with premature ejaculation and their partners. *Archives of Sexual Behavior, 42*(1), 51–66.

Laumann, E. O., Nicolosi, A., Glasser, D. B., Paik, A., Gingell, C., Moreira, E., et al. (2005). Sexual problems among women and men aged 40–80 years: Prevalence and correlates identified in the Global Study of Sexual Attitudes and Behaviors. *International Journal of Impotence Research, 17,* 39–57.

Laumann, E. O., Paik, A., Glasser, D. B., Kang, J.-H., Wang, T., Levinson, B., et al. (2006). A cross-national study of subjective sexual well-being among older women and men: Findings from the Global Study of Sexual Attitudes and Behaviors. *Archives of Sexual Behavior, 35,* 143–159.

Lewis, L. J. (2004). Examining sexual health discourses in a racial/ethnic context. *Archives of Sexual Behavior, 33,* 223–234.

Lim, T. O., Das, A., Rampal, S., Zaki, M., Sahabudin, R. M., Rohan, M. J., et al. (2003). Cross-cultural adaptation and validation of the English version of the International Index of Erectile Function (IIEF) for use in Malaysia. *International Journal of Impotence Research, 15,* 329–336.

Lo, H. T., & Fung, K. P. (2003). Culturally competent psychotherapy. *Canadian Journal of Psychiatry, 48,* 161–170.

Mercer, C. H., Fenton, K. A., Johnson, A. M., Wellings, K., Macdowall, W., McManus, S., et al. (2003). Sexual function problems and help seeking behaviour in Britain: National probability sample survey. *British Medical Journal, 327,* 426–427.

Meston, C. M., & Ahrold, T. (2008). Ethnic, gender, and acculturation influences on sexual behaviors. *Archives of Sexual Behavior, 39,* 179–189.

Moreira, E., Brock, G., Glasser, D., Nicolosi, A., Laumann, E., Paik, A., et al. (2005). Help-seeking behaviour for sexual problems: The Global Study of Sexual Attitudes and Behaviors. *International Journal of Clinical Practice, 59,* 6–16.

Mosher, D. L., & Cross, H. J. (1971). Sex guilt and premarital sexual experiences of college students. *Journal of Consulting and Clinical Psychology, 36,* 27–32.

Oberg, K., Fugl-Meyer, A. R., & Fugl-Meyer, K. S. (2004). On categorization and quantification of women's sexual dysfunctions: An epidemiological approach. *International Journal of Impotence Research, 16,* 261–269.

Puzek, I., Stulhofer, A., & Bozicevic, I. (2012). Is religiosity a barrier to sexual and reproductive health? Results from a population-based study of young Croatian adults. *Archives of Sexual Behavior, 41*(6), 1497–1505.

Quirk, F. H., Heiman, J. H., Rosen, R. C., Laan, E., Smith, M. D., & Boolell, M. (2002). Development of a sexual function questionnaire for clinical trials of female sexual dysfunction. *Journal of Women's Health and Gender-Based Medicine, 11,* 277–289.

Ramanathan, V., & Weerakoon, P. (2012). Sexuality in India: Ancient beliefs, present-day problems, and future approaches to management. In K. S. K. Hall & C. A. Graham (Eds.), *The cultural context of sexual pleasure and problems: Psychotherapy with diverse clients* (pp. 173–196). New York: Routledge.

Rellini, A. H., Nappi, R. E., Vaccaro, P., Ferdeghini, F., Abbiati, I., & Meston, C. M. (2005). Validation of the McCoy Female Sexuality Questionnaire in an Italian sample. *Archives of Sexual Behavior, 34,* 641–647.

Robinson, B. E., Munns, R. A., Weber-Main, A. M., Lowe, M. A., & Raymond, N. C. (2011). Application of the sexual health model in the long-term treatment of hypoactive sexual desire and female orgasmic disorder. *Archives of Sexual Behavior, 40,* 469–478.

Rosen, R. C., Cappelleri, J. C., & Gendrano, N. (2002). The International Index of Erectile Function (IIEF): A state-of-the-science review. *International Journal of Impotence Research, 14,* 226–244.

Rosen, R. C., Riley, A., Wagner, G., Osterloh, I. H., Kirkpatrick, J., & Mishra, A. (1997). The international index of erectile function (IIEF): A multidimensional scale for assessment of erectile dysfunction. *Urology, 49*(6), 822–830.

Ryder, A. G., Alden, L. E., & Paulhus, D. L. (2000). Is acculturation unidimensional or bidimensional?: A head-to-head comparison in the prediction of personality, self-identity, and adjustment. *Journal of Personality and Social Psychology, 79,* 49–65.

Savage, N. (2012). The multi-cultural complexity of sexuality in Cameroon. In K. S. K. Hall & C. A. Graham (Eds.), *The cultural context of sexual pleasure and problems: Psychotherapy with diverse clients* (pp. 113–134). New York: Routledge.

Seth, V. (1993). *A suitable boy.* London: Phoenix.

Shifren, J. L., Monz, B. U., Russo, P. A., Segreti, A., & Johannes, C. B. (2008). Sexual problems and distress in United States women: Prevalence and correlates. *Obstetrics and Gynecology, 112*(5), 970–978.

So, H. W., & Cheung, F. M. (2005). Review of Chinese sex attitudes and applicability of sex therapy for Chinese couples with sexual dysfunction. *Journal of Sex Research, 42,* 93–101.

Stulhofer, A., & Arbanas, G. (2009). Sex therapy in a cultural context. *Archives of Sexual Behavior, 38,* 1044–1045.

Sue, S., & Zane, N. (2009). The role of culture and cultural techniques in psychotherapy: A critique and reformulation. *Asian American Journal of Psychology, S*(1), 3–14.

Sungur, M. (2012). The role of cultural factors in the course and treatment of sexual problems: Failures, pitfalls, and successes in a complicated case from Turkey. In K. S. K. Hall & C. A. Graham (Eds.), *The cultural context of sexual pleasure and problems: Psychotherapy with diverse clients* (pp. 308–332). New York: Routledge.

Temkina, A., Rotkirch, A., & Haavio-Mannila, E. (2012). Sex therapy in Russia: Pleasure and gender in a new professional field. In K. S. K. Hall & C. A. Graham (Eds.), *The cultural context of sexual pleasure and problems: Psychotherapy with diverse clients* (pp. 221–248). New York: Routledge.

Thakker, J., & Ward, T. (1998). Culture and classification: The cross-cultural application of the DSM-IV. *Clinical Psychology Review, 18,* 501–529.

Uberoi, P., & Palriwala, R. (2008). *Marriage, migration and gender.* New Delhi: Sage.

Verma, K. K., Khaitan, B. K., & Singh, O. P. (1998). The frequency of sexual dysfunctions in patients attending a sex therapy clinic in North India. *Archives of Sexual Behavior, 27,* 309–314.

Waldinger, M. D., McIntosh, J., & Schweitzer, D. H. (2009). A five-nation survey to assess the distribution of the intravaginal ejaculatory latency time among the general male population. *Journal of Sexual Medicine, 6,* 2888–2895.

Waldinger, M. D., Quinn, P., Dilleen, M., Mundayat, R., Schweitzer D. H., & Boolell, M. (2005). A multinational population survey of intravaginal ejaculation latency time. *Journal of Sexual Medicine, 2,* 492–497.

Williams, R. (1983). *Culture and society, 1780–1950.* New York: Columbia University Press.

Witting, K., Santtila, P., Varjonen, M., Jern, P., Johansson, A., von der Pahlen, B., et al. (2008). Female sexual dysfunction, sexual distress, and compatibility with partner. *Journal of Sexual Medicine, 5,* 2587–2599.

Woo, J. S. T., Morshedian, N., Brotto, L. A., & Gorzalka, B. B. (2012). Sex guilt mediates the relationship between religiosity and sexual desire in East Asian and Euro-Canadian college-aged women. *Archives of Sexual Behavior, 41*(6), 1485–1495.

World Health Organization. (2005). *Multi-country study on women's health and domestic violence against women: Initial results on prevalence, health outcomes and women's responses.* Geneva, Switzerland: Author.

Wright, W. K. (2006). The tide in favour of equality: Same-sex marriage in Canada and England and Wales. *International Journal of Law, Policy and the Family, 20*, 249–285.

Yasan, A., & Gurgen, F. (2009). Marital satisfaction, sexual problems and the possible difficulties on sex therapy in traditional Islamic culture. *Journal of Sex and Marital Therapy, 35*, 68–75.

Youn, G. (2012). Challenges facing sex therapy in Korea. In K. S. K. Hall & C. A. Graham (Eds.), *The cultural context of sexual pleasure and problems: Psychotherapy with diverse clients* (pp. 156–169). New York: Routledge.

Zargooshi, J., Rahmanian, E., Motaee, H., Kohzadi, M., & Nourizad, S. (2012). Culturally based sexual problems in traditional sections of Kermanshah, Iran. In K. S. K. Hall & C. A. Graham (Eds.), *The cultural context of sexual pleasure and problems: Psychotherapy with diverse clients* (pp. 136–154). New York: Routledge.

CHAPTER 16

Body Image and Sexuality

Michael W. Wiederman and Sabina Sarin

Being distracted during sex diminishes pleasure and contributes to a variety of sexual dysfunctions. Performance anxiety has been identified as a common distraction, but body image concerns may be as prevalent. In this chapter, Wiederman and Sarin integrate the growing empirical social psychological literature on body image and sexuality into clinical sex therapy practice. "The aspect of body image most relevant for sexual functioning appears to be the experience of anxious self-consciousness during sexual intimacy with a partner. . . . [T]he important question appears to be how much body image concerns are on the mind of the individual during sex." Wiederman and Sarin suggest that evaluating body image concerns while taking a sexual history should be standard, as available research clearly shows that body image is only weakly correlated with attractiveness as judged by others. In addition to standard cognitive techniques (e.g., reframing), they also emphasize the utility of exercise, yoga, mindfulness, and body work in order to help individuals overcome "anxious self-consciousness" about their bodies.

Michael W. Wiederman, PhD, is professor of psychology at Columbia College, an all-women's college in Columbia, South Carolina. A former Assistant Editor and Book Review Editor for the *Journal of Sex Research*, he is the author of *Understanding Sexuality Research* and co-editor of the *Handbook for Conducting Research on Human Sexuality*. Currently Dr. Wiederman serves as one of a few psychologists answering questions at *www.askthepsych.com*.

Sabina Sarin, MS, MPhil, is completing her PhD in Clinical Psychology at McGill University. Her research examines the psychophysiology of sexual desire, arousal, and the factors that influence and distinguish these experiences in healthy and clinical populations. Also a psychotherapist and yoga teacher, Sabina has specialized in the treatment of sexual disorders, eating disorders, trauma, mood and anxiety problems, and couple/relationship difficulties.

Sexual activity requires bodies, or at least one. Yet perceptions, thoughts, and emotions are at least as important as bodies for understanding variation in human sexual functioning. So therapists must consider the intersection of the body and the individual's perceptions, thoughts, and feelings about that body (i.e., *body image*). Before considering the intersection of body image and sexual functioning, it is necessary to deconstruct the multifaceted concept of body image.

Often the term "body image" is used to refer to an individual's self-assessment of overall appearance, or the extent to which a person is satisfied with how his or her body looks. Of course that is only one definition, albeit a popular one. "Body image" also could refer to self-assessment of the appearance of particular body parts or even self-assessment of bodily *functioning* as opposed to appearance. Then there is the issue of how important these self-assessments are to the individual; what they *mean* to the person, or how invested the individual is in his or her body image.

When it comes to the relevance of body image for sexual functioning, there are numerous aspects of body image to consider. Which ones are most relevant for sexuality? What are the mechanisms or mediating variables by which body image affects sexual functioning? Do the answers to these and other questions vary across different types of people? Hopefully continued research will provide increasingly accurate answers. For now, what do we know?

RESEARCH ON BODY IMAGE AND SEXUALITY

Research on body image and sexuality has grown steadily since about 1990. However, the existing research is limited in several ways. For example, Woertman and van den Brink (2012) performed a comprehensive review of the research on body image and sexual functioning and behavior. However, they limited their focus to women because of a relative lack of corresponding research on males. Many researchers have assumed that, because body image concerns generally are associated more with women than with men, the same would be true for sexuality-related body image.

Woertman and van den Brink (2012) found 57 relevant studies published since 1990 but noted that these studies were based predominantly on European American college students from the United States and Canada. Indeed, very little research has been published on body image and sexuality outside of Western cultures. Of the 57 studies Woertman and van den Brink (2012) reviewed, only two included non-Western samples (one from China, one from South Africa). Although the samples that make up the relevant research have been relatively homogeneous (young women from Western cultures), a variety of body image measures have been administered. As a result, some general conclusions have emerged across studies.

General Body Image

One consistent finding across studies is that global body satisfaction is the type of body image *least* predictive of sexual activity and functioning. More relevant are measures of body image as experienced during sexual activity and measures assessing perceptions of those body parts most relevant to sexual activity or sexual appeal (e.g., breasts, genitals). In other words, global body satisfaction is not synonymous with body image in the bedroom, and understandably it is the latter that is most relevant for understanding sexuality. The overall prevalence of body image concerns during sexual activity is difficult to assess, but in college student samples approximately one-third of women have reported experiencing such concerns at least some of the time (Woertman & van den Brink, 2012). The prevalence in clinical settings is unknown, but presumably greater.

The aspect of body image most relevant for sexual functioning appears to be the experience of anxious self-consciousness during sexual intimacy with a partner. Regardless of whether those concerns are focused on physical attractiveness (e.g., Pascoal, Narciso, & Pereira, 2012; Sanchez & Kiefer, 2007; Yamamiya, Cash, & Thompson, 2006) or appearance of the breasts or genitals (e.g., Schick, Calabrese, Rima, & Zucker, 2010), the important question appears to be how much body image concerns are on the mind of the individual during sex. To the extent that a person is focused on body image concerns, he or she may focus less on aspects of the sexual interaction that should be arousing and enjoyable.

Another consistent finding across several studies is that respondents who report experiencing greater body image self-consciousness during physical intimacy with a partner also report more problems with sexual functioning (e.g., Cash, Maikkula, & Yamamiya, 2004; La Rocque & Cioe, 2011; Sanchez & Kiefer, 2007). The forms of self-reported sexual problems identified in these studies included greater aversion to sex, less desire for sex, decreased arousal, increased anxiety during sexual activity, and, ultimately, less frequent orgasm. Also, research has demonstrated that those with negative body image report less motivation to avoid risky sexual behavior (Schick et al., 2010) and more experiences of unsafe and unwanted sexual activity (e.g., Littleton, Breitkopf, & Berenson, 2005). The proposed explanation has been that such individuals feel less able to assert their own desires and boundaries due to the perception that their relatively lower sexual attractiveness exalts the sexual partner to the position of greater power.

Genital and Breast Body Image

As erogenous zones, self-perceptions of genitals, as well as women's breasts, seem especially relevant for understanding sexual functioning. However, relatively little data exist on these aspects of body image. In a survey of college students in Canada, males indicated more positive genital body image overall compared with females (Morrison, Bearden, Ellis, & Harriman, 2005). The most common genital concerns for males involved the size and appearance of their nonerect penises (indicated by approximately one-quarter of respondents), whereas for females vaginal odor and the amount and texture of pubic hair were the most common concerns (again indicated by approximately one-quarter of respondents). Approximately 10% of females reported dissatisfaction with the size and/or shape of their labia.

The largest survey regarding genital body image involved more than 52,000 heterosexual respondents (ages 18–65 years) who responded online to questions pertaining to their perception of penises (Lever, Frederick, & Peplau, 2006) and breasts (Frederick, Peplau, & Lever, 2008). Most men (66%) reported that they believed their penises to be of average size (22% rated their penises as large; 12% as small), yet 45% of the men wanted to have larger penises. Apparently, men's desire for a larger penis did not translate into shame or partner dissatisfaction: Only 3.5% of the men reported concealing their penises from sexual partners, and 85% of the women indicated being satisfied with the size of their male partners' penises. Unfortunately, a single survey item assessed perceptions of penile size, with no distinction between length and circumference.

Although the extent to which dissatisfaction with penis size results in surgery to increase penis size is unknown, men who seek such surgery typically have penises of average size (Vardi, Har-Shai, Gil, & Gruenwald, 2008). Perhaps because the gain in penile size from such surgeries is typically minimal (1–2 cm increase in length and 2–3 cm in girth) and rates of complications relatively high, patient satisfaction tends to be low (Vardi et al., 2008).

In some cases, congenital deformity or physical trauma may be the catalyst for negative genital body image. Consider the case of Jason:

> Jason, a single 36-year-old Jamaican male, sought treatment for low desire and erectile dysfunction during partnered sexual activity. Exploration of his concern quickly revealed negative genital image. Jason explained that he had always believed his penis was not large enough and claimed to have been told as much by previous partners. His concerns became markedly worse after he suffered injury to his penis during intercourse. He had been only partially erect at the time but continued to let his partner "ride him" until he felt severe pain as his penis bent inside her. Not long after, he noticed that his penis became "deformed." Jason did nothing, hoping it would heal, but as the months passed, the downward curvature worsened, and scar tissue (plaques) began to form. He felt like a "monster."
>
> Jason soon stopped initiating sexual activity, and when unavoidable he would have sex in the dark to try to conceal the appearance of his penis. Still, Jason had become so afraid that his partners would notice or comment on his "deformity" that he found he was unable to focus on his sexual experiences and would promptly lose his erection. As Jason's

erectile difficulties progressively worsened over time, his fears of losing his erections led to avoidance of sexual activity altogether. Jason had consulted various medical practitioners without success. His only remaining option was an invasive surgery that would almost certainly shorten the length of his penis. For Jason, this was an unacceptable option, and so he decided to seek counseling. By that point, Jason was ridden with shame and self-loathing.

Whereas males who are dissatisfied with the size of their penises virtually always desire larger ones, there is less consistency among women who are dissatisfied with their breasts. In the large online survey noted earlier (Frederick, et al., 2008), most (70%) of the women were dissatisfied with their breasts, whereas a slight majority (56%) of the men were satisfied with their female partners' breasts. Younger and thinner women were most likely to desire larger breasts than they had, whereas older and heavier women were most likely to indicate dissatisfaction with droopiness or sagging of their breasts. Apparently the ideal breasts hold the contradictory distinctions of being relatively large and full yet gravity-defying and perky. Despite the high rate of breast dissatisfaction, only 9% of the women overall reported hiding their breasts during sex.

The high prevalence of breast dissatisfaction among women corresponds to the fact that, according to the American Society of Plastic Surgeons, breast augmentation surgery is the most common form of cosmetic surgery performed in the United States (*www.plasticsurgery.org*). In 2011, more than 300,000 such surgeries were performed, a 4% increase from 2010 and a 45% increase from the year 2000. More than 90,000 breast lift operations were performed in the United States in 2011, a 72% increase from the year 2000. Research on the effects of cosmetic breast surgery on women's sexuality is sparse, although one survey of 26 women who had undergone breast augmentation surgery revealed that 46% reported having sex more frequently after the surgery, 39% reported being more willing to experiment sexually, and 31% reported an increased ability to experience orgasm (Stofman, Neavin, Ramineni, & Alford, 2006).

Data on the extent to which dissatisfaction with women's genitals results in surgery or other procedures are severely lacking. However, it appears that at least awareness of such surgery has grown, as in 2010 an entire special issue of the professional journal *Reproductive Health Matters* (Vol. 18, No. 35) was devoted to the topic of genital cosmetic surgery and the related controversies, and in 2011 Goodman performed a review of the available research reports. For women, these surgeries most commonly include reducing the size of the labia minora (labiaplasty) and/or the clitoral hood or "tightening" of the vagina so that it "feels" or functions like a much younger, prematernity version.

Beyond concerns about the appearance of one's labia, another motivation for labiaplasty may be to correct excessively long or thick labia that cause pain during vaginal penetration. How often is the motivation for surgery functional versus cosmetic? In one study from a private gynecology practice in a large U.S. city, of the 131 women who underwent the surgery during a period of 27 months, 32% did so strictly to correct functional impairment, 31% because of both functional impairment and aesthetic concerns, and the remaining 37% indicated strictly appearance-related concerns (Miklos & Moore, 2008). Perhaps more surprising were the results from a similar study conducted in the United Kingdom involving 33 women who had been referred to gynecologists by their general physicians because of a stated desire for labiaplasty (Crouch, Deans, Michala, Liao, & Creighton, 2011). Surprisingly, the women averaged only 23 years of age, and all had labia minora of normal size (although three were offered surgery to correct significant asymmetry). Follow-up data on the effects of labiaplasty on women's sexuality are sparse (Berer, 2010), but rates of satisfaction appear high and incidence of complications low (Goodman, 2011). See Veale et al. (2013) for discussion of how to screen for body dysmorphic disorder among women seeking labiaplasty.

Potential Influences on Sexual Body Image

Although the combination of influences on body image is unique to each client, research points to a few general risk factors for body image concerns during sexual activity. One such variable is gender, or at least gender roles. Traditionally, concerns about appearance have been considered feminine. Traditional masculine ideologies prescribe a cool indifference to one's physical features as a source of sex appeal; instead, masculine sexual appeal rests on confidence, achievement, status, and experience. Although there are indications that males are increasingly concerned about physical appearance as a source of their sexual appeal, there still appears to be a marked male-female discrepancy in this regard (e.g., Owens, Allen, & Spangler, 2010; Pascoal et al., 2012). Also, when body image concerns are present, males may be more concerned about their degree of muscularity (e.g., Filiault, 2007), whereas females may be more concerned about their degree of fat (e.g., Pujols, Meston, & Seal, 2010). However, this apparent gender difference may be exaggerated due to the research being focused typically on young adults (college students).

A gender difference in the nature of concerns during sexual activity also has been demonstrated by multiple researchers, at least based on college-student samples. For example, Meana and Nunnink (2006) found that college males reported more frequently being concerned about their sexual performance than their bodily appearance during sexual activity with a partner. Compared with their male peers, female college students reported more frequently being concerned about bodily appearance during sexual activity. However, among the women, concerns about appearance versus performance were equal in frequency.

Some factors influencing body image concerns during sexual activity are more developmental or experiential in nature. Perhaps the most obvious factor is actual physical appearance. However, appearance changes over the lifespan, and indeed sexual body image may as well (Montemurro & Gillen, 2013). Even an individual who approximates the cultural ideal of sexual attractiveness currently may continue to be influenced by a history of having been overweight or deemed less attractive in some way (Annis, Cash, & Hrabosky, 2004). Also, physical disability or changes in bodily appearance or function due to illness, accident, or surgery may profoundly influence an individual's body image during physical intimacy with a partner (e.g., Moin, Duvdevaney, & Mazor, 2009).

Other important factors in the development of body image concerns during sex include specific comments, criticism, or teasing regarding one's sexual appeal, appearance, or bodily functioning (Annis et al., 2004). Such messages could be general or highly specific. For example, an individual may have been raised in a sociocultural environment in which genitals and their sexual functions were deemed dirty, shameful, and a source of anxiety. Conversely, a person may have had an unremarkable upbringing, yet have been traumatized by the negative reactions, verbal or otherwise, of one or more specific sexual partners

An individual's body image also may be influenced by current life circumstances aside from his or her sexual partners. For example, particular occupations such as modeling, dancing (erotic or otherwise), athletics, and sex work may facilitate either body confidence or anxious self-consciousness, depending on numerous factors. For example, physical exercise and body competence inherent in an occupation may facilitate comfort and confidence with one's body that then extends into the bedroom. Receiving continual positive feedback regarding one's attractiveness and sexual appeal at work may facilitate a positive body image during sexual activity. Conversely, work-related criticism, interpersonal comparison, or competitiveness based on appearance or body competence may undermine body image during sexual activity.

Other risk factors for body image concerns include exposure to unrealistic standards or images of what is implied to be normal. Research on what psychologists refer to as "contrast effects" has shown that exposure to images of very attractive people tends to leave the viewer less satisfied with his or her own appearance, especially when the viewer already has low self-esteem (Jones & Buckingham, 2005). So repeated exposure to professional models in various media may foster a negative body image for some. Similarly, repeated exposure to professionally produced erotica, with its digitally altered images, scripted sexual poses, and highly edited finished product, may lead the viewer to judge his or her sexual appeal and functioning as inadequate. These contrast effects may be insidious, affecting self-perceptions even when viewers are aware that the models and actors are professionals and the media based on fantasy.

ASSESSMENT

Researchers use numerous scales and inventories to measure various aspects of body image, so it may be tempting to ask which ones would be useful in a clinical context. However, most such measures are not specific to body image in a sexual setting. Even those that are may generate a score designed for use by researchers interested in correlating the score with other variables. Clinically, however, the scores lack interpretative meaning for the individual test-taker. Without an established cutoff score indicating substantial problems, what does a particular client's score indicate? For the individual, phenomenology is more important than a numerical score.

Clinicians who ask new clients to complete a packet of self-report materials may choose to include some specific questions pertaining to body image concerns. Rather than using a formal scale per se, directly asking about body image concerns that interfere with sexual functioning is much less ambiguous. Consider this sample set of questions a clinician might pose to a client either in an intake packet or during an interview: Does how you think or feel about your body ever interfere with your sex life? *If yes*, in what ways? For example, does it affect your frequency of sexual activity, your ability to ask for what you want and set limits with your partners, or distract you from focusing on your pleasure during sex? What have you tried before to work around the problem? What happened?

The initial query casts a broad net, with the follow-up questions aimed at better understanding the phenomenology of the body image concerns as experienced by the client. What are the specific characteristics of the body image concerns? In what ways do they affect the client's sexuality? What has the client attempted as a means of coping or remediation?

It also may be productive to investigate ways in which the client uses body image concerns to make sense out of negative sexual outcomes. In other words, does the client attribute his or her sexual problems to those aspects of body image over which he or she is dissatisfied, regardless of whether those attributions are accurate? As long as sexual problems are attributed to deficits in appearance or bodily functioning, the client is unlikely to have considered solutions other than alteration of the body, which may not be realistic or helpful.

It may be good practice to routinely include for all clients a broad screening question pertaining to body image during sexual activity. Otherwise the clinician might fall into using implicit stereotypes or assumptions about the types of clients most likely to experience such problems. For example, if a client appears sexually attractive, it might be easy to assume that the client does not experience body image concerns (and vice versa). In reality, research has revealed that body image is only weakly correlated with attractiveness as judged by others (e.g., Weeden & Sabini, 2007).

Assessment may be more complex when working with couples. In addition to the sheer number of issues to assess, some pertain to the individual members of the couple, whereas others to their joint interactions. In that regard, consider the case of Stefan and Maria:

> Stefan and Maria were in their mid-40s and had been married 15 years, during most of which they had been raising their two children. Although they sought treatment for Maria's low sexual desire and lifelong anorgasmia, both admitted that their sexual relationship had been lacking almost since its onset. Maria typically avoided sex, engaging in it once every few weeks, "just to please her husband." Maria was able to become lubricated and experience some arousal during sex, but reported that her arousal quickly plateaued and then tapered off. Maria and Stefan agreed that this had been the case throughout their relationship and that, despite some experimentation, nothing seemed to help.
>
> The assessment revealed that both Maria and Stefan held conservative sexual attitudes deriving from their Italian Catholic backgrounds and lacked knowledge of female sexual functioning. Indeed, Maria had never even looked at her genitals, had a strong aversion to them, and consequently had never allowed her husband to perform oral sex on her. Stefan noted that each also had gained weight over the years and that neither felt attractive or comfortable in their bodies, although both denied decreased attraction to the other. Whereas Stefan's negative body image had not affected his interest in sexual activity, Maria dreaded having sex. Typically she would "lie there and hope he would quickly get it over with," all the while distracted by her hatred of her body. Not only did Maria never ask for things that might give her more pleasure, but she was also mostly unaware of what might do so and reported feeling few sensations she would call "enjoyable." Sensing her detachment during sex, Stefan felt insecure and would try to rush sex for her sake. With the focus on their negative body images and sex as a chore to get through, neither Stefan nor Maria attended to what they could do to make it more satisfying.

APPROACHES TO TREATMENT

Currently there are no published reports on the assessment of interventions to improve body image concerns during sexual activity. Accordingly, clinicians addressing body image concerns in the bedroom are left to "bootstrap" techniques shown to be effective at improving body image generally, which tend to fall along cognitive-behavioral lines. Therapists must also factor in comorbid psychopathology and whether the client has a steady sexual partner who may be affected by, and willing to work on, the problematic body image.

Because body image interference with sexual functioning frequently has its roots in anxious self-consciousness and resulting distraction from sexual stimuli, addressing thoughts experienced by the client during sexual activity is a prime place to start. Making such thoughts explicit may be enough to reveal their inherent irrationality, and client anxiety decreases. In other cases, however, the client may readily recognize the irrationality of the problematic thoughts, yet still react to such thoughts as though they were valid. Depending on the nature of these irrational or inaccurate thoughts, the clinician and client may collaborate on developing "experiments" so that the client can empirically test the validity of his or her assumptions. One such experiment may involve seeking explicit feedback from the client's sexual partner.

Clients with body image concerns frequently engage in "mind reading" about what partners believe, think, and feel. Clinicians working with the couple have the opportunity to facilitate detailed discussion of each partner's perceptions of, and reactions to, the body-image-related concerns. This seemingly obvious step toward possible resolution of the concerns may not have occurred to the client due to assumptions that the partner's beliefs, thoughts, and feelings are "obvious" or simply the same as the cultural norm or stereotype. One risk, however, is that the partner will agree with the client or exacerbate the client's negative body image through criticism. In such cases, couple counseling is warranted. The body image concerns involve both members and may be a symptom of larger relationship problems.

Even when a client's partner is very supportive, positive feedback may be discounted by the client, thereby maintaining the negative self-schema, through rationalizing that the partner is being polite or conflict avoidant. It may be necessary to engage the client in an ongoing process of cognitive restructuring, emphasizing that undoing these ingrained thoughts and assumptions will not occur suddenly or completely but takes practice, with resulting incremental improvement. Such a process entails repeated awareness of problematic cognitions and explicit self-refutation of those thoughts and beliefs.

When discussion of client versus partner perceptions does not appear to be effective at decreasing client anxious self-consciousness, homework might entail massage or sexual activity during which the client's partner verbalizes his or her thoughts and feelings about the client's body and sexual appeal. By tying expression of partner perceptions to actual experiences of physical intimacy, such expressions become more valid and can be based on specifics (e.g., "I love how your _____.") versus generalities that may or may not be true (e.g., "I think you're as sexy as when we first met").

Being massaged or pleasured by one's partner is an aspect of sensate focus, and the same approach may be helpful for learning to focus on the immediate sensual experience rather than cognitive distraction over body image concerns. Similarly, mindfulness training and practice may help clients learn to be aware and focused on the present moment—their immediate sexual experience—and thus be inoculated against disruptive body image distractions (de Jong, 2009).

Any strategies that facilitate decreased anxiety while engaging in sexual activity with a partner will likely have the positive effect of reducing future anxiety through the well-established process of systematic desensitization. Consideration of antianxiety medication may be warranted in some cases to facilitate that process. Intentional use of systematic desensitization also may be a primary intervention to disrupt body image anxiety during sexual activity. For example, explicit relaxation training and practice may be paired with viewing, or allowing the client's partner to view or touch, those body parts that prompt body image anxiety. Past avoidance of viewing or revealing problematic body parts simply reinforced body image anxiety and must be reversed. Consider the previously introduced case of Stefan and Maria:

> Early treatment with Maria and Stefan concentrated on education about the female and male sexual response cycles, with an emphasis on the importance of "sexy" thoughts and adequate sexual stimulation. Connections among thoughts (e.g., interpretations, expectations, attitudes, and beliefs), feelings, behaviors, and physiological response were explained, particularly with respect to Maria's negative body image and her ensuing sexual difficulties. Relaxation exercises were introduced, and the couple was instructed to practice these before engaging in self-examination exercises. In a relaxed setting, Maria used a mirror to examine her genitals for the first time and to sketch what she saw. She was asked to then describe what she saw, using neutral or positive terms, and if comfortable, to discuss her drawing with Stefan. Both were encouraged to practice the same exercise on their own, noticing and describing their entire bodies. Maria admitted surprise at enjoying the experience of genital examination, although she felt shy and uncomfortable sharing the experience with Stefan. Stefan, too, was surprised to discover that he could think of his body in new, positive ways.
>
> Next, an alternative model of sexuality was presented, one based on valuing intimacy and pleasure rather than goal-directed sex (i.e., reaching orgasm). A temporary ban was placed on sexual intercourse, and for the next month, Stefan and Maria were encouraged to engage in sensate focus exercises while telling each other authentically what they enjoyed about specific aspects of the other's body. They were encouraged to explore and discuss what turned them on, both during masturbation and together (e.g., types of touch, activities, scenarios), and to reinforce each other for touch they found arousing. Maria was instructed to practice asking for what she wanted. It was agreed that the ban on intercourse would end on Maria's initiative.
>
> Maria and Stefan initially found this assignment quite challenging. Stefan worried that they would never have sex again. Maria, while reassured by the intercourse restriction, still felt indirect pressure to initiate and anxiety about the vulnerability that came from a more intimacy-based model of sexuality. However, after weeks of exploring resistances and ongoing practice of direct communication between them about their fears and expectations, their sexual relationship opened up. Maria began to take the lead and found it arousing to do so; in fact, she found that once things got started, it was not always easy to stop, and the ban on

intercourse soon became a seductive boundary they had fun taunting each other to cross. With this increased intimacy, both began to take better care of their bodies: They went for walks together, exercised more, ate less out of boredom, and soon felt more comfortable with themselves and each other. In subsequent months they experienced more sexual intimacy and pleasure. Maria had not yet attained orgasm but was experiencing more desire and arousal than ever before.

As with Stefan and Maria, particular forms of body work may facilitate increased comfort with the client's own body. Regular physical exercise may improve body image, even in the absence of weight loss. Rather than simply enhancing physical attractiveness, exercise may affect body image through an increased sense of body competence and connection to one's body. Exercise may facilitate a sense of personal ownership of one's body and increased awareness of bodily sensations. Although research on the topic is needed, particular forms of exercise may be most beneficial for addressing body image concerns pertaining to sexuality. For example, yoga combines physical exercise with relaxation (breath work) and mindful awareness, thereby addressing both physical and cognitive aspects of body image concerns.

In some cases clients have developed unrealistic standards for the appearance or functioning of bodies generally or the genitals specifically. Particularly in cultures with a high degree of personal privacy, seeing naked bodies and genitals representative of one's age, gender, and ethnicity may be very rare. Instead, images of professional models and actors may have filled that void, leaving the client feeling inadequate by comparison. Intervention in such cases may involve homework entailing online searches for images demonstrating the range of bodies and genitals that characterize the population (e.g., amateur erotica, medical photos).

Human nature is such that we more readily compare our circumstances with those who are better off than us (upward comparison) rather than those who are worse off (downward comparison). Part of the value in exposing particular clients to a wide range of images of bodies and genitals is to make explicit that not *everyone* is thinner, more muscular, or more attractive. Rather than focusing on what could always be better, the therapist may help the client consider what could be worse.

CASE DISCUSSION

Claire, a slim and attractive 28-year-old white woman, was initially referred for complaints of vaginal numbness and soreness during intercourse, infrequent orgasms, poor lubrication and mental arousal, and clitoral hypersensitivity. Claire was single but engaged somewhat regularly in casual, often unprotected, sex—generally under the influence of alcohol so as to "get out of her head." Claire was consumed by negative thoughts about how her partners might evaluate her body and "sex appeal" and navigated each sexual encounter in ways to appear as attractive as possible. Rather than avoid sex entirely, Claire frequently had unwanted sex because it was easier than saying "no."

Claire had struggled with poor body image since her early teens. With numerous younger siblings she had to take care of, Claire reported feeling that it was not okay for her to take up any space, physically or mentally. Not surprisingly, Claire's discomfort with "taking up space" had migrated to the realm of her sexuality. As a result, Claire had learned to disconnect from her own body, both its needs and its pleasurable sensations.

Claire's first experience of sexual intercourse had occurred against her will; he had penetrated without her consent, and she felt she couldn't stop him. This initial experience set the stage for her subsequent pattern of "passive consent" with men. Claire seduced men as a means to feel attractive, then went through the motions of having sex to avoid saying "no," all the while feeling little connection to her own bodily experience.

Early in treatment Claire was surprised to learn how her problematic issues with body, self, and sex were connected. She learned about the detrimental effects of focusing on "unsexy" thoughts and feelings, such as her hatred of parts of her body or fears of her partner's reactions, and that she missed many informative signals (e.g., bodily cues of pleasure and arousal, or signs of anxiety suggesting that she should not engage in the activity at all). Although Claire was aware of intense bodily sensations, she was devoid of accompanying feelings of pleasure—instead she felt numbness or overwhelming hypersensitivity. Lacking the assertiveness skills to improve her situation (e.g., by using lubricants, directing the sexual activity, or stopping altogether), Claire typically experienced vaginal pain and soreness and a lack of interest in sexual activity. Consequently, Claire used alcohol or drugs to get over the "hump" of anxiety-related reluctance in the face of an impending sexual encounter and to dull her self-conscious thoughts and fears while engaging in sex.

In addition to helping her build a more defined sense of herself, as well as skills in asserting that self, relaxation and mindfulness exercises were taught and practiced as a way of easing her into becoming reacquainted with her own body. Claire was asked to start attending to her bodily sensations (e.g., hunger, anxiety, arousal) as informational signals and not problems to be avoided or smothered. She was encouraged to trust her body, her needs, and her instincts and ultimately to pursue behaviors that represented self-care. Claire found this very difficult and showed much resistance, reporting that she would prefer to be taken care of by others.

Through exploration of her resistance, Claire eventually became more aware of the connections among how she felt about herself, how she treated her body (with regard to drugs and alcohol, food, sex, and sleep), and the kinds of men she attracted. Gradually, Claire began to see that the more she engaged in self-care, the better she felt about herself, and the easier it became to act in her own self-interest in the future. She started to "say no" to sexual activity with men who saw her as little more than their "catch for the night" and began to build meaningful relationships with men who valued her thoughts and feelings. Claire began to see that her body image had very little to do with how she looked.

As Claire became more self-accepting and assertive, her thoughts about her body became less punitive and all-consuming. She began to experience more pleasure during sex. She asked for more of what she wanted, and she focused more on how it felt to receive it. Her pain disappeared entirely, her arousal levels increased, and she found that she was more orgasmic than ever before. By the end of treatment, Claire had begun to crave *real* intimacy in the context of a committed relationship, although she still struggled with the inherent vulnerability. Although not there yet, Claire was on the road toward autonomy and loving self-care.

Claire's case illustrates the problems when clients are more focused on *analyzing* their bodies than actually being *in* them. Although aspects of Claire's treatment were focused on sexual activity, treatment more generally included bolstering her general self-worth and restructuring her beliefs about herself and her body so that her body was not viewed as her enemy to be avoided or subdued. Direct attempts at behavioral change were met with resistance initially, but creating the safe and supportive space needed to take new steps resulted in slow yet steady progress.

CONCLUSIONS

Although body image concerns do not constitute a specific clinical diagnosis, the role of such problems in understanding and improving sexual functioning can be of utmost importance. Research has demonstrated some general factors and issues related to body image concerns during sexual activity, but numerous questions remain. For example, the prevalence of such concerns, in both clinical and community samples, is unclear. Also, research is needed on the mechanisms and dynamics through which body image concerns affect sexual functioning, including the effects of bodily alteration. More important for clinicians, empirical evaluation of therapeutic strategies and techniques to address body image concerns in the bedroom is lacking entirely. The ultimate goal, of course, is to better serve those clients who seek to improve their sexual lives and require more positive body images to do so.

REFERENCES

Annis, N. M., Cash, T. F., & Hrabosky, J. I. (2004). Body image and psychosocial differences among stable average weight, currently overweight, and formerly overweight women: The role of stigmatizing experiences. *Body Image, 1*, 155–167.

Berer, M. (2010). Cosmetic surgery, body image and sexuality. *Reproductive Health Matters, 18*(35), 4–10.

Cash, T. F., Maikkula, C. L., & Yamamiya, Y. (2004). "Baring the body in the bedroom": Body image, sexual self-schemas, and sexual functioning among college women and men. *Electronic Journal of Human Sexuality, 7.*

Crouch, N., Deans, R., Michala, L., Liao, L., & Creighton, S. (2011). Clinical characteristics of well women seeking labial reduction surgery: A prospective study. *British Journal of Obstetrics and Gynecology, 118,* 1507–1510.

de Jong, D. C. (2009). The role of attention in sexual arousal: Implications for treatment of sexual dysfunction. *Journal of Sex Research, 46,* 237–248.

Filiault, S. M. (2007). Measuring up in the bedroom: Muscle, thinness, and men's sex lives. *International Journal of Men's Health, 6,* 127–142.

Frederick, D. A., Peplau, A., & Lever, J. (2008). The Barbie mystique: Satisfaction with breast size and shape across the lifespan. *International Journal of Sexual Health, 20,* 200–211.

Goodman, M. P. (2011). Female genital cosmetic and plastic surgery: A review. *Journal of Sexual Medicine, 8,* 1813–1825.

Jones, A. M., & Buckingham, J. T. (2005). Self-esteem as a moderator of the effect of social comparison on women's body image. *Journal of Social and Clinical Psychology, 24,* 1164–1187.

La Rocque, C. L., & Cioe, J. (2011). An evaluation of the relationship between body image and sexual avoidance. *Journal of Sex Research, 48,* 397–408.

Lever, J., Frederick, D. A., & Peplau, L. A. (2006). Does size matter?: Men's and women's views on penis size across the lifespan. *Psychology of Men and Masculinity, 7,* 129–143.

Littleton, H., Breitkopf, C. R., & Berenson, A. (2005). Body image and risky sexual behaviors: An investigation in a tri-ethnic sample. *Body Image, 2,* 193–198.

Meana, M., & Nunnink, S. E. (2006). Gender differences in the content of cognitive distractions during sex. *Journal of Sex Research, 43,* 59–67.

Miklos, J. R., & Moore, R. D. (2008). Labiaplasty of the labia minora: Patients' indications for pursuing surgery. *Journal of Sexual Medicine, 5,* 1492–1495.

Moin, V., Duvdevany, H., & Mazor, D. (2009). Sexual identity, body image and life satisfaction among women with and without physical disability. *Sexuality and Disability, 27,* 83–95.

Montemurro, B., & Gillen, M. M. (2013). Wrinkles and sagging flesh: Exploring transformation in women's sexual body image. *Journal of Women and Aging, 25,* 3–23.

Morrison, T. G., Bearden, A., Ellis, S. R., & Harriman, R. (2005). Correlates of genital perceptions among Canadian post-secondary students. *Electronic Journal of Human Sexuality, 8.*

Owens, T. E., Allen, M. D., & Spangler, D. L. (2010). An fMRI study of self-reflection about body image: Sex differences. *Personality and Individual Differences, 48,* 849–854.

Pascoal, P., Narciso, I., & Pereira, N. M. (2012). Predictors of body appearance cognitive distraction during sexual activity in men and women. *Journal of Sexual Medicine, 9,* 2849–2860.

Pujols, Y., Meston, C. M., & Seal, B. N. (2010). The association between sexual satisfaction and body image in women. *Journal of Sexual Medicine, 7,* 905–916.

Sanchez, D. T., & Kiefer, A. K. (2007). Body concerns in and out of the bedroom: Implications for sexual pleasure and problems. *Archives of Sexual Behavior, 36,* 808–820.

Schick, V. R., Calabrese, S. K., Rima, B. N., & Zucker, A. N. (2010). Genital appear-
    ance dissatisfaction: Implications for women's genital image self-consciousness,
    sexual esteem, sexual satisfaction, and sexual risk. *Psychology of Women Quar-
    terly, 34*, 394–404.

Stofman, G. M., Neavin, T. S., Ramineni, P. M., & Alford, A. (2006). Better sex from
    the knife?: An intimate look at the effects of cosmetic surgery on sexual prac-
    tices. *Aesthetic Surgery Journal, 26*, 12–17.

Vardi, Y., Har-Shai, Y., Gil, T., & Gruenwald, I. (2008). A critical analysis of penile
    enhancement procedures for patients with normal penile size: Surgical proce-
    dures, success, and complications. *European Urology, 54*, 1042–1050.

Veale, D., Eshkevari, E., Ellison, N., Cardoza, L., Robinson, D., & Kavouni, A.
    (2013). Validation of Genital Appearance Satisfaction scale and the Cosmetic
    Procedure Screening scale for women seeking labiaplasty. *Journal of Psychoso-
    matic Obstetrics and Gynaecology, 34*, 46–52.

Weeden, J., & Sabini, J. (2007). Subjective and objective measures of attractiveness
    and their relation to sexual behavior and sexual attitudes in university students.
    Archives of Sexual Behavior, 36, 79–88.

Woertman, L., & van den Brink, F. (2012). Body image and female sexual functioning
    and behavior: A review. *Journal of Sex Research, 49*, 184–211.

Yamamiya, Y., Cash, T. F., & Thompson, J. K. (2006). Sexual experiences among col-
    lege women: The differential effects of general versus contextual body images on
    sexuality. *Sex Roles, 55*, 421–427.

CHAPTER 17

The Treatment of Sexual Dysfunctions in Survivors of Sexual Abuse

Alessandra H. Rellini

Sexual abuse is not uncommon in the history of sex therapy clients. However, "a therapist should not assume that the sexual dysfunction of an individual with a history of sexual abuse is the result of abuse." With this caveat in mind, Rellini suggests that the possibility of sexual abuse should be treated as a "working hypothesis," and she counsels clinicians to collect sufficient information to determine whether the pattern of sexual difficulties presented by a patient matches the commonly discussed clinical profiles of sexual difficulties in sexual abuse survivors. Rellini critically reviews the literature and notes that the heterogeneity in sexual outcomes as a result of sexual abuse makes generalizations difficult. She also notes that the experience of other forms of abuse (physical and emotional maltreatment and neglect) are perhaps just as important to consider when formulating a treatment plan. While noting that there is little empirical support for the efficacy of the existing various treatment approaches, her review provides important guidelines for conducting sex therapy with men and women who have experienced sexual abuse in childhood.

Alessandra H. Rellini, PhD, is Associate Professor in Psychology at the University of Vermont. Dr. Rellini is a Fulbright Scholar, and her research on the psychophysiological responses of women and their treatment implications has been funded by competitive private and government grants. She has over 40 publications, and her work has received numerous awards from the International Society of Women's Sexual Health, the International Society of Sexual Medicine, the Scientific Society for the Study of Sexuality, the Society for Sex Therapy and Research, and the International Society for the Study of Traumatic Stress. Currently, Dr. Rellini serves on the editorial board of the *Archives of Sexual Behavior* and the *Journal of Sexual Medicine,* and she is part of the Standardization Committee for the International Society of Sexual Medicine.

Sexual abuse is a common experience among individuals seeking treatment (Sickel, Noll, Moore, Putnam, & Trickett, 2002), and, therefore, it is an experience that we are likely to find in the histories of our sex therapy clients. For example, among 412 married women seeking psychological counseling at a sexual dysfunction clinic, 20% reported a history of childhood sexual abuse (Sarwer & Durlak, 1996). In the larger population, nonpenetrative sexual abuse (i.e., fondling) was reported by 12% of men and 23% of women, and penetrative sexual abuse (i.e., vaginal penetration, anal penetration, and oral sex) was reported by 4% of men and 13% of women (Najman et al., 2005). The experience of abuse among clients varies in terms of age at which the abuse occurred, the relationship with the perpetrator, the types of behaviors that occurred, the frequency of these behaviors, and the clarity of the patients' memories (Rellini & Meston, 2007). The symptoms that emerge after sexual abuse are heterogeneous, varying greatly between clients and showing a constellation of possible outcomes rather than a specific syndrome (Schloredt & Heiman, 2003). Research has found a significant association between sexual abuse and sexual dysfunctions in both women and men, with sexual dysfunctions being reported by double the number of men who had been abused as compared with nonabused men (Najman et al., 2005). Other disorders are common among these clients, including depression, borderline personality disorder, eating disorders, posttraumatic stress disorder, and other anxiety disorders (Polusny & Follette, 1995). The great variety in types of abuse and in their long-term sequelae creates a challenge in identifying a specific approach that can address the complexity of sexual dysfunctions following sexual abuse. Despite the heterogeneity of symptoms and experiences, accumulating evidence points to overarching themes, risk factors, and mechanisms that are common in the sexual lives of many sexual abuse survivors and that can be used as guiding points when conducting sex therapy with this population.

To facilitate the treatment of sexual dysfunction among individuals with a history of sexual abuse, this chapter reviews the empirical evidence on the types of sexual dysfunction most commonly experienced, the most appropriate assessment methods, and the potential mechanisms of action that link the abuse to sexual functioning. There is only scarce information on the treatment of sexual dysfunction in sexual abuse survivors, but a comprehensive review of the extant literature on clinical studies and on potential malleable targets for treatment will provide guidance to the clinician treating this population. Finally, two case studies that illustrate the complexity of sexual dysfunction in sexual abuse survivors will showcase the limitations of our current understanding of sex therapy with sexual abuse survivors.

DEFINITION OF SEXUAL ABUSE

Researchers have adopted a number of different operationalizations of sexual abuse, mostly based on *activity-specific* criteria (Peters, Wyatt, & Finkelhor, 1986), that is, definitions that rely on an objective description of the abuse, such as behavior(s) that occurred during the abuse, the age of the abuse onset, and the relationship with the perpetrator. Comparing results from studies using different definitions is complicated because it is currently unclear whether sexual abuse can be considered on a continuum, with some types of abuse representing more severe forms, or if some types of abuse are qualitatively different from others. Independently from the categorical–continuum argument, the variance in definitions adopted by researchers makes it hard for clinicians to know when the results can be applied to their clients.

Defining sexual abuse in the therapy room follows different parameters. For the therapist, the patient's perception that he or she was sexually abused is the cornerstone of the definition. This requires the individual to recognize the event as abusive and to label it. This is a *relationship-specific* definition (Peters et al., 1986). The difference between *activity-* and *relationship-specific* definitions is noteworthy because not all individuals who experienced sexual abuse based on behavioral definitions will self-identify as sexual abuse survivors (Rellini & Meston, 2007). Women endorsing the sexual abuse label are more likely to have experienced more chronic and invasive sexual behaviors (i.e., vaginal penetration from a parent or a parental figure) and tend to have lower sexual functioning than individuals who respond positively to more commonly used activity-specific definitions (Rellini & Meston, 2007). For men, research has shown the tendency to redefine, retrospectively, the abusive experience as normative (Holmes & Slap, 1998). Both men and women who have been exposed to childhood sexual abuse are stigmatized in our society; they are perceived as victims, weak, and damaged. It is likely that the burden of this stigma may explain the reticence of individuals to identify as sexual abuse survivors. To overcome these limitations, the therapist needs to pay particular attention to using both definitions of abuse when collecting the sexual history of patients: Relationship-specific definitions allow for a more client-centered assessment, whereas the activity-specific definition enables a more detailed review of the important sexual experiences that may have affected the patient's sexuality.

EPIDEMIOLOGY OF SEXUAL ABUSE AND SEXUAL DYSFUNCTIONS

Because of the tendency for people not to report sexual abuse, prevalence estimates are conservative (Green, 1996). Rates reported by community studies tend to indicate that approximately 28% of women and 10% of men have a history of sexual abuse prior to age 14 (Loeb et al., 2002; Leonard & Follette, 2002). These rates are slightly lower than they were prior to 1998 but remain alarmingly high (U.S. Department of Health and Human Services, 2003).

The estimate of sexual dysfunction among sexual abuse survivors is complicated to interpret. It is not possible to directly test whether sexual abuse caused the development of sexual problems. Clients who identify as sexual abuse survivors are likely to believe that the abuse has indeed caused sexual dysfunction. However, the fact that child sexual abuse preceded the development of sexual dysfunction and the ethical limitations precluding an experimental study using randomization make inferences based on semiexperimental data the only tool available to understand this relationship. Correlational studies consistently point to a significant relationship between sexual abuse and adult sexual functioning (Loeb et al., 2002). For example, a review of 38 studies reported that across methodologies, samples, and measures, childhood sexual abuse is a risk factor for adult sexual dysfunction (Neumann, Houskamp, Pollock, & Briere, 1996). Variance in effect sizes is noteworthy, with studies conducted with college students showing smaller effects than studies conducted on the community samples (for a review, see Rellini, 2005). A recent summary of epidemiological studies reported that among a population-based sample across different countries, sexual abuse is positively associated with greater sexual difficulties (Lewis et al., 2010). In a random community sample, 40% of women with a history of childhood sexual abuse had experienced lack of sexual desire in the previous year (Laumann, Gagnon, Michael, & Michaels, 1994). American women who felt forced to have sex by a man reported lower desire and greater sexual arousal disorder than women with no history of forced sex. For Swedish women, a history of sexual abuse predicted higher numbers of sexual dysfunctions, and the strongest effects were observed for orgasmic dysfunction. For these women, sexual abuse that occurred more than once (chronic) was specifically associated with greater sexual dissatisfaction. In Moroccan women, sexual abuse negatively predicted sexual interest. The data on men recruited from the community showed small effects of sexual abuse on sexual function (Elliott, Mok, & Briere, 2004; Laumann et al., 1994). A study on college students confirmed the small effects and also reported that more severe forms of abuse (i.e., rape) were more strongly associated with sexual dysfunction (Turchik, 2012).

It is important to note that a statistical significance does not mean that all individuals with a history of sexual abuse will develop sexual dysfunctions. Indeed, the effect sizes of these studies are modest, suggesting that many women who experienced abuse are able to develop satisfying sexual relationships and do not experience sexual dysfunctions (Watson & Halford, 2010). In a study conducted on women seeking sex therapy, 37% of women with a history of sexual abuse did not have sexual dysfunctions, and 48% of women with no history of sexual abuse had sexual dysfunctions, highlighting the fact that sexual abuse is neither sufficient nor necessary for the development of sexual dysfunction (Sarwer & Durlak, 1996). Thus a therapist should not assume that the sexual dysfunction of an individual with a history of sexual abuse is the result of the abuse. Moreover, accumulating evidence is pointing to the negative effects of other forms of childhood maltreatment on adult sexual functioning, such as physical abuse and emotional neglect (Schloredt & Heiman, 2003; Rellini, 2005). Sexual abuse is an important aspect of the patient's history that needs to be assessed, and, for individuals who have experienced sexual abuse, the case conceptualization should include sexual abuse. However, the therapist should consider the abuse as part of a working hypothesis while continuing to collect data to assess whether the pattern of sexual difficulties observed in the patient matches the most commonly discussed profiles of sexual abuse survivors. Embracing in haste the assumption that sexual abuse is the problem underlying the sexual dysfunction may cause a negative reaction from the patient, who may not feel understood. Also, this hasty decision may obfuscate other important factors of the sexual dysfunction. For example, a recent study on sexual abuse survivors reported that everyday hassles predicted lower sexual functioning better than the severity of the abuse and the development of posttraumatic stress disorder symptoms, suggesting that daily problems can have more serious effects on sexual function than moderate symptoms of posttraumatic stress disorder caused by the abuse (Zollman, Rellini, & Desrocher, 2013).

Some sexual dysfunctions and sexual problems are associated with sexual abuse more strongly than others. Low sexual desire is one of the most commonly reported sexual dysfunctions in women with a history of childhood sexual abuse. Among women seeking therapy, hypoactive sexual desire disorder was experienced more frequently by those women who had experienced more invasive forms of childhood sexual abuse, such as forced vaginal penetration and the presence of physical force during the abuse (Sarwer & Durlak, 1996). Difficulties in becoming sexually aroused occur frequently in survivors of childhood sexual abuse recruited from the community (Becker, Skinner, Abel, & Treacy, 1982; Fergusson & Mullen, 1999) and from clinical populations (Westerlund, 1992; Becker, Skinner, Abel, & Cichon, 1986). In particular, sexual arousal problems secondary to childhood sexual abuse have been positively correlated with fear of being out of control, with guilt or shame regarding the abuse (Westerlund), with guilt during sexual arousal (Heiman, Gladue, Roberts, & LoPiccolo, 1982), with younger age at the time of the abuse, with repeated incidents of abuse, and with knowing the assailant (Becker et al.). Epidemiological studies indicate that difficulty reaching an orgasm is often reported by women who have experienced sexual abuse (Lewis et al., 2010). A rigorous epidemiological study that utilized a representative random sample of the population reported that both physical and sexual abuse prior to age 12 were associated with sexual pain and that the association was particularly strong when the perpetrator was a parent or parental figure or a sibling (Harlow & Stewart, 2005).

The association between a history of sexual abuse and sexual satisfaction tends to be stronger than the association with sexual function (Leonard, Iversone, & Follette, 2008; Rellini & Meston, 2007), suggesting that clinicians should inquire about sexual satisfaction even if patients report no sexual problems. The fact that sexual satisfaction has stronger effects than sexual dysfunction also has been suggested as evidence that the sexual difficulties of sexual abuse survivors may not be completely captured by the currently available definitions of sexual abuse (Rellini & Metson, 2007). Indeed, sexual abuse survivors report concerns related to their sexuality for which there is no clear DSM diagnosis. Examples of such concerns include promiscuous risky sexual activities that are perceived as out of the patient's control, unwanted sexual abuse fantasies (Maltz, 1992; Wilson & Wilson, 2008), and difficulty trusting one's partner (DiLillo et al., 2009).

The sexual dysfunctions for men who experienced sexual abuse have received limited attention in the literature, partially because only recently have studies have focused on men. Among 302 male college students, 21.7% reported unwanted sexual contact, 12.4% experienced sexual coercion, and 17.1% reported rape[1] (Turchik, 2012). Men who reported rape experienced more sexual dysfunctions than men who did not experience any type of unwanted sex; however, the measurement of sexual dysfunction was quite primitive (one item not previously validated), which prevents any inference of the type of sexual dysfunction experienced by these men.

ASSESSMENT

Because of the negative connotations associated with the "sexual abuse" label, assessment may be more effective if the therapist is careful about the words utilized. In our research and clinical work we use one of the following opening sentences to begin the discourse: "Have you ever been in situations in which you were forced or coerced to engage in sexual activities?" or "Have you ever engaged in sexual activities against your will?" No matter how careful the wording selected to begin this conversation, some clients will adamantly deny any unwanted sexual experiences in the beginning of the interviews but will end up disclosing sexual abuse by the end of the interview. To provide an illustration, a woman was almost done with her assessment interview when she revealed that her first orgasm occurred when she was 10 years old through manual stimulation initiated by her uncle, who was 30 years old at the time. When asked whether she felt forced or coerced at the time, she paused and then answered positively (despite having previously denied experiencing abuse).

There are several reasons why clients may not reveal sexual abuse in the beginning interview. First, they may not see the experience as abusive, and this may be particularly true for men, who are socialized to interpret any sexual

---

[1]Rape was defined as being engaged in unwanted oral, vaginal, or anal sex with someone because he or she (1) took advantage of the person being drunk or high, (2) purposely gave the person drugs or alcohol, (3) blocked the person's retreat, (4) used physical restraint, (5) threatened to physically harm the person.

offer as a confirmation of their masculinity. Also, men are likely to report that the abuse led to pleasant physical sensations, and this may add to the confusion (Najman et al., 2005). For the woman in the preceding example, the fact that she reached orgasm during the event precluded her from labeling the event as abuse, because she experienced pleasure. Second, the perpetrator may have seduced the child and convinced him or her that the sexual behavior was a form of love. Usually, this dynamic is most common in intrafamilial abuses. Third, the patient may not feel comfortable talking about these events with the interviewer, who is still a stranger. For this reason, we ask about sexual abuse toward the end of the assessment interview, after the client has had the opportunity to see us respond in a supportive and nonjudgmental way.

Asking questions about past abuse is an important step in the history taking for all clients, independently from the response, because it sends the message that the therapist is open to listen and that it is okay to bring this information into the therapy room. A thorough assessment should also include questions about forms of abuse other than sexual (i.e., physical abuse, physical neglect, emotional abuse, and emotional neglect). Given that childhood sexual abuse is often accompanied by other forms of abuse and that these types of abuse can affect sexuality, a comprehensive assessment should include, at minimum, questions about the family environment in which the patient grew up. Interview questions can be supplemented with the Childhood Trauma Questionnaire (CTQ; Bernstein, Fink, Handelsman, & Foote, 1994), a widely utilized scale that offers clinical cutoffs to identify the severity of abuse that is considered clinically meaningful. The CTQ is composed of six subscales, five of which are reliable and valid for clinicians and researchers: Physical Abuse, Sexual Abuse, Emotional Abuse, Physical Neglect, and Emotional Neglect.

Important details of the abuse that could explain underlying patterns of the sexual dysfunction include the following: age of abuse onset, type of behaviors during the abuse (e.g., penetration behaviors), age of and relationship with the perpetrator (e.g., family member or parental figure, acquaintance, boyfriend, or stranger), frequency of the abuse (e.g., isolated incident or chronic). Other details that may have an impact on the experience of the patient include the following: Was the patient the only one who was victimized? Did the patient reveal the abuse to someone he or she trusted? What was the response of the person who was told about the abuse?

Although less discussed in the literature, sexual abuse during adulthood perpetrated by a partner can also have negative effects on sexual function. Thus questions about unwanted or forced sexual experiences within a dating or committed relationship are important. In cases when the patient reveals forced sexual activities by a partner, the therapist should inquire about experiences of physical abuse, because sexual abuse often occurs along with physical abuse within a relationship, and studies have shown that the negative effects of combined physical and sexual abuse are more severe than the effects of physical or sexual abuse alone (Katz, Moor, & May, 2008).

Assessment of sexual function in sexual abuse survivors should follow

the normal protocol that is utilized for all clients. In my clinic, we assess severity of the main sexual dysfunction symptoms and sexual satisfaction using
questionnaires such as the Female Sexual Functioning index (FSFI; Rosen et
al., 2000), and the Sexual Satisfaction Scale (SSS; Meston & Trapnell, 2003).
In addition, we measure the mechanisms targeted in therapy, such as the Cues
of Sexual Desire (McCall & Meston, 2006) and the Sexual Excitation and
Sexual Inhibition Index—Women (SESI-W; Graham, Sanders, & Milhausen,
2006). The Dyadic Adjustment Scale (DAS; Spanier, 1976) is also an important scale that we monitor throughout treatment to ensure that improvements
in sexual function are corresponding to improvements in dyadic adjustment.
A complete review of questionnaires for the assessment of sexual dysfunction is available (Giraldi et al., 2011). In compliance with our goal to provide
evidence-based practice, the assessment does not end after the first two sessions. We ask clients to complete the scales assessing targeted mechanisms
on a monthly basis, and every 4 months we administer the scales assessing
symptoms and sexual satisfaction. We utilize these tools to redirect the treatment goals in case we fail to see the expected changes in symptoms or in case
the client is showing a significant drop in other areas we are monitoring. In
particular, for sexual abuse survivors, it is important to continue monitoring
psychiatric symptoms that are comorbid with sexual dysfunction.

COMORBIDITY

The high comorbidity of sexual abuse with psychiatric conditions requires a
comprehensive understanding of the overall picture of the disorders and dysfunctions affecting the individual. A complete description of trauma-related
problems goes beyond our scope; however, it is important to acknowledge
the value of a comprehensive assessment of all psychiatric disorders. At this
time, it remains unclear whether psychiatric disorders, such as depression,
posttraumatic stress, and eating disorders, should be addressed before sexual
dysfunctions. To date, only one study reported data relevant to this question
(Schnurr et al., 2009). In this randomized clinical outcome study, 246 women
received either prolonged exposure or supportive therapy (present-centered
therapy) to treat posttraumatic stress disorder. Unfortunately the sexual measure was not specific to sexual dysfunction (i.e., the scale included items on
negative thoughts during sex, feelings of shame and guilt during sex, and no
items addressing sexual desire or difficulties becoming sexually aroused or
reaching orgasm); thus interpretations of the findings need to be cautious.
Prolonged exposure significantly reduced posttraumatic stress disorder symptoms and sexual problems at posttreatment, but only when all participants
were included in the analyses. When only those individuals who reported
significant sexual problems at pretreatment were included in the analyses,
the treatments showed no improvements in the sexuality of these women.
Thus, for individuals with posttraumatic stress disorder and with mild sexual

problems, alleviating posttraumatic stress symptoms may be enough to allevi-ate their sexual symptoms. However, for individuals with more severe sexual problems, simply reducing nonsexual symptoms may not be enough. More studies are needed on individuals with other types of psychiatric conditions and different levels of severity of symptoms, as well as on individuals both in relationships and single, to provide a more comprehensive picture of the best way to approach the treatment of sexual dysfunctions comorbid to other psychiatric diagnoses in women with a history of child sexual abuse (CSA).

THEORETICAL MODELS

Although a number of articles and books have been written on how to treat sexual dysfunctions in sexual abuse survivors, very little empirical evidence is available on the efficacy of such approaches. In response to the scarce infor-mation available on this topic, researchers have gone back to the drawing board and focused on proposing and testing theoretical models to identify treatment-malleable factors that influence sexual function in survivors of sex-ual abuse. Among the theoretical models proposed to explain the sexuality of sexual abuse survivors, Finkelhor and Browne's (1985) four traumagenic dynamics model has accumulated the most evidence. The four dynamics pro-posed are traumatic sexualization, betrayal, stigmatization, and powerless-ness. Although this model has been mostly proposed to explain the hyper-sexuality of women exposed to childhood sexual abuse, it is feasible that each of these dynamics alters a child's cognitive-emotional orientation to the world, which may affect the view of the sexual self (i.e., sexual self-schema). The first dynamic, traumatic sexualization, refers to conditions of the abuse under which a child's sexuality is shaped in developmentally inappropriate and inter-personally dysfunctional ways. For example, sexually abused children are often rewarded by their offenders for engaging in sexual behavior. Through this, the child may have learned to use sexual behavior as a means for manip-ulating others to get their own needs met. The second dynamic, betrayal, affects developing sexual schemas by teaching children that they cannot trust people, even those on whom they depend. Stigmatization, the third dynamic, can affect sexual schemas via the negative messages that lead to a sense of the self as evil, worthless, and shameful. The fourth dynamic, powerlessness, occurs when the child experiences having her or his body space repeatedly invaded against her or his wishes. This intrusion affects the ability to be asser-tive, which can lead to an imbalance in power in future romantic relationships and may translate into dysfunctional relationship dynamics. The traumatic sexualization model by Finkelhor and Browne (1985) has been shown to be associated with promiscuous sexual behaviors and the high HIV/STI infection rates among individuals with a history of childhood sexual abuse. However, to date, the ability of this model to explain problems with low desire, difficul-ties becoming sexually aroused, and reaching orgasm remain speculative.

Trauma-focused models have also been utilized as a conceptualization frame for several approaches to the treatment of sexual dysfunction in survivors of sexual abuse. These models are based on the assumption that sexual abuse at an early age teaches individuals to respond to sex with fear. The fear response, conceptualized as the reexperiencing of emotional, physiological, and cognitive responses that occurred during the trauma (including dissociation), may be specific to aspects of the situation or the perpetrator—for example, a woman who experiences fear during sex with partners who have beards but who is comfortable with men who are well shaved. The reexperiencing of the fear, typical of posttraumatic stress disorder, may also be associated with internal sensations so that the trigger for the fear response may be feeling sexually aroused. The underlying assumption is that a fear response is expected to inhibit normal sexual function.

Despite the potential usefulness of a trauma model, some major limitations need to be acknowledged. First, the underlying assumption that, for all individuals, the sexual abuse was traumatic does not apply to all survivors of CSA. Trauma is defined as an experience that caused sudden feelings of horror, fear for one's life or integrity, and hopelessness. Although many CSA survivors often report such feelings, many do not (Rellini & Meston, 2007). Especially for individuals with whom coercion was used, the conceptualization of the abuse as traumatic may not apply. Second, this model assumes that anxiety and fear may inhibit sexual responses. Research has shown mixed results on the effects of negative affect on sexual responses, with some studies showing that anxiety actually facilitates sexual arousal (Peterson & Janssen, 2007). A study found that negative affect prior to exposure to sexual stimuli was indeed higher in women with a history of CSA as compared with women with no history of abuse. Also, women with a history of CSA have lower physiological sexual arousal responses to sexual stimuli shown in the laboratory. However, negative affect did not predict sexual responses in women with a history of CSA (Rellini, Elinson, Janssen, & Meston, 2008). Despite these limitations, it is feasible that some adult women with a history of CSA may experience a stress response during sex. Indeed, female CSA survivors showed an increase in cortisol responses (a hormone released during stress) during exposure to sexual stimuli (Rellini, Hamilton, DelVille, & Meston, 2008), suggesting that, for these women, sexual stimuli acted as stressors. It is important to note, however, that the increase in cortisol was not found in all women with a history of CSA and that it remains unclear why some did and others did not show the cortisol response.

An important factor that emerged from this study is that the increase in cortisol was independent from self-reports of anxiety or fear experienced during exposure to the sexual stimuli. Thus women showing a physiological response that suggests an anxiety response did not necessarily report subjective feelings of anxiety or fear. This may indicate that not all dysfunctional sexual processes may operate at the conscious level. A woman may report feeling comfortable and open about sexuality, but her body may carry the scars of her past experiences, and this may cause her physiology to reject sexual activities. Other evidence that the impairment experienced by women with a history of CSA may occur underneath the consciousness level comes from a study on implicit associations (Rellini, Ing, & Meston, 2011). Women with a history of CSA showed a weaker association between sex and pleasure as compared with women with no history of abuse. Interestingly, both women with and without a history of sexual abuse visualized romance (e.g., a candle-light dinner) as pleasant. Also, both groups reported having positive feelings toward sex. The discrepancy between implicit (i.e., automatic) and explicit (i.e., conscious) attitudes toward sex is an obviously important point to take into consideration during therapy, as approaches designed to modify cognitive distortions or dysfunctional beliefs may not be useful when the impairment occurs at the implicit level. On the other hand, behavioral approaches designed to expose the woman to sexual stimuli and experience positive and pleasant sexual responses may be more effective at teaching more functional sexual responses.

APPROACHES TO TREATMENT

As previously indicated, despite the existence of many psychological interventions to treat sexual dysfunction in sexual abuse survivors, very few have empirical support for their efficacy. Most of these interventions focus on helping the client becoming more assertive, on relaxation training, on stopping the "reenactment" of the abuse during sex with the partner, and on challenging beliefs about the abuse (Bolen, 1993). Recently, mindfulness-based programs have shown promising results for the treatment of sexual arousal dysfunction in women, and effects are particularly strong for individuals with a history of sexual abuse (Brotto, Basson, & Luria, 2008). Mindfulness is an approach rooted in the Eastern tradition of meditation. The main goal of mindfulness is to teach the individual to be present in the moment, fully and nonjudgmentally. Brotto and colleagues were the first to test the efficacy of this treatment for sexual dysfunction in women, and they specifically selected exercises that helped patients to practice focusing on sensations in the present moment (Brotto et al., 2008). For example, one of the exercises asked women to hold a raisin in their mouths for 5 minutes while focusing on the sensations associated with the raisin. Another exercise instructed women to perform a body scan, carefully focusing on the sensations first in their toes and then slowly up their bodies to their heads. During these exercises, distracting thoughts are likely to intrude and affect the ability to be in the present moment. The main directions provided by the therapist are to notice the distracting thoughts and to redirect one's attention to the task, without judgment. It is indeed this constant redirection of the mind to the present moment that helps individuals become more aware of the here and now and more in tune with their sensations in the moment (for more information on this approach, see Brotto &

Luria, Chapter 1). In a recent study, mindfulness was compared with cognitive-behavioral therapy (CBT) for the treatment of sexual dysfunction in women with a history of CSA (Brotto, Seal, & Rellini, 2012). Mindfulness increased subjective sexual responses during a laboratory sexual psychophysiological assessment and also modified the relationship between physiological and subjective sexual responses to the erotic videos used in the assessment. Specifically, after treatment, a lower physiological arousal was needed to achieve a higher subjective state of sexual arousal. To the extent that physiological sexual responses can facilitate sexual arousal by providing feedback to the individual, the fact that less physiological sexual arousal was needed to reach higher levels of subjective sexual arousal indicates that mindfulness increased the sensitivity of the sexual response.

Theoretically, mindfulness in the bedroom could positively affect sexual arousal through two paths. First, it could reduce distracting thoughts, which can have an inhibitory effect on sexual arousal. Second, it could increase focus on physical sensations, thereby increasing arousability. These hypothesized paths are in line with the dual-control model of sexual arousal proposed by Bancroft and Janssen (2000), purporting that sexual arousal is the product of the balance between inhibitory and excitatory forces.

Larger studies with control groups are needed to test whether this promising treatment is more effective in survivors of sexual abuse. It is feasible that one of the inhibiting factors affecting sexuality in women with a history of sexual abuse is distraction caused by intrusive thoughts about the abuse. Clinicians have indeed reported that many survivors of sexual abuse report dissociation symptoms during sex. To provide an example, a patient explained that she felt like she was floating above the bed during sexual activities with her partner. Another, revealed she would "get out" of her body and hide in the corner of the room, leaving her body behind. For other women, the dissociating aspect may not be as extreme. For example, many women with a history of sexual abuse mention that they cannot focus on the present moment and become distracted, but cannot pinpoint the thoughts that distract them. To date, it is unknown whether these distractions and tendencies to dissociate during sex are more pronounced in survivors of sexual abuse as compared with women with no history of abuse and whether dissociation is directly affecting sexual responses in these women. In my laboratory, a recent study showed that, although dissociative symptoms were more prevalent in survivors of sexual abuse, these symptoms were not associated with greater sexual arousal problems in individuals with a history of sexual abuse (Bird, Seehuus, Clifton, & Rellini, 2012). More studies are needed to investigate the complex relationship between dissociation, distractions, and sexuality before we can have a good understanding of the impact of sexual abuse on these cognitive processes.

No study, apart from Brotto, Seal, and Rellini's (2005) recent investigation, has compared the efficacy of different treatments for sexual dysfunction in sexual abuse survivors. However, a number of studies have pointed to treatment-malleable factors specific to sexual dysfunction in sexual abuse survivors. In particular, studies have focused on sexual self-schemas, and more recent studies have addressed emotion dysregulation and experiential avoidance.

Scholars have purported that trauma affects one's sense of self (Dutton, Burghardt, Perrin, Chrestman, & Halle, 1994), a construct commonly referred to as self-schema. Self-schemas are conceptualized as blueprints utilized by the individual to filter, organize, and understand self-relevant information. Schemas also play a key role in the regulation of cognitions, affect, and behaviors (e.g., Kihlstrom & Cantor, 1983; Markus & Zajonc, 1985). The role of sexual self-schemas in sexual problems can be understood within the theoretical model proposed by Barlow (1986) and previously introduced to explain mindfulness and sexual arousal functioning. In this model, the distraction from sexually arousing stimuli is caused by anticipatory anxiety, which is the product of negative expectations (e.g., "My partner will think there is something wrong with me because I cannot become aroused"). The anxiety causes the attention to shift away from sexually relevant cues (the distraction addressed during mindfulness treatment). Eventually, a belief that the experience is doomed to fail may be transformed into a belief about the self, which becomes a part of the sexual self-schema (e.g., "I am sexually inadequate"). Empirical studies identified three main categories of schemas: romantic/passionate, open/direct, and embarrassed/conservative.

Studies have shown that women with a history of childhood sexual abuse hold significantly different schemas than do women with no history of abuse. Specifically, sexual abuse survivors perceive themselves as less romantic/passionate and more embarrassed/conservative (Meston, Rellini, & Heiman, 2006; Rellini & Meston, 2011). Studies on the implicit (nonconscious) association between schemas and sex have corroborated that women with a history of sexual abuse perceive sex as less pleasant than women with no history of abuse (Rellini, Ing, & Meston, 2011), providing further support for the idea that expectations and attitudes toward sex are different for survivors of sexual abuse.

The effects of schemas on sexual function may be mediated by the impact of schemas on mood. For example, initial evidence indicates that feeling less romantic and passionate is associated with greater depressive symptoms and that these symptoms mediate the lower sexual satisfaction observed in sexual abuse survivors compared with women with no history of abuse (Meston et al., 2006). Moreover, it was a combination of less romantic/passionate and more embarrassed/conservative sexual self-schemas that mediated the relationship between a history of sexual abuse and greater negative affect in anticipation to sexual stimuli (Rellini & Meston, 2011). From these findings, we can deduce that therapy might be more effective with sexual abuse survivors if it addressed sexual self-schemas. Especially an approach aimed at increasing the perception of the self as passionate and romantic and reducing a sense of embarrassment and conservative attitudes toward sex may be most effective for these women.

Unfortunately, to date, no information is available on the benefits of a treatment targeting sexual self-schemas in sexual abuse survivors; although a number of validated manuals are available for the modifications of schemas, such as schema-focused therapy. Briefly, this approach is a modification of cognitive-behavioral therapy and was developed to treat individuals with symptoms that are characterological and therefore more stable and harder to modify (for a comprehensive description see Young, Klosko, & Weishaar, 2003). The treatment is divided into two stages: assessment (further divided into identification, activation, and conceptualization) and change. Cognitive techniques within this approach are utilized to allow the patient to explore new ways to respond to targeted situations. The underlying assumption of this therapeutic approach is that acting against a set schema allows the individual to accumulate information about herself that contradicts the original schema, thereby promoting a change in her self-view.

In addition to self-schemas, emotion dysregulation is becoming the center of attention of many scholars studying and testing treatments for a variety of psychiatric conditions. Emotion dysregulation is commonly referred to as difficulties in recognizing and tolerating negative emotions and in self-regulating affective states and lacking of self-control over affect-driven behaviors (Carver, Lawrence, & Scheier, 1996; Gross, 1998). The ability to recognize, tolerate, and modulate negative affect has been the core of exposure treatments and, more recently, the focus of acceptance-based treatments, including dialectical behavior therapy (Linehan, 1993), mindfulness-based cognitive therapy (Segal, Williams, & Teasdale, 2001), acceptance and commitment therapy (ACT; Hayes, Strosahl, & Wilson, 1999), and integrative couple therapy (Jacobson & Christensen, 1996). The underlying assumption is that difficulty regulating emotions leads to experiential avoidance, or the willingness to engage in potentially harmful or dysfunctional behavior to avoid experiencing internal states, including emotions, physical sensations, thoughts, memories, and so forth. Specific to sexuality, initial studies have shown evidence for a significant relationship between low sexual satisfaction and high emotional dysregulation, including the tendency to avoid experiences, in trauma survivors (Rellini, Vujanovic, Gilbert, & Zvolensky, 2011; Rellini, Vujanovic, & Zvolensky, 2010; Staples, Rellini, & Roberts, 2012). Specifically for women with a history of childhood sexual abuse but not for women with no history of abuse, the tendency to avoid interpersonal closeness and avoid emotional involvement predicted orgasm functioning (Staples et al., 2012). The lack of longitudinal data on the development of sexual problems in relation to the tendency to avoid experiences prevents specific directional interpretation of these findings. However, one plausible interpretation is that trauma survivors who allow themselves to have corrective sexual experiences and do not shield themselves from the emotional experiences that occur during sexual activities are able to develop satisfying sexual experiences. To this end, it may be a helpful treatment goal to teach clients with a history of sexual abuse to be more in touch with their emotions, reduce avoidance of internal sensations, and increase satisfying sexual activities with partners.

It is also interesting to note that studies on the ability to understand and modulate emotions showed that lower sexual satisfaction but not lower sexual function was correlated with higher emotion dysregulation (Rellini et al., 2010; Rellini, Vujanovic, Gilbert, & Zvolensky, 2011). It is feasible that trauma survivors with emotion dysregulation may negatively interpret sexual experiences, even if their ability to become sexually aroused, have an orgasm, and experience sexual desire is normal. Alternatively, it is also feasible that the low sexual satisfaction experienced by trauma survivors may not be captured by the currently available diagnoses for desire, arousal, orgasm, and pain disorders (Rellini & Meston, 2007). Clinical experience and the literature suggest that individuals with a history of sexual abuse frequently report hypersexuality (i.e., numerous sexual partners, one-night stands, and unprotected sexual relations; Loeb et al., 2002). Indeed, hypersexuality is more strongly associated with a history of sexual abuse than any other sexual dysfunction (Rind, Tromovich, & Bauserman, 1998). It is possible that a feeling of being sexually out of control may cause distress to individuals with a history of sexual abuse. This may explain why it is not just the difficulties in experiencing desire, becoming sexually aroused, or reaching orgasm that preoccupies these patients but mostly the feeling that sex is out of their control. Although there is no empirical evidence in support of this hypothesis, the case study of Louise and Frank, described later, provides an illustration of how avoidance of sexual activities and hypersexuality coexist in patients with a history of sexual abuse seeking sex therapy. The first case (Myla) shows how sexual abuse can affect all relationships of the client, including the trusting relationship with the therapist.

CASE DISCUSSIONS

Case 1: Myla

Myla's case is a good illustration of the importance of considering how the abuse may affect the patient's ability to develop not only romantic relationships but also therapeutic ones. Myla was referred to individual therapy from our clinical outcome study because she did not meet inclusion criteria but was distressed by what she defined as low sexual desire. Myla was a slim, attractive woman in her 30s. She was a stay-at-home mom, although her children (5 and 8 years old) were now old enough so that she was considering starting a career again. She had been married for 12 years to a successful businessman. Myla had experienced a drop in sexual desire ever since her first child was born, but she had decided to remain with her husband for the sake of her children. However, now that her children were older, she was considering alternatives, and this was her "last attempt to make things work." Myla felt that the core of her marital problems was a feeling of distance from her husband and believed that reintroducing sexual activities with him would fix the problem. Myla had had sex with her husband only once in the previous 12 months. She scored below the clinical cutoff on the Female Sexual Functioning Index (FSFI-Total = 20), and on the Cues of Sexual Desire scale (McCall & Meston, 2006), she scored very high in the romantic/implicit (R/I), love/ emotional bonding (L/E) and visual/proximity (V/P) factors (R/I = 3.4; L/E = 3.5; V/P = 3.6) as compared with the norm of individuals with and without hypoactive sexual desire disorder. However, her score on Erotic/Explicit (E/E = 3.4) was in the range of the hypoactive sexual desire disorder population. These scores suggest that Myla identified a number of things that activated her sexual desire, with cues in the relational realm captured by R/I and L/E (e.g., *Feeling a sense of security in your relationship, Having a romantic dinner with a partner*) being particularly important for her. The first working hypothesis was that the lack of romantic and love-related cues in her daily life could be a factor in her low desire. Myla did not find explicit sexual cues (e.g., *Sensing your own or your partner's wetness, lubrication, or erection; You experience genital sensations—e.g., increased blood flow to genitals*) to be arousing. Her scores on the SESI-W (Graham, Sanders, & Milhausen, 2006) were all within one standard deviation from the norms provided by the authors, except for the factor Relationship Importance (e.g., *If I think that a partner might hurt me emotionally, I put the brakes on sexually*).

During a semistructured clinical interview, Myla reported that she found her husband attractive and felt love toward him, although she was unhappy with her relationship and did not feel she could trust him. On the DAS (Spanier, 1976), her scores showed that she felt that she and her husband agreed on many areas of their lives, including finances, parenting, and how to handle the in-laws (DAS consensus = 49). However, the scores for cohesion and satisfaction were very low, 10 and 25, respectively. Moreover, the total score on the DAS was 90. Considering that the cutoff for couples experiencing distress is 101 (Spanier, 1976), Myla showed a relatively low score. The average DAS among divorced couples is 70.7, and for married couples it is 114.8; thus Myla fell right in the middle, indicating that, although her marital difficulties caused much distress, they were not quite at the level of individuals who have sought a divorce. An encouraging sign was Myla's response to the last item of the DAS: *Which of the following statements best describes how you feel about the future of your relationship?* To which she answered, "I want very much for my relationship to succeed, and will do my fair share to see that it does."

Myla's problem was not just low sexual desire; Myla engaged in masturbation once a week and also experienced feelings of sexual desire when in the presence of other attractive men or when watching sensual movies. During masturbation, she felt sexually aroused, noticed an increase in lubrication, and 7 out of 10 times she masturbated to orgasm.

Myla denied any history of sexual abuse during the semistructured interview and on questionnaires specifically geared toward the assessment of abuse. As therapy progressed, it became evident that Myla's decision to with-hold information about her past abuse had common roots with her current sexual problems.

Based on these data, I proposed to Myla to start couple therapy to address the underlying relationship blocks that affected her desire, but she was ada-mantly against this option because she had already completed 6 months of couple therapy and felt it did not help. Myla believed that increasing her ability to experience sexual desire would lead to more sexual activities, and this would solve their inability to feel connected. Psychoeducation was intro-duced to help Myla understand that, in the presence of relationship problems, increasing sexual functioning in one of the partners does not necessarily lead to greater sexual satisfaction (Stephenson, Rellini, & Meston, 2013). How-ever, Myla insisted that she wanted to have individual sex therapy to fix her level of sexual desire.

The therapy selected for this case was a combination of mindfulness and schema work. Treatment goals included a greater sense of desire for sexual activities with her husband, greater awareness of and ability to express sexual likes and dislikes during sex with him, and greater frequency of partnered sexual activities initiated by the client. After two sessions dedicated to psycho-education on the sexual dual-control model (Janssen & Bancroft, 2007) and the female sexual response, the therapy moved toward exploration of sexual self-schemas.

One of the assignments designed to increase Myla's awareness of her schemas consisted of writing her sexual and relationship history. One year after giving birth to her second child, she started masturbating more, but, right when she was considering initiating sex again with her husband, she discovered that he had lied to her about his use of alcohol. Myla and her hus-band had decided to give up alcohol to raise their children in an alcohol-free environment. This decision was important for Myla and her husband because of the history of alcoholism in both families. Myla felt betrayed and insulted when she found that her husband had been drinking behind her back. She felt angry at him for thinking she was so "stupid" to not notice. They had an explosive argument (7 years before therapy), and Myla never forgave her husband.

Her narrative of her sexual development was otherwise unremarkable, which made her report of sexual abuse a few sessions later even more shock-ing. Although the treatment plan called for work on problematic schemas, Myla's schemas did not need this intervention; thus we went back to assess-ment mode to determine whether the problem was in the lack of sexual plea-sure experienced during sex or due to difficulty communicating sexual likes and dislikes (after all, Myla had not had sex with her husband in a long time). At the session following the assignment, Myla reported that she had not completed the sensate focus exercises. Through a behavioral analysis of the obstacles encountered in completing the exercise, it emerged that she never fully committed to engage in the sexual activities. Indeed, she knew she was not going to complete the exercise the minute she left the therapy room. After much exploration, Myla realized that she really did not want to engage in sexual activities with her husband because having sex with him and experiencing pleasure during sex with him would have meant that she forgave him and that it was OK for him to think she was "so stupid" as not to find out he was drinking. This is the point in therapy where her history of abuse emerged: She had been sexually abused by an uncle when she was 12 years old. When asked to explain the reasons for not coming forward with this information earlier on, she said that she may have forgotten or did not recall any direct question about this. Myla felt that men cannot be fully trusted, and she felt that the reason that she was abused by her uncle was that she was "too stupid" not to know that all men want is sex. She spent years telling herself that, although it was not her fault, she should have known better then to trust her uncle. After being asked to compare her feelings toward her husband with her feelings toward her uncle, Myla realized that her fear of being taken advantage of by a man was preventing her from forgiving her husband. Shortly after this realization, Myla voiced her feeling that she needed to go back to couple therapy before she could address her sexual problems and that her feeling distant from her husband was not something that sex could solve. Given the already established relationship between the therapist and Myla, the couple was referred to another therapist who could address both sexual and relationship problems concerning trust.

This case is not unusual; sexual symptoms often occur as a sign that something is not working in the relationship. Because it is often useless to force a patient to seek a treatment goal different from the one she or he perceives as being the cause of her or his distress, allowing patients to face incongruences between their treatment goals and their behavior can be an effective way to help them redirect their attention toward the real underlying problem. Utilizing a systematic approach to the assessment of the case is very useful; it was clear since the beginning that Myla was not having a problem of sexual desire per se. All measures and interviews pointed to something else brewing under the low desire for sex with her husband. The client was not receptive to directly addressing the relational problem; thus this is an example of client and therapist disagreeing on the best line of action. It would have not been useful to force the client to proceed with the treatment goals identified by the therapist. Instead, we began therapy and utilized the treatment as an opportunity for the client to identify, on her own, the underlying problems that resulted in the low desire.

Case 2: Louise and Frank

Louise and Frank were 52 and 58 years old, respectively. Their couple therapist referred them for sex therapy after it appeared that the communication problems they were experiencing were specifically related to sexual matters. Louise was a realtor, and Frank was an engineer working for a small company. They had been together for 10 years and married for 3. Frank was Louise's fourth husband, and Louise was Frank's third wife. Louise was highly engaged in art projects and workshops focused on being connected with nature, whereas Frank was more reclusive and liked spending time reading physics books. This difference between them was what attracted them to each other in the first place and what kept them together at the time of therapy. Frank said that Louise brought "color" to his life, and Louise felt Frank was her "rock" when things become too emotionally labile. Their presenting problem was discrepancy in sexual desire, with Louise feeling that she did not want to have sex because it took away from her personal energy and Frank wanting more sex and wanting for Louise to be satisfied during sex, because he felt she was no longer enjoying sex with him. Louise met criteria for hypoactive sexual desire disorder, and Frank did not meet diagnostic criteria for any sexual dysfunction.

During a semistandardized assessment interview, it emerged that Louise and Frank used to have frequent and passionate sex before they decided to get married. Louise mentioned that she had noticed a similar pattern in previous relationships: She felt very passionate when not in a committed relationship, but, as soon as she made a commitment, she became sexually withdrawn.

Louise was open about the sexual abuse she experienced as a child, inflicted by her biological father, and again as a young teenager, perpetrated by her stepfather. Louise was not new to psychotherapy and had seen a number of therapists to work through her traumatic experiences. She had met criteria for depression and posttraumatic stress disorder in the past (age 20–25 years) but denied any present symptoms and did not meet criteria for any other disorders. She was emotionally engaged but not overwhelmed while telling her story, a sign that she had done extensive work on this topic and was now able to be in touch with her emotions associated with the trauma while feeling sufficiently detached not to become overwhelmed. In situations in which a patient has had the opportunity to work extensively on her or his trauma, it may be useful to inquire about the things that helped her or him overcome the difficulties. For Louise, art and spirituality played a large role in her ability to overcome adversities. She found a small artist community composed mostly of women who integrated art and spirituality in their work.

Frank appeared as the prototypical engineer: very practical, attentive to details, very controlled in his expression of emotions. He sat rigidly in the chair during the sessions, and it was not until the third or fourth session that he started opening up and talking about his emotions. He started trusting the therapeutic process after clear treatment goals were set and I had explained the evidence behind the theoretical models we used for the treatment. Frank denied any abuse but described a childhood deprived of emotional support. He did not have any memories of his parents giving him positive feedback. Dinner always occurred in a darkly lit room, and children were not allowed to talk.

When he or his brothers were upset about something, they were instructed to go to their rooms and come back after they were no longer "bothered" by their emotions.

At the beginning of therapy, the couple was instructed not to engage in sexual activity, and a series of sensate focus exercises was prescribed to help Louise focus on pleasurable experiences during sensual touch. The couple struggled with the exercises, and, after three sessions spent brainstorming on how to overcome obstacles to practicing the exercises, I reconceptualized the situation as a lack of commitment and readiness for therapy. We moved back to orientation and commitment work, during which we focused on treatment goals. Although both Louise and Frank wanted to increase their sexual pleasure and satisfaction, Louise was having a negative reaction toward this goal. She vocalized the problem as a clash between the goal and her art. She believed that she had a finite amount of energy that could translate to either sexual or artistic pursuits. Engaging in sexual activities meant taking away from her art, which was something she was doing for herself.

Each partner was instructed to complete a writing exercise designed to help them reflect on what a "more satisfying sexual relationship" would be like and the pros and cons of developing such a relationship. It emerged that Louise was concerned about giving up her autonomy and was feeling powerless because she was afraid that her sexual satisfaction was going to be controlled by her partner. Frank's main goal was Louise's satisfaction, not his own, further fueling Louise's fears. Louise felt she no longer had the right to feel "unsatisfied." In the following 2 months our work led to a sexual script that included choosing to *not* reach an orgasm and taking responsibility for one's own sexual pleasure. Louise felt more in control of the situation and felt freer to express and experience pleasure. Frank did not feel responsible for Louise's pleasure, and therefore he stopped worrying about failing her. We resumed the sensate focus assignment, during which it appeared that the couple needed to improve their ability to communicate. Exercises in which they used nonverbal communication were added to the sensate focus. Also, given that communication problems also occurred outside the bedroom, the couple identified projects they could perform together on which they needed to collaborate. The couple started a yard project. With practice, the new sexual script became familiar, and their improved communication skills allowed them to reach greater levels of sexual satisfaction. Also, the frequency of sexual activities was significantly improved (twice a month compared with once every 3–4 months).

This is a case in which knowing how to improve communication is not enough. Being able to implement efficacious interventions requires full commitment from the clients. The orientation and commitment work that preceded the therapy had a profound effect on the willingness of the couple to fully engage in therapy. Also, the use of a behavioral analysis to identify the reasons for not completing the assignment can cut down on time spent trying to make the couple complete an assignment. A behavioral analysis should attempt to determine whether the assignment was not completed because of lack of motivation, lack of skills, or lack of understanding. In this case, I initially wrongly assumed that the problem was lack of skills and focused on solving the problems for them. An early utilization of a behavioral analysis would have revealed the real underlying problem earlier on.

CONCLUSIONS

It is important to include assessment of a history of sexual abuse in all clients presenting with a sexual dysfunction and to ask about sexual function in clients reporting a history of sexual abuse. However, it is equally important to avoid assumptions that a history of abuse will always lead to sexual dysfunctions. Treatment for sexual abuse survivors may be more effective if it includes behavioral techniques such as mindfulness and exposure designed to break avoidance and introduce patients to sexually satisfying experiences. Finally, therapists should strive to integrate partners in both assessment and treatment, as sexual abuse may have affected the ability to form intimate connections, and the sexual problems may be a symptom of this larger problem.

REFERENCES

Bancroft, J., & Janssen, E. (2000). The dual control model of male sexual response: A theoretical approach to centrally mediated erectile dysfunction. *Neuroscience and Biobehavioral Reviews, 24,* 571–579.

Becker, J. V., Skinner, L. J., Abel, G. G., & Treacy, E. C. (1982). Incidence and types of sexual dysfunction in rape and incest victims. *Journal of Sex and Marital Therapy, 8,* 65–74.

Bernstein, D. P., Fink, L., Handelsman, L., & Foote, J. (1994). Initial reliability and validity of a new retrospective measure of child abuse and neglect. *American Journal of Psychiatry, 151*(8), 1132–1136.

Bird, L., Seehuus, M. O., Clifton, J., & Rellini, A. (2012). *Dissociation and sexual function in women with and without a history of sexual abuse.* Poster presented at the annual conference of the International Academy of Sex Research. Lisbon, Portugal.

Brotto, L. A., Basson, R., & Luria, M. (2008). A mindfulness-based group psychoeducational intervention targeting sexual arousal disorder in women. *Journal of Sexual Medicine, 5,* 1646–1659.

Brotto, L. A., & Heiman, J. R. (2007). Mindfulness in sex therapy: Applications for women with sexual difficulties following gynaecologic cancer. *Sexual and Relationship Therapy, 22,* 3–11.

Carver, C. S., Lawrence, J. W., & Scheier, M. F. (1996). A control-process perspective on the origins of affect. In L. L. Martin & A. Tesser (Eds.), *Striving and feeling: Interactions among goals, affect, and self-regulation* (pp. 11–52). Hillsdale, NJ: Erlbaum.

DiLillo, D. A., Peugh, J., Walsh, K., Panuzio, J., Trask, E., & Evans, S. (2009). Child maltreatment history among newlywed couples: A longitudinal study of marital outcomes and mediating pathways. *Journal of Consulting and Clinical Psychology, 77*, 680–692.

Elliott, D. M., Mok, D. S., & Briere, J. (2004). Adult sexual assault: Prevalence, symptomatology, and sex differences in the general population. *Journal of Traumatic Stress, 17*, 203–211.

Exton, N. G., Truong, T. C., & Exton, M. S. (2000). Neuroendocrine response to film-induced sexual arousal in men and women. *Psychoneuroendocrinology, 25*, 187–199.

Finkelhor, D., & Browne, A. (1985). The traumatic impact of child sexual abuse: A conceptualization. *American Journal of Orthopsychiatry, 55*, 530–541.

Graham, C. A., Sanders, S. A., & Milhausen, R. R. (2006). The Sexual Excitation/Sexual Inhibition Inventory for Women: Psychometric properties. *Archives of Sexual Behavior, 35*, 397–409

Green, A. H. (1996). Overview of child sexual abuse. In S. J. Kaplan (Ed.), *Family violence: A clinical and legal guide* (pp. 73–104). Washington, DC: American Psychiatric Press.

Gross, J. J. (1998). The emerging field of emotion regulation: An integrative review. *Review of General Psychology, 2*, 271–299.

Hayes, S. C., Strosahl, K., & Wilson, K. (1999). *Acceptance and commitment therapy: Understanding and treating human suffering.* New York: Guilford Press.

Jacobson, N. S., & Christensen, A. (1996). *Integrative couple therapy: Promoting acceptance and change.* New York: Norton.

Janssen, E., & Bancroft, J. (2007). The dual-control model: The role of sexual inhibition and excitation in sexual arousal and behavior. In E. Janssen (Ed.), *The psychophysiology of sex* (pp. 197–222). Bloomington: Indiana University Press.

Katz, J., Moore, J., & May, P. (2008). Physical and sexual covictimization from dating partners: A distinct type of intimate abuse? *Violence Against Women, 14*, 961–980.

Laumann, E., Gagnon, J., Michael, R., & Michaels, S. (1994). *The social organization of sexuality: Sexual practices in the United States.* Chicago: University of Chicago Press.

Lewis, R. W., Fugl-Meyer, K. S., Corona, G., Hayes, R. D., Laumann, E. O., Moreira, E. D., et al. (2010). Definition/epidemiology/risk factors for sexual dysfunction. *Journal of Sexual Medicine, 7*, 1598–1607.

Linehan, M. M. (1993). *Cognitive-behavioral treatment of borderline personality disorder.* New York: Guilford Press.

Maltz, W. (1992). *Sexual healing journey: A guide for survivors of sexual abuse.* New York: Harper Perennial.

McCall, K., & Meston, C. M. (2006). Cues resulting in desire for sexual activity in women. *Journal of Sexual Medicine, 3*, 838–852.

Meston, C. M., Rellini, A. H., & Heiman, J. (2006). Women's history of sexual abuse, their sexuality, and sexual self-schemas. *Journal of Consulting and Clinical Psychology, 74*, 229–236.

Neumann, D., Houskamp, B., Pollock, V., & Briere, J. (1996). The long-term sequelae of childhood sexual abuse in women: A meta-analytic review. *Child Maltreatment: Journal of the American Professional Society on the Abuse of Children, 1*, 6–16.

Peters, S. D., Wyatt, G. E., & Finkelhor, D. (1986). Prevalence. In D. Finkelhor (Ed.), *Sourcebook on child sexual abuse* (pp. 15–59). Newbury Park, CA: Sage.

Peterson, Z., & Janssen, E. (2007). Ambivalent affect and sexual response: The impact of co-occurring positive and negative emotions on subjective and physiological sexual responses to erotic stimuli. *Archives of Sexual Behavior, 36,* 793–807.

Polusny, M. A., & Follette, V. M. (1995). Long-term correlates of childhood sexual abuse: Theory and review of the empirical literature. *Applied and Preventative Psychology, 4,* 143–166.

Rellini, A. H. (2005). Psychological factors of sexual abuse on women's sexual functioning. In I. Goldstein, C. Meston, S. Davis, & A. Traish (Eds.), *Women sexual function and dysfunction: Study, diagnosis and treatment* (pp. 98–104). London: Taylor & Francis Group.

Rellini, A. H., Ing, A. D., & Meston, C. M. (2011). Implicit and explicit cognitive sexual processes in survivors of childhood sexual abuse. *Journal of Sexual Medicine, 8,* 3098–3107.

Rellini, A. H., & Meston, C. M. (2007). Sexual function and satisfaction in adults based on the definition of child sexual abuse. *Journal of Sexual Medicine, 4,* 1312–1321.

Rellini, A. H., & Meston, C. M. (2011). Sexual self-schemas, sexual dysfunction, and the sexual responses of women with a history of childhood sexual abuse. *Archives of Sexual Behavior, 40,* 351–362.

Rellini, A. H., Vujanovic, A. A., Gilbert, M., & Zvolensky, M. J. (2011). Childhood maltreatment and difficulties in emotion regulation: Associations with sexual and relationship satisfaction among young adult women. *Journal of Sex Research, 19,* 1–9.

Rellini, A. H., Vujanovic, A. A., & Zvolensky, M. J. (2010). Emotional dysregulation: Concurrent relation to sexual problems among trauma-exposed adult cigarette smokers. *Journal of Sex and Marital Therapy, 36,* 137–153.

Rind, B., Tromovitch, P., & Bauserman, R. (1998). A meta-analytic examination of assumed properties of child sexual abuse using college samples. *Psychological Bulletin, 124,* 22–53.

Robinson, B. E., Munns, R. A., Weber-Main, A. M., Lowe, M. A., & Raymond, N. C. (2011). Application of the sexual health model in the long-term treatment of hypoactive sexual desire and female orgasmic disorder. *Archives of Sexual Behavior, 40,* 469–478.

Sarwer, D. B., & Durlak, J. A. (1996). Childhood sexual abuse as a predictor of adult female sexual dysfunction: A study of couples seeking sex therapy. *Child Abuse and Neglect, 20,* 963–972.

Schloredt, K. A., & Heiman, J. R. (2003). Perceptions of sexuality as related to sexual functioning and sexual risk in women with different types of childhood abuse histories. *Journal of Traumatic Stress, 16,* 275–284.

Schnurr, P. P., Lunney, C. A., Forshay, E., Thurston, V. L., Chow, B. K., Resick, P. A., et al. (2009). Sexual function outcomes in women treated for posttraumatic stress disorder. *Journal of Women's Health, 18,* 1549–1557.

Segal, Z. V., Williams, J. M. G., & Teasdale, J. D. (2001). *Mindfulness-based cognitive therapy for depression: A new approach to preventing relapse.* New York: Guilford Press.

Sickel, A. E, Noll, J. G., Moore, P. J., Putnam, F. W., & Trickett, P. K. (2002). The long-term physical health and healthcare utilization of women who were sexually abused as children. *Journal of Health Psychology, 7,* 583–598.

Spanier, G. B. (1976). Measuring dyadic adjustment: New scales for assessing the quality of marriage and similar dyads. *Journal of Marriage and the Family, 38*, 15–28.

Staples, J., Rellini, A. H., & Roberts, S. P. (2012). Avoiding experiences: Sexual dysfunction in women with a sexual abuse history in childhood. *Archives of Sexual Behavior, 41*, 341–350.

Stephenson, K. R., Rellini, A. H., & Meston, C. M. (2013). Relationship satisfaction as a predictor of treatment response during cognitive behavioral sex therapy. *Archives of Sexual Behavior, 42*, 143–152.

Turchik, J. A. (2012). Sexual victimization among male college students: Assault severity, sexual functioning, and health risk behaviors. *Psychology of Men and Masculinity, 13*(3), 243–255.

U.S. Department of Health and Human Services, Administration on Children, Youth and Families. (2003). *Child maltreatment 2001*. Washington, DC: U.S. Government Printing Office. Retrieved from *www.acf.hhs.gov/programs/cb*.

Watson, B., & Halford, K. W. (2010). Classes of childhood sexual abuse and women's adult couple relationships. *Violence and Victims, 25*, 518–535.

Wilson, J. E., & Wilson, K. M. (2008). Amelioration of sexual fantasies to sexual abuse cues in an adult survivor of childhood sexual abuse: A case study. *Journal of Behavior Therapy and Experimental Psychiatry, 39*, 417–423.

Young, J. E., Klosko, J. S., & Weishaar, M. E. (2003). *Schema therapy: A practitioner guide*. New York: Guilford Press.

Zollman, G., Rellini, A. H., & Desrocher, D. (2013). The mediating effect of daily stress on the sexual arousal function of women with a history of childhood sexual abuse. *Journal of Marital and Sex Therapy, 39*(2), 176–192.

CHAPTER 18

Infidelity

Stephen B. Levine

Infidelity is not a sexual dysfunction. In fact, it is not a mental disorder. Although infidelity is often described as a betrayal of trust, it is more accurately described as a sexual betrayal whose underlying motivation may be obscure. But when infidelity brings an individual or couple into therapy, it is usually a crisis. Noting that research on infidelity is sorely lacking or plagued by methodological flaws and inconsistencies, Levine exhorts us to listen to the experts, that is, the three people involved. Unless sexual dysfunction was present before the affair, Levine asserts that understanding and working with the couple regarding the meaning of the affair will offer the best chance of restoring sexual intimacy for those couples seeking that outcome. Levine's approach is devoid of technique and exercises and focuses on process. He cautions therapists to be aware of "the appearance of an uncharacteristic authoritative voice" and advises us that "our role is to be interested in the person's dilemmas, to clarify the options, to focus on what the person is thinking and feeling about the present, past and future; it is not to tell the person what to do."

Stephen B. Levine, MD, is Clinical Professor of Psychiatry at Case Western Reserve University School of Medicine and Co-Director of the Center for Marital and Sexual Health in Beachwood, Ohio. His 40 years of therapeutic experience in individual and conjoint therapy is the basis for his two decades of writing about love and infidelity. In 2005 he was recipient of the Masters and Johnson Lifetime Achievement Award from the Society for Sex Therapy and Research. His most recent book is *Barriers to Loving: A Clinician's Perspective.*

Happily married people, particularly those with young children and a pleasing family life, find it difficult to imagine that they or their spouses could want to have an affair. As the children grow older, however, particularly after a spouse has sensed the limitations of marriage and wondered what an affair might be like, a transient dread of being a victim of infidelity may appear. This psychological shift happens at different moments for each partner. A spouse can only hope that the partner remains happy enough or committed enough to resist temptation.

An affair is both an affect-laden event and a process for all concerned. The first unfaithful act immediately creates a set of emotions, a series of thoughts and subtle shifts in identity. These evolve as the sexual behaviors continue. The behaviors create new psychological and social complexities involving the unfaithful person, the partner, and the paramour. The marriage subtly changes. The partner may attribute the change to some other life process, may not notice it, or may not want to consider this unsettling explanation.

What the clinician learns about an affair will depend on which of the three protagonists tells the story. If the couple tells the story together, a fourth version unfolds.

AMANDA HAS AN AFFAIR

Adam's calm, pleasant, happily married life changed in an instant. He went from unemotional stability to panicky uncertainty as he faced the first major problem in his life. He became suffused with the pain of betrayal and the humiliation of failing as a husband.

The couple appeared to be a physically healthy, athletic, educated pair who had been together for 19 years, almost half of their lives. They said that they had nothing major to complain about. Adam had trusted Amanda implicitly despite the fact that he perceived that they never fully clicked sexually. Amanda never complained about their sexual life. Each was devoted to the children. Their first son had been a challenge because of his attention, learning, and social problems. Their younger son had been easier to parent. The couple had friends and cordial relationships with each of their families. Each partner took short breaks from the family to pursue separate interests with friends. Money was not a concern.

Amanda had been on a stable dose of a selective serotonin reuptake inhibitor (SSRI) since several months after the birth of their first son 12 years before. When she stopped the medication 4 years later, she developed mysterious abdominal symptoms, which disappeared a week after resuming it. Two years ago she took up a new sport. Her skills progressed rapidly under the guidance of an instructor, who previously was teaching her son. Their growing 8-month friendship was transformed by the pro's declared wish to kiss her. During these months, she began to think that her husband was preoccupied with his career and seemed distant from her. "Just this once" gradually led to sexual intercourse. Amanda was astounded by how exciting all this was. Sex with her paramour was much more compelling than her quieter, four to six times per month, regularly orgasmic sexual life with Adam, until then her only sexual partner. Guilt led her to end the relationship after 4 months, but she quickly resumed the arrangement for another 7 months.

Amanda and her paramour had no interest in leaving their families, never said they loved each other, and communicated by texting almost daily. They saw each other several times a week at the sports club and had intercourse weekly. Adam began to notice that Amanda frequently seemed to be in a different room when he was home. She often preferred reading in the bedroom. He began to feel alone. After he dreamed that she was having an affair, he checked her cell phone records and confronted her.

She immediately confessed, told him who it was, cried in grave, shameful embarrassment, promised to end the relationship, and said that she wanted to stay married. She apologized repeatedly. She thought that no one else knew about the relationship. The couple agreed to tell no one about this. The next day, Adam visited the instructor, who nervously corroborated Amanda's story, apologized, said he would not contact her again, and asked Adam not to tell his wife. After 3 tumultuous days of mutual despair, intense communication, numerous "when," "what," and "why" questions, and taking turns being overwhelmed in tears, they decided to ask Amanda's psychiatrist, whom she saw annually, for a referral for "a marital issue."

I saw them together for an hour three times in the first week and saw her once alone. Adam was the most distressed person in the room. He said he was devastated, could not sleep, experienced anxiety all day long, felt pressure in his chest, and could not eat. I prescribed a hypnotic for him, which he never took. I asked them to tell me what was important for me to know about their marriage. ("It was fine until the affair," they agreed.) He emphasized how much he loved Amanda because she was sincere, honest, and without pretense. She loved him for his accepting, friendly-to-all nature and kindness. He originally felt much sexual ardor for her, but she was uncomfortable during their early sexual behaviors, so he held himself back. He told himself that keeping her comfortable was required because he loved her. Amanda found sex to be messy and dirty.

After 10 sessions over 4 weeks, including separate ones with each partner, Adam told me that he had recommitted to Amanda. He emphasized that he clearly was, by far, the better man. He felt that he understood as much as could be understood about what happened. He was convinced that she really did love him. He perceived that she was getting over the other man. After refusing to have sex with Amanda for 10 days and then tentatively resuming sex while they were out of town, they eventually had the best sex of their lives after Adam returned from a 5-day business trip.

In this first month I was consistently interested in each of their viewpoints, concerns, and wishes for the future. Adam remained uncommitted about how things would work out until Amanda patiently answered all his questions and maintained a consistent concern about his recurring emotional breakdowns. Initially, he could not understand how she could love him and sleep with another man and why she did not agree that it was a poor idea to continue to take their son for lessons from "this guy." At the end of the month, knowing that "Amanda truly loves me," he concluded that "she had made a very big mistake in judgment to get involved." Still, Amanda's reasoning that she should not interrupt their son's progress because of her problem did not sit well with Adam.

Only when the crisis seemed past did Adam speak of his use of methylphenidate for his attention-deficit disorder and previous learning disorders. Amanda also spoke at greater length about her parents' divorce when she was a toddler, her mother's cancer death when Amanda was 8, her father's second wife, and her obsessive–compulsive disorder during high school. She attributed her chronic anxiety to her stepmother's favoritism toward her new biological daughter. Amanda's florid symptoms largely disappeared when she went away to college, where she did not have a serious boyfriend until she met Adam. Amanda had been in therapy off and on since her adolescence.

A very calm week ensued, but when I saw Adam alone, he expressed his concern that Amanda seemed too ready to sweep the affair under the rug. She did not want him to mention it. She floated the idea of going to a group class taught by the pro. Adam, still disturbed that she did not think it reasonable to move the family to another sports facility, did not want to speak of this to her yet another time. I gave him an analogy to coping with cancer chemotherapy: Both partners are suffering anxieties but choose to lighten each other's burden by not fully discussing their subjective experience. Adam then wondered whether the affair was just the most dramatic manifestation of something else that had been going on for the last few years—that Amanda felt she had the right to do what she wanted. She was far more self-centered than she had been in the past. I wondered whether this was a natural response to their baby growing up—that is, whether she was making up for the period of sacrificing her wishes for the children's needs. Adam asked whether he should talk to her about his impression of her growing sense of entitlement. I inquired whether he thought that Amanda's style of coping with the loss of her mother—pushing it under the rug—was being repeated with her paramour. I told Adam about Freud's concept that an adult's sense of entitlement may derive from early life adversity (Freud, 1916). I said that I did not know whether it was a good idea to bring up the subject.

Another calm "normal" week occurred, complete with the couple's weekend lovemaking. There was no discussion of the affair, lessons, or entitlement. Each was busy with his or her usual tasks. He said the cancer analogy helped him protect her from his deepest worries. Adam was pleased that Amanda was putting 100% of herself into him and the children again. He worried that the affair was a response to a problem that she felt in the relationship that might cause trouble again in the future. He feared that "the shadow of another person would always be intoxicating to her." Amanda worried about the meaning of her always having to initiate their sexual opportunities. Adam replied, "Yes, but once you do, everything flows normally and we are both pleased." "But why won't you initiate it?" she asked.

That evening Adam was very sad, had difficulty sleeping, and felt that Amanda wanted sexual things from him that he could not provide. "I only want you to indicate that you really want me sexually!" she told him. They had a long talk. He awakened in the morning feeling better, but she was sad, worried, and confused. "I thought we had made progress, but last night he was like he was a while ago," she told me. After one of Amanda's athletic events, she cried in gratitude for his support during this event and the more trying previous 6 weeks. Adam was pleased. Before the athletic event, they had the best sex of their lives.

MONOGAMY

An affair is but one of many forms of infidelity. Whether or not they involve physical interaction with a person, online communication, or an intense emotional attachment in anticipation of physical intimacy, all infidelities imply a violation of a prior agreement to be monogamous (Brand, Markey, Mills, & Hodges, 2007). Infidelity is a hidden but much discussed transgression of this internalized value system. The faithful partner often refers to the lingering consequence of infidelity as a "loss of trust." Monogamy is the dominant sexual arrangement in the current Western world. Its violation is the most often cited reason for divorce (Betzig, 1989). Monogamy is not, however, a universal organizing feature of marital relationships (Solstad & Mucic, 1999). Many societies support polygamy. Some individuals organize themselves into social groups that practice consensual nonmonogamy (Anapol, 2010). Because relationships evolve in their sexual, social, economic, and psychological circumstances, every form of sexual arrangement brings its own potential problems.

Nonnegotiated Nonmonogamy

The commitment to monogamy is not always made verbally. Some individuals decide to be monogamous and erroneously assume that their partners have made the same decision. Other individuals insincerely agree. Yet others, like Amanda, do not maintain the commitment over time. Clinicians should not assume that every person has an internalized prohibition against infidelity (Solstad & Mucic, 1999). If a person does, however, the clinician can infer that the unfaithful person gave in to a temptation. Temptations abound in social and work environments. Legal and illegal businesses sell sexual opportunities. Convention cities cultivate the expectation of sexual opportunities. Power differentials of teacher–student, doctor–nurse, lawyer–client, and supervisor–subordinate often carry erotic temptations. A long monogamous partnership represents the mastery of numerous mental and behavioral temptations.

Infidelity can occur at any adult age. Homosexual and transgendered persons experience it. Reactions to its discovery range from the poles of devastation, which may create a clinical intervention, to indifference, which usually does not. How the partner regards the unfaithful person before the discovery of the infidelity may be the most important determinant of the reaction. Responses can be overshadowed by one of its complications: pregnancy, an arrest, a sexually transmitted disease, violence, a suicide attempt, or media coverage or by the need to simultaneously deal with a weightier matter—such as a new life-threatening diagnosis, a personal criminal indictment, a suicide attempt, or a bankruptcy.

RESEARCH FINDINGS

Prevalence

Researchers use personal interviews, telephone or Internet surveys, or questionnaires to study infidelity. Some studies focus on undergraduate students, others on cohabitating individuals, and still others on married couples. Some ask about extradyadic sexual intercourse only, whereas others ask about infidelity in a manner that allows the participant to decide what infidelity is. The questions focus on infidelity in the preceding year, lifetime infidelity within the current relationship, or lifetime infidelity in any relationship. Studies emanate from different countries. As a result of these variations, prevalence estimates range between 1.2% and 85.5% (Luo, Cartun, & Snider, 2010).

Prior to the 1990s American men admitted to infidelity more frequently than women in a 3:2 ratio. This statistic should not be generalized to other countries, because many cultures are organized around male privilege, and many men (and some women) surreptitiously take this right as their own. In surveys from the 1980s and 1990s, less than half of American men said that they had been unfaithful, but the prevalence varied between 24 and 44% (Weiderman, 1997; Thompson, 1984). In the largest representative sample of Americans from 18 to 59 years old, 20–25% of men and 10–15% of women acknowledged infidelity (Laumann, Gagnon, Michaels, & Michaels, 2001). These figures are usually quoted to the public (Snyder, Baucom, & Gordon, 2007). These data were generated before the Internet gained ascendancy. It is impossible to ascertain the role of lying in research studies (Mark, Janssen, & Millhausen, 2011; Luo et al., 2010). Scientists tend to study the infidelities of heterosexuals. Sexual minority communities may have far different prevalence rates and attitudes toward nonmonogamy.

Motivation

In research, motivation for unfaithful acts rests heavily on the correlates of infidelity. Male gender, low relationship and sexual satisfaction, and opportunity (urban location, and employment) are frequently cited (Havlicek,

Husarova, & Rezacova, 2011). Among dating couples, low conscientiousness and neuroticism also predict infidelity (Barta & Kiene, 2005). Among cohabitating couples, infidelity on the part of men's fathers increased the likelihood of the sons' unfaithfulness. This was not true for daughters (Havlicek et al., 2011). Some modern studies report a similar prevalence for men and women (Traen, Holmen, & Sigum, 2008; Havlicek et al., 2011), whereas others still find a male predominance (Luo et al., 2010).

The clinical study of motivation is limited by selection bias and the assumptions that a clinician may have about causes (Allen et al., 2008). Brown posits five types of affairs, each with its separate motivations (Brown, 2007). Clinicians rarely have much experience with the infidelities of the poor and of the vast majority of ethnic groups. Clinical and research findings seem to agree that most women's affairs are associated with their perception of low relationship quality (Havlicek et al., 2011; Mark et al., 2011). I am impressed that there is a particularly high incidence of undiscovered extramarital sexual experience in the 3 years preceding divorce.

To learn about the motives for infidelity, clinicians can usefully focus on the thinking process that occurred prior to a person's stepping outside of monogamy. Although it is important to inquire about motives, clinicians should not expect that the reasons will or can be initially fully revealed. The patient is much more likely than the therapist to know what the motivations were. When a therapist authoritatively explains the motives for the infidelity to the patient, the wrong person is doing the teaching.

Two Treatment Models

Models of treatment are marvels of clinical synthesis. They reduce the complexity of individual characteristics, personal history, interpersonal life, communication patterns, sexual experience, and working-through processes into therapeutic steps. Authors emphasize their models as research-supported, but only a small fraction of the work has been empirically tested. Nonetheless, two models are thought to be helpful to those who are beginning their work with infidelity.

The *intersystems approach* asserts that infidelity is a relationship issue: Partners suffer together and must heal together (Gambescia, Jenkins, & Weeks, 2003). Conjoint therapy simultaneously focuses on multiple interrelated problems of the individuals and their relationship. This approach aims to optimize the relationship as the couple passes through five phases: (1) crisis of discovery; (2) discovery of the individual and relationship susceptibilities; (3) facilitation of forgiveness; (4) treating the previously identified risk factors; and (5) improving intimacy through communication.

The *integrated approach* describes three phases of recovery: (1) dealing with the initial impact; (2) developing a shared understanding of the contributing factors; and (3) reaching an informed decision as to how to move on—separately or together (Baucom, Snyder, & Gordon, 2009). This model assumes that infidelity has had a traumatic impact and that recovery is brought about through the promotion of skills and understanding by using both cognitive-behavioral and insight-oriented techniques. Forgiveness may occur even though a decision may be made to end the relationship.

All modern models, however, emphasize individual pathways through the processes of therapy and the importance of empathy. They warn against having a uniform approach (Peluso, 2007). Hertlein and Weeks (2011) have provided an extensive review of the evolution of these models.

Treatment Outcome

There are three often-quoted outcome studies of therapy with couples with infidelity. They have a number of limitations. Sample sizes varied (n = 6, 19, and 145); they were done in three countries; they are missing follow-up data; they are hampered by the inability to ascertain secrets kept from therapists; they lack descriptions of the type and extent of infidelity; and they have limited age ranges and few parameters of measurement. Nevertheless, three findings converge: (1) Unfaithful couples do as well over a 1-year period as couples who present with other marital problems; (2) the affected spouse is more depressed and anxious than the one who has been unfaithful; and (3) infidelity does not invariably end marriages (Gordon, Baucom, & Snyder, 2004) (Atkins, Baucom, Eldrich, & Christensen, 2005) (Atkins, Klann, Marin, Lo, & Hahlweg, 2010). The therapists in these studies had different therapy ideologies. The studies were not designed to compare approaches. Recent reviews of research have concluded that "There is a large gap between research findings and treatment models" (Hertlein & Weeks, 2011, p. 3) and "There has been an incredible disconnect between clinical reality and research focus" (Kessel, Moon, & Adkins, 2007).

CLINICAL CONSIDERATIONS

The Type of Infidelity Matters

The contexts of infidelity vary, and therefore interventions must also (Baucom et al., 2009). The most egregious circumstances of infidelity are excluded from research and model building. A factor analysis of 29 types of infidelity in face-to-face or online emotional attachments and online sexual activities did not conceptualize a partner's use of a child or stepchild for sexual gratification (Luo et al., 2010). Such events create the most horrified reactions to relationship infidelity and are typically treated as both crimes and profound moral failings. Other criminal infidelities involve exhibitionistic, voyeuristic, and pedophilic paraphilic patterns, prostitute dependence, and masturbation to child pornography. Such activities make the infidelity per se seem a minor aspect of a more basic problem. They often lead to divorce. In many clinical settings, clinicians hear about infidelities but focus their interventions on the alcoholism, sexual addiction, bipolar disorder, character pathology, or psychosis.

Expectations for the Clinician

Clinicians have to be comfortable discussing this topic. Comfort can be attained without any training in sex therapy and requires no particular allegiance to a mental health ideology. Therapists have to act, however, as though they know that infidelity is part of many individuals' lives at some time. Some individuals in the midst of infidelity are hesitant to discuss their situation, even when they present for assistance. The comfortable clinician can transform dialogue about mysterious anxiety, depression, or somatic complaints by asking about infidelity. The therapist has to maintain clear boundaries, to provide skillful listening to the feelings and concerns of the individual or the couple, to understand the predicaments that relationships bring (Baucom et al., 2009) and to remain a humble lifelong student of the topic (Levine, 2006b).

It can be difficult to attain these six capacities if strong feelings are stirred up by the patient's situation. Private intensely negative or positive reactions increase the risk of therapeutic blunders (Weeks, 2003). Consider the therapist's negative affect if his or her marriage has been harmed and restructured by infidelity or if a past personal affair is regretted; consider the positive feelings if the therapist has long participated in a satisfying affair or if infidelity catalyzed a decision to leave an unsatisfying union.

A common boundary crossing is the appearance of an uncharacteristic authoritative voice: Don't have an affair! End the affair now! Your partner is scum! You must divorce! You should have an affair of your own! Our role is to be interested in the person's dilemmas, to clarify the options, to focus on what the person is thinking and feeling about the present, past, and future; it is not to tell the person what to do. We all must watch our countertransference reactions.

Culture and Language

Although textbooks treat infidelity as a dramatic independent topic, it does not actually stand alone. It is an aspect of the personal lifelong developmental struggle with love, entitlement, and responsibility to others (Levine, 2006a). Infidelity is a ripe topic of gossip between friends and in media outlets. The latter readily become preoccupied with the "inappropriate" sexual activities of the rich, powerful, or famous. Wider ranging, often more profound, perspectives are found in fiction, movies, polemics, biographies, and humor (Kipnis, 2003; Shanahan, 2007).

In the United States the dominant public position concerning marital infidelity is that it is wrong, destructive, and a personal moral failing (Smith, 1994). There is no term for the person who is unfaithful that does not connote a negative social judgment—cheater, womanizer, adulterer, slut, tart, and so forth. It is easier to employ the term "infidelity" than "nonnegotiated non-monogamy," even though "infidelity" has a negative connotation. Because mental health professionals begin their training within a disorders paradigm, problematic behaviors tend to be viewed through a lens of psychopathology that assumes that the behavior is a symptom of individual or relationship psychopathology. Eventually, we come to see that it is a decision that is frequently made in a relationship after balancing the benefits and the dangers.

Assessment

Although there are potentially many things to assess when the initial complaint is infidelity, this process is best accomplished by simply letting the individual or couple tell the story. The patient and the clinician notice what the story consists of, how it is told, affects that accompany the narrative, and what questions the therapist asks. Though clinicians may think of the first session as an assessment, we should realize that the patient is also assessing the clinician. Sometimes we flunk our audition; the patient never returns. There is no one correct way to conduct the early process. The goal is have the patient return to continue the discussion based on his or her realistic belief that therapy can be of assistance. Some clinicians see the couple first and then see the partners separately, and others continually see the couple together, but many people come alone to discuss their or their partners' infidelity. Seeing the individuals separately poses the dilemma of what to do about a history that a partner does not want to be disclosed. This is one of the major reasons that some therapists only see the couple together in the early phases of working together. Every approach has its advantages and disadvantages. Although some therapists use psychometric testing during evaluation and have a formal process of evaluation before making recommendations, clinicians need to recognize that clients may perceive this as delaying assistance with their painful dilemmas. Baucom and colleagues (2009) use two chapters to discuss assessment, but I am inclined to let the story flow and to allow myself to respond to the concerns that surface.

RETURNING TO AMANDA AND ADAM

The Crisis of the Betrayed

The mind of a person who has recently discovered a partner's infidelity swirls with questions and disturbing feelings; patients often feel like they are "going crazy." This "craziness" is merely the struggle to answer four questions:

1. "What is the personal meaning of the infidelity to me?"
2. "What is the best way I can respond to it?"

3. "Will I be abandoned?"
4. "Why did this happen?"

I listened to Adam struggle with these questions over 6 weeks. At times I rephrased his concerns in terms of a specific question. Various affects accompanied his numerous questions, of course, and I made sure that he labeled them accurately. I did this with him in a relaxed fashion, gently repeating that the answers to the questions and his feelings would evolve.

When he asked, staccato fashion, in Amanda's presence, "Does anyone ever get over this? Will I be able to trust her again? Will I be able to ever forget this?" I explained that the Chinese write the character for "crisis" by combining the words "danger" and "opportunity." I had seen that they were in grave danger. I was there to help them work through the danger in order to create a better life of their choosing. I asserted that many people get over a spouse's affair, but that I did not want to mislead them into thinking that there was no possibility of future unhappiness. "Why would anyone aspire to forget that an affair occurred?" I asked rhetorically. I told them that I often dramatically pointed to my patients and accused them of being "meaning makers." "Amanda's affair has different meanings to each of you. We all should act as though we know that over time meanings change, behaviors are viewed from a different perspective, and that which is painful can sometimes eventually become discussed more lightly." I neither wanted to trivialize what had happened nor to regard this as the worst possible thing that can happen in life. I certainly did not think that any self-respecting betrayed person should act in some prescribed way.

The Crisis of the Discovered

Frequently changing questions and affects dominate the mind of the unfaithful person, too. He or she may also feel unstable and uncertain about what to say. Having already caused intense distress in the partner, the unfaithful person tries to minimize further damage by being discreet about what is revealed. But a dilemma quickly appears. To share more details is to immediately increase pain in the partner and to risk the spouse's decision to divorce; to refuse to answer questions is to increase the partner's preoccupation with what has transpired. To get annoyed at the questions may inhibit the partner, but it also reflects a lack of empathy for the pain of the betrayed, which can prevent any progress. It is our responsibility to help the person think through the matter (Levine, 2006b). I do this by focusing on the five questions that swirl in the mind of the discovered partner.

1. "What do I want the outcome of this crisis to be?"
2. "Can I give up my relationship with the other person?"
3. "Why did I engage in this affair?"

4. "Is it wise to explain my motives?"
5. "What do I privately feel about this experience? Am I regretful? Happy? Justified? Disgraced?"

Amanda never wavered about wanting to stay married. The possibility that Adam ultimately would choose to divorce her made her sad and frightened. She did not want them to temporarily separate. Although she said she could give up the relationship immediately, she longed to communicate with her ex-lover. I explained to them at the end of the first session that both should realize that, having been involved for over a year, Amanda was quite attached to this man. Grief was to be expected. I didn't expect Adam to be solicitous about her grief. But I thought it was a dangerous mistake to act as though it were not happening. Adam quickly reversed his initial firm position by telling Amanda and her paramour that they could talk in order to help Amanda to end their relationship. The former lovers then spoke briefly on the telephone, texted each other for 2 days, and stopped. When specifically asked, Amanda revealed that she missed her paramour. After 1 month, she reported that she was thinking about him far less and did not miss him during Adam's 5-day absence. She missed Adam! This development preceded their passionate weekend of lovemaking during which Adam emotionally reattached to his wife.

Amanda tried to explain why she engaged in the affair. She acknowledged that she had grown comfortable with sex over the course of her marriage and no longer found it to be germ-ridden. She nodded in agreement when I asked her whether their pattern of marital sexual behavior left her somewhat bored despite her dependable orgasms. She was curious what it might be like to be sexually involved with another person. The excitement of this relationship was far greater than she ever imagined—"I loved being pursued!" She told herself that she would be disciplined and discreet, that one day the relationship would end of its own accord and her husband would never know. She was shocked to discover how easy it was for her to conduct the affair. She had thought that she was not the kind of person who would do such a thing. She was mortified that her husband found out and profoundly guilty about the pain she caused him. When she spoke of her shame, she looked ashamed. She worried about whether he could ever be calm again. She had always known him to be centered, quietly confident, and warm toward her. He was anything but these things now. His symptoms lessened session by session. He began to be able to concentrate at work, to stay there longer, and to return to his sport. Amanda was more concerned about him than about answering the painful question of "why."

Amanda told Adam that she was telling the whole truth, but it was apparent to me that she minimized the frequency of sexual contact with her paramour and that she withheld from Adam much of the process of missing her lover.

SEARCHING FOR NEW LIFE POSSIBILITIES

Physical and mental illness, treatment of disease, developmental misfortune, or poor intimacy often render a marriage asexual far before old age. What is a spouse to do when a partner becomes sexually incapacitated by any of these forces? Whether it is a wife who deteriorates from amyotrophic lateral sclerosis or a husband with a low sex drive who sticks to his word, without warmth or affection, for a decade that he does not want to have sex again, the more details a clinician is entrusted with, the greater one's interest becomes in what motivates fidelity and infidelity.

When a strongly homoerotic person takes a heterosexual mate, longings to be sexually involved with a same-gender person may recur over time. When a homosexual experience occurs, the person often feels that he or she does not want to or cannot possibly give up such an opportunity. The long-suppressed homosexual experiences feel so natural, exciting, and satisfying, unlike the infrequent and far less passionate marital sex. Although the world is used to hearing about marriages that end because a spouse is gay or lesbian, many such marriages continue (Friedman & Downey, 2010). A therapist's role may be to help the couple or simply one of the individuals to negotiate how they are going to deal with this in the future. Will it be surreptitious or open by agreement? Will one or both choose to be abstinent. Will they seek help for sexual addiction or something else? The needs and wishes of the heterosexual partner are of equal importance to those of the homosexual partner. The therapist needs to offer continuing discussions of possibilities until the couple gets beyond their crisis stage. Then they may be in a better position to decide what to do.

> A 60-year-old man, who had had intensifying homosexual desire since his last child moved out, was tempted to engage in homosexual behavior with a new, uneducated acquaintance who he thought might be gay. This would be something he had not done since two drunken episodes in college. Married to an anorgasmic wife who never seemed to like sex, he sought my assistance for depression and anxiety. What he wanted to talk about was his discovery of the Internet gay community and the opportunities this represented for him away and in town. His explorations eventually led to homosexual behavior within several evolving but brief personal relationships. These delighted him. He and his wife periodically had conversations about his homosexual desire, and she realized he was no longer depressed. He told her that he had had some very enjoyable homosexual encounters. She became distressed during each of these conversations and issued ultimatums. Her distress was assuaged by his reassurance that he was not interested in leaving the marriage or humiliating her at church. He refused to give up his friendships. Several times she agreed to see therapists—including me—but four times she found reasons

not to. Their newfound capacity to be married and unilaterally unfaithful lost its equilibrium when he fell in love with a divorced man of his age and educational level. When he acknowledged his wish to live with his paramour, she decided to divorce.

INFIDELITY AS THE CAUSE OF SEXUAL DYSFUNCTION

An affair can produce an array of new sexual dysfunctions in either partner. When the chief complaint is a dysfunction that began in the aftermath of infidelity, I try to reprocess the infidelity rather than to focus exclusively on the dysfunction. This works best when the couple was sexually adequate prior to the infidelity. The new empathic psychological intimacy created by the discussion of each partner's inner experiences can yield more intense sexual pleasures than the couple ever had. Psychological intimacy is, after all, an aphrodisiac!

In those couples with dysfunctional pre-affair sexual adaptations, the clinician has to deal with the affects related to the affair and recognize their mutual disappointment over their previous sexual life. Before the focus shifts to trying to alleviate the dysfunction, attention should be paid to creating a secure sense of attachment. The dysfunctional person will have a more difficult time improving if divorce is likely to be the consequence of continuing dysfunction. When the empathic reattachment that occurs in a therapy does not improve the dysfunction, specific techniques discussed in other chapters of this book can be judiciously employed, as long as the commitment to each other seems genuine. One should not expect all couples to have a lasting improved sexual life after therapy.

The simplest way of providing help for a man who has been dysfunctional prior to a wife's affair is to provide him with an effective medication for the problem—for example, premature ejaculation. Occasionally the use of a PDE5i will assist a couple whose pre-affair erectile dysfunction was problematic. Long-standing male sexual desire deficiencies are far more difficult. As previously dysfunctional women use the new psychological intimacy brought about during therapy, they may be able to overcome their previous dysfunction or at least have more pleasure in and desire for sex. Some individuals may elect to have individual sessions to focus on their sexual anxieties.

During an initial evaluation for a new sexual dysfunction, clinicians should ask about remote infidelity. The professional should understand that the couple may choose not to reveal it for a host of reasons. The unfaithful partner may not be aware that the spouse knows. The spouse feels it is not in his or her best interest to reveal their knowledge of the past. The couple may have previously dealt with it and does not want to rehash its pain. The couple believes or *knows* there is another cause of the presenting symptom. If the couple fails to make progress, the topic can be readdressed in individual sessions with each partner to learn about the patient's perspective.

CONCLUSIONS

Infidelity is not a psychiatric diagnosis. DSM-5 (American Psychiatric Association, 2013) does not have a category for it. Its assessment and treatment are processes. This chapter does not emphasize techniques, because research and clinical experience converge to suggest that the understanding of the evolving experience of the partners is more vital than an organizing ideology, a particular sequence of assessment, or what a particular therapist may call an approach. The kind, interested, calm, knowledgeable therapist can make a significant difference to the couple by generating a respectful attitude of three people learning together. The therapist may know more about the facts of infidelity, but the betrayed and the betrayer know far more about their background, motivations, and meanings than the therapist does. Therapy is a cooperative venture that is modified imperceptibly session by session.

Although there are degrees of infidelity, even lesser violations may be overwhelming, because people have their own standards for what their partners are permitted to do and their unique coping capacities. New clinicians can quickly grow comfortable with these problems, knowing that dealing with infidelity requires dealing with patients' meanings. Because there is no absolute meaning of infidelity, we witness patients' interpretations over time. Many patients can profit from our knowledge, experience, demeanor, and mastery of our countertransference as we attempt to help the parties to absorb, understand, and tolerate their new relationship situation. In helping patients deal with their painful new realizations, we inadvertently help ourselves to mature as clinicians.

REFERENCES

Allen, E. S., Rhoades, G. K., Stanley, S. M., Markman, H. J., Williams, T., Melton, J., et al. (2008). Premarital precursors of marital infidelity. *Family Process, 47,* 243–259.

American Psychiatric Association. (2013). *Diagnostic and statistical manual of mental disorders* (5th ed.). Arlington, VA: Author.

Anapol, D. (2010). *Polyamory in the 21st century: Love and intimacy with multiple partners.* Lanham, MD: Rowman & Littlefield.

Atkins, D. C., Baucom, D. H., Eldrich, K. A., & Christensen, A. (2005). Infidelity and couples behavioral therapy: Optimism in the face of betrayal. *Journal of Counseling and Clinical Psychology, 73*(1), 144–150.

Atkins, D. C., Klann, N., Marin, R. A., Lo, T. T. Y., & Hahlweg, K. (2010). Outcome of couples with infidelity in a community-based sample of couples therapy. *Journal of Family Psychology, 24*(2), 212–216.

Barta, W. D., & Kiene, S. M. (2005). Motivations for infidelity in heterosexual dating couples: The roles of gender, personality differences, and socio-sexual orientation. *Journal of Social and Personal Relationships, 22,* 339–360.

Baucom, D. H., Snyder, D. K., & Gordon, K. C. (2009). *Helping couples get past the affair: A clinician's guide.* New York: Guilford Press.

Betzig, L. (1989). Cause of conjugal dissolution: A cross-cultural study. *Current Anthropology, 30,* 654–676.

Brand, R. J., Markey, C. M., Mills, A., & Hodges, S. D. (2007). Sex differences in self-reported infidelity and its correlates. *Sex Roles, 57,* 101–109.

Brown, E. M. (2007). The affair as a catalyst for change. In P. R. Peluso (Ed.), *Infidelity: A practitioner's guide to working with couples in crisis* (pp. 149–165). New York: Routledge.

Freud, S. (1916). Some character types met with in psychoanalytic work. In J. Strachey (Ed. & Trans.), *The standard edition of the complete psychological works of Sigmund Freud* (Vol. 14, pp. 311–315). London: Hogarth Press.

Friedman, R. C., & Downey, J. I. (2010). Male and female homosexuality in heterosexual life. In S. B. Levine, C. B. Risen, & S. E. Althof (Eds.), *Handbook of clinical sexuality for mental health professionals* (pp. 369–381). New York: Routledge.

Gambescia, N., Jenkins, R. E., & Weeks, G. R. (2003). *Treating infidelity: Therapeutic dilemmas and effective strategies.* New York: Norton.

Gordon, K. C., Baucom, D. H., & Snyder, D. K. (2004). Integrative intervention for promoting recovery from extramarital affairs. *Journal of Marital and Family Therapy, 30,* 213–231.

Havlicek, J., Husarova, B., & Rezacova, V. (2011). Correlates of extra-dyadic sex in Czech heterosexual couples: Does sexual behavior of parents matter? *Archives of Sex Behavior, 40,* 1153–1163.

Hertlein, K. M., & Weeks, G. L. (2011). The field of infidelity: Past, present, and future. In J. L. Wetchler (Ed.), *Handbook of clinical issues in couples therapy* (pp. 145–161). New York: Routledge.

Kessel, D. E., Moon, J. H., & Adkins, D. C. (2007). Research in couples therapy for infidelity: What do we know about helping couples when there has been an affair? In P. R. Peluso (Ed.), *Infidelity: A practitioner's guide to working with couples in crisis* (p. 56). New York: Routledge

Kipnis, L. (2003). *Against love: A polemic.* New York: Pantheon.

Laumann, E. O., Gagnon, J. H., Michaels, R. T., & Michaels, S. (2001). *Sex, love, and health in America: Private choices, and public policies.* Chicago: University of Chicago Press.

Levine, S. (2006a). *Demystifying love: Plain talk for the mental health professional.* New York: Routledge.

Levine, S. (2006b). Infidelity: Basic concepts. In S. Levine (Ed.), *Demystifying love: Plain talk for the mental health professional.* New York: Routledge.

Luo, S., Cartun, M. A., & Snider, A. G. (2010). Assessing extradyadic behavior: A review, a new measure, and two new models. *Personality and Individual Differences, 49,* 155–163.

Mark, K., Janssen, E., & Millhausen, R. R. (2011). Infidelity in heterosexual couples: Demongraphic, interpersonal, and personality-related predictors of extradynadic sex. *Archives of Sexual Behavior, 40*(5), 971–982.

Peluso, P. R. (Ed.). (2007). *Infidelity: A practitioner's guide to working with couples in crisis.* New York: Routledge.

Shanahan, D. (2007). *Bad sex.* New York: Abrams Image.

Smith, T. W. (1994). Attitudes towards sexual permissiveness: Trends, correlates, and behavioral connections. In A. S. Rossi (Ed.), *Sexuality across the life course* (pp. 63–97). Chicago: Chicago University Press.

Snyder, D. K., Baucom, D. H., & Gordon, K. C. (2008). An integrative approach to treating infidelity. *Family Journal, 16,* 300–307.

Snyder, D. K., Baucom, D. H., & Gordon, K. C. (2007). *Getting past the affair: A program to help you cope, heal, and move on—together or apart.* New York: Guilford Press.

Solstad, K., & Mucic, D. (1999). Extramarital sexual relationships of middle-aged Danish men: Attitudes and behaviors. *Marturitas, 32,* 51–59.

Thompson, A. P. (1984). Emotional and sexual components of extramarital relations. *Journal of Sex Research, 46,* 35–42.

Traen, B., Holmen, K., & Sigum, H. (2008). Extradyadic activity in a random sample of Norwegian couples. *Journal of Sex Research, 45,* 319–328.

Weiderman, M. W. (1997). Extramarital sex: Prevalence and correlates in a national survey. *Journal of Sex Research, 34,* 167–174.

Medical Problems

CHAPTER 19

Sexuality and Infertility

Judith C. Daniluk, Emily Koert, and Erin Breckon

Infertility can change the meaning of sex. For many infertile couples, sex is no longer a joyous or intimate connection; instead, it is associated with disappointment or failure. Depending upon one's culture, religion, or upbringing, infertility can challenge one's virility or femininity, not to mention one's marriage. Sex therapists are not usually part of the team of experts that is involved in infertility treatment. Perhaps they should be. Daniluk, Koert, and Breckon argue that sex therapy has an important role to play but that the nature of the intervention will likely depend on the stage of infertility treatment. Early in treatment, sex therapy is directed to helping couples overcome a dysfunction (e.g., erectile dysfunction) that may interfere with achieving a pregnancy or to help increase compliance with timed intercourse. After treatment, couples may want and require interventions focused on restoring pleasure. Above all, Daniluk and colleagues admonish us that "recognition of the common experience of shame, guilt, and inadequacy regarding infertility and sexuality is paramount in providing sensitive support and intervention."

Judith C. Daniluk, PhD, is Professor of Counselling Psychology at the University of British Columbia. Her areas of clinical and research expertise include women's sexuality and reproductive health and the psychosocial consequences of infertility and involuntary childlessness.

Emily Koert, MA, is a PhD candidate in Counselling Psychology at the University of British Columbia. Her area of clinical practice and research is women's reproductive health. She is conducting research on the psychosocial consequences of permanent, unintentional childlessness for women who delayed childbearing.

Erin Breckon, BA, is a master's student in Counselling Psychology at the University of British Columbia. She is interested in exploring the effectiveness of psychotherapeutic interventions for improving quality of life and sexual health for couples receiving medical interventions for infertility.

Infertility is defined as the inability to achieve and sustain a viable pregnancy after 12 months of regular, unprotected intercourse for women under 35 years of age and after 6 months for women 35 and over. It is estimated that approximately 15–20% of both men and women of reproductive age experience fertility problems. These problems in women are generally caused by endocrine imbalances or anatomical impairments such as blocked fallopian tubes, ovulatory difficulties, advanced reproductive age, or endometriosis. Male fertility problems are primarily caused by a deficiency in the number, quality, or motility of sperm. For both men and women, fertility problems are exacerbated with age (Keye, 2006). The assisted reproductive technologies available to treat these conditions include fertility drugs, *in vitro* fertilization (IVF), intracytoplasmic sperm injection (ICSI), egg freezing, donated sperm, eggs, or embryos, and gestational or traditional surrogacy. Due to the rapid advances and changes in reproductive technologies, it may be best to suggest that clients regularly visit *www.asrm.org/patient_resources* for current and accurate information on the latest fertility treatments and family planning options.

The psychosocial impact of infertility and medical treatment is well documented in the literature. Episodes of grief, depression, low self-esteem and diminished self-worth, relationship difficulties, and both episodic and long-term sexual dysfunction and dissatisfaction have been reported for infertile women and men (Daniluk & Tench, 2007; Möller, 2001; Wischmann, 2010). The focus of this chapter is the impact of infertility and related treatment on men's and women's sexual satisfaction and functioning.

EPIDEMIOLOGY

A significant body of literature provides evidence for temporary or permanent sexual impairment during and following infertility and related medical treatments (e.g., Marci et al., 2012; Möller, 2001; Nelson, Shindel, Naughton, Ohebshalom, & Mulhall, 2008; Pepe & Byrne, 2005). Sexual concerns are commonly cited by men and women, particularly during the often-invasive and protracted medical fertility investigations and treatments—with estimates ranging from 10 to 60% of couples reporting these concerns (Möller, 2001; Wischmann, 2010).

While in rare cases sexual dysfunction can be the cause of fertility impairments (e.g., vaginismus, dyspareunia, erectile and ejaculatory dysfunction), the preponderance of sexual complaints occur subsequent to a diagnosis of infertility (Hammer Burns, 2006; Leiblum, 1997). For men, common sexual complaints include erectile dysfunction, ejaculatory problems, loss of libido, and decreased frequency of intercourse (Lenzi, Lombardo, Saladone, Gandini, & Jannini, 2003; Shindel, Nelson, Naughton, Ohebshalom, & Mulhall, 2008). In a sample of 244 men with couple infertility, erectile dysfunction and premature ejaculation were reported by one in six men (Lotti et al., 2012). For women, problems with arousal, diminished desire, inability to achieve orgasm, and painful intercourse are the most common sexual complaints (Leiblum, 1997; Keskin et al., 2011; Millheiser et al., 2010).

Some sexual concerns may be the consequence of fertility impairments, as in the case of dyspareunia caused by endometriosis (uterine adhesions and scarring). In others, *medical conditions* (e.g., diabetes, high blood pressure, thyroid disorders, low testosterone, uterine fibroids, prostatitis, pelvic inflammatory disease [PID]), *fertility medications* (e.g., clomid, gonadotropins), *cancer treatments* (radiation, chemotherapy), *lifestyle factors* (e.g., excessive alcohol and drug use, excessive exercise, poor nutrition or eating disorders, obesity), *psychological conditions* (e.g., depression, anxiety), *relationship distress*, or *environmental toxins* are implicated in the sexual complaints and impairments reported by infertile individuals (Hammer Burns, 2006). In some situations, these sexual concerns can impede successful treatment—such as when erectile or ejaculatory dysfunctions impede a man's ability to produce a fresh semen sample for an IVF cycle or when vaginismus obstructs intrauterine insemination, egg retrieval, or embryo transfer.

Sexual problems are generally more pronounced for couples whose sexual dissatisfaction and difficulties predate the onset of a diagnosis of infertility, with the reported incidence of sexual complaints increasing among the infertile population with prolonged treatment (Daniluk & Frances-Fischer, 2009; Hammer Burns, 2006; Leiblum, 1997). In terms of comorbidity, sexual complaints are commonly reported secondary to depression and anxiety (Keskin et al., 2011; Lotti et al., 2012; Nelson et al., 2008), although it is not clear whether the incidence of sexual dysfunction is higher for infertile individuals versus their fertile counterparts who have been diagnosed with depression or anxiety. Partner dynamics also play a role, with infertile individuals' sexual satisfaction and functioning being highly correlated with those of their partner (Nelson et al., 2008; Shindel et al., 2008).

In terms of gender differences, when comparing men's and women's sexual difficulties during treatment, Lenzi et al. (2003) and Marci et al. (2012) found that men had higher frequencies of sexual difficulties and negative impact on their sexuality than women. However, other research findings (e.g., Nelson et al., 2008; Wischmann, 2010) suggest that women are equally, if not more, affected by sexual problems during infertility and related treatment, especially given that women and their bodies bear the primary burden during fertility investigations and treatments.

Basson's model of sexual desire (Basson, Brotto, Laan, Redmond, & Utian, 2005) helps to explain the way in which mental and physical factors are implicated in and affect sexual desire for women, with intimate contact often preceding the experience of sexual arousal or desire, particularly for women in longer term relationships. Basson and her colleagues (2005) have adapted the model to account for the experiences of infertile women to assist in understanding the sexual sequelae of the diagnosis and treatment of infertility for many women. The stresses associated with fertility treatments reduce a woman's motivation and receptivity to sexual intimacy. Depression and poor self-image decrease a woman's subjective arousal and subsequent desire response, resulting in diminished desire and sexual satisfaction. There are fewer nonsexual rewards, such as emotional intimacy and closeness; thus the infertile woman is less motivated to repeat the experience. The shift in the purpose of sex from pleasure to procreation and the monthly pairing of sex with reproductive failure further diminishes the infertile woman's desire for sexual intimacy and adds considerably to the incidence of sexual difficulties and dissatisfaction reported by infertile women and their partners (Daniluk & Frances-Fischer, 2009; Leiblum, 1997).

Similar models have not been adapted to explain the impact of a diagnosis of infertility on men. However, the prevalence of sexual complaints and episodes of sexual dysfunction reported by infertile men, particularly during the demands of medical treatment (Lenzi et al., 2003; Lotti et al., 2012), would suggest that the burden of being unable to produce a child and the stresses of medical testing and treatment may take a similar toll on the sexual self-esteem, desire, and functioning of men—particularly those diagnosed with male factor infertility (Marci et al., 2012).

What is clear is that sexual difficulties and dissatisfaction appear to persist for many infertile women and men, long after medical treatments have ended (e.g., Lenzi et al., 2003; Sundby, Schmidt, Heldaas, Bugge, & Tanbo, 2007; Wirtberg, Moller, Hogstrom, Tronstad, & Lalos, 2007). For example, in a longitudinal, mixed-methods study of 38 infertile couples following failed fertility treatments, despite increases in positive self-evaluations and perceptions over time, a persistent decrease in sexual satisfaction was evidenced throughout the 33 months following treatment termination (Daniluk & Tench, 2007). Sexual satisfaction was also reported to decline for 101 men and 113 women 5 years following fertility treatments (Schanz et al., 2011). In a 20-year follow-up study of 14 women following unsuccessful fertility treatments, participants reported a persistent negative impact on their sexual desire and satisfaction (Wirtberg et al., 2007). Nine of these women said that their sexual desire was lost forever subsequent to the diagnosis and treatment of infertility and lamented that mental health support was not made available during or following fertility treatment to address their sexual and relationship concerns. It remains to be determined whether the negative sexual aftermath of infertility similarly persists over many years for men.

ASSESSMENT AND DIAGNOSTIC ISSUES

Sex therapists are not routinely included in the initial medical fertility workup, which typically is conducted by a nurse and gynecologist or reproductive endocrinologist. Although some questions in the medical assessment focus on the frequency and timing of intercourse and previous sexual history (i.e., sexually transmitted infections [STIs], therapeutic abortion), psychosexual assessment or intervention typically is recommended by the medical team only in cases in which a sexual dysfunction is implicated in the couple's fertility problem (e.g., inability to engage in intercourse due to impotence or vaginismus) or is impeding fertility treatment.

In Figure 19.1 we present a psychosexual assessment and treatment decision algorithm to guide decision making when working with infertile individuals or couples. Assessment and diagnosis require assessing the presence, frequency, and severity of an individual's or couple's sexual complaint (e.g., vaginismus, dyspareunia, impotence and erectile difficulties, lack of interest/ desire) and determining whether a sexual dysfunction is impeding the implementation or successful outcome of fertility treatments. If the sexual problem is impeding fertility or successful medical intervention, it is necessary to consult with the patients' fertility specialist and ascertain whether, based on factors such as the patients' age and fertility status, taking time out from treatment will reduce their chances of a successful pregnancy. In cases in which the sexual dysfunction is contributing to the couple's inability to conceive, a hiatus from fertility treatments is warranted while the sexual dysfunction is addressed only if time permits.[1]

If time does not permit taking a break from medical treatment or if the sexual concern is not impeding the couple's fertility or successful treatment, it is imperative to ascertain whether the sexual problem is viewed as problematic by the infertile couple (Hammer Burns, 2006; Leiblum, 1997). For many infertile couples, concerns related to sexual satisfaction or functioning are *not a high priority* when engaged in the all-consuming process of fertility treatments and trying to achieve a pregnancy (Daniluk, 1998). Although early intervention is always recommended (particularly given that sexual problems are very likely to be further exacerbated by prolonged fertility investigations and treatments), unless the sexual dysfunction is contributing to a couple's inability to conceive, they may not be willing to invest the time and energy in addressing these problems until after they have terminated, and emotionally recovered from, medical treatment (Hammer Burns, 2006). In these cases, couples should be provided with psychosocial support to help them cope with and to reduce the sexual and performance stresses associated with medical treatment. Couples can be given strategies to manage challenging situations, such as the use of erotic material and partner assistance when producing a sperm sample or the use of visualizations and progressive relaxation to cope with the insertion of a speculum, catheter, or probe. The sexual concern should be monitored on an ongoing basis to assess changes in severity and impact, and if the couple is receptive to the idea, it can be helpful to develop a tentative future treatment plan to address their sexual concern(s) after fertility treatments have ended.

Psychosexual intervention should be initiated when sexual dysfunctions

---

[1]In the case of patients dealing with age-related fertility declines and women diagnosed with premature ovarian failure, polysystic ovarian syndrome, or primary ovarian insufficiency, there will be greater urgency to continue with medical treatment.

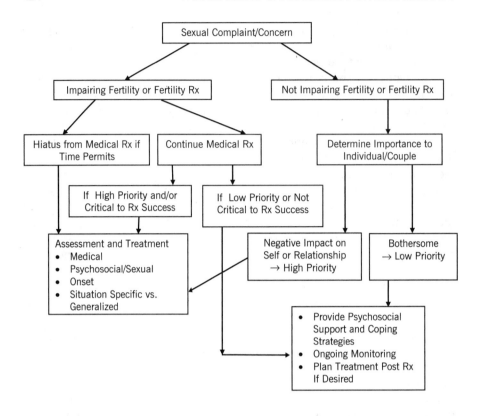

FIGURE 19.1. Assessment and treatment algorithm for infertility.

are impeding fertility or successful medical intervention (if time permits), or when the dysfunctions are having a negative impact on one or both members of the couple or threatening the stability of their relationship and/or are identified as being a high priority by one or both members of the couple. In conducting a thorough psychosexual assessment, it is necessary to ascertain whether the sexual problems are secondary to infertility and whether they are generalized or situation specific (e.g., whether problems commonly occur when having to perform on demand to produce a sperm sample or during times of the month when the woman is ovulating). It is particularly important to determine whether medical conditions or medications are implicated in the dysfunction (e.g., endometriosis resulting in dyspareunia; retrograde ejaculation caused by prostatitis, diabetes, multiple sclerosis or nerve damage or disease; diminished sexual responsiveness and desire due to fertility medications such as clomiphene or gonadotropins; other health conditions such as cystic fibrosis or Turner syndrome). Mental health (e.g., depression), lifestyle (e.g. alcohol and drug use; use of steroids), and relationship issues should also be included in a thorough psychosexual assessment. With the strong link between fertility and femininity–masculinity in most cultures and religions worldwide, particular attention should be paid to the impact of infertility on the sexual self-perceptions and body image of both members of the couple—factors that can have a considerable impact on reducing sexual responsiveness and desire (Daniluk & Frances-Fischer, 2009).

In terms of assessing sexual functioning and satisfaction, currently there are no existing assessment measures that have been developed or adapted for specific use with an infertile population. The most frequent measures cited in the research literature examining the incidence or prevalence of sexual distress or dysfunction within the infertile population are the Female Sexual Function Index (FSFI; Rosen et al., 2000), the International Index of Erectile Function (IIEF; Rosen et al., 1997), and the short form of the Derogatis Interview for Sexual Functioning (DSFI-SR; Derogatis, 1997). The Golombok–Rust Inventory of Sexual Satisfaction (GRISS; Rust & Golombok, 1985) might be a good adjunct to these standard sexual functioning measures in that it assesses both the sexual and nonsexual aspects of the relationship between a couple, with scores for both men and women. We also recommend the Comprehensive Psychosocial History for Infertility developed by Burns (1993), which provides a framework for a comprehensive psychosocial assessment of infertile individuals, including questions focused on sexual dysfunction and marital adjustment.

When conducting a sexual assessment with couples who are dealing with infertility, therapists must be *acutely sensitive* to context and appreciate that through the medical treatment process, infertile men and women have had the most intimate and private aspects of their lives and bodies laid bare and scrutinized. A significant toll will have been taken on each individual's sexual self-esteem, based on the man's "failure" to impregnate his partner and the woman's inability to achieve a pregnancy. Understandably, they will want to maintain what little privacy and dignity they can (Daniluk, 1998). Wischmann (2010) and Daniluk and Frances-Fischer (2009) underscore the value of normalizing the experience of sexual distress and episodic sexual dysfunction during fertility treatments. For example, a man is more likely to acknowledge his difficulties in being able to produce a semen sample "on demand" during an IVF cycle if he is told that bouts of impotence are extremely common under these circumstances.

It is also important to be very sensitive to gender and cultural differences—particularly as these are related to beliefs about fertility and masculinity–femininity—and to infertile individuals' levels of comfort in discussing their sexual difficulties, in general and with a therapist of the opposite sex.

DSM-5 Diagnostic Protocols

DSM-5 includes a new diagnosis, female sexual interest/arousal disorder (FSIAD). This revision reflects mounting empirical evidence that female sexual desire and subjective sexual arousal overlap—a reconceptualization that more accurately reflects the experiences of many infertile women. Male hypo-active sexual desire disorder addresses the parallel experience of low sexual desire among men—a commonly reported experience among infertile men, particularly in cases of male factor infertility.

DSM-5 (American Psychiatric Association, 2013) omits the diagnosis of sexual dysfunction due to general medical condition. If a thoroughly conducted assessment determines that an infertile woman or man is experiencing sexual difficulties exclusively accounted for by medical or biological factors, then she or he would not receive a DSM diagnosis. However, under some of the sexual disorders such as female orgasmic disorder, a medical condition may be noted as a differential diagnosis. In this case, the specifier of "with medical factors relevant to prognosis, course, or treatment" should be used. Because short-term sexual problems are common among couples experiencing difficulties conceiving, the recommendation that problems must persist for a minimum of 6 months will be useful in avoiding any inappropriate diagnosis (although treatment should still be made available).

It is important to note that the psychosexual aftermath of infertility is often distressing enough that an additional diagnosis of sexual dysfunction may serve to further damage the sexual self-esteem and agency of infertile men and women (Daniluk, 1998; Hammer Burns, 2006; Leiblum, 1997). As a consequence, such diagnostic labels should be applied with sensitivity and caution.

EFFICACY OF TREATMENT APPROACHES

The growing body of literature evaluating psychosocial interventions for infertility-related distress is reviewed briefly here. Within these studies, sexual functioning is also a focus of intervention and measured as an outcome variable, along with variables such as marital satisfaction and psychological well-being (e.g., Haemmerli, Znoj, & Berger, 2010; Tuschen-Caffler, Florin, Krause, & Pook, 1999). Psychosocial treatments frequently include cognitive-behavioral interventions to reduce stress and anxiety, modules on enhancing communication, strategies for accessing social support, and skills for managing work and familial relationships (e.g., Haemmerli et al., 2010; Schmidt, Holstein, Christensen, & Boivin, 2005).

Two large meta-analyses conducted within the past 10 years evaluating the most recent research on psychosocial interventions for infertility-related distress show mixed support for the usefulness of these forms of treatment (Boivin, 2003; de Liz & Strauss, 2005). Boivin (2003) evaluated 25 studies that described psychosocial interventions and evaluated their effect on at least one outcome measure. De Liz and Strauss (2005) examined 22 studies that assessed the efficacy of psychosocial intervention in the reduction of negative affect, depressive symptoms, and pregnancy rates. Overall, Boivin (2003) and de Liz and Strauss (2005) found that psychosocial interventions focused on emotional expression, psychosocial support, and discussion of feelings and thoughts about their infertility were effective in reducing the negative distress related to infertility. However, there was little unequivocal research support for changes in other areas of psychosocial functioning or interpersonal behavior. According to Boivin, "the way that people related to their partners and other members of their social network was rarely affected by these interventions" (2003, p. 2234). Similar conclusions were reached by de Liz and Strauss (2005) who found that group, individual and couple psychotherapy were effective only in reducing symptoms of anxiety and depression for this population. The effect of these interventions on pregnancy rates was equivocal.

Tuschen-Caffler et al. (1999) conducted one of the few studies of a 6-month cognitive-behavioral therapy group for 17 infertile couples focused specifically on improving sexual functioning and satisfaction, reducing thoughts of helplessness, and enhancing marital communication. The intervention involved the use of daily diaries to track the effect of sex therapy interventions on frequency of sexual intercourse during fertile times. Pre- and posttreatment scores were compared within the treatment group and across a control group. Before the group intervention only 50% of couples in the treatment group were actively scheduling intercourse during their fertile times in the month. Posttreatment, this rose to 100%. However, although the intervention was effective in increasing compliance with the timing of intercourse, levels of sexual pleasure and satisfaction remained low for these couples, even during the nonfertile times of the month. Although dated, this study demonstrates that a planned intercourse schedule can improve couples' chances of becoming pregnant when frequency of intercourse is an issue.

More recently, early intervention was found to be effective in somewhat mitigating the negative sexual and relational aftermath of fertility treatments (Vizheh, Pakgohar, Babaei & Ramezanzadeh, 2013). In a randomized controlled study with 100 infertile couples in Iran, 50 couples were assigned to the counseling intervention group consisting of three weekly 60- to 90-minute counseling sessions. The other 50 couples were assigned to the no-intervention group. Those couples who received the counseling intervention demonstrated significantly higher levels of marital and sexual satisfaction when measured 3 months after the intervention compared with those who did not receive the intervention. These findings highlight the impact that medical treatment may have on the sexual and marital satisfaction of infertile couples and underscore the value of early intervention.

Given that many patients are reluctant to access psychosocial support during fertility treatments—perhaps due to the emotional and physical burdens of the treatment process—more targeted psychosexual approaches may be warranted to mitigate or remediate the sexual toll taken on infertile individuals and couples (Boivin, Scanlan, & Walker, 1999; Vizheh et al., 2013). However, the literature suggests that interventions need to move beyond compliance and adequate sexual functioning to the broader realm of maintaining and even enhancing sexual pleasure and intimacy throughout, and subsequent to, the often protracted course of medical treatment (Millheiser et al., 2010; Schanz et al., 2011). That said, when working on relationship and sexual issues is a priority for the couple, a more holistic and integrative therapeutic approach focused on enhancing intimacy and communication, on reducing the focus on timed intercourse (i.e., "work sex"), and on disrupting the link between intercourse and reproductive failure is necessary to improve sexual satisfaction and pleasure (Daniluk & Frances-Fischer, 2009; Leiblum, 1997).

INTEGRATION OF SEX THERAPY INTO PSYCHOSOCIAL INTERVENTION FOR INFERTILITY

Effective treatment requires careful assessment and diagnosis of the particular sexual problem and the extent to which the problem is causing the couple distress or impeding the success of their fertility treatments (see Figure 19.1). There is considerable evidence for the effective treatment of the sexual difficulties that most commonly impede pregnancy and successful fertility treatments (e.g., erectile dysfunction, ejaculation difficulties, vaginismus, dyspareunia) that can be applied to working with infertile couples whose sexual problems are impeding spontaneous pregnancy or successful medical intervention. As treatment effectiveness will be directly related to the couple's motivation and readiness to address their sexual concern(s), it is essential to determine the extent to which sex therapy is a priority for both members of the couple before proceeding with treatment (Hammer Burns, 2006; Leiblum, 1997).

An awareness of, and sensitivity to, cultural and religious diversity related to the meaning of infertility and what is considered appropriate sexual expression is critical when working with people from different cultures and religions (Hammer Burns, 2006). As well, recognition of the common experience of shame, guilt, and inadequacy regarding infertility and sexuality is paramount in providing sensitive support and intervention (Daniluk, 1998; Leiblum, 1997). It is important to challenge rigidly held beliefs, such as that a woman's worth is tied to her fertility and that a man's worth is tied to his ability to sexually perform or to the quality of his sperm. However, therapists must be sensitive to the extent to which these views are embedded in the clients' cultural and religious beliefs. For example, after six failed IVF attempts, a highly educated and very successful Muslim woman with whom Daniluk was working, said in anguish, "If I am not a mother I am nothing . . . my husband will take another wife and in my culture he has every right to do so."

In her review of the literature and discussion of sexual counseling and infertility, Hammer Burns (2006) summarizes the basic behavioral strategies within psychosocial counseling that are most commonly employed with infertile patients in the treatment of their sexual difficulties. These include (1) anxiety reduction techniques (e.g., progressive relaxation, assertiveness training); (2) directed masturbation (for men or women who are unable to achieve orgasm); (3) orgasmic reconditioning (i.e., directed fantasy in relation to masturbation to shift arousal stimuli); (4) imagery techniques (i.e., assessment and rehearsal of sexual response); (5) explicit homework assignments (e.g., massage, communication exercises); and (6) sensate focus exercises (Hammer Burns, 2006, pp. 228–229).

In general, approaches to treatment involve an individualized combination of interventions that address the unique sexual problems and contributing factors of each couple (Hammer Burns, 2006; Leiblum, 1997). They may include medication, the use of devices (e.g., vibrators), and medical or surgical intervention. Hypnosis (e.g., Araoz, 2005) has also been integrated into treatment with some success. Psychosocial interventions are more commonly used in treating fertility-related distress (and, by extension, the sexual difficulties and dissatisfaction that frequently accompany the inability to produce a child) and medical fertility investigations and treatment (e.g., Wischmann, 2010). We turn now to a case example to highlight the complexities of assessing and working with sexual complaints of couples who are undergoing fertility treatments.

CASE DISCUSSION

Lynn, 39, and Bill, 56, a European-American couple, were referred for therapy by the medical team of a local fertility clinic. Both were well-educated professionals. The couple had been diagnosed with primary infertility based on Lynn's fertility status and had been pursuing a pregnancy for 36 months. This was a second marriage for Bill, who had two children from his previous marriage, both now in their early 20s. Lynn had always been ambivalent about having children while pursuing her MBA and building her investment consulting business. However, when she reached her mid-30s and things started to stabilize in her business, Lynn found her thoughts turning to having children. She and Bill had originally agreed that they would not have children, and Bill was looking forward to retirement in the next 10–12 years. They went through 10 sessions of couple counseling to work through their deadlock on this issue and agreed that they would attempt to have only one child.

After several months of trying to conceive without success, Lynn and Bill's general practitioner referred them to a fertility specialist, and they underwent a standard medical investigation. Lynn was found to have a slightly elevated day 3 FSH (follicle-stimulating hormone)—indicating diminishing ovarian reserve—and, to the surprise of the couple, Bill's sperm parameters were found to be highly problematic (low count, poor motility, compromised morphology). They were informed that their only viable treatment option was IVF with ICSI. Given Bill's poor sperm parameters, the couple were encouraged by the clinic to select an anonymous sperm donor to use as backup for their treatment cycle in the event that Bill's sperm sample was inadequate for fertilization on the day of egg retrieval. Bill was unable to produce a fresh sperm sample the morning of Lynn's egg retrieval, so Lynn's five eggs were fertilized with the sperm of the anonymous donor they had previously selected. Only two of the fertilized eggs resulted in viable embryos. Given the caliber of the embryos and Lynn's age, the doctors were recommending that both embryos be transferred to Lynn's uterus. However, the day before the embryos were to be transferred, the couple found themselves in a dilemma—with Bill insisting that only one embryo be transferred and Lynn feeling emotionally unprepared to go through with the transfer of embryos created with the DNA of a "complete stranger." The couple was unable to resolve their dilemma and time was of the essence, so they requested an emergency appointment with the clinic's consulting psychologist.

Three issues were identified at the outset of this session: Bill's impotence that resulted in the need to use donor sperm, Bill's reticence to transfer two embryos in case this resulted in a twin pregnancy, and Lynn's reluctance to go ahead with the transfer of the embryos created with anonymous donor sperm. To reduce the urgency of the decision regarding the transfer of the embryos, the therapist recommended that the two embryos be cryopreserved (frozen), thereby defusing the immediate emotional intensity of the situation and giving Bill and Lynn time to unpack and work through the various issues that were creating a dilemma for them. Although they were aware that frozen embryos are often not as successful as fresh embryos, they reluctantly agreed that they were not prepared to make such an important and potentially life-altering decision under pressure and were willing to accept the potentially reduced viability of the frozen embryos.

With the pressure off in terms of making an immediate decision about transferring the embryos, the therapist was able to assist the couple in prioritizing their treatment goals. An assessment of Bill's impotence—which was a concern for him—indicated that although he had previously experienced brief periods of erectile difficulties during times of severe stress (e.g., during his divorce), the onset of Bill's current erectile dysfunction followed his surprising diagnosis of male factor infertility. Considering the frequency with which men experience such episodic difficulties during the stresses of medical fertility testing and treatment (Moller, 2001; Shindel et al., 2008; Wischmann, 2010), the prognosis for successful treatment was good. However, given Lynn's age and her rising FSH levels, the couple agreed that addressing Bill's impotence was not a priority at this time.

The therapist reassured them that reduced sexual desire and episodic, situational bouts of impotence are a common consequence of the pressures experienced during the course of dealing with infertility and medical treatment (Hammer Burns, 2006; Leiblum, 1997; Wischmann, 2010). Bill and Lynn agreed to pursue sexual and relationship therapy in the future following termination of their fertility treatments if impotence continued to be problematic for Bill. Both members of the couple acknowledged the toll infertility and medical treatment had taken on their sexual pleasure and desire and were keen to invest energy and time in rekindling their sexual passion once the issue of having children was resolved.

Treatment then turned to addressing the couple's reluctance to use the two embryos created with Lynn's eggs and anonymous donor sperm. Lynn wondered about her desire to become a mother and questioned Bill's commitment to becoming a parent again. For his part, Bill said he felt comfortable fathering a child that was not genetically his own, having already fathered two children, but he was not comfortable with the implications of a possible twin pregnancy if both embryos were successfully transferred to Lynn's uterus and resulted in a viable pregnancy.

The therapist created a validating, empathic, and safe space within which Bill and Lynn could talk openly to each other about their feelings and concerns related to their inability to produce a child together. Within this space, Lynn was able to acknowledge that as desperately as she wanted to have a child, that desire was inextricably linked to wanting to have Bill's child. She wanted to be a mother, but not at the price of Bill's having no genetic link to this child. When pressed by the therapist about why she agreed to select a donor as backup for IVF, she admitted that she honestly never felt that they would need to turn to that option—believing that on the day of retrieval, Bill's sperm would be sufficient to proceed with ICSI. She also acknowledged that she was "extremely disappointed" and "devastated" when Bill was unable to produce a sperm sample the day of the retrieval.

In exploring Bill's commitment to being a father again, it became clear that he felt considerable guilt and responsibility for the couple's infertility and for the fact that his impotence forced them to turn to donor sperm. Not surprisingly, given the social and cultural links between masculinity and fertility (Daniluk, 1998), Bill's inability to produce a child with Lynn inevitably had a negative impact on his sexual self-esteem and sexual performance. Bill acknowledged that he felt he "owed it to Lynn" to go ahead with donor sperm as backup during their IVF treatment cycle and with the transfer of one of the two embryos. However, with deeper exploration it became apparent that he, too, was not comfortable fathering a child to whom he had no genetic connection. When challenged, Bill was able to see that his resistance to transferring the two embryos was less about the possibility of a twin pregnancy and more about being a genetic outsider in the family that he and Lynn were trying to create. As is common in cases in which the man's reproductive capacity is the source of the couple's infertility (Leiblum, 1997; Lotti et al., 2012; Wischmann, 2010), Bill took comfort in hearing from Lynn that she still perceived him as masculine and sexually desirable and in knowing that she wanted their relationship to continue more than she wanted to have a child that was not genetically his.

Within six therapy sessions, Lynn and Bill were able to work through their feelings about parenthood and concluded that they would attempt one more IVF–ICSI cycle, using only Bill's sperm. During the 4 weeks while they awaited the start of their next treatment cycle, Bill and Lynn were encouraged not to refrain from intercourse, as a way of separating "work sex" from sex for pleasure (Hammer Burns, 2006) and extinguishing the pairing of intercourse with reproductive failure (Daniluk & Frances-Fischer, 2009). The therapist used hypnosis to help Bill manage his anxiety about his ability to get an erection and provide a sperm sample at the time of treatment. Lynn and Bill were encouraged to select an erotic video and together to practice pairing the video with masturbation—so that Bill could use the video to assist him in producing a fresh sperm sample on the day of Lynn's egg retrieval. Arrangements were also made to use electro-ejaculation as a backup option, should the stress of the situation preclude Bill from being able to produce a sperm sample on the day of the retrieval.

Bill was able to produce a sperm sample, and embryos were created, but unfortunately these did not result in a viable pregnancy. Bill and Lynn terminated their fertility treatment efforts and took time to emotionally recover from their treatment ordeal. As is common when treatment has not been successful, Lynn in particular went through a period of intense grief during which any acts of intimacy were impossible for her for several months after treatment termination (Daniluk, 2001). As would be expected after the loss of a child, Bill and Lynn needed time to heal before they were able to reconnect with their own sense of sexuality separate from the process of procreation.

Approximately 18 months later, they sought therapy to help restore their sexual pleasure and intimacy and to resuscitate their sex life. Basson et al.'s (2005) model of the sexual responses of infertile women was a very useful tool in normalizing Lynn's diminished sexual desire as a consequence of infertility. Bill's impotence was no longer an issue, so treatment was focused on helping Lynn and Bill "explore and indulge sensuality for its own sake" (Leiblum, 1997, p. 163). Sensate focus exercises were used to help enhance their sexual intimacy and closeness while reducing the emphasis on all sexual encounters having to lead to, and end in, intercourse (Hammer Burns, 2006; Wischmann, 2010). As their comfort levels increased, Lynn and Bill were encouraged to incorporate fantasy, massage, erotic films, and toys into their sexual play. Also, they were asked to reflect on the activities and settings that resulted in sexual pleasure before their experience of infertility and were encouraged to incorporate some of these into their sexual lives again.

EARLY INTERVENTION

In light of the often negative, pervasive sexual legacy of infertility and medical treatment (Daniluk & Tench, 2007; Lenzi et al., 2003; Lotti et al., 2012; Marci et al., 2012; Sundby et al., 2007; Wirtberg et al., 2007), early intervention efforts might help to assuage the sexual toll of infertility (Vizheh et al., 2013). It would seem prudent to prepare couples for the potential strain this invasive, time-consuming, and protracted process will likely place on their sexual relationship and to normalize common difficulties encountered during treatment. Psychoeducation about ways a couple can keep their sex life fulfilling and intimate during infertility treatment may help to prevent more serious sexual problems from developing (Hammer Burns, 2006). Although we were unable to find any group or individual intervention programs focused specifically on the sexual health and well-being of infertile couples, it may be useful to offer infertile individuals and couples an adapted version of Brotto, Basson, and Luria's (2008) mindfulness group intervention for treating sexual arousal disorders in women prior to beginning medical treatment. Such an approach, which attends to both the psychological and physiological reactions to the considerable stresses of infertility and involuntary childlessness, would provide a holistic and integrative way to potentially mitigate the sexual aftermath of infertility and can be used with individuals or couples.

CONCLUSIONS

There is no evidence that, prior to a diagnosis of infertility, couples have any higher rates of sexual dysfunction or distress than those in the general population (Leiblum, 1997). However, the stress of infertility and the invasiveness of medical treatments, the physical and emotional investment in having a child, the life-altering significance of treatment failure, the social and cultural associations between fertility and both masculinity and femininity, the shift in the purpose of sex from pleasure to procreation, and the pairing of intercourse with repeated reproductive failures will inevitably take a toll on individuals' feelings about themselves, their bodies, and their sexual self-esteem. The experience will challenge all aspects of a couple's relationship and most certainly will affect their sexual desire and satisfaction. Sexual concerns and difficulties are reported by upward of 50–60% of men and women during medical fertility treatment (Möller, 2001). For many couples, the sexual aftermath can continue to play itself out in their relationships for many years following the termination of treatment (Daniluk & Tench, 2007; Schanz et al., 2011). Mental health professionals must understand the complex layers of the experience of being unable to produce a child and the lifelong implications of permanent involuntary childlessness if medical treatment fails. With time and our support, many couples can heal and move forward with renewed and even deeper intimacy and closeness after infertility.

REFERENCES

American Psychiatric Association. (2013). *Diagnostic and statistical manual of mental disorders* (5th ed.). Arlington, VA: Author.

Araoz, D. (2005). Hypnosis in human sexuality problems. *American Journal of Clinical Hypnosis, 47*, 229–242.

Basson, R., Brotto, L. A., Laan, E., Redmond, G., & Utian, W. H. (2005). Assessment and management of women's sexual dysfunctions: Problematic desire and arousal. *Journal of Sexual Medicine, 2*, 291–300.

Boivin, J. (2003). A review of psychosocial interventions in infertility. *Social Science and Medicine, 57,* 2325–2341.

Boivin, J., Scanlan, L. C., & Walker, S. M. (1999). Why are infertile patients not using psychosocial counselling? *Human Reproduction, 14,* 1384–1391.

Brotto, L. A., Basson, R., & Luria, M. (2008). A mindfulness-based group psycho-educational intervention targeting sexual arousal disorders in women. *Journal of Sexual Medicine, 5,* 1646–1649.

Burns, L. H. (1993). An overview of the psychology of infertility: Comprehensive psychosocial history of infertility. *Infertility and Reproduction Medicine Clinics of North America, 4,* 433–454.

Daniluk, J. C. (1998). *Women's sexuality across the lifespan: Challenging myths, creating meanings.* New York: Guilford Press.

Daniluk, J. C. (2001). Reconstructing their lives: A longitudinal, qualitative analysis of the transition to biological childlessness for infertile couples. *Journal of Counseling and Development, 79,* 439–449.

Daniluk, J. C., & Frances-Fischer, J. E. (2009). A sensitive way to approach your infertile patients' concerns. *Journal of Sexual and Reproductive Medicine, 7,* 3–7.

Daniluk, J. C., & Tench, E. (2007). Long-term adjustment of infertile couples following unsuccessful medical intervention. *Journal of Counseling and Development, 85,* 89–100.

de Liz, T. M., & Strauss, B. (2005). Differential efficacy of group and individual/couple psychotherapy with infertile patients. *Human Reproduction, 20,* 1324–1332.

Derogatis, L. R. (1997). The Derogatis Interview for Sexual Functioning (DISF, DISF-SR): An introductory report. *Journal of Sex and Marital Therapy, 23,* 291–304.

Haemmerli, K., Znoj, H., & Berger, T. (2010). Internet-based support for infertile patients: A randomized controlled study. *Journal of Behavioral Medicine, 33,* 135–146.

Hammer Burns, L. (2006). Sexual counseling and infertility. In S. N. Covington & L. Hammer Burns (Eds.), *Infertility counseling: A comprehensive handbook for clinicians* (2nd ed., pp. 212–235). New York: Cambridge University Press.

Keskin, U., Coksuer, H., Gungor, S., Ercan, C. M., Karasahin, K. E., & Baser, I. (2011). Differences in prevalence of sexual dysfunction between primary and secondary infertile women. *Fertility and Sterility, 96,* 1213–1217.

Keye, W. R. (2006). Medical aspects of infertility for the counselor. In S. N. Covington & L. Hammer Burns (Eds.), *Infertility counseling: A comprehensive handbook for clinicians* (2nd ed., pp. 20–36). New York: Cambridge University Press.

Leiblum, S. R. (1997). Love, sex and infertility: The impact of infertility on couples. In S. R. Leiblum (Ed.), *Infertility: Psychological issues and coping strategies* (pp. 149–166). New York: Wiley.

Lenzi, A., Lombardo, F., Saladone, P., Gandini, L., & Jannini, E. A. (2003). Stress, sexual dysfunctions, and male infertility. *Journal of Endocrinological Investigation, 26,* 72–76.

Lotti, F., Corona, G., Rastrelli, G., Forti, G., Jannini, E. A., & Maggi, M. (2012). Clinical correlates of erectile dysfunction and premature ejaculation in men with couple infertility. *Journal of Sexual Medicine, 9,* 2698–2707.

Marci, R., Graziano, A., Piva, I., Lo Monte, G., Soave, I., Giugliano, E., et al. (2012). Procreative sex in infertile couples: The decay of pleasure? *Health and Quality of Life Outcomes, 10,* 140–146.

Millheiser, L. S., Helmer, A. E., Quintero, R. B., Westphal, L. M., Milki, A. A., & Lathi, R. B. (2010). Is infertility a risk factor for female sexual dysfunction?: A case-control study. *Fertility and Sterility, 94,* 2022–2025.

Möller, A. (2001). Infertility and sexuality: An overview of the literature and clinical practice. *Scandinavian Journal of Sexology, 4*, 75–87.

Nelson, C. J., Shindel, A. W., Naughton, C. K., Ohebshalom, M., & Mulhall, J. P. (2008). Prevalence and predictors of sexual problems, relationship stress, and depression in female partners of infertile couples. *Journal of Sexual Medicine, 5*, 1907–1914.

Pepe, M. V., & Byrne, T. J. (2005). Women's perceptions of immediate and long-term effects of failed infertility treatment on marital and sexual satisfaction. *Family Relations, 40*, 303–309.

Rosen, R., Brown, C., Heiman, J., Leiblum, S., Meston, C. M., Shabsigh, R., et al. (2000). The Female Sexual Function Index (FSFI): A multidimensional self-report instrument for the assessment of female sexual function. *Journal of Sex and Marital Therapy, 26*, 191–208.

Rosen, R. C., Riley, A., Wagner, G., Osterloh, I. H., Kirkpatrick, J., & Mishra, A. (1997). The International Index of Erectile Function (IIEF): A multidimensional scale for assessment of erectile dysfunction. *Urology, 49*, 822–830.

Rust, J., & Golombok, S. (1985). The Golombok–Rust Inventory of Sexual Satisfaction (GRISS). *British Journal of Clinical Psychology, 24*, 63–64.

Schanz, S., Reimer, T., Eichner, M., Hautzinger, M., Hafner, H. M., & Fierlbeck, G. (2011). Long-term life and partnership satisfaction in infertile patients: A 5-year longitudinal study. *Fertility and Sterility, 96*, 416–421.

Schmidt, L., Holstein, B., Christensen, U., & Boivin, J. (2005). Does infertility cause marital benefit?: An epidemiological study of 2250 women and men in fertility treatment. *Patient Education and Counseling, 59*, 244–251.

Shindel, A. W., Nelson, C. J., Naughton, C. K., Ohebshalom, M., & Mulhall, J. P. (2008). Sexual function and quality of life in the male partner of infertile couples: Prevalence and correlates of dysfunction. *Journal of Urology, 179*, 1056–1059.

Sundby, J., Schmidt, L., Heldaas, K., Bugge, S., & Tanbo, T. (2007). Consequences of IVF among women: 10 years post-treatment. *Journal of Psychosomatic Obstetrics and Gynecology, 28*, 115–120.

Tuschen-Caffler, B., Florin, I., Krause, W., & Pook, M. (1999). Cognitive-behavioral therapy for idiopathic infertile couples. *Psychotherapy and Psychosomatics, 68*, 15–21.

Vizheh, M., Pakgohar, M., Babaei, G., & Ramezanzadeh, F. (2013). Effect of counseling on quality of marital relationship of infertile couples: A randomized, controlled trial (RCT) study. *Archives of Gynecology and Obstetrics, 287*, 583–589.

Wirtberg, I., Moller, A., Hogstrom, L., Tronstad, S. E., & Lalos, A. (2007). Life 20 years after unsuccessful infertility treatment. *Human Reproduction, 22*, 598–604.

Wischmann, T. H. (2010). Sexual disorders in infertile couples. *Journal of Sexual Medicine, 7*, 1868–1876.

Self Help Books/Resources For Patients

Daniluk, J. C. (2004). *Keeping your sex life alive while coping with infertility.* Available at *www.inciid.org/article.php?cat=&id=263.*

Nelson, T. (2008). *Getting the sex you want.* Beverly, MA: Quayside.

Weiner Davis, M. (2003). *The sex-starved marriage.* New York: Simon & Schuster.

CHAPTER 20

Sexuality in the Context of Chronic Illness

Paul Enzlin

Enzlin tells us "Chronic illness often requires those afflicted, and their partners, to cope with restrictions and/or changes in their sexual functioning and therefore necessarily alters the meaning and significance of their sexual experiences." Enzlin cautions sex therapists not to contribute to the "waiting-room culture" regarding sexual problems in the chronically ill, in which both patients and therapists wait for each other to raise the topic. Whereas much of the literature deals with the sexual consequences of specific illnesses, Enzlin takes on the ambitious challenge in this chapter of providing a conceptual model for understanding the association between chronic illness and sexuality. Noting that not every disease will affect every patient the same way, Enzlin's model identifies sexual consequences of illness that extend beyond the dysfunctions listed in DSM-5. These consequences include substantial changes in both the physical and interpersonal experience of sex. These experiential changes are often accompanied by other significant life changes, making the coping process difficult. Enzlin points out that sexuality may not be a high priority during the early and often intensive stages of treatment; however, at the appropriate time, sexuality may become an important contributor to quality of life. In addition to practical advice and guidelines, Enzlin encourages therapists and patients alike to focus on what is still possible, rather than what once was.

Paul Enzlin, MSc, PhD, is Associate Professor of Sexology and the Program Director of the Institute for Family and Sexuality Studies of the Department of Neurosciences at KU Leuven. Additionally, he is Head of the Sex Therapy Team at Context: Center for Couple, Family and Sex Therapy at UPC KU Leuven, in Leuven, Belgium.

Sexuality contributes to the quality of life for many individuals, and for many couples, it contributes to the quality and preservation of their relationship. However, chronic illness often requires those afflicted and their partners to cope with restrictions and/or changes in their sexuality and so alters the meaning and significance of their sexual experiences. Although sexuality should be an important topic in clinical care, both clinical experience and research show that in medical and rehabilitation care it too often remains a neglected aspect of human health (Verschuren, Enzlin, Geertzen, Dijkstra, & Dekker, 2013).

The association between chronic illness and sexuality is complex. Much of the literature in this area offers descriptions of how and how often specific diseases may (negatively) affect sexual functioning (e.g., Comfort, 1978; Schover & Jensen, 1988; Sipski & Alexander, 1997; Gianotten, Meihuizen-de Regt, & Sons-Schoones, 2008; Stevenson & Elliott, 2007; Incrocci & Gianotten, 2008; Bancroft, 2009; Basson & Weijmar Schultz, 2007; Basson, Rees, Wang, Montejo, & Incrocci, 2010). However, the long list of sexual dysfunctions and problems that may occur in the context of illness makes it impossible to completely review this literature in a chapter of this length (Basson & Weijmar Schultz, 2007; Gianotten et al., 2008; Verschuren, Enzlin, Dijkstra, Geertzen, & Dekker, 2010). Instead, this chapter offers a conceptual framework for understanding the association between illness and sexuality, both broadly defined. This conceptual framework is based on two premises: First, human sexuality is a complex phenomenon involving biological, psychological, relational and sociocultural factors (Bancroft, 2009). Second, illness not only refers to biological symptoms but also entails psychological, relational, and/or psychosocial pressures (see, e.g., Rolland, 1994).

PREVALENCE OF SEXUAL DYSFUNCTION IN PEOPLE WITH CHRONIC ILLNESS

The available data on the prevalence of sexual dysfunction in chronic illness vary widely due to important methodological drawbacks (Verschuren et al., 2010). Research has largely focused on the prevalence of DSM-defined "sexual dysfunctions" (typically disorders of desire, arousal, and orgasm and pain disorders), usually without taking into account the distress criterion of the DSM. Historically, the literature has concentrated on erectile dysfunction (ED), ignoring other aspects of male sexuality and almost completely neglecting female sexual dysfunction. Furthermore, prevalence data are often based on uncontrolled studies that do not use standardized definitions or validated measurement of sexual dysfunction, thus limiting the conclusions that can be reached and hampering comparisons across studies. Importantly, the studies in this area typically address inadequately described populations in terms of degree, severity, and progression of disease, medication use, and psychological adjustment. Most, if not all, of the studies utilize retrospective designs, preventing conclusions about the temporal sequence between chronic disease and sexual problems. Unfortunately, research in this area has probably been hindered by a societal taboo that supports the idea that patients with a chronic disease are not "sexual beings" (Sipski & Alexander, 1997). The continuing dearth of sound research may perpetuate this notion.

SEXUAL PROBLEMS IN CHRONIC ILLNESS

Understanding sexuality in the context of illness necessitates expanding our definitions. Sexual dysfunctions as defined in the DSM do not adequately encompass the range of sexual issues and concerns of individuals with chronic illnesses. In DSM-5 (American Psychiatric Association, 2013), a diagnosis of sexual dysfunction cannot be made if the problem (e.g., erectile dysfunction) is attributable to a medical condition. Medication-induced sexual dysfunction is, however, recognized as a distinct diagnosis and refers to the development of a sexual dysfunction subsequent to the use, change, or discontinuation of medication. The categorical nature of the DSM-defined sexual dysfunctions does not allow for sexual problems to be partially caused by medical conditions or medications. As I discuss later in the chapter, it is unlikely that there is a single cause of a sexual dysfunction in a person with chronic illness.

An important caveat is that sexual dysfunctions and sexual problems may occur independently. To clarify this, we give two examples. A man with diabetes having ED clearly has a sexual dysfunction, but when he and/or his partner experience this ED as very disturbing and problematic (e.g., because of their continued desire for penetrative sex), he also has a sexual problem. A young woman with breast cancer confronted with medication-induced premature menopause and consequent estrogen deficiency that leads to vaginal atrophy and dyspareunia who develops secondary vaginismus clearly has a sexual dysfunction, but when she and her partner enjoy other—non-penetration-based—forms of sexual stimulation, her vaginismus is not a sexual problem. The situation in which someone is sexually unhappy but has no apparent sexual dysfunction is referred to as "sexual dissatisfaction"—for example, sexual dissatisfaction can be due to the fact that the frequency of intercourse is too low (e.g., due to fatigue after chemotherapy), because the sexual contact does not meet expectations (e.g., due to inability to orgasm after a hysterectomy) or because the partner has extramarital affairs. In short: not everyone with a sexual dysfunction has a sexual problem, and not everyone with a sexual problem has a sexual dysfunction, but they can also occur together (Fugl-Meyer & Sjögren, 1999, Fugl-Meyer, Hendrickx, Gijs, & Enzlin, 2012).

The following classification of sexual problems affecting individuals with chronic illness is by no means exhaustive, but it may serve as a starting point for discussion.

1. *Disruption in the experience of sexual pleasure.*
   a. Due to physical factors (e.g., diminished sensation during sexual

intercourse as a result of neuropathy; hypersensitivity as a result of multiple sclerosis [MS]).

   b. Due to emotional factors (e.g., sex provokes feelings of sadness or mourning instead of pleasure and lust).

2. *Disruption of the sexual relationship.* Although the overall quality of the relationship may be only slightly changed by the illness, the sexual relationship suffers from the consequences of the disease (e.g., uncertainty about the partner's interest or desire for sex).

3. *Sexual adjustment problems.* Couples may experience difficulty adjusting to the changes needed for satisfying sex (e.g., a previously passive partner needs to become more active during sexual activity due to his/her partner's reduced mobility);

4. *Practical sexual problems* (e.g., incontinence, fatigue) for which a couple may need help and/or an outside perspective to find a practical solution (e.g., encourage the couple to plan sex at a moment when the patient is most fit and is least impacted by a sedating medication; use pillows or bolsters to position the patient for intercourse).

5. *Disruption in sexual development.* A disease may interrupt or interfere with a crucial stage of sexual maturation (e.g., puberty), resulting in deferred or delayed development of sexuality and sexual relationships (e.g., stunted growth due to Crohn's disease, overprotective attitude of parents during adolescence; Bender, 2003).

A CONCEPTUAL MODEL

Each illness or chronic disease may have a direct and/or indirect impact on sexual functioning and sexual experiences (Bancroft, 2009; Stevenson & Elliott, 2007; Verschuren et al, 2010). The nature and course of the disease will partly determine whether, how and to what extent there will be an impact on sexuality. According to this model, a disease—whether congenital or acquired, whether physical or mental—may affect sexuality by affecting physical, psychological, and/or relational factors. Physical, psychological, and relationship factors also affect the disease in a reciprocal and constantly evolving dynamic that includes treatment and treatment compliance. Each component of the model is briefly described and discussed in the following subsections. A detailed discussion of this model may be found in Verschuren et al. (2010).

Physical Condition

It is important to note that the link between illness and sexuality is not an inevitable one-to-one relationship: Not every patient with a particular disease will have the same problem(s). However, the impact of any illness or disease on sexuality is largely mediated by the impact of the disease on the physical condition of the patient. Disease-specific symptoms can have direct or indirect impacts on sexual function. For example, vulvar or penile cancer will directly affect sexual functioning, as will other diseases that affect the basic physiology required for sexual function (e.g., disease states that affect vasocongestion, such as congestive heart failure or hypertension; diseases that affect the central nervous system, such as multiple sclerosis or Parkinson's disease; illnesses that affect the musculoskeletal function, such as rheumatoid arthritis or muscular dystrophy; diseases that affect hormone functioning, such as prolactinoma). Examples of indirect impacts of diseases on sexual function include general comorbid consequences of a disease, such as chronic pain or fatigue, spasticity, or incontinence. Furthermore, patients are expected to adhere to (prescribed) treatment regimens in order to get control over the disease and to prevent potentially life-threatening complications (compliance). Patients who do not succeed in following the prescribed regimen (noncompliance) run the risk that the disease or complications will worsen, thus exacerbating the disease condition and its impact on sexuality. The treatments themselves may alter the physical condition of the individual and thus affect sexuality. For example, removal of the prostate gland may directly affect the ability to ejaculate, whereas the removal of a testicle due to cancer may indirectly affect sexuality by its impact on body image. Pain, either from the disease itself or from the treatment, may be distracting or may induce severe fatigue, which might reduce sexual desire or even take sexuality out of the picture. When the body constantly needs to avoid pain, the sufferer is distracted from sexual pleasure. Pain medication may also interfere with sexual function, pleasure, or both.

Psychological Well-Being

In this model, it is assumed that a person's physical condition has an influence on his or her psychological functioning, and vice versa. Aspects of psychological functioning with the most relevance to this model include acceptance of the disease, body image, self-esteem, and mood disorders. Each is considered separately here, with the understanding that the effects may be interactive.

Acceptance

The extent to which patients experience psychological distress is dependent on the extent to which they succeed (or fail) in accepting the disease as a part of their lives (McCracken, 1998; Van Damme, Crombez, Van Houdenhove, Mariman, & Michielsen, 2006). The process of acceptance is complex and is not a linear progression to an endpoint of absolute acceptance. Acceptance of a chronic disease is a process in which patients come to accept not only the diagnosis but also the course and treatment regimen of the disease, including expected complications and limitations. Acceptance thus heavily relies on the strength of an individual and his or her ability to cope with the required changes in life. Acceptance has been hypothesized to be associated with sexuality (Rolland, 1994; Sipski & Alexander, 1997; Gianotten et al., 2008). It has been suggested that patients who have accepted their disease may have less trouble accepting the sexual sequelae of the disease and that the absence of sexual side effects may have a positive influence on the acceptance of the disease (e.g., Casier et al., 2008; Jensen et al., 1990).

Body Image

A chronic illness will often give rise to questions about one's own attractiveness (Helms, O'Hea, & Corso, 2008; Walker, 2009). In this respect, a distinction can be made between changes in appearance (e.g., mutilation after burns, trauma, amputations, operations) and changes in functioning (e.g., loss of control of movements in case of spasms), including impairments in basic bodily functions (e.g., incontinence with fear of "accidents"). Given the association between body image and sexual functioning (Pujols, Meston, & Seal, 2009; Woertman & van den Brink, 2012), it is not surprising that some patients and/or partners may partially or totally avoid sexual activity due to changes in body image.

Impaired attraction due to physical changes may interfere with a patient's sexual functioning and also with that of the partner. Factors that disrupt attractiveness (real or perceived) range from small but visible scars from surgery to full limb amputation, from the reduced mobility of an arthritic individual to the rigid movements of a patient with Parkinson's disease or the half-paralyzed body of the stroke patient, or from the increase in weight and sweat of patients who are taking antidepressants to incontinence or a leaking stoma.

For the individual with chronic illness, a diminished sense of attractiveness may make it more difficult to find or engage in an intimate relationship and/or may hinder the resumption of sexual activity in an existing relationship. Patients with distorted facial features (e.g., from muscle diseases, cerebral palsy, or burns) and with speech problems (e.g., cerebral palsy, cardiovascular accident (CVA), throat cancer) feel especially pessimistic regarding their chances to find a partner. But people with less severe disturbances in appearance also believe it is less likely that someone will fall in love with them.

Self-Esteem

In addition to the impact on attractiveness, the limitations imposed by the disease (e.g., immobility, fatigue, pain) may require a patient to surrender some of his or her responsibilities and tasks to the partner, which may seriously affect the patient's self-esteem (Rolland, 1994). Very often this involves changes in social roles (e.g., roles as father, mother, spouse, partner, breadwinner, lover). The need to give up personal responsibilities can provoke feelings of loss of control and cause a feeling of dependence. In these situations, two quite different reactions are possible. A number of patients will continue to embrace and fight for the preservation of some or all of these personal responsibilities, whereas others completely let go and surrender all responsibility and control to their caregiver(s). The fact that one is less able to take up certain roles may give rise to a degree of uncertainty regarding self-worth that may contribute to the development or maintenance of sexual problems. Moreover, when sexual dysfunctions and/or fertility problems result from the illness, more fundamental doubts and questions about sexual identity and desirability may occur.

Mood Disorders

Confrontation with a chronic illness often initiates a grief reaction as patients take leave of their healthy bodies and pace of life and must rethink and/or give up a number of plans they had in their lives. In other words, a chronic disease often compels people to make changes in their identities, inducing a shift in priorities and necessitating finding new meaning in their lives. They must gradually learn to accept what they can and cannot do and learn to live with changed bodies that are less reliable and less controllable.

Patients with chronic diseases often develop mood disorders, including depression and anxiety disorders (Roy & Lloyd, 2012; Walker et al., 2013; Ziemssen, 2009). It has been estimated that depression and anxiety disorders are 1.5 to 4 times more common in people with a chronic disease (Rodin, 2007). It is important to note that the association between illness and depression–anxiety may vary per type of illness and treatment protocol. As depression and anxiety affect quality of life in general, they also affect sexuality both in terms of functioning and experience. Psychotropic medications used to treat mood disorders often have sexual side effects. It will be difficult to tease apart the cause of sexual problems in patients with chronic illness and comorbid mood disorders.

Relationship Factors

In terms of the impact of illness on a relationship, it is important to distinguish between relationships that started before and after the onset of the disease. The individual who opts for an ill partner accepts the "person-with-the-disease." This person will learn from the beginning of the relationship how the disease and its treatment may affect daily life—including sexuality—and can prepare for a life with an ill partner. However, when the diagnosis of a chronic illness is made in someone in an existing relationship, the couple is confronted with something unexpected, something for which no one could prepare him- or herself. From one moment to the next, one is no longer married to the healthy partner he or she chose but to a partner with an illness. This requires from both partners not only some grief and mourning work—to say good-bye to the healthy body and/or the healthy partner—but also high adaptability to the new situation with changed responsibilities and roles (sexual and otherwise).

The extent to which a chronic illness is experienced as limiting within a relationship also depends on the couple's position in the lifecycle. When illness strikes a young person just starting a career and a family, the impact and the adjustment required will be significantly different from those of the retired or elderly person struck by disease (Dracup et al., 2004). The impact of illness on a relationship is also determined by the nature of the disease. In the case of a stable condition (e.g., lower limb amputation), a couple may learn to adapt and may experiment with new possibilities in terms of sexuality. The unpredictable nature of progressive diseases (e.g., multiple sclerosis, dementia, Parkinson's disease, Huntington's disease) is a source of uncertainty for both patients and partners. Progressive chronic diseases create uncertainty not only regarding the timing of the next breakthrough or step but also about the implications of renewed disease activity, such as functional limitations or pain that may negatively influence sexual functioning and sexual experience.

In couples in which one partner has an illness or disability, it is almost inevitable that at least some care will be given at home by the partner. The possibility, chance, or obligation to care for someone may have both negative and positive effects for the patient, the partner, and the relationship (see, e.g., Harrison, Stuifbergen, Adachi, & Becker, 2004). Caring for a partner with an illness involves a loss of personal freedom and time, which may lead to the experience of a "limited life" (Lukkarinen & Kyngäs, 2003). Feeling helpless and hopeless about the situation may lead to depression in the well partner. It is also not uncommon for the well partner to experience fatigue and poor health as a result of taking on additional responsibilities. Partners who are well frequently report that they do not dare discuss their own concerns (e.g., about the drop in sexual frequency) with their partners lest they hurt them. Partners may also stop initiating sexual activity to spare the partner who is ill. Often this leads to a narrowing and rigidity of roles in the relationship, with the role of the partner being reduced to one of caregiver and that of the partner with an illness being restricted to feelings and behaviors associated with "being ill." If this type of polarization occurs in a couple, it may increase emotional distance between them, and a feeling of alienation may arise. Consequently, passion and feelings of sexual attraction may disappear.

Partners often feel anxious when dealing with partners who are newly ill (see, e.g., Miller & Timson, 2004). A heightened sensitivity to the patient's experience of physical pain, emotional problems, and depressed or anxious mood may blind them to their partners' continued sexual interest. However, the well partner's estimation of the situation is not always accurate. A misjudgment of the circumstances or the mood of the ill partner may exacerbate the uncertainty about the best way of interacting. In the long run, this may give rise to conflicts in the couple that may hinder their sexual expression.

Sometimes patients and/or partners use the chronic illness as an alibi or justification to end an existing unsatisfying sexual relationship. Sometimes a chronic disease is the starting point of an extramarital affair. The way couples cope with the changes necessitated by the disease will depend on their relational skills, including communication, social and problem-solving and conflict-management skills. These relational qualities may be protective against the development of sexual problems. The prognosis for sexual well-being is improved when the partner is better able to cope with the consequences of the disease (Brotto & Kingsberg, 2010).

SEXUALITY AND SEXUAL DEVELOPMENT IN THE CONTEXT OF CONGENITAL DISEASE

Typically, people with a history of chronic illness that required extensive physical care (e.g., from parents, nurses, doctors) have learned to experience their own bodies as objectified, sexless, and genderless "things" that must be cared for (by others). In the end, this experience may induce a kind of "learned sexlessness" such that when sexual feelings occur, they may no longer be recognized (Meihuizen-de Regt, Wiegerink, & van der Doef, 2008; Veldman, 2004). Moreover, parents may be more reluctant to promote independence and autonomy in children with chronic illness. As a result, these children may have less opportunity to develop contacts with (healthy) peers, to experiment with all kinds of sexual behavior, or to independently discover the world (of dating relationships). Indeed, a clearly visible illness or disability may lead to uncertainty about one's attractiveness to potential partners and may act as a further barrier to establishing relationships. An invisible illness, however, may also raise uncertainty and questions about when—in a new or growing relationship—it is best to communicate about the disease and its (sexual) consequences. Even if the illness has been resolved (treated, stabilized, or cured) in adulthood, a history of childhood or adolescent illness may affect later sexual relationships.

BREAKING THE CONSPIRACY OF SILENCE

In medical and rehabilitation centers there is often a "waiting-room culture" based on a "conspiracy of silence" between both patients and professionals. Patients remain silent out of shame or fear of rejection. Professionals remain silent for several reasons: fear of not being able to answer eventual questions about sexuality or a belief that it is not necessary to talk about sexuality if a patient does not ask or when the patient has no partner. In the first therapeutic encounter, patients or couples may not readily discuss sexual concerns because the recent diagnosis of a serious illness has relegated sexuality to a lesser priority. Based on their clinical experience, Ramakers and Jacobs (2008) describe four stages typical of many couples. The first is a phase of absence, in which patient and partner are not thinking about sexuality. This is followed by a phase of uncertainty about sexuality (e.g., "What is still possible?"; "What do I want in this respect?"; "Am I still attractive/attracted to my partner?"). The third phase is one of sexual opportunities during which partners try to reshape their sexual relationship. Finally, a phase of sexual stability in which a new—active or inactive—homeostasis is achieved. Because both partners may not progress through the stages at the same pace, it is important to determine whether the patient and partner have the same expectancies regarding the resumption of sexual interaction. However, when the topic of sexuality is raised at the beginning of therapy, both patients and partners will be more comfortable raising sexual concerns when relevant.

ASSESSMENT

In clinical practice, the central diagnostic question in sex therapy for couples confronted with chronic illness is "Which potentially modifiable behavioral, psychosocial, physical, and treatment factors are involved in the beginning, course, and maintenance of sexual dysfunctions, problems, and worries?" In addition to a generic sexual history, relevant questions might include the following:

1. Are the sexual dysfunctions and/or impaired sexual experiences
   a. the direct result of physical aspects of the disease (e.g., ED secondary to Peyronie's Disease);
   b. the indirect result of physical complications of the disease (e.g., paralysis, contractures, spasticity, incontinence, or pain);
   c. the indirect result of illness-related psychological mechanisms (e.g., depression, anxiety, low self-esteem);
   d. iatrogenic in origin (e.g., due to surgery, medication, chemo- or radiotherapy, prescribed behavior)?
2. Are there any other relevant factors resulting from the disease such as physical appearance, cognitive disturbances, impaired fertility, and so forth, that may affect sexual functioning and/or sexual experiences?
3. Were there already disturbances in sexual functioning and sexual experiences before the onset of the chronic illness? (Premorbid sexual functioning is the best indicator of the possibility or quality of sexuality after the diagnosis or treatment of an illness or disability.)
4. Because not every sexual dysfunction is perceived as problematic by patients and their partners, it is important to ask for whom the dysfunction really is a problem (e.g., is the reduced mobility of a patient with rheumatoid arthritis a problem for the patient and/or the partner, who may enjoy being more active?).

Apart from this "narrative" history, additional physical examinations (e.g., to exclude a vaginal infection in the diagnosis of pain during intercourse or to assess pelvic floor muscle tension) and laboratory testing (e.g., to investigate hormonal parameters) may be needed. It is important to discuss the necessity of the additional tests with the patient, as in most cases patients have already undergone numerous medical investigations (Van Lunsen, Weijenborg, Vroege, Brewaeys, & Meinhardt, 2004).

The use of standardized questionnaires (e.g., Female Sexual Function Index [FSFI], Female Sexual Distress Scale [FSDS], Golombok–Rust Inventory of Sexual Satisfaction [GRISS], International Index of Erectile Function [IIEF/IIEF-5], Sexual Self-Consciousness Scale [SSCS]), with a population with a chronic illness is of questionable utility. The psychometric qualities of most, if not all, of these measures have been studied in a healthy population, so there is a lack of normative information for the chronically ill. At present, a thorough sexual history, obtained through clinical interview, is the most appropriate diagnostic tool for the population with chronic illness.

TREATMENT

Validating and Revalidating Sexuality

A distinction should be made between "validating sexuality" and "revalidating sexuality" (Bender & Gianotten, 2008). "Validating sexuality" refers to helping patients whose sexual development was hindered by chronic illness. Often these patients have had little or no sexual experience. Thus, in a validating approach, the aim is to help the patient gain a more positive view of his or her possibilities for relationships and sexuality. The goal of therapy is the development of a positive sexual identity such that the patient may achieve his or her optimal level of sexual functioning, given the constraints of his or her illness (Bender & Gianotten, 2008).

Case Vignette (Validating Sexuality)

Jane was a 24-year-old engineer with the presenting complaint of anxiety about her sexuality. She had never been in a sexual relationship. Jane had been diagnosed with diabetes mellitus Type I at the age of 4. Throughout her childhood and adolescence, Jane's mother was extremely anxious about controlling her daughter's diabetes, as she had witnessed her own mother's health deteriorate due to the same illness. As a consequence, Jane's mother was extremely overprotective; Jane was not allowed to go to birthday parties, to play at friends' houses, or to date. Not surprisingly, Jane often felt lonely. However, Jane compensated for her lack of social interaction by working hard and excelling at school. Being an only child, Jane was accustomed to creating her own world into which she often withdrew. However, when finishing her studies at the school of engineering, she noticed many of her classmates starting to cohabit or even marry, and she "suddenly" became aware of her social isolation. Jane felt sad and uncertain about the possibility of ever having a partner. In the sessions, we discussed her lost opportunity to experiment with relationships and sexuality. After an initial phase in which we focused on her sadness (about that lost opportunity) and anger (at her mother, her illness, and her own lack of pubertal opposition), she slowly came to accept the importance and value of a partner relationship and came to view sexuality as a normal part of life. She felt more confident about her ability to enter into a relationship, even though she was reluctant to have to explain "the whole issue about diabetes again and again." Finally, after 18 months of therapy and discussion about how and where to find a partner, Jane succeeded in having her first relationship.

"Revalidating sexuality" is what is most often recognized as sex therapy in the context of chronic illness. It refers to helping individuals—whose sexual development occurred prior to their illness—overcome the sexual limitations they experienced subsequent to their diagnosis and/or treatment. This perspective is aimed at helping people cope with the changes needed to regain a satisfying sex life. This approach aims at an optimal adjustment to the illness or at finding a solution for a particular sexual concern.

Case Vignette (Revalidating Sexuality)

Linda, age 50, and Peter, age 55, had been married for 27 years. They were referred to me after a follow-up visit with the physiotherapist of the rehabilitation center where Linda had been a patient. Linda was experiencing continuous chronic back pain and fatigue secondary to spinal stenosis. Due to Linda's increasing pain over the preceding year, the couple had stopped having sex, hoping that surgery to correct the stenosis and the subsequent rehabilitation would allow them to resume sexual activity. However, when the couple attempted to have sex, they discovered that Linda had both dyspareunia and back pain. Peter had never had an orgasm during partnered sex without penetration, and so the couple continued to have intercourse—although the frequency of sexual activity declined to once every 3 or 4 months. As they discussed with the physiotherapist, they found that this was "not enough" at their ages, but they did not know how to change this pattern, and they were referred to me. In our meetings, I found that they had a warm relationship but that they were not really able to communicate about sexuality. When I told them that I could understand their difficulty and asked whether they had ever tried alternative, non-penetration-based ways to have sex, a long silence occurred during which they looked at each other in an embarrassed but also cheerful way. In the following three sessions, we explored their options. The couple learned to revalidate their sexuality by focusing on what was still possible instead of on what was no longer achievable.

In order to help couples determine what is still possible sexually, it may be necessary in the course of treatment to:

1. Provide psychoeducation about how this illness or disability may affect sexual functioning and sexual experience (e.g., how diabetic

neuropathy may influence ED; how post-breast cancer aromatase inhibitor treatment may affect vaginal atrophy and induce dyspareunia).

2. Address negative attitudes (e.g., discuss body image issues with patients with a stoma).

3. Help couples dare to take up sexuality again (e.g., invite partners to "experiment" with touching the "breast area" after a mastectomy).

4. Explore how the physical limitations due to the illness can be overcome (e.g., invite partners to "explore" how the vagina reacts after a hysterectomy).

5. Be attentive and seek solutions for relational tensions (e.g., initiate a frank and open discussion about the feelings of loneliness, shame, anger, and disappointment and discuss how they can cope with these (Sipski & Alexander, 1997).

The therapist can provide an overview of the inhibiting factors on the physical, psychological, and practical levels and can discuss with the patient and his or her partner which factors are modifiable (e.g., feelings of attractiveness, anxiety) and which are not (e.g., damage to nerves, movement restrictions).

PRINCIPLES OF STEPPED CARE

In general, when treating the sexual concerns of patients with chronic illness and their partners, it is important to follow the principles of "stepped care" (Van Lunsen et al., 2004). These principles stipulate that the least intensive treatment (both in terms of effort and costs) of which sufficient benefit is expected should be chosen (Van Lunsen et al., 2004). In a first step, patients and/or couples are provided with information and tools that will allow them to come up with their own solutions to their sexual problems. This step can strengthen their self-esteem and avoid overdependence on professional care (Weijmar Schultz, Incrocci, Weijenborg, van de Wiel, & Gianotten, 2004). In the context of illness and sexuality, this means providing information regarding the sexual consequences of the disease and its treatment(s) and about sexual aids and medical devices that might be helpful. In these consultations, attention should be given to the attitudes and expectations that the individual and his or her partner have about sexuality. Patients and partners should be advised that a return to the "normal" situation before the disease is not always possible. How they can and will handle these changes should be discussed, again drawing on the couple's own problem-solving and adaptive capacities. This process of acceptance can be furthered through contact with other patients, either informally or in actual or virtual groups (e.g., Kroll & Klein, 1992; Sipski & Alexander, 1997; Blackburn, 2002; Roszler & Rice, 2007). When these basic interventions are insufficient, a couple may need more specialized help. In a second step, consultations are focused on providing solutions for the specific problem of a patient or couple (e.g., use of a lubricant, specific sexual techniques, medications). The suggestions in this second step are based on the needs identified by a comprehensive sexual history taking. Finally, when the previous interventions are inadequate, more intensive sex and/or couple therapy may be indicated.

MODIFICATIONS TO SEX THERAPY

Patients with chronic illness and their partners may suffer from the same sexual dysfunctions that occur in the general population. When this is the case, sex therapy in the context of chronic illness does not significantly differ from its practice in "healthy" patients. However, special attention should be paid to two important points. First, in patients with chronic illness, multidisciplinary discussion and collaboration is indispensable. The basis for efficient multidisciplinary cooperation is that all involved caregivers know what to expect from each other (Bergeron, Meana, Binik & Khalifé, 2010). It is often helpful to discuss the importance of a multidisciplinary approach with patients and partners so that they understand and embrace its usefulness (Weijmar Schultz et al., 2004). A comprehensive sexual history is not only a necessary condition but also an instrument to help patients and partners to appreciate the interdependence of various factors and thus the need for a multidisciplinary approach. Second, because illness makes sexuality less "easy" or "straightforward," some modifications of standard sex therapy practices may be necessary. For example, it may be necessary to give direct suggestions for overcoming practical problems (e.g., the use of pillows for positioning or sexual toys and aids to intensify stimulation).

Sensate focus exercises used in classic sex therapy (Masters & Johnson, 1970), supplemented with elements from systemic and cognitive-behavioral therapy, are central to the treatment of sexual problems for people with chronic illness. The goal of these homework assignments is to learn to refocus on the experience of touch and bodily sensations and to again dare to explore the body, which has changed and/or reacts differently due to the disease. These exercises often have an anxiety-reducing effect and re-create the possibility of having positive sexual experiences (Van Lunsen et al., 2004). In psychotherapeutic consultations, the focus is often on changing the cognitions that maintain the negative feelings and behavior surrounding the sexual difficulties. Finally, there should be attention given to the relationship and restoring a balance between care and autonomy, intimacy and connectedness.

Medical/Technical Aspects

In the context of chronic illness, the impact of physical factors is often either underestimated or overestimated. Nevertheless, medical interventions are an important element in treating the sexual dysfunctions and problems of patients with chronic illness. Many of the same options for medical treatment of sexual dysfunction in otherwise healthy men and women can be used with people suffering from chronic illness (e.g., phosphodiesterase-5 inhibitors, intracavernosal injections or an erection prosthesis implant for ED). However, it is also important to be knowledgeable about "technical" tools and to be able to give practical advice such as discussing different positions (e.g., due to restricted movement), how to limit depth of penetration (e.g., after a hysterectomy), and when to attempt intercourse (e.g., in order to avoiding extreme fatigue). In cases in which problems with posture and movement occur, advice can be given regarding learning to make ergonomic transfers (e.g., use of a bed ladder that can help turning in bed) and on positions that facilitate sex; for example, after total hip replacement surgery, there is a risk of dislocating the hip when the legs are spread, so the couple may consider using a different position (e.g., the partner with the hip replacement lying on her side and being approached behind). In cases of neurological disturbances, often the area just above the level of the lesion becomes more sensitive to stimulation, so patients may be encouraged to discover these new erogenous zones. For problems with arousal based on sensory deficits or when sexual arousal sensation is below a certain threshold, the use of a vibrator may be proposed. In the case of incontinence, various methods for collecting can be talked about, such as specific absorbent material in underwear or for the bed.

CASE DISCUSSIONS

Case 1

Martin, age 34, and his wife, Kathleen, age 32, had two daughters, ages 5 and 3 years. At the age of 32, Martin was diagnosed with MS. After the initial shock of the diagnosis, the couple decided to seek information about the impact, progress, and prognosis of the disease, including its effect on sexuality. They consulted with a specialist nurse who referred the couple for sex therapy. In the first session, we discussed their premorbid level of sexuality, and I learned that sexuality had always been very important and satisfying for both of them. This helped to explain their interest in sex therapy, as they were not "willing to completely lose this aspect of their relationship." During the initial session, I provided psychoeducation on the possible direct impact of MS on sexual functioning (e.g., less and/or changed sensibility of body parts, fatigue, and in the long run decreased muscle strength, tremor, spasms, and eventual incontinence); the psychological burden (e.g., coping, anxiety, uncertainty about one's own body, roles), and we discussed the unpredictable and uncertain outcomes of exacerbations of the disease and how this might affect both partners differently.

Indeed, as Martin was losing his personal health, Kathleen was losing her "healthy partner" in a very busy period of life (building a family and a career).

Because there were not yet actual problems, we ended the session by discussing the necessity of courage and creativity to cope with potential problems in the future. Once or twice a year, the couple came for follow-up sessions in order to share their emotional uncertainties, to discuss the changes they experienced, and to seek help in finding solutions. During the first 6 years, there were not too many problems, and they were able to overcome most of the issues they encountered, sometimes with and sometimes without therapy. For example, Martin frequently suffered from fatigue and muscle pain during sex. They found they could minimize these problems by first taking a hot shower together in the morning. When the time came that the number of sexual positions and activities had to be limited, the couple was encouraged to continue to experiment and discover what worked for them.

When Martin was almost 40 years old, he began to suffer from ED resulting from the progression of the disease and the use of muscle relaxants and corticosteroids. While I encouraged the couple to find nonpenetrative ways to enjoy and share physical intimacy, Martin became depressed and wanted Kathleen to leave him as he could "no longer be her man." Kathleen's initial reaction was to reassure Martin and to deny the importance of penetration. After some discussion she was able to admit that she also missed having intercourse. As a result, I referred them to a urologist who prescribed a PDE5 inhibitor, which was very helpful.

When Martin was 42, the couple made a new appointment because Martin's physical condition had progressively deteriorated (e.g., walking difficulties, muscle spasms, incontinence). As a result, he had to leave his job, which he loved very much. Martin required more physical care from Kathleen and others, which made him feel insecure about his future and affected his self-confidence about his role as a breadwinner, good husband, father, and lover. As a result, Martin became depressed, and the antidepressant he had been prescribed affected his ability to orgasm.

Kathleen said that although she was taking up the care of her husband with love, she was having a hard time. The combination of a full-time job with caring for her husband and two teenage daughters left only a little time for herself. Moreover, she found it difficult to continue to see Martin as an attractive sexual partner. Martin confirmed that Kathleen was withdrawing from the sexual relationship and that sometimes he found himself snapping at her for no apparent reason. The couple began quarrelling more frequently, and both felt that they had started to lose each other and grow apart. The sexual component of the relationship was temporarily put aside, and the focus was redirected to their relationship.

I saw Martin and Kathleen individually for two sessions each. During the following conjoint session, I facilitated an open discussion of the uncertainties and difficulties both partners were confronted with. These sessions enabled the couple to create a new "we"-ness. Kathleen was able to negotiate some personal time, which she spent with her friends. Although Martin was afraid of losing his wife to someone else, he actually felt loved by her again. The couple resumed being sexually intimate—being naked together, kissing, caressing, and sexually stimulating each other without penetration. They reported great satisfaction with their new connection.

Case 2

Steve and Ann were, respectively, 58 and 56 years old when they entered my consultation room for the first time. He was a teacher in a primary school for children with learning disabilities. He was experiencing burnout and was looking forward to early retirement at the age of 60. Ann was working in the administration of a big company, where she was responsible for several projects, a job that she still enjoyed very much. They had been married for 30 years and had two adult sons, one of whom still lived at home. When I asked them with what I could help them and who took the initiative to make an appointment, Steve immediately jumped in and shared his frustration about the lack of sex in their relationship. Ann looked at him, smiled at me, but did not otherwise react to what he said. I learned that since the first time they had sex with each other—more than 30 years ago—it did not work well between them and that this never changed. Steve was quite frustrated about that aspect of their relationship and was especially angry about the fact that Ann had never been willing to "experiment" more to find a solution. Ann grew up with a very negative idea about sex and could never find a positive meaning connected to sexuality for herself. On the other hand, Steve placed great value on sex, as his idolized father had been considered a "ladies' man." Earlier in their marriage, Ann acquiesced to sex in an effort to be a good wife. However, she never fully participated in or enjoyed the sex they had. After the children were born, the frequency of sex declined to four or five times per year. As Ann aged, intercourse became painful due to a lack of genital (and mental) excitement. As a consequence, her willingness to allow Steve to have sex with her further diminished. This made him even more reproachful and angry at her. Ann felt humiliated by the extramarital affairs Steve had during their marriage, something he did not deny and justified by "being a healthy man who got elsewhere what he did not get at home: love and sex."

The reason this couple came to therapy now was that Ann had been diagnosed with and treated for breast cancer. When I first met them, she was completely recovered from the illness and the necessary treatments (i.e., lumpectomy and chemotherapy). Steve had not pushed for sex during her treatment but now wanted to resume and even increase the frequency of their sexual interactions. In the session, Ann identified strongly as a breast cancer survivor. She said that her illness had caused her to confront the finiteness of life and made her decide that she would no longer do anything she did not want to do. As a consequence, she stopped agreeing to have sex with Steve, and that was frustrating him even more. In the five sessions I had with them, I tried to have them listen to each other's perspectives on their marriage, as well as their sexual relationship. However, their animosity was so great that they were not willing to listen to the other's perspective. Both Ann and Steve felt such resentment and pain regarding their failing relationship that I was not able to discuss any sexual issue or attempt to make a change in that respect. After the fifth session, Steve decided to stop the therapy as "nothing was coming out of it in terms of sexuality." I had the impression that Ann was happy that nothing was or had to be changed in terms of sexuality. Because divorce was not an option due to financial issues, I suppose that they are still "living together apart."

This case illustrates how the premorbid level of sexual functioning is an important factor in determining what is possible after an illness and also how an illness can be used as a reasonable alibi to stop "unsatisfying" sex.

CONCLUSIONS

Despite the growing focus on evidence-based sexology, the scientific evidence for the effectiveness of sex-therapeutic approaches to sexual dysfunction in general—and certainly in the context of chronic diseases—is very limited (see Rowland, 2007, and Basson et al., 2010, for reviews). Nevertheless, as patients with chronic illness are living longer and desiring care that is directed not only at treating the illness but also improving quality of life, addressing the sexual concerns of patients with chronic illnesses and their partners will be increasingly necessary and important. At present, the conceptual model of interacting physical, psychological, and relational factors could and should guide treatment.

In this era of sexual medicine, it seems reasonable to recommend the further development of "medical sexology" or "rehabilitation sexology," in which sex therapists play a central educational, caring, or coordinating role. After all, intimacy and sexuality between partners can be an important source of support in times of emergency, as they may offer comfort, provide confirmation that someone is lovable, be an adequate remedy for pain, facilitate relaxation, and provide a way to cope with difficult and confusing emotions (Gianotten et al., 2008). These are all good reasons to restore sexuality as soon as possible in relationships that are already under pressure due to non-sexual factors.

REFERENCES

American Psychiatric Association. (20113). *Diagnostic and statistical manual of mental disorders* (5th ed.). Arlington, VA: Author.

Bancroft J. (2009). Sexual aspects of medical practice. In J. Bancroft (Ed.), *Human sexuality and its problems* (3rd ed., pp. 381–412). London: Elsevier.

Basson, R., Rees, P., Wang, R., Montejo, A. L., & Incrocci, L. (2010). Sexual function in chronic illness. *Journal of Sexual Medicine, 7*(1, Pt. 2), 374–388.

Basson, R., & Weijmar Schultz, W. (2007). Sexual sequelae of general medical disorders. *Lancet, 369*(9559), 409–424.

Bender, J. (2003). Seksualiteit, chronische ziektes en lichamelijke beperkingen: Kan seksualiteit gerevalideerd worden [Sexuality, chronic illnesses and physical disabilities: Can sexuality be rehabilitated?] *Tijdschrift voor Seksuologie, 27*(4), 169–177.

Bender, J., & Gianotten, W. (2008). Aspecten van seksuologische hulpverlening [Aspects of sexological care]. In W. L. Gianotten, M. J. Meihuizen-de Regt, & N. van Son-Schoones (Eds.), *Seksualiteit bij ziekte en lichamelijke beperking* (pp. 394–420). Assen, The Netherlands: Van Gorcum.

Bergeron, S., Meana, M., Binik, Y. M., & Khalifé, S. (2010). Painful sex. In L. B. Stephen, C. B. Risen, & S. E. Althof (Eds.), *Handbook of clinical sexuality for mental health professionals* (pp. 193–214). New York: Routledge.

Blackburn, M. (2002). *Sexuality and disability*. Oxford, UK: Butterworth Heinemann.

Brotto, L. A., & Kingsberg, S. A. (2010). Sexual consequence of cancer survivorship. In L. B. Stephen, C. B. Risen, & S. E. Althof (Eds.), *Handbook of clinical sexuality for mental health professionals* (pp. 329–347). New York: Routledge.

Casier, A., Goubert, L., Huse, D., Theunis, M., Franckx, H., Robberecht, E., et al. (2008). The role of acceptance in psychological functioning in adolescents with cystic fibrosis: A preliminary study. *Psychology and Health, 23*(5), 629–638.

Comfort, A. (Ed.). (1978). *Sexual consequences of disability*. Philadelphia: Stickley.

Dracup, K., Evangelista, L. S., Doering, L., Tullman, D., Moser, D. K., & Hamilton, M. (2004). Emotional well-being in spouses of patients with advanced heart failure. *Heart and Lung: The Journal of Critical Care, 33*(6), 354.

Fugl-Meyer, A., & Sjogren, K. (1999). Sexual disabilities, problems and satisfaction in 18–74 year old Swedes. *Scandinavian Journal of Sexology, 2*, 79.

Gianotten, W. L., Meihuizen-de Regt, M. J., & Sons-Schoones, N. (2008). *Seksualiteit bij ziekte en lichamelijke beperking* [Sexuality in illness and physical disability]. Assen, The Netherlands: Van Gorcum.

Harrison, T., Stuifbergen, A., Adachi, E., & Becker, H. (2004). Marriage, impairment, and acceptance in persons with multiple sclerosis. *Western Journal of Nursing Research, 26*(3), 266–285.

Helms, R. L., O'Hea, E. L., & Corso, M. (2008). Body image issues in women with breast cancer. *Psychology, Health and Medicine, 13*(3), 313–325.

Hendrickx, L., Gijs, L., & Enzlin, P. (2013). Distress, sexual dysfunctions and DSM: Dialogue at cross purposes? *Journal of Sexual Medicine. 10*(3), 630–641.

Incrocci, L., & Gianotten, W. L. (2008). Disease and sexuality. In D. L. Rowland & L. Incrocci (Eds.), *Handbook of sexual and gender identity disorders* (pp. 284–324). Hoboken, NJ: Wiley.

Jensen, P., Jensen, S. B., Sørensen, P. S., Bjerre, B. D., Rizzi, D. A., Sørensen, A. S., et al. (1990). Sexual dysfunction in male and female patients with epilepsy: A study of 86 outpatients. *Archives of Sexual Behavior, 19*(1), 1–14.

Kroll, K., & Klein, E. L. (1992). *Enabling romance: A guide to love, sex and relationships for the disabled*. New York: Harmony Books.

Lukkarinen, H., & Kyngäs, H. (2003). Experiences of the onset of coronary artery disease in a spouse. *European Journal of Cardiovascular Nursing, 2*(3), 189–194.

Masters, W. H., & Johnson, V. E. (1970). *Human sexual inadequacy*. Boston: Little, Brown.

McCracken, L. M. (1998). Learning to live with the pain: Acceptance of pain predicts adjustment in persons with chronic pain. *Pain, 74*, 21–27.

Meihuizen-de Regt, M. J., Wiegerink, D. J. H. G., & van der Doef, S. (2008). De psychoseksuele ontwikkeling en beleving verstoord [The psychosexual development and experience disturbed]. In W. L. Gianotten, M. J. Meihuizen-de Regt, & N. van Son-Schoones (Eds.), *Seksualiteit bij ziekte en lichamelijke beperking* (pp. 154–164). Assen, The Netherlands: Van Gorcum.

Miller, J., & Timson, D. (2004). Exploring the experiences of partners who live with a chronic low back pain sufferer. *Health and Social Care in the Community, 12*(1), 34–42.

Pujols, Y., Meston, C. M., & Seal, B. N. (2009). The association between sexual satisfaction and body image in women. *Journal of Sexual Medicine, 7*(2, Pt. 2), 905–916.

Ramakers, M. J., & Jacobs, E. A. M. (2008). Bevordering van seksuele gezondheid [Improvement of sexual health]. In W. L. Gianotten, M. J. Meihuizen-de Regt, & N. van Son-Schoones (Eds.), *Seksualiteit bij ziekte en lichamelijke beperking* (pp. 127–134). Assen, The Netherlands: Van Gorcum.

Rodin, G., Nolan, R. P., & Katz, M. R. (2007). Depression. In J. L. Levenson (Ed.), *The American Psychiatric Publishing textbook of psychosomatic medicine* (pp. 193–218). Washington, DC: American Psychiatric Publishing.

Rolland, J. (1994). *Families, illness, and disability: An integrative treatment model.* New York: Basic Books.

Roszler, J., & Rice, D. (2007). *Sex and diabetes: For him and her.* New York: American Diabetes Association.

Rowland, D. L. (2007). Will medical solutions to sexual problems make sexological care and science obsolete? *Journal of Sex and Marital Therapy, 33*(5), 385–397.

Roy, T., & Lloyd, C. E. (2012). Epidemiology of depression and diabetes: A systematic review. *Journal of Affective Disorders, 142*, S8–S21.

Schover, L. R., & Jensen, S. B. (1988). *Sexuality and chronic illness: A comprehensive approach.* New York: Guilford Press.

Sipski, M., & Alexander, C. (1997). Impact of disability or chronic illness on sexual function. In *Sexual function in people with disability and chronic illness: A health professional's guide* (pp. 3–12). Gaithersburg, MD: Aspen.

Stevenson, R. W. D., & Elliott, S. L. (2007). Sexuality and illness. In S. R. Leiblum (Ed.), *Principles and practice of sex therapy* (4th ed., pp. 313–349). New York: Guilford Press.

Van Damme, S., Crombez, G., Van Houdenhove, B., Mariman, A., & Michielsen, W. (2006). Well-being in patients with chronic fatigue syndrome: The role of acceptance. *Journal of Psychosomatic Research, 61*, 595–599.

Van Lunsen, R., Weijenborg, P., Vroege, J., Brewaeys, A., & Meinhardt, W. (2004). Diagnostiek in interventies [Diagnostics in interventions]. In L. Gijs, W. Gianotten, I. Vanwesenbeeck, & P. Weijenborg (Eds.), *Seksuologie* (pp. 333–357). Houten, The Netherlands: Bohn Stafleu Von Loghum.

Veldman, F. (2004). *Haptonomie, amour et raison.* Paris: Presse Universitaire de France.

Verschuren, J. E., Enzlin, P., Dijkstra, P. U., Geertzen, J. H., & Dekker, R. (2010). Chronic disease and sexuality: A generic conceptual framework. *Journal of Sex Research, 47*(2–3), 153–170.

Verschuren, J. E., Enzlin, P., Geertzen, J. H., Dijkstra, P. U., & Dekker, R. (2013).

Sexuality in people with a lower limb amputation: A topic too hot to handle? *Disability and Rehabilitation, 35*(20), A698–A706.

Walker, A. (2009). The role of body image in pediatric illness: Therapeutic challenges and opportunities. *American Journal of Psychotherapy, 63*(4), 363.

Walker, J., Holm Hansen, C. H., Martin, P., Sawhney, A., Thekkumpurath, P., Beale, C., et al. (2013). Prevalence of depression in adults with cancer: A systematic review. *Annals of Oncology, 24*(4), 895–900.

Weijmar Schultz, W., Incrocci, L., Weijenborg, P., van de Wiel, H., & Gianotten, W. (2004). Ziekte, handicap en medische interventies [Illness, handicap and medical interventions]. In L. Gijs, W. Gianotten, I. Vanwesenbeeck, & P. Weijenborg (Eds.), *Seksuologie* (pp. 533–559). Houten, The Netherlands: Bohn Stafleu Von Loghum.

Woertman, L., & van den Brink, F. (2012). Body image and female sexual functioning and behavior: A review. *Journal of Sex Research, 49*(2–3), 184–211.

Ziemssen, T. (2009). Multiple sclerosis beyond EDSS: Depression and fatigue. *Journal of the Neurological Sciences, 277*, S37–S41.

CHAPTER 21

Sexuality and Disability

A Disability-Affirmative Approach to Sex Therapy

Linda R. Mona, Maggie L. Syme, and Rebecca P. Cameron

Mona and her coauthors exhort sex therapists to increase their level of "disability-related cultural competence" because "people with disabilities have become the largest minority group in the world." Viewing disability as a cultural issue challenges the traditional medical approach, which has conceptualized it as a condition that exists within an individual—that is, the problem is the dis-abled body. In this chapter, disability is framed as the product of an individual impairment interacting with the limitations of the social and physical environment. Effective treatment of sexual problems among people with disabilities will therefore target both the individual and the environment. Physical factors associated with sexually related disability may include pain, discomfort, reduced sensory response, and limited mobility. Sex toys and other assistive devices might be useful in overcoming these limitations. Socioenvironmental factors that need to be challenged in therapy include ableist models of beauty or societal expectations of asexuality in the disabled. Cooperation with other health care providers will likely be necessary. Above all, Mona and her colleagues challenge us to view sexual pleasure as a universal right, not a privilege of the able-bodied.

The number of authors was limited to three by editorial guidelines. However, the following individuals contributed significantly to this chapter: Colleen Clemency Cordes, Sarah S. Fraley, Linda R. Baggett, Kimberly Smith, and Vincenzo G. Roma.

Linda R. Mona, PhD, is a licensed clinical psychologist who serves as the Director of Psychology Postdoctoral Training at the VA Long Beach Healthcare System. Her research and clinical work focuses on providing sexual health education and psychotherapy services for people with disabilities. Dr. Mona has received numerous nationally based awards for her work focusing on sexuality and disability, in addition to publishing over 50 articles in academic-related publications and delivering over 100 workshops and seminars on this topic. She received her doctorate in Clinical Psychology from Georgia State University in 1998.

Maggie L. Syme, PhD, MPH, is a Research Assistant Professor at San Diego State University. Her research examines older adult sexuality and focuses on sexual consent capacity in an aging population and sexual well-being across the lifespan. She received her doctorate in Counseling Psychology from the University of Kansas in 2009 and her master's in Public Health from San Diego State University in 2012.

Rebecca P. Cameron, PhD, is Professor of Psychology at California State University, Sacramento, and a licensed psychologist in California. Her research and scholarly interests include the relationships of stress and social support to psychological, physical, and sexual well-being among diverse populations. She received her doctorate in Clinical Psychology from Kent State University in 1997.

People with disabilities (PWD) have become the largest minority group in the world, with the number of PWD increasing to approximately 10% of the world's population (World Health Organization [WHO], 2011). Thus PWD are no longer a specialty population of care but instead a group of clients to whom clinicians are likely already providing services. Over the past decade, the experience of disability has begun to be conceptualized as more than a medical condition. Clinicians now readily see disability as a multicultural variable important in the assessment and treatment of sexual health issues. Understanding disability as a minority experience invites clinicians to utilize a cultural strengths-based model for working with PWD.

As this shift in perspective occurs around disability, people living with impairments are increasingly understood to be limited by social and environmental constraints that interact with their individual characteristics—physical, mental, or psychiatric conditions—to produce disablement (WHO, 2011; National Institute on Disability and Rehabilitation Research [NIDRR], 1999). This socioecological view values person-centered interactions and calls for changes to the traditional approach to diagnosis, assessment, and treatment planning in sex therapy.

The prevailing view of sexuality in our society has been limited, dominated by a heterocentric, ableist definition that best parallels a medical model of disability (Olkin, 1999). A more expansive definition of sexuality that includes disability-relevant variations in sexual expression and incorporates a broader range of sensual experience is needed. In addition, any conceptualization of sexuality among PWD should incorporate an inclusive understanding of the intersection of multiple identities relevant to PWD (e.g., addressing the experiences of people of color; lesbian, gay, bisexual, and transgender [LGBT] individuals). A diversity framework provides a cultural lens through which to view sexuality for PWD and their families, partners, and caregivers (Higgins, 2010) and encourages those providing services for PWD to move beyond difference to create an atmosphere of inclusion.

Providers may feel some trepidation about treating PWD, as it is common to question existing skills in novel situations. It is important for sexual health clinicians to keep in mind that the nature of their work necessitates tolerance for discomfort and the ability to address topics that may be experienced as taboo. Increasing one's level of disability-related cultural competence is crucial for successful treatment outcomes with PWD. This chapter addresses the experiences of PWD and provides strategies that clinicians can use in working with their clients with disabilities.

CULTURE OF DISABILITY

Disability has historically been represented variously as a moral consequence, a source of shame, a medical anomaly, or a tragic condition associated with the need for rehabilitation. As interpretations of disability have evolved, a medical and eventually sociomedical–rehabilitative viewpoint emerged (Mona, Cameron, & Fuentes, 2006). Both of these approaches locate disability within the individual, and both regard the disabling condition as an affliction that separates the PWD from "normal" functioning. In contrast, the social model of disability emphasizes the strengths of PWD (e.g., humor, acceptance of variation, a matter-of-fact orientation toward assistance, tolerance for unpredictability and ambiguity, a flexible, adaptive approach to tasks; Gill, 1995) and identifies the physical and social barriers that obstruct PWD's ability to thrive.

In 1999, the NIDRR's new paradigm of disability was introduced, which attempts to bridge both individual-level and environmental-level conceptualizations of disability (NIDDR, 1999) by framing disability as the product of impairment possessed by the individual *interacting with* the limitations of the environment. Accordingly, there has been a shift toward viewing PWD as persons existing in interpersonal, social, political, and environmental contexts that vary in how much they enable or disable people with widely variable functional statuses (Mona et al., 2006). By considering multiple levels, clinicians become more effective in identifying treatment foci, in advocating for and empowering clients, and in engaging the client's strengths in the treatment process.

Once we begin to consider disability from a multiplicity of perspectives, both the importance and complexity of sexual expression for PWD become more visible. Sexual expression need not be defined by sexual majority or nondisabled norms. Challenges facing PWD in achieving sexual expression are no longer purely a function of medical condition, and goals for sexual expression become more open to creative discovery rather than convention. Importantly, when the experiences of PWD are viewed from the perspective of healthy functioning and resilience, sexual expression begins to be seen as a right versus a privilege and barriers to sexual expression crystallize as problems rather than natural, expected sequelae of individual inadequacy.

Case Vignette

Consider Don and Jodi, a heterosexual couple in their 40s, who had a creative, nontraditional sexual script. Jodi, who had lived with cerebral palsy since birth, met Don, a nondisabled man, while on a cruise 7 years before. Don described their sex life as "different and yet very satisfying." Before meeting Jodi, Don had experienced sexual interactions only with nondisabled women. Early in their sexual relationship, they found that engaging in penile–vaginal intercourse was difficult for Jodi due to significant leg muscle spasms that at times prevented her from opening up her pelvic area. After exploring alternative positions, the couple decided to shift their focus away from intercourse to other sexual activities. To gain support and information, they consulted a sex therapist to address adaptive sexual techniques. The therapist challenged the couple's beliefs about penile–vaginal intercourse being the only "grand finale" activity and focused them on creating non-penile–vaginal intercourse activities, such as vaginal penetration with fingers or sexual toys, in positions that lessened Jodi's leg spasms. Also, they experimented with oral sexual activity, with Jodi remaining in a sitting position while she provided oral and manual stimulation for Don. They began to focus on the fun and creative aspect of enhancing their sexual repertoire and were able to mourn the loss of their prior sexual expectations. Don and Jodi continued experimenting with their sexual script by using positioning cushions and massage to decrease the potential of Jodi's leg spasms. These mutually pleasing intimate experiences helped increase and maintain the couple's sexual well-being.

Sexual Health Care

Accessing quality sexual health care is difficult for many PWD. Given the multifaceted needs of PWD, the emphasis has been on the utility of interdisciplinary care (Collins, Hewson, Munger, & Wade, 2010; Walker, 2008). However, sexual health care and sex therapy are often specialty services that require an outside referral. Sexual health clinicians are uniquely positioned to provide care to PWD, as issues of sexuality and sexual activity for PWD are often overlooked by medical providers, due in part to discomfort (Rubin, 2005; Walker, 2008).

Additional challenges to quality care include environmental and structural limitations that impede access to sexual and reproductive health care (e.g., pap smears, colorectal and prostate exams, labor and delivery services) and attitudinal and informational barriers, all of which may lead to misconceptions and insensitivities about patient needs (Prilleltensky, 2003; Rubin, 2005; Schopp, Sanford, Hagglund, Gay, & Coatney, 2002). Also, the prototypical 15-minute appointment may not be appropriate for PWD, as they may require more time to undress for an exam or additional time during the appointment to accommodate necessary changes in positioning to alleviate pain (Piotrowski & Snell, 2007). Advocacy for appropriate and timely sexual health care may be a key role for sexual health clinicians, and this can be addressed by researching disability-informed resources in the local health care system, providing that information to PWD, empowering clients to advocate for their own care, and educating providers on improving accessibility to clinical settings (e.g., making architectural modifications, repositioning furniture, making materials available in a variety of formats).

DIAGNOSTIC AND ASSESSMENT CONSIDERATIONS

Diagnostic Considerations

The clinician does not diagnose in a cultural vacuum but in a society in which PWD are often marginalized, thought of as asexual, and otherwise stigmatized within a culture that is highly ableist about sexuality. Sexual health care is dominated by the biomedical model, which results in diagnostic categories that are based on deficits in the sexual response cycle (Olkin, 1999). Clients with disabilities may experience changes in the sexual response cycle; these changes may be disability-linked or independent of disability, and they may or may not be appropriate targets of treatment. The physiological deficits inherent in a specific disability may overshadow key psychosexual and relationship-oriented symptoms that need to be addressed. Clinicians diagnose sexual disorders for PWD in order to assist in the pursuit of interventions that may improve quality of life (e.g., designating an issue as worthy of clinical attention rather than an expected consequence of disability), but we need to exercise caution to avoid misdiagnosis, overdiagnosis, and overpathologizing.

DSM-5

When utilizing the fifth edition of the *Diagnostic and Statistical Manual of Mental Disorders* (DSM-5; American Psychiatric Association, 2013) for diagnosis of sexual disorders, keep in mind that this calls for a careful attention to symptoms in PWD that may be either related to a specific disability—not necessarily a sexual disorder—or due to societal assumptions about PWD. For example, the new diagnostic categories related to lack of interest in sexual activities—both female sexual interest/arousal disorder and male hypoactive sexual desire disorder—are based on symptoms (low sexual desire) that are commonly attributed to PWD due to societal myths that they are asexual and lack sexual desire (Olkin, 1999). Furthermore, heightened awareness of negative sexual stereotypes about PWD in women with disabilities (WWD) has been linked to low sexual desire (Nosek, Howland, Rintala, Young, & Chanpong, 2001). Thus clinicians need to consider the impact of biases about sexuality in PWD in order to avoid misunderstanding and misdiagnosis.

Of note, the current criteria for the sexual disorders in DSM-5 incorporate consideration of medical contributions, which do not specifically delineate but would include disabilities. Although the sexual disorders do not specifically include medical specifiers, each sexual disorder describes the importance of taking into account medical contributions to symptoms (e.g., sexual pain, low desire), which may be particularly important when diagnosing PWD. Clinicians should also recognize that PWD may not be best served by emphasizing erection/penetration/orgasm-focused sexual activities. Attending to the cultural and contextual situations in which sexual symptoms are manifested is key.

Assessment Considerations

Approach

In assessing sexual difficulties among PWD, clinicians need to attend to an array of factors beyond symptomatology or diagnosis. We also need to be mindful of our own potential for bias toward negative or dismissive attitudes about sexuality of PWD that can arise from a cultural milieu that stigmatizes and often infantilizes PWD. Maintaining an empowering, sex-positive stance will help to build rapport and guide assessment toward sources of resilience and creativity that may aid treatment efforts.

Tools

Clinical tools specifically for assessment of sexuality among PWD have not been well-developed. However, there are tools that can be adapted and utilized to facilitate a thorough clinical history, presenting concerns, and relevant contextual influences that provide a comprehensive conceptualization of sexuality for the client with a disability. Zeiss, Zeiss, and Davies (1999) offer a model of interview-based assessment of sexual functioning for older adults, expanded on by Mona and colleagues (2010). This model lends itself well to adaptation for use with PWD due to its comprehensiveness and sensitivity to diversity factors and to the ways in which these intersect with sexual concerns. Zeiss and colleagues (1999) emphasize creating an alliance through sensitivity to the client's comfort and readiness to discuss sexual concerns. They provide a framework that includes an in-depth approach to gathering background information, sexual functioning across the sexual response cycle, and relevant beliefs, goals, and behaviors. Traditional existing measures for sexual functioning may be useful in the assessment process with PWD; however, the clinician should be mindful of the population the measure was developed for, the existing norms available, and inherent biases that may exist in these measures. For example, the Female Sexual Functioning Index (FSFI; Rosen et al., 2000) assesses several areas of functioning (desire, arousal, lubrication, orgasm, satisfaction, and pain) with a clinical cutoff suggested to be indicative of dysfunction. However, it was normed on nondisabled women, and though it provides very useful information about potential sexual difficulties, using the clinical cutoff for diagnostic purposes should be approached with caution, as scores may be inflated due to symptoms that can be related to a physical or sensory disability (e.g., inability to orgasm, sexual pain, low desire).

Content

When conducting a comprehensive clinical interview, clinicians should consider the unique physiological, behavioral, cognitive, psychological, sociorelational, and cultural aspects of sexuality and intimacy to form a comprehensive conceptualization of sexual health and well-being of PWD. The following sections discuss these areas, providing a foundation for understanding of key issues of sexuality for PWD and informing the clinical interview.

PHYSIOLOGICAL FACTORS

Although the physiological nature of a person's disability is relevant to her or his sexual experiences, it is important to note that its impact is not essentially negative and that it does not inherently inhibit the potential for sexual enjoyment (Chance, 2002). The willingness of PWD to look beyond traditional cultural emphases on heterosexual penile–vaginal intercourse and instead focus on intimacy as mutual pleasure and enjoyment allows more PWD to experience thriving sexual lives, in the context of any challenges in sexual functioning that may occur secondary to disability.

Differences in sexual functioning may occur throughout the sexual response cycle for PWD and may vary based on the specific nature of the individual's disability. For example, among individuals living with spinal cord injury (SCI), a woman's experience of physiological pleasure related to genital or other stimulation varies depending on the nature and severity of her injury (Mona et al., 2009), as does a man's ability to ejaculate and/or have an orgasm (Cardoso, Savall, & Mendes, 2009). Despite reductions in genital sensation in people living with SCI, most individuals continue to be able to experience orgasm in alternative ways (e.g., through fantasy, stimulation of other body parts, use of erotic imagery), though the experience may be different than it was preinjury (Cardoso et al., 2009; Chance, 2002).

Mobility limitations and pain must also be assessed. Understanding the parameters of mobility will inform the conceptualization and treatment process, such as constructing adaptive sexual scripts. Additionally, the clinician should inquire about pain symptoms, which may be experienced during sexual activities as a result of either organic (e.g., inflammatory disorder, urinary tract infection, or other identifiable physical cause), nonorganic (e.g., anxiety and other psychological factors), or both (Clemency Cordes, Mona, Syme, Cameron, & Smith, 2013) factors.

COGNITIVE FACTORS

Research on the sexual lives of PWD has increasingly examined the intimate activities of persons with cognitive and intellectual disabilities (McGuire & Bayley, 2011; Ward, Bosek, & Trimble, 2010). Of particular importance is the notion of sexual consent capacity, the capability for sexual decision making (McGuire & Bayley, 2011; Mona et al., 2010). Much of the focus has historically been on individuals with developmental disabilities (Mona et al., 2010); work is needed to expand the existing knowledge base to individuals with acquired cognitive impairments, such as traumatic brain injury (TBI) or stroke. Deficits in planning and problem-solving abilities, communication, or social skills and changes in behavior, such as disinhibition or apathy, can affect consent capacity and pose challenges to intimacy (Cameron et al., 2011). Although capacity to consent to sexual activities has not yet been defined for PWD beyond those with developmental disabilities, clinicians must be aware of the legal and ethical issues surrounding an individual's ability to consent to intimate sexual contact and the potentially fluid nature of this capacity (McGuire & Bayley, 2011).

PSYCHOLOGICAL FACTORS

Positive sexual experiences for PWD involve psychological factors related to self-image. Body image is of particular relevance to PWD, especially in light of our society's devaluation of the disabled body, which may lead to internalized negative body images in PWD and even to lowered sexual desire in WWD (Nosek et al., 2001; Taleporos & McCabe, 2002). This internalized ideal may also affect how PWD view potential partners, leading PWD to reject those who have physical characteristics that are seen as potentially limiting to sexual enjoyment (Leibowitz & Stanton, 2007). Notably, body image and its centrality to the sexual well-being of PWD is variable and may change over time; thus ongoing assessment is warranted.

Sexual self-esteem (or sexual esteem) is the understanding of oneself as a sexual being and may include a personal evaluation of both sexual competence and attractiveness (Mayers, Heller, & Heller, 2003). Sexual esteem encompasses the cognitive, behavioral, and emotional facets of one's sexuality (Mayers et al., 2003) and is a predictor of sexual adjustment after SCI (Mona et al., 2000). The experience of disability can negatively affect sexual esteem (Moin, Duvdevany, & Mazor, 2009); however, effective coping, such as keeping the disability in perspective, can protect against loss of sexual esteem among PWD (Taleporos & McCabe, 2001).

SOCIAL AND RELATIONAL FACTORS

The current sociocultural environment in the United States chronically exposes PWD to narrow definitions of attractiveness, virility, and beauty. The myth that PWD are asexual contributes to disablement (Olkin, 1999), as this misperception is often perpetuated by individuals closest to the PWD who may actively discourage them from dating (Esmail, Darry, Walter, & Knupp, 2010; Ward et al., 2010). When PWD do initiate intimate relationships, this stereotype may lead nondisabled peers to dismiss them as potential sexual partners (Howland & Rintala, 2001).

PWD also report practical issues as a barrier to successfully dating and establishing long-term relationships. Higher rates of poverty for PWD (She & Livermore, 2009) may affect access to partners by limiting the affordability of transportation and leisure pursuits conducive to meeting prospective partners. Living situations may be constrained by financial concerns and need for personal assistance, resulting in relatively less privacy for intimacy. For example, women have reported having to rely on their parents for accessible transportation to dates (Howland & Rintala, 2001).

For PWD who acquire their disabilities after establishing long-term relationships with partners, there may be a unique set of challenges. In one study examining the intimate lives of persons living with TBI and their partners, role changes and role strain left the nondisabled partner with limited energy for intimate acts (Gill, Sander, Robins, Mazzei, & Struchen, 2011). An examination of the sexual lives of persons with Parkinson's disease has revealed that as the condition progresses and functioning declines, the quality of the marital and sexual relationship tends to decline (Hand, Gray, Chandler, & Walker, 2010). Clinicians are encouraged to work with PWD and their partners to address the unique experiences of partnerships following an acquired disability, as effective communication can be helpful when facing the challenges of a new-onset disability (Esmail, Munro, & Gibson, 2007).

An additional consideration about the relational context is the increased risk of abuse or trauma for the PWD. Research has indicated that PWD, and particularly WWD and individuals with intellectual disabilities (Ward et al., 2010), are at risk of intimate partner violence, with approximately 60% of WWD reporting some sort of abuse (Nosek et al., 2001). When WWD find themselves in abusive relationships, they have fewer options for leaving than women without disabilities, due to lack of accessible services (Nosek et al., 2001). Poverty and its interaction with disability may also affect power issues within relationships, compounding the risk of abuse for the PWD due to challenges in leaving a problematic relationship. Clinicians need to be alert to the potential for abuse, to the practical consequences to a PWD when a relationship ends, and to the difficulties of seeking help for abuse due to lack of privacy, transportation, or other facilitators of help-seeking behavior.

DIVERSITY FACTORS

Viewing disability as a minority cultural experience helps to conceptualize the context of clients' sexual functioning concerns (Olkin, 1999). Assessment should include stigma and discrimination, access to or isolation from disability culture, and degree of identification with values of disability culture. Beyond a disability cultural lens, clients' frames of reference include multiple identity statuses that affect treatment. Hays (2008) developed a useful mnemonic, ADDRESSING, for the key areas of identity. ADDRESSING highlights the need to attend to Age, Disability (Developmental), Disability (Acquired), Religion, Ethnicity, Socioeconomic status, Sexual orientation, Indigenous heritage, National origin, and Gender as domains that affect our experience of identity, social realities, well-being, therapeutic relationships, and treatment goals and processes. Often, these identity areas intersect in ways that are not simply additive. For example, generational status may interact with disability and sexual orientation in complex ways. An older gay male with a disability who came of age during a time of severe intolerance of and discrimination against LGBT individuals may have had a very different history of interactions with his social milieu and health care providers than a younger gay man with a disability. Assessing multiple sources of identity will help to understand the context within which sexuality is experienced for PWD.

Summary

A comprehensive assessment of sexual health concerns among PWD will involve diagnosis when relevant and helpful but will avoid an overreliance on diagnosis at the expense of context and resilience. Culturally competent sexual health clinicians will integrate information about physiological, cognitive, psychological, social/relational, and diversity-related factors affecting the PWD. In addition to barriers and challenges, clinicians will be alert for information about adaptive coping (e.g., perspective taking), individual and culturally based areas of strength (e.g., military veteran status, religious affiliations, ethnic ties), and other sources of resilience that may aid in treatment.

TREATMENT APPROACHES TO SEXUAL ENHANCEMENT FOR PWD

Sexual enhancement for PWD is a collaborative endeavor among health care disciplines to address multiple facets of sexual well-being. Medical treatments have historically dominated sexual health care—especially following the advent of PDE5s to treat erectile dysfunction (ED). However, as sexual health care has advanced, key intimate and psychosocial aspects of sexuality, as well as the need for a more comprehensive treatment approach, have been acknowledged (Basson, Wierman, van Lankveld, & Brotto, 2010; Consortium for Spinal Cord Medicine, 2010; McCabe et al., 2010). The following section provides an overview of the evidence base and recommended treatments for PWD with sexual concerns and offers an integrated approach to sex therapy with PWD that incorporates established and emerging therapies for sexual well-being.

Medical Approaches

The majority of research regarding treatment for sexual symptoms in PWD has focused on medical treatments (i.e., pharmaceutical, surgical), predominantly for individuals with an SCI or multiple sclerosis (MS), leaving much to be learned about the diverse disability community. Of note, medical treatment for sexual concerns in PWD can be very complex—requiring an in-depth understanding of an often-complicated medical history and treatment regimen—and the following treatments are general guidelines represented in the literature.

The clinical practice guidelines for adults with SCI (Consortium for Spinal Cord Medicine, 2010) represent a pivotal move toward evidence-based sexual rehabilitation for PWD. For treatment of sexual functioning, they recommend reviewing the evidence-based options with men and women with an SCI, prioritizing treatment with least invasive option(s), and providing comprehensive resources for the decision-making process (the recommendations are available for download at *www.pva.org*). General treatment recommendations for males with an SCI include testosterone replacement for hypogonadism, PDE5 medications and intracavernosal injections for ED, vacuum devices and penile rings for ED, and penile implants as a last option due to the invasive nature and irreversible damage to tissue. The guidelines for women are very limited, with one recommendation for an external stimulating device to increase ability to orgasm (Sipski et al., 2001). Medical treatments for individuals with MS are very similar to those for individuals with SCI and include PDE5 medications, intracavernosal injections, and vacuum devices for the management of neurogenic ED (Fletcher et al., 2008).

Metatheoretical Approaches

When considering medical and/or psychosocial treatment options for a client with a disability, the clinician should consult evidence-based practices for the particular presenting symptom(s) and keep in mind the unique experience of living with a disability and how that may affect therapy (Sue et al., 2006). Many evidence-based models of treatment are overly focused on individual disease and deficit. However, evidence-based treatment can be adapted to disability-affirmative approaches that emphasize interactions among physical, environmental, and social factors, with a particular focus on the removal of social and political barriers to well-being (NIDRR, 1999; Sue et al., 2006).

Disability-affirmative therapy (DAT; Olkin, 1999) is a metatheoretical perspective that provides a disability-positive context wherein specific treatment interventions can be applied. The DAT model encompasses several components: (1) empowerment and acknowledgment of social marginalization and environmental barriers, (2) appreciation of the dynamic nature of disability, (3) consideration of the medical realities of PWD and recognition of personal coping strategies, and (4) provision of a therapeutic environment that provides affirmative goal setting and an integrated view of the self and encapsulates the values of flexibility and creativity that are prized in the disability community. Embedding established therapeutic practices (e.g., cognitive-behavioral therapy [CBT], behavioral therapy, relaxation techniques) into a disability-affirmative framework will allow for a truly integrated approach that includes addressing the individual's symptoms (e.g., physical discomfort, distress due to lowered sexual self-esteem), as well as the facilitating social and political factors (e.g., inadequate sexual health care, myth of asexuality, ableist models of beauty). Accounting for these multiple levels will aid the clinician in effectively empowering clients and promoting sexual health and well-being for PWD.

An additional treatment approach for working with PWD that can be applied across therapeutic modalities is feminist sex therapy. Key to this type of therapy is the process of addressing and deconstructing socially created messages about sex and understanding that sex and gender (and many would say disability) are social constructions (Tiefer, 1996). Also relevant for PWD is the feminist concept of defining sex in terms of the whole person in the context of a relationship, rather than individual-level terms such as dysfunction, disorder, pathology, or disability (Mona et al., 2009). The feminist conception is an excellent complement to well-established therapies, such as CBT, that challenge dysfunctional cognitions related to sexuality.

Established Psychosocial Approaches: Cognitive and Behavioral Therapies

To date there are no well-defined or empirically established models of psychosocial treatment to address sexual well-being for PWD (Mona et al., 2009). In fact, randomized controlled trials examining the effectiveness of psychological interventions for sexual functioning in general are few and far between, though a small number of studies have illustrated the importance of an integrated approach to sex therapy—pharmaceutical, surgical, and psychological (Banner & Anderson, 2007; Meana & Jones, 2011; Melnik, 2008; Melnik, Glina, & Rodrigues, 2009). These studies primarily address ED and premature ejaculation in the general adult population—on either the individual or the dyad level—and combine the use of PDE5s or other pharmacotherapy with CBT techniques that include communication skills training, addressing maladaptive cognitions, decreasing performance anxiety, and behavioral techniques such as sensate focus and relaxation (Banner & Anderson, 2007; Meana & Jones, 2011; Melnik et al., 2009).

Several well-established and emerging therapeutic modalities provide useful tools that can be integrated into a sex-positive approach to treatment. CBT techniques are foundational to sex therapy (Heiman & Meston, 1997; Meana & Jones, 2011), and, when utilized in a disability- and sex-positive framework, they can assist in the successful achievement of therapeutic goals through increasing cognitive and behavioral flexibility (Mona et al., 2009). For example, specific goals and strategies may include overcoming myths about disability and sexuality via psychoeducation and bibliotherapy, decreasing performance anxiety using relaxation techniques (e.g., sensate focus), decreasing maladaptive cognitions and negative sexual self-schemas, and increasing stimulus control (Nezu, Nezu, & Lombardo, 2004; for psychoeducational resources, see Kaufman, Silverberg, & Odette, 2003, and the National Sexuality Resource Center online at *http://cregs.sfsu.edu/issues/sex-and-disability*).

When working with PWD, treatment goals for attaining and maintaining intimate relationships may include social empowerment, which can be achieved through techniques such as normalizing, validation, Socratic questioning about personal and societal sexual values, and psychoeducation about enhancing sexual enjoyment. Also, the use of cognitive restructuring can help to increase flexible thinking and behavior by replacing maladaptive cognitions with more adaptive ones to facilitate sexual confidence and performance. Increased cognitive flexibility can lead to more creativity and experimentation, as well as a focus on pleasure and intimacy rather than on physiologically based performance. Stimulus control may be particularly salient for PWD, including optimizing environmental (e.g., temperature, lighting), temporal (e.g., time of day, post-bowel and bladder care), biological (e.g., fatigue, painful positioning), psychological (e.g., mood), and interpersonal (e.g., attractiveness to partner) factors to further enhance the intimate experience (Nezu et al., 2004). The emphasis on cognitive flexibility and behavioral skill building may make CBT particularly effective in empowering PWD to enhance their sexual and intimate experiences and relationships.

Emerging Psychosocial Approaches: Third-Wave CBTs

Third-wave CBTs (TWCBTs) such as acceptance and commitment therapy (ACT) have emerged as effective treatments for various presenting problems (Pull, 2009). Though the empirical foundation for TWCBTs is developing, few studies have adapted and evaluated these innovative treatments for sexuality issues (Brotto, Basson, & Luria, 2008; Carson, Carson, Gil, & Baucom, 2004), and none have specifically addressed the use of TWCBT for sexuality issues among PWD. Mindfulness—purposeful and nonjudgmental attention to the present moment—was successfully applied to a small sample of gynecological cancer survivors with female sexual arousal disorder (FSAD) as a psychoeducational and behavioral homework tool to increase desire and intimacy (Brotto et al., 2008; Brotto & Heiman, 2007). Also, preliminary evidence for the application of ACT principles to couples' intimate and sexual lives has been found in a small number of studies, with behavioral and mindfulness techniques such as couples yoga, relaxation, and loving-kindness mindfulness meditation (Carson et al., 2004; Honarparvaran, Tabrizy, Navabinejad, Shafiabady, & Moradi, 2010). Several elements of TWCBT approaches may benefit PWD. For example, ACT utilizes mindfulness, along with cognitive and behavioral techniques that facilitate psychological flexibility, emphasize value-driven behavior, and increase awareness and acceptance. The present-focused, nonjudgmental stance that ACT promotes appears well-suited for improving sexual health.

Sensual Mindfulness

Mindfulness has wide application for sex therapy and may be particularly helpful for PWD (Mona et al., 2009). For example, integrating mindfulness with traditional techniques, such as sensate focus, can enhance an already effective strategy to include the ACT goal of experiencing something fully without defense. A sensual mindfulness approach includes the traditional sensate focus—emphasis on staged practice of intimate touch—and integrates the goal of accepting any uncomfortable feelings or thoughts that might arise during intimacy while intentionally remaining in the present moment (i.e., not looking ahead to increasing levels of intimacy). As intimacy increases—whether that is advancing sexual experiences or becoming more emotionally intimate with a dating partner—the client may subsequently experience heightened distress or anxiety. Mindfulness practice is rooted in a nonjudgmental stance and openness to all emotional experiences, and through practice it can aid in accepting anxious thoughts and reducing subsequent distress and avoidance behaviors during intimacy. As the client continues to practice mindfulness, he or she can become fully aware of present experiences and learn to accept his or her emotional experiences in the face of fear and/or anxiety while continuing to engage in value-driven behavior. For the clinician, mindfulness techniques and meditations can be found throughout the ACT literature, and specific resources are available through an online community at *www.contextualpsychology.org*.

Values Clarification

ACT emphasizes engaging in behavior that reflects personal values and promotes values clarification—the process of articulating and exploring personal beliefs and core values. This lends itself to sex therapy by allowing clients to generate questions about how their values affect their experiences of sexual and intimate relationships (Mona et al., 2009). Examples of values for romantic and intimate relationships may include being intimate and honest, sharing similar interests, being trustworthy, experiencing new things, and being physically affectionate. Examples of sexual-expression values may include being open in sexual communication, being focused on the present moment in sexual interactions, being able to satisfy a partner, prioritizing sexual expression in relationships, and being willing to think broadly about sex and intimacy.

Clients with disabilities may benefit from clarifying their values that underlie sexuality, which can be facilitated by asking questions about sexuality (e.g., "How important is sex in my life?"), relationships (e.g., "What do relationships mean to me?"), and beliefs (e.g., "What exactly do I believe sex and intimacy to be like for me?"). Some attitudes and beliefs regarding sexuality reflect early teachings that may interfere with optimal sexual functioning (e.g., "individuals with a disability are asexual") or may be in the form of negative self-statements (e.g., "I'm not as attractive as other women"; "my penis doesn't get hard easily, so I might not be able to please my partner"). The ACT literature provides several values-clarification tools that may be particularly useful for PWD who are exploring sexual and intimate values in therapy. The following is a brief example of values clarification utilizing the tool adapted from *ACT for Depression* (Zettle, 2007).

Case Vignette

Ted was a 38-year-old divorced white male with a T_{10} incomplete SCI following an automobile accident 3 years before. Ted used a wheelchair, lived in an accessible apartment, and had minimal assistance for activities of daily living (i.e., help with dressing and transferring from wheelchair to bed and bed to wheelchair). He presented for treatment stating that he "hadn't felt like himself" sexually since his accident and was not sure how he felt about pursuing sexual experiences as a man with a disability. He had been casually dating a few different women over the past year, but had difficulties coming to terms with his own sexuality and was not sure what an intimate relationship would be like for him. Ted reported no significant past mental health history with the exception of "being depressed" approximately 2 years before, after he and his former wife were divorced. After discussing his treatment goals, he and his therapist agreed that he might benefit from clarifying his values concerning sexuality and intimacy.

Before Ted was given the values clarification exercise, his clinician provided him with information about core values, differentiating them from goals or feelings, and about the importance of living in accordance with his personal values. His clinician explained that values were what were most important to him—the deepest, most meaningful aspects of his life—and that living these values daily instead of avoiding valued experiences would help him achieve his goals. The clinician assisted Ted with identifying intimate and sexual-expression values through questioning (i.e., "How important is my sex life to me?"; "What do I think sex will be like for me?"; "Do I feel sexual?"). Ted identified the values he wanted to explore as (1) prioritizing sexual experiences in his life, (2) pleasing his partner, and (3) having open communication about sex and intimacy with his partner. The values clarification exercise was explained to Ted. It consisted of nine statements to be asked for each value, and included questions such as "I value this because someone else wants me to," "I value this because I would be ashamed or guilty or anxious if I didn't," and "I value this because doing this makes my life better, more meaningful, and/or more vital," and questions related to the importance Ted placed on the value and his intentions to live accordingly. During the next session, Ted and his clinician discussed his responses to this exercise, allowing Ted to continue to develop his thoughts about his own sexual needs and wishes for the future and to express any worries or distress that arose as a result of this process. Ted affirmed that having an intimate and sexual relationship was a core value of his and that he was motivated to work on relationship goals. Further areas of interest for Ted included discussing the challenges of dating as a PWD and getting a referral to sexual medicine or urology to discuss the physiological aspects of his sexual functioning.

Practical/Experiential Approaches to Enhance Sexual Expression

When conducting sex therapy with a person with a disability, practical issues may emerge as part of the treatment plan, including the use of sexual enhancement products, aspects of sexual positioning, preparation for sexual experiences, self-stimulation, and seeking relationships. An overall philosophical stance that may be helpful to PWD is one of creativity, humor, and experimentation, as suggested by Kaufman and colleagues (2003) in their consumer guide to sexuality and disability.

The use of sexual enhancement products, or "sex toys," is a potentially helpful intervention. In terms of what a clinician might suggest for an individual or couple, several variables might be relevant, including functional or physical limitations, the person's comfort level and desire to try a certain product, and whether or not assistance would be needed for that person to use the product. In some cases, personal assistance services (PAS) or caregiving services can be incorporated to help facilitate sexual encounters. For example, PAS services can be utilized to assist the PWD with preparations, such as setting up a device (e.g., vibrator) or positioning the person prior to a sexual act (Earle, 1999; Mona, 2003). However, given that caregiver assistance for sexual activity may not be readily available to some PWD, sexual products can lessen or change the ways that assistance is needed—or provide additional privacy for sexual activity (e.g., a privacy pillow with a storage pocket for erotica or a vibrator). For PWD, sexual products that provide better and safer positioning (e.g., sex cushions), increased lubrication for women (e.g., lubricating gels), or increased genital or other erogenous zone stimulation for those with decreased nerve sensation (e.g., ergonomically designed vibrators or extender toys) may be useful. It is also important to consider the acceptability of this option and to approach it with sensitivity. Also, individuals who are unfamiliar with the use of sexual aids will benefit from education about safety (e.g., cleaning instructions) and specific goals for use. For a review of adaptive sexual devices, see *www.mypleasure.com/education/disability.*

Physical and functional limitations for PWD may call for increased preparation for sexual experiences and present the need to adapt sexual scripts. This includes attending to bowel and bladder functioning, timing sexual activity to follow regular bowel and bladder care, and making potential modifications in sexual positioning for catheters or other assistive equipment. Also, for individuals whose daily pain levels may vary, scheduling sexual acts during times that are associated with less pain can be helpful but may require a new way of thinking about how to incorporate sexuality and intimacy into a daily routine. It can be helpful for PWD to develop communication skills that involve partners and/or PAS in avoiding or minimizing pain during sexual activity. Experimenting with a range of intimate acts can help a PWD develop a repertoire of options beyond intercourse, such as kissing and skin-to-skin contact, that may be less likely to result in pain (Welner, 1997). The clinician can assist the client by talking through the sexual script, planning for potential challenges, and emphasizing preparation of the sexual environment (i.e., stimulus control).

Some PWD may be concerned with the limited availability of intimate partners. Depending on individual values, beliefs, and goals, self-stimulation may be an appropriate behavioral intervention for PWD with or without available intimate partners. Self-stimulation can be a positive way of expressing sexuality that is less likely to be impeded by physical and social limitations (Fraley, Mona, & Theodore, 2007). Sensitive intervention strategies may include behavioral approaches (e.g., utilizing sexual aids to achieve stimulation), cognitive work (e.g., exploring core beliefs about solitary sexual behaviors and increasing cognitive flexibility about stimulation activities), and experiential homework (e.g., mindfulness during stimulation exercises).

For those who are uncomfortable with self-stimulation or who simply prefer to seek a relationship for sexual expression, identifying opportunities for meeting people may become the primary goal of treatment. Clients with disabilities may seek partners in the "usual" places, including through work, friends, religious communities, and so forth. Others may choose to seek partners in disability-friendly environments, such as events in the disability community (e.g., wheelchair sporting events), in which individuals may be more open to difference. Internet resources are increasingly utilized by disabled and nondisabled individuals looking for romantic relationships (and sometimes purely sexual relationships), and this may be a potential avenue to explore. The internet also affords opportunities to "practice" being comfortable with flirting and talking with potential partners before making a commitment to meet in person. Preparing to meet potential partners face-to-face may include identifying ways to feel sexually desirable, such as prioritizing attractive clothing and engaging in personal grooming strategies such as wearing makeup and using scented products. Given the physical vulnerability of many PWD and the higher rates of trauma and abuse that have been reported for this population (Ward et al., 2010), clinicians should be sure to educate clients about safety precautions when meeting prospective partners.

CASE DISCUSSION

The following is a case discussion of Tony, a composite of clinical and research experiences with PWD presented to illustrate many of the suggestions made here. We suggest that readers consider how they might respond to Tony. What does this trigger in terms of fears, assumptions, values, and confidence level in developing treatment goals and strategies? How might therapists go about developing greater awareness of disability in order to move beyond problematic responses (e.g., pity, infantilization, and idealization)?

Tony was a 27-year-old cisgender Latino male Marine Corps combat veteran of Operation Iraqi Freedom (OIF) who had recently returned from two successive deployments. Tony, working in infantry as a rifleman, fought on the front lines during both deployments. He returned from military service with several combat-related injuries as a result of stepping on an improvised explosive device. This damaged many areas of Tony's body, leading to a moderate hearing loss in his left ear, two above-the-knee amputated legs, and the loss of his penis and testicles. He was triaged for immediate medical care in Iraq and then transferred through a series of treatment sites prior to reaching his local Veterans Medical Center. Tony spent most of the first 3 months after being discharged from the Marines as an inpatient at the Veterans Administration (VA) hospital and then began outpatient medical treatment.

Tony had no history of mental health concerns prior to entering the service; however, he had had a very positive experience with an LGBT support group in his late teens that helped him to be receptive to mental health care as part of his rehabilitation process. At his VA hospital, he met with a rehabilitation psychologist regularly until discharge to discuss issues related to adjustment, adaptive skills, and the use of assistive devices—prosthetic legs, crutches, and occasionally a manual wheelchair. Working with this therapist, he began to address issues about his sexuality and sexual identity in the context of the changes to his body. At the time, however, he acknowledged that he had much to learn about caring for and working with his new body, and sexuality was not the immediate priority.

Approximately a year and a half after sustaining his injuries, Tony decided to seek assistance from a psychotherapist at a well-known LGBT-affirmative psychotherapy practice to work through his adjustment to his genital loss. Tony had selected his therapist because she seemed open and comfortable with his disclosed body changes, as demonstrated by her willingness to discuss ways in which she might adapt her office environment to accommodate Tony's disability-related limitations. Specifically, Tony had difficulty hearing her at first, given the acoustics in her office. She was able to reduce noise interference by turning down her ceiling fan and moving her white noise machine further from their sitting area. She also positioned her chair so that her voice could carry more directly to his right ear and so that he could see her lips more clearly as she was speaking to him.

During their first meeting, Tony stated that after acquiring his injuries, he felt a profound sense of discontinuity from his preinjury life and experienced ongoing uncertainty and worry about his future. He had envisioned having a military service career and felt that being a Marine was a major part of his identity as a man, personally and also within his family of origin, for whom military service was a highly prized aspect of masculinity. Also of increasing importance to Tony were the issues of retaining his identity as a gay man with a strong sexual drive and pursuing his goal of being romantically and sexually partnered with another man. His therapist validated the importance of this disclosure and employed reflective listening and Socratic questioning to encourage Tony to further discuss how his identity as a gay Latino male related to his current sexual concerns. Tony recalled always being aware of his attraction to other males. His involvement in his first long-term sexual relationship in his late teens prompted him to join the LGBT support group that focused on coming-out issues and developing a positive identity. Tony had found it empowering and eventually disclosed his sexual orientation to his parents, who acknowledged that a maternal uncle was also gay and supported Tony as a gay male. While in the Marines, he reported having shorter term sexual partners, finding it difficult to pursue a serious relationship.

Over the course of their work together, Tony readily disclosed his fears about his viability as a romantic and sexual partner given the degree to which his body—especially his genitals—had been altered. The therapist became aware of her own challenges in visualizing a hopeful, partnered future for her client given the severity of his injuries. She obtained consultation and was encouraged to examine her own worldviews further. This was facilitated by a self-awareness exercise her consultant led her through, examining her own identities, personal experiences of being included or excluded, and times she had treated others unequally. This raised her awareness of her tendency to stereotype male sexuality, and it helped her reconnect empathically with Tony's dilemma from a stronger, advocacy-centered position. She also led Tony to identify his own assumptions and values about disability, masculinity, attractiveness, and sexuality. He found that many of his beliefs were still relevant (e.g., "Feeling desirable is important to me"), whereas others required modification (e.g., "Sex should be spontaneous") or needed to be challenged (e.g., "Gay men have to live up to certain ideals of physical beauty and sexual performance").

The therapist did have previous experience working with transgender people and had some knowledge of genital changes and the functional issues that may follow genital surgery. This background helped her detach more completely from a culturally ingrained conceptualization of sexuality that was ableist in its reliance on typical genital structure and function. She found it helpful to draw upon her knowledge of creative strategies for sexual pleasure that her transgender clients had utilized in order to expand Tony's sense of sexual possibility. Fortunately, Tony's sex-positive worldview helped him to be open to exploring sexual activities. His therapist discussed different enhancement options, including sex toys and positioning pillows, that expanded the options for stimulation. Initially, Tony experimented with these sexual enhancement aids in solo sexual activity. Sensual mindfulness helped him to tolerate and eventually reduce the feelings of anxiety that initially arose during sexual activity and fantasy. With practice, he found that he could experience a great deal of erotic stimulation and satisfaction, often enhanced by fantasy of his preinjury or postinjury self. But he longed for partnered activity and to provide pleasure and experience mutual enjoyment.

As he and his therapist discussed the risks in meeting men and initiating dating, Tony identified disclosure of his physical differences as the next challenge in establishing a romantic and sexual relationship. Tony and his therapist role-played conversations in which he broached the topic of intimacy and disclosed the nature of his genital changes. His experiences with dating provided much clinical material for them to work with. At times, they found that leveraging Tony's gentle sense of humor provided perspective and leavened the painfulness of disappointment in those initial encounters. Ultimately, he found that he was better able to identify with men who were less tied to conventional sexual expressions and who might be open to exploring a sexual connection with him. It remained easier for him to connect with veterans, whether nondisabled or disabled, because they understood the risks of combat that had led to the changes in his body. Over time, his volunteer involvement with disabled veterans' organizations led him to connect with other gay veterans, and his outgoing personality helped to attract the attention of some of these men.

By the end of treatment, Tony had achieved many of his goals. He claimed his identity as a disabled veteran, was proud he had served his country, and felt connected to veterans who also had major changes in bodily functioning. Tony's self-esteem was further enhanced as he embraced disability cultural strengths, such as flexibility, humor, and pragmatism. Behaviorally, Tony had developed a sexual repertoire that included solo and partnered activity that was sensuous, pleasurable, and emotionally rewarding, and he was confident in his ability to both receive and provide pleasure. At times, popular media, gay culture, or mainstream assumptions about what it means to be a virile man still caught him off guard, and he felt hurt or angry about the insensitive, narrow portrayals of male desirability. But he would typically regain perspective through talking things over with members of his support network.

Tony benefited from his therapist's attention to diversity and her willingness to modify practical aspects of her therapy and engage in her own learning process. His therapist utilized both traditional CBT (cognitive restructuring and role playing) and TWCBT strategies (values clarification and sensual mindfulness) in the context of a disability- and gay-affirmative approach to psychotherapy. She encouraged practical strategies for developing a sexual repertoire through the use of sexual aids. Finally, she retained a sense of Tony as a person within the context of multiple intersecting identities, rather than distancing from him by either pitying or idealizing him.

CONCLUSIONS

Working with PWD concerning issues of sexuality can be challenging given the unique culture of disability. It involves a comprehensive assessment process that goes beyond identifying biomedical symptoms and dysfunction and includes key areas of concern for PWD and cultural contributions. It culminates in a treatment process that integrates evidence-based CBT and TWCBT with a sex-positive and disability-affirmative approach. Continuing education (self-directed reading, workshops, and consultation) and a willingness to challenge dominant, ableist assumptions are important aspects to working effectively with PWD.

REFERENCES

American Psychiatric Association. (2013). *Diagnostic and statistical manual of mental disorders* (5th ed.). Arlington, VA: Author.

Banner, L., & Anderson, R. (2007). Integrated sildenafil and cognitive-behavior sex therapy for psychogenic erectile dysfunction: A pilot study. *Journal of Sexual Medicine, 4,* 1117–1125.

Basson, R., Wierman, M., van Lankveld, J., & Brotto, L. A. (2010). Summary of the recommendations on sexual dysfunction in women. *Journal of Sex Medicine, 7,* 314–326.

Brotto, L. A., Basson, R., & Luria, M. A. (2008). Mindfulness based group psychoeducational intervention targeting sexual arousal disorder in women. *Journal of Sex Medicine, 5,* 1646–1659.

Brotto, L. A., & Heiman, J. (2007). Mindfulness in sex therapy: Applications for women with sexual difficulties following gynecologic cancer. *Sex Relationship Therapy, 22*(1), 3–11.

Cameron, R. P., Mona, L. R., Syme, M., Clemency Cordes, C., Fraley, S. S., Chen, S. S., et al. (2011). Sexuality among wounded veterans of Operation Enduring Freedom (OEF), Operation Iraqi Freedom (OIF), and Operation New Dawn (OND): Implications for rehabilitation psychologists. *Rehabilitation Psychology, 56,* 289–301.

Cardoso, F. L., Savall, A., & Mendes, A. K. (2009). Self-awareness of the male sexual response after spinal cord injury. *International Journal of Rehabilitation Research, 32,* 294–300.

Carson, J. W., Carson, K. M., Gil, K. M., & Baucom, D. H. (2004). Mindfulness-based relationship enhancement. *Behavior Therapy, 35*, 471–494.

Chance, R. S. (2002). To love and be loved: Sexuality and people with physical disabilities. *Journal of Psychology and Theology, 30*, 195–208.

Clemency Cordes, C., Mona, L., Syme, M., Cameron, R., & Smith, K. (2013). Sexuality and sexual health among women with physical disabilities. In D. Castaneda (Ed), *An essential handbook of women's sexuality: Diversity, health, and violence introduction* (Vol. 2, pp. 71–92). Santa Barbara, CA: Praeger..

Collins, C., Hewson, D. L., Munger, R., & Wade, T. (2010). *Evolving models of behavioral health integration in primary care.* New York: Milbank Memorial Fund.

Consortium for Spinal Cord Medicine. (2010). *Sexuality and reproductive health in adults with spinal cord injury: A clinical practice guideline for healthcare professionals.* Washington, DC: Paralyzed Veterans of America.

Earle, S. (1999). Facilitated sex and the concept of sexual need: Disabled students and their personal assistants. *Disability and Society, 14*, 309–323.

Esmail, S., Darry, K., Walter, A., & Knupp, H. (2010). Attitudes and perceptions toward disability and sexuality. *Disability and Rehabilitation, 32*, 1148–1155.

Esmail, S., Munro, B., & Gibson, N. (2007). Couple's experience with multiple sclerosis in the context of their sexual relationship. *Sexuality and Disability, 25*, 163–177.

Fletcher, S., Castro-Borrero, W., Remington, G., Treadaway, K., Lemack, G., & Frohman, T. (2008). Sexual dysfunction in patients with multiple sclerosis: A multidisciplinary approach to evaluation and management. *Nature Clinical Practice Urology, 6*, 96–107.

Fraley, S. S., Mona, L. R., & Theodore, P. S. (2007). The sexual lives of lesbian, gay, and bisexual people with disabilities: Psychological perspectives. *Sexuality Research and Social Policy, 4*, 15–26.

Gill, C. J. (1995). A psychological view of disability culture. *Disability Studies Quarterly, 15*(4), 16–19.

Gill, C. J., Sander, A. M., Robins, N., Mazzei, D., & Struchen, M. A. (2011). Exploring experiences of intimacy from the viewpoint of individuals with traumatic brain injury and their partners. *Journal of Health Trauma Rehabilitation, 26*(1), 56–68.

Hand, A., Gray, W. K., Chandler, B. J., & Walker, R. W. (2010). Sexual and relationship dysfunction in people with Parkinson's disease. *Parkinsonism and Related Disorders, 16*, 172–176.

Hays, P. A. (2008). *Addressing cultural complexities in practice: Assessment, diagnosis, and therapy* (2nd ed.). Washington, DC: American Psychological Association.

Heiman, J. R., & Meston, C. M. (1997). Empirically validated treatment for sexual dysfunction. *Annual Review of Sex Research, 8*, 148–194.

Higgins, D. (2010). Sexuality, human rights and safety for people with disabilities: The challenge of intersecting identities. *Sexual and Relationship Therapy, 25*(3), 245–257.

Honarparvaran, N., Tabrizy, M., Navabinejad, S., Shafiabady, A., & Moradi, M. (2010). Acceptance and commitment therapy training with regard to reducing sexual satisfaction among couples. *European Journal of Social Sciences, 15*, 166–172.

Howland, C., & Rintala, D. (2001). Dating behaviors of women with physical disabilities. *Sexuality and Disability, 19*, 41–70.

Kaufman, M., Silverberg, C., & Odette, F. (2003). *The ultimate guide to sex and disability.* San Francisco, CA: Cleis Press.

Leibowitz, R. Q., & Stanton, A. L. (2007). Sexuality after spinal cord injury: A conceptual model based on women's narratives. *Rehabilitation Psychology, 52*, 44–55.

Mayers, K. S., Heller, D. K., & Heller, J. A. (2003). Damaged sexual self-esteem: A kind of disability. *Sexuality and Disability, 21*, 269–282.

McCabe, M., Althof, S. E., Assalina, P., Chevret-Meason, M., Leiblum, S. R., Simonelli, C., et al. (2010). Psychological and interpersonal dimensions of sexual function and dysfunction. *Journal of Sex Medicine, 7*, 327–336.

McGuire, B. E., & Bayley, A. A. (2011). Relationships, sexuality and decision-making capacity in people with an intellectual disability. *Current Opinion in Psychiatry, 24*, 398–402.

Meana, M., & Jones, S. (2011). Developments and trends in sex therapy. *Advances in Psychosomatic Medicine, 31*, 57–71.

Melnik, T. (2008). The effectiveness of psychological interventions for the treatment of erectile dysfunction: Systematic review and meta-analysis, including comparisons to sildenafil treatment, intracavernosal injection, and vacuum devices. *Journal of Sexual Medicine, 5*, 2562–2574.

Melnik, T., Glina, S., & Rodrigues, O. M., Jr. (2009). Psychological interventions for premature ejaculation. *Nature Reviews Urology, 6*(9), 501–558.

Moin, V., Duvdevany, I., & Mazor, D. (2009). Sexual identity, body image and life satisfaction among women with and without physical disability. *Sexuality and Disability, 27*, 83–95.

Mona, L. R. (2003). Sexual options for people with disabilities: Using personal assistance services for sexual expression. In M. E. Banks & E. Kaschak (Eds.), *Women with visible and invisible disabilities: Multiple intersections, multiple issues, multiple therapies* (pp. 211–222). Gloucestershire, UK: Hawthorn Press.

Mona, L. R., Cameron, R. P., & Fuentes, A. J. (2006). Broadening paradigms of disability research to clinical practice: Implications for conceptualization and application. In K. J. Hagglund & A. Heinemann (Eds.), *Handbook of applied disability and rehabilitation research* (pp. 75–102). New York: Springer.

Mona, L. R., Cameron, R. P., Goldwaser, G., Miller, A. R., Syme, M., & Fraley, S. S. (2009). Prescription for pleasure: Exploring sex-positive approaches in women with spinal cord injury. *Topics in Spinal Cord Injury and Rehabilitation, 15*, 15–28.

Mona, L. R., Goldwaser, G., Syme, M., Cameron, R. P., Clemency, C., Miller, A. R., et al. (2010). Assessment and conceptualization of sexuality among older adults. In P. A. Lichtenberg (Ed.), *Handbook of assessment in clinical gerontology* (2nd ed., pp. 331–356). New York: Elsevier.

Mona, L. R., Krause, J. S., Norris, F., Cameron, R. P., Kalichman, S., & Lesondak, L. M. (2000). Sexual expression following spinal cord injury. *NeuroRehabilitation, 15*, 121–131.

National Institute on Disability and Rehabilitation Research. (1999). *NIDRR long-range plan.* Washington, DC: Office of Special Education and Rehabilitative Services.

Nezu, A., Nezu, C., & Lombardo, E. (2004). *Cognitive-behavioral case formulation and treatment design: A problem-solving approach.* New York: Springer.

Nosek, M., Howland, C., Rintala, D., Young, M., & Chanpong, G. F. (2001). National study of women with physical disabilities: Final report. *Sexuality and Disability, 19,* 5–39.

Olkin, R. (1999). *What psychotherapists should know about disability.* New York: Guilford Press.

Piotrowski, K., & Snell, L. (2007). Health needs of women with disabilities across the lifespan. *Journal of Obstetric, Gynecologic, and Neonatal Nursing, 36,* 79–87.

Prilleltensky, O. (2003). A ramp to motherhood: The experiences of mothers with physical disabilities. *Sexuality and Disability, 21,* 21–47.

Pull, C. B. (2009). Current empirical status of acceptance and commitment therapy. *Current Opinion in Psychiatry, 22,* 2255–2260.

Rosen, R., Brown, C., Heiman, J., Leiblum, S., Meston, C, Shabsigh, R, et al. (2000). The Female Sexual Function Index (FSFI): A multidimensional self-report instrument for the assessment of female sexual function. *Journal of Sex and Marital Therapy, 26,* 191–208.

Rubin, R. (2005). Communication about sexual problems in male patients with multiple sclerosis. *Nursing Standard, 19*(24), 33–37.

Schopp, L. H., Sanford, T. C., Hagglund, K. J., Gay, J. W., & Coatney, M. A. (2002). Removing service barriers for women with physical disabilities: Promoting accessibility in the gynecologic care setting. *Journal of Midwifery and Women's Health, 47,* 74–79.

She, P., & Livermore, G. A. (2009). Long-term disability and poverty among working-age adults. *Journal of Disability Policy Studies, 19*(4), 244–256.

Sipski, M. L., Alexander, C. J., & Rosen, R. C. (2001). Sexual arousal and orgasm in women: Effects of spinal cord injury. *Annals of Neurology, 49,* 35–44.

Sue, S., Zane, N., Levant, R. F., Silverstein, L. B., Brown, L. S., Olkin, R., et al. (2006). How well do both evidence-based practices and treatment as usual satisfactorily address the various dimensions of diversity? In J. C. Norcross, L. E. Beutler, & R. F. Levant (Eds.), *Evidence-based practices in mental health: Debate and dialogue on the fundamental questions* (pp. 329–374). Washington, DC: American Psychological Association.

Taleporos, G., & McCabe, M. (2001). The impact of physical disability on body esteem. *Sexuality and Disability, 19,* 293–308.

Taleporos, G., & McCabe, M. (2002). The impact of sexual esteem, body esteem, and sexual satisfaction on psychological well-being in people with physical disability. *Sexuality and Disability, 20,* 177–183.

Tiefer, L. (1996). Towards a feminist sex therapy. *Women and Therapy, 19*(4), 53–64.

United Nations. (n.d.). *Fact sheet on persons with disabilities.* Retrieved January 8, 2012, from *www.un.org/disabilities/default.asp?id1/418.*

Walker, W. O., Jr. (2008). Primary care providers and medical homes for individuals with spina bifida. *Journal of Pediatric Rehabilitation Medicine, 1,* 337–344.

Ward, K. M., Bosek, R. L., & Trimble, E. L. (2010). Romantic relationships and interpersonal violence among adults with developmental disabilities. *Intellectual and Developmental Disabilities, 48*(2), 89–98.

Welner, S. L. (1997). Gynecologic care and sexuality issues for women with disabilities. *Sexuality and Disability, 15,* 33–40.

World Health Organization. (2011). *World report on disability*. Geneva, Switzerland: Author.

Zeiss, A. M., Zeiss, R. A., & Davies, H. (1999). Assessment of sexual function and dysfunction in older adults. In P. Lichtenberg (Ed.), *Handbook of assessment in clinical gerontology* (pp. 270–296). New York: Wiley.

Zettle, R. (2007). *ACT for depression: A clinician's guide to using acceptance and commitment therapy in treating depression*. Oakland, CA: New Harbinger.

CHAPTER 22

Suppose They Gave an Epidemic and Sex Therapy Didn't Attend?

Sexually Transmitted Infection Concerns in the Sex Therapy Context

William A. Fisher and Stephen Holzapfel

In this chapter we are reminded that sexual behavior may take place in the context of the risk of contracting or actually having a sexually transmitted infection (STI). STIs may play an important role in the etiology and maintenance of sexual and relationship dysfunction, such as in cases in which an infidelity is revealed through the acquisition or transmission of an STI. Fear of acquiring or transmitting an STI, as well as shame, blame, and guilt, may complicate sexual pleasure and contribute to problems with sexual performance. Fisher and Holzapfel argue that in order to provide competent care, sex therapists should have not only knowledge of the sexual and relationship consequences of an STI but also a foundation of knowledge regarding STI prevalence, prevention, testing, and treatment. Included in this chapter, therefore, is a primer of common STIs. Fisher and Holzapfel observe that sex therapists are generally skilled at coaching clients on how to communicate about sensitive sexual and relationship issues and about how to integrate novel sexual practices in order to improve sexual satisfaction. The authors note that these skills may be similarly employed to coach clients about how to communicate about, negotiate, and integrate safer sexual practices in their ongoing or new sexual relationships.

William A. Fisher, PhD, is Distinguished Professor in the Department of Psychology and the Department of Obstetrics and Gynaecology at the University of Western

Ontario in London, Ontario, Canada. Professor Fisher's work focuses broadly on sexual and reproductive health behavior change, and he has published more than 200 papers in this area. Professor Fisher serves on the editorial boards of five academic journals, is a Fellow the Society for the Scientific Study of Sexuality and the Canadian Academy of Health Sciences, and has been a National Health Scientist (AIDS) for Health Canada. His research on HIV/AIDS prevention has been supported by the U.S. National Institute of Mental Health for the past two and a half decades.

Stephen Holzapfel, MD, is Director of the Sexual Medicine Counseling Unit in the Family Practice Health Centre at Women's College Hospital in Toronto, Ontario, Canada. Dr. Holzapfel is an academic Family Physician and registered Sex Therapist and Supervisor member of BESTCO (Board of Examiners in Sex Therapy and Counseling of Ontario) and Associate Professor in the Department of Family and Community Medicine and the Department of Obstetrics and Gynaecology at the University of Toronto.

Dear Dr. Fisher,

I'm using this e-mail for now instead of my usual e-mail to try to keep this anonymous. I feel a little more comfortable writing you from my ancient e-mail.

I was recently diagnosed with genital herpes HSV-1. I have a lot of questions and have tried researching them but have not been able to get many answers. I'm hoping you may know some of these answers or know someone I may be able to ask.

I was diagnosed in June. I'm not sure who I contracted it from. I have told my boyfriend and being a great guy he stood by me through everything and has decided to remain with me. According to the doctors it is most likely I got it from him even though he has never had symptoms.

Going forward he and I are using condoms to prevent the risk of transmission. We are not ruling out the chance that he is infected as well and also not putting him at risk for infection in case he isn't.

1. Previously my partner and I enjoyed oral sex. We haven't done it at all since the diagnosis and it's a constant reminder to me that I am infected.

2. The doctors had briefly mentioned to me suppressive therapy but scared me out of considering it. They basically said if I use it I'm going to suffer liver failure. My sex life hasn't been nearly the same since this happened and it has really upset me. Any way to try to reduce the risk of transmission and return things to how they were before would be a bonus.

3. Eventually someday I'd like to have children. I realise that I can have kids if I'm pregnant just that I'd have a C-section if I had an outbreak during delivery. BUT what about getting pregnant in the first place? Because I'm doomed to using a condom for the rest of my life how am I supposed to get pregnant? With a turkey baster?

4. It would be EXTREMELY helpful to know if my boyfriend does or does not have the virus and if he does already have the antibodies in his system does this mean that he is less likely to become infected by me? Every time we've asked to get tested doctors have denied us. If he is negative then we know for sure we need to be 100% careful.

Before I got diagnosed I thought I was being careful and I was definitely uninformed about herpes even though I assumed I was educated about STD's. . . . I was very careful about sex and have only had 2 sexual partners in my history, one of several years that I had tested before I agreed to do anything with, and the other we were committed to each other before we agreed to any sexual activity. My partners had only had one or two other sexual partners themselves. I sort of always assumed more promiscuous girls were more likely to get it or guys with lots of sexual partners. I didn't know that herpes can lie dormant for many years. I didn't know that STD tests don't test for herpes and I didn't know that a condom is not effective in preventing the spread of herpes.

—ANONYMOUS (personal communication, 2011)

Sex therapists are in the business of restoring sexual function and enabling sexual behavior. Sexual behavior, however, may take place in the context of the risk of contracting a sexually transmitted infection (STI), the subjective fear of contracting an STI, the acute acquisition of an STI, or the chronic carriage of an STI, each of which may result in a cascade of negative effects on an individual's sexual and relationship health. Sex therapists must acquire a foundation of knowledge concerning STI prevention, prevalence, natural history, testing, treatment, and sexual and medical sequelae in order to be able to provide competent care in relevant situations, but this has not been the traditional standard of training or care in sex therapy. This chapter reviews situations in which STIs may play an important role in the etiology and maintenance of sexual and relationship dysfunction, reviews relevant medical, psychological, and relationship impacts of STIs, and outlines general counseling principles that may prove useful in working with clients who have STI-related sexual and relationship concerns.

THE WORRIED WELL

Case Illustrations

"I just got back from vacation. I need to get tested for *all* the STIs. *Now.*"

A middle-aged gay male who has recently "come out" and left a heterosexual marriage consults a sex therapist about his erectile dysfunction (ED). It emerges that he is very fearful of contracting HIV. His fear of infection has interfered with efforts to treat his ED with traditional sex therapy techniques and has contributed to his rejection of the therapist's suggestion that he try PDE5 inhibitor treatment.

Sex therapists will often be dealing with the "worried well," whose sexual and relationship functioning is adversely affected by clinically evident or background concerns about STI risk. Accordingly, sex therapists should be able to knowledgeably provide effective counseling to the "worried-well" client concerning STI risk and STI prevention. Such counseling, which we have provided often enough to name—"How to be reasonably sexual in the new millennium"—can touch on a number of issues, articulated to a specific client's STI risk, with the aim of guiding effective STI prevention practices and providing appropriate reassurance that can reduce risk of STI and its sequelae, help control STI-related anxieties, and assist in improving sexual health.

Following a familiar permission–limited information–specific suggestions–intensive therapy (PLISSIT) model (Annon, 1976), counseling for the "worried well" whose sexual functioning is compromised by STI-related anxieties might address the following issues.

STI Prevalence

An individual's STI risk is a function of his or her specific risky sexual behaviors, the prevalence of a given pathogen in a given epidemiological niche, and the infectivity of specific pathogens, among other factors, and assessment of a client's risk and decisions about counseling emphasis can be approached from this perspective (see Canadian STI Guidelines, 2012a, for discussion of assessment of STI risk).

For the individual who has just returned from vacation and is seeking testing for " . . . *all* the STIs. *Now,*" information about the prevalence of various STIs and the behavior that is thought to have posed risk can guide risk assessment and counseling. For example:

> "I'm glad you brought that up. And you should know that, having met a new partner on a seniors cruise, with whom you engaged in mutual masturbation, your risk of most STIs is pretty low."

> "I'm glad you brought that up. Since, as you say, you were in the Caribbean, and some people at the bar shared some kind of pills with you, and you woke up in a bed with naked men and women sleeping around you, and you don't remember exactly what happened, yes, getting tested for STIs might be a good idea."

For the individual who has just left a heterosexual marriage and "come out," who is experiencing ED, and whose treatment seems complicated by HIV-related fears, the clinical interaction might include the following:

"I'm glad you brought that up. You've said that you are distressed about the changes you've noticed in your erection, that the things we've tried so far haven't helped much, and that you're not too interested in the 'little blue pill.' You've also said that you're looking forward to being openly involved in the gay scene, but that you're very apprehensive about the whole HIV story. There are a couple of reasonable things you might want to do to minimize your risk. Let's talk."

Condoms

Most lay persons and many professionals equate condom use with safer sex, and most assume that condom use may be safely abandoned when an individual is in a monogamous relationship with a known and trusted partner. Although latex condoms are a highly effective STI-preventive measure—as are polyethylene condoms for those with latex allergy and female condoms for use by women—there are important limitations concerning condom use for STI prevention. (Note that natural "lambskin" condoms, made from sheep intestines, are not effective in preventing infection.)

First, it is critical to use condoms consistently to prevent STIs. However, inconsistent condom use is common, as is discontinuation of condom use without the benefit of STI testing as relationships become more intimate, despite the fact that intimacy cannot eliminate sexually transmitted pathogens that may have been brought into a relationship by an individual's or a partner's sexual history (Black et al., 2009; MacDonald et al., 1990; Misovich, Fisher, & Fisher, 1997).

Second, it is essential to note that condoms prevent some, but not all, STIs. Counseling concerning condoms needs to take into account the fact that condoms are effective in preventing transmission of some STIs, including HIV, chlamydia, gonorrhea, and syphilis, but not others, such as herpes or human papillomavirus (HPV) infection (Centers for Disease Control and Prevention, 2012a). Moreover, unless condoms are used as a barrier in oral sexual contacts, they cannot prevent the oral transmission of STIs, including herpes, chlamydia, gonorrhea, and HPV. In general, counseling can emphasize that consistent condom use can be an effective and reassuring means of preventing HIV and a number of other sexually transmitted pathogens and should be maintained at least until mutual STI testing, mutual agreement on monogamy, and discussion of how to handle any unintended breach of mutual monogamy (e.g., disclosure to partner, reversion to consistent condom use) have taken place. Counseling should also acknowledge that consistent condom use cannot prevent all STIs, including herpes and HPV.

Sexual History Taking and Monogamy

Many laypersons and professionals assume that reviewing a partner's sexual history and entering into a monogamous relationship with a known and trusted partner can be effective in reducing STI risk. Counseling must take into account the fact that known and trusted partners may be completely unaware that they are asymptomatic carriers of an STI (Centers for Disease Control and Prevention, 2012b; Canadian STI Guidelines, 2012a), or they may minimize or lie about their sexual or drug use history (Cochran & Mays, 1990). Counseling also needs to take into account the likelihood that a currently monogamous individual may have been serially monogamous, with a history of faithful one-partner relationships that have succeeded one another and that have involved the unnoticed accumulation of STI risk with each serially monogamous partner. Extramarital and extrarelationship sexual activity is also not uncommon (Laumann, Gagnon, Michael, & Michaels, 1994). For these reasons, STI testing and discussion of monogamy, or maintenance of consistent condom use, may be quite relevant for those who have a sexual history and who are in or entering a monogamous relationship.

STI Testing

STI testing is often regarded as a nearly foolproof method of STI prevention if testing takes place before sexual contact with a partner. Although STI testing is advisable and appropriately reassuring in many cases, the sex therapist should keep a number of limitations of STI testing in mind. First and foremost, STI testing generally covers only a subset of STIs, including HIV, chlamydia, gonorrhea, and perhaps syphilis and hepatitis. STI testing generally does not test for herpes or HPV infection. Second, many individuals assume, incorrectly, that they have been tested for STIs in the course of routine medical care (e.g., "I had a blood test when I had my annual physical," or "I've donated blood"), whereas in fact STI testing may not have taken place. In addition, STI testing is retrospective in that it tests which of a subset of STIs an individual may have been exposed to in the past, but it is not informative about STI status if the individual or the partner has engaged in risky sexual behavior since the STI test. Finally, the sex therapist should be aware of the "window period" in HIV, syphilis, and viral hepatitis (A, B, C) testing. That is, testing may not be accurate or definitive for a period of time after infection has taken place. For example, HIV testing assesses the presence or absence of antibodies to HIV, which take time to develop following a risky sexual contact. Thus the apprehensive individual who wants to be tested "now," soon after a risky exposure, should be tested for HIV and retested following the HIV window period, some 3 months after his or her last possible exposure to the virus (Canadian STI Guidelines, 2012b).

Coaching Communication about Condom Use, STI Testing, and Posttest Monogamy

The sex therapist is generally skilled at coaching clients concerning how to communicate effectively with partners about sensitive sexual and relationship issues and about how to integrate novel sexual practices that have the potential to improve sexual outcomes. These skills may be employed to coach clients about how to bring up and negotiate safer sexual practices, such as condom use, STI testing, and maintenance of posttest monogamy, in their relationships, employing assertive but not aggressive communication strategies. The sex therapist may also need to work with clients to foster partner communication about safe sex issues; counseling approaches such as Motivational Interviewing may be used to support client consistency in condom use (Canadian STI Guidelines, 2012a; Rollnick, Miller, & Butler, 2008).

Specific Suggestions

The sex therapist may wish to make specific suggestions concerning STI prevention when appropriate to a client's situation. For example, an HPV vaccine is now available for the prevention of cervical cancer and genital warts, and it may be effective in reducing risk of anal cancers as well, which can be of special relevance to gay men and to individuals who engage in anal intercourse (Fisher, 2012). Finally, not to be ignored are routine Pap tests, which serve as secondary prevention of HPV infection-related precancerous and cancerous conditions of the cervix. And, as hepatitis A, B and C may be sexually transmitted diseases, vaccination against hepatitis A and B (no vaccine is available for hepatitis C) may be suggested as well.

THE BLISSFULLY IGNORANT

Case Illustrations

A successful 30-something bisexual man consults a sex therapist about a persistent and embarrassing problem with rapid ejaculation that has deterred him from seeking sexual and romantic partnerships. The client reports a new sexual encounter in which the strategies you have taught him have been quite successful.

"The treatment really helped with my vulvar pain—but it didn't save my marriage. Anyway, I'm really looking forward to starting to date again—at the age of 45! Thank you, doctor."

Sex therapists who successfully address a client's sexual problem may unintentionally facilitate their client's acquisition of an STI. Competent clinical practice may include addressing a presenting sexual problem, assessing STI risk of which the client may be aware or completely unaware, and providing effective counseling to minimize STI risk. Consider the prevalence of HIV infection in the United States in connection with the successful 30-something bisexual male whose distressing problem with rapid ejaculation has been addressed and who is reentering the social and sexual scene (see Figure 22.1). As a result of the successful introduction of antiretroviral therapy for HIV-infected individuals in the mid-1990s, HIV mortality has

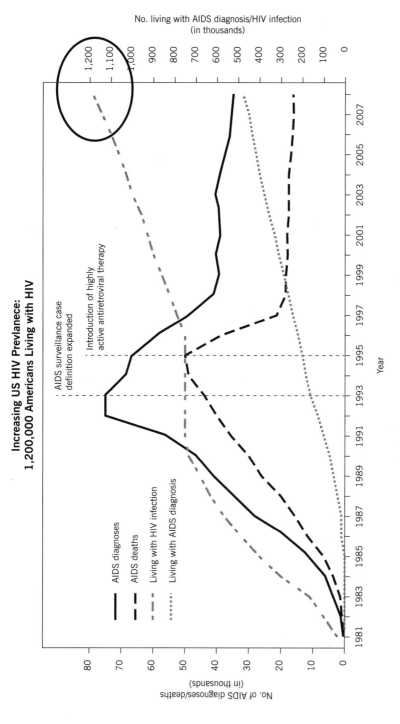

FIGURE 22.1. HIV prevalence in the United States, 1981–2008. From Centers for Disease Control and Prevention (2012c).

dramatically declined. At the same time, HIV prevalence—the number of persons now living with HIV and potentially infectious—has dramatically increased. Despite the fact that adherence to antiretroviral therapy reduces transmission of HIV from infected to uninfected individuals (Granich, Gilks, Dye, De Cock, & Williams, 2009) and despite the fact that HIV prevalence in the United States is far from exclusive to gay and bisexual men, HIV prevalence information provides a basis for some sensitivity to STI risk in this clinical scenario.

Consider as well findings for age-specific prevalence of high-risk potentially cancer-causing types of HPV in connection with the 45-year-old woman whose vulvar pain has been successfully treated and who is anticipating returning to the dating scene following her marriage breakup. Roughly 13% of women in this age range show evidence of high-risk cancer-causing HPV infection (Dunne et al., 2007).

In the case of the 30-something bisexual male who is more confidently returning to social and romantic relationships, the sexuality clinician may consider counseling HIV risk-reduction principles, some of which have been articulated in the preceding section of this chapter. Discussion of condom use, consideration of the advantages of STI testing and monogamous relationships, and HPV and hepatitis A and B vaccination may all be relevant subjects of discussion about tactics that can provide protection and reassurance. Discussion of risk-reduction practices, including serosorting (restricting sexual contact to HIV-negative partners only), strategic positioning (being the insertive, not the receptive, partner may reduce risk), and even use of rapid home HIV antibody tests to screen oneself and one's sexual partner may be relevant as well (Fisher, 2012; Golden, Stekler, Hughes, & Wood, 2008; Parsons et al., 2005). Similarly, in the case of the 45-year-old woman who is returning to the dating scene, counseling concerning STI prevention may be relevant, including condom use, discussion of the advantages and limitations of monogamy, and consideration of HPV vaccination (despite the fact that the woman in question is outside the HPV vaccine target age), hepatitis A and B vaccination, and continuation of routine Pap tests. The aim of such counseling, of course, is to avoid a situation in which, as noted, successful sex therapy results in the inadvertent enabling of risky sexual behavior.

THE AFFECTED INDIVIDUAL AND COUPLE

Case Illustrations

A heterosexual couple presents with hypoactive sexual desire disorder (HSDD; female partner) and frequency dissatisfaction (male partner). In their history it emerges that these issues have been of concern during the course of the relationship but have been getting worse, and the sex therapist is advised that she is the "last stop" before a divorce lawyer. History also reveals that the female partner was treated for chlamydia and pelvic inflammatory disease in her early 20s, a decade prior to the beginning of the current relationship.

A heterosexual couple presents with a sexual and relationship crisis after the female partner reads about the advantages of HPV DNA testing over traditional Pap tests and requests and receives an HPV DNA test from her gynecologist. She tests positive for HPV, and the couple is in crisis. "He gave me an STD!" "She won't touch me!"

Sex therapists will encounter clients and couples who have experienced the sexual and relationship consequences of acquiring an STI. Some clients will shy away from sexual contact because of the residual psychological effects of a past STI of which they have been cured; some will have residual physical effects of a past STI of which they have been cured; and some will experience personal and relationship crises when an STI occurs or appears to occur within the context of a relationship.

In the case of the couple experiencing HSDD and frequency dissatisfaction, their history revealed that past experience with a fertility-endangering STI (chlamydia and pelvic inflammatory disease) may represent a predisposing factor for current sexual distress that is being maintained and exacerbated by couple arguments about sexual frequency. It is possible that individual therapy to process anxieties about the past STI and its sequelae (for the female partner) and providing some insight into partner history as a predisposing factor (for the male partner), as well as therapeutic focus on the HSDD and the argumentation—exacerbation cycle, may prove helpful to this couple. It is also essential to determine whether the previously "cured" STI has left residual physical effects, such as chronic pelvic pain, provoked by sexual intercourse, that may contribute to the presenting problems of HSDD and frequency dissatisfaction. Such clarification may involve referral to a gynecologist with experience in pelvic pain.

In the case of the couple experiencing a cascade of sexual and relationship distress following an HPV diagnosis, the sex therapist must be knowledgeable about the natural history of HPV infection in order to effectively counsel the couple. Adopting nothing more complicated than an initial PLISSIT approach, the therapist may provide "permission" for the upset ("Many people would indeed be distressed by this") and address the limited information that has permitted the couple to assume that the HPV diagnosis represents a newly imported STI from an unfaithful partner. The natural history of HPV infection and its prevalence at midlife suggests the possibility of reactivation of a long latent infection that does not represent introduction of an STI by an adulterous partner ("This is *not* necessarily a new infection"). What is more, the sex therapist can consider exploiting this crisis to begin processing past and emerging sexual issues with the couple, who—after addressing the HPV crisis—may be interested and open to such couple enhancement approaches.

We wish to emphasize that sex therapists will see couples in whom an

STI infection *has* occurred as the result of extrarelationship sexual activity. In such cases, the individual involved in extrarelationship sex may have disclosed the occurrence of his or her STI to the partner, or, worse, the individual may have infected his or her partner with an STI. Situations such as these can constitute primary relationship crises owing to unfaithfulness, violated trust, and attachment wounds, exacerbated by the impact of the STI on one or both partners. In addition to skill in managing a primary relationship crisis occasioned by infidelity, the sex therapist will need to act knowledgeably in respect to the STI itself by ensuring that the affected individuals have received appropriate testing and treatment and undertaken appropriate preventive actions.

THE INDIVIDUAL AND COUPLE CONFRONTING A CHRONIC STI

Case Illustrations

An HIV-serodiscordant couple (one partner is HIV infected, one partner is not), both experiencing sexual aversion and both distressed by the years-long disturbance to their relationship that this has occasioned, consult a sex therapist.

A committed heterosexual couple in which the man has recurrent herpes outbreaks and the woman is presumed to be uninfected have significant concerns about sex and marriage and seek assistance from a sex therapist.

In view of the prevalence of chronic viral STI (see the following discussion), sex therapists may encounter individuals and couples who have chronic STIs, including herpes, HPV, and HIV. Sex therapists can acquire knowledge of the acquisition, natural history, consequences, management, and prevention of these chronic STIs and can integrate this knowledge in providing supportive sex therapy for such clients. Sex therapists may find the biomedical aspects of these situations to be challenging and may elect to comanage them with knowledgeable and supportive medical providers who can contribute to comprehensive care for those experiencing sexual and relationship consequences of a chronic STI. For example, in the case of the HIV-serodiscordant couple, the sex therapist and medical comanagement team might provide comprehensive information about HIV transmission and HIV prevention, including discussion of the effectiveness of condoms in preventing HIV transmission and adherence to HIV antiretroviral therapy as a means of reducing HIV transmission risk, that permits partners to make informed decisions about their desired level of sexual contact and prevention. In the case of the couple considering marriage but distressed and sexually limited by one partner's recurrent herpes outbreaks, sex therapy and medical comanagement can also provide information about safer sexual practices, possible suppressive therapies, and realistic appraisal of the risk and the consequences of transmission of herpes as a basis for decision making and action. Following is a case illustration of a relatively complex couple sexual dysfunction that required both intensive therapeutic intervention and comanagement by a sex therapist and a physician experienced in the treatment of HPV infection.

CASE DISCUSSION: GENERALIZED ANXIETY, UNREALISTIC PORNOGRAPHY, FEELINGS OF INFERIORITY, AND COUPLE SEXUAL DYSFUNCTION

Mark was a 42-year-old newly married man with a history of generalized anxiety disorder. Treatment for Mark's anxiety allowed him to be able to meet and marry Elena, a 40-year-old divorced woman. Mark considered himself inferior to Elena, as he had never had a relationship, whereas she was previously married. Mark generally deferred to Elena on decisions regarding their marriage (where to live, what to do for the holidays). However, Mark felt that Elena was "bossy," and he resented her "control" over him. Mark also felt that Elena was sexually deficient. Comparing Elena to the women he viewed in pornography and who occupied his fantasies, Mark found Elena overweight, unattractive, and sexually undesirable. Mark's previous sexual experiences involved masturbation with pornography, a few "one-night stands," and infrequent visits to prostitutes. As a result of these experiences, Mark has HPV and recurrent outbreaks of genital warts.

Mark and Elena were referred to sex therapy by Mark's individual therapist. The couple's presenting complaint was that Elena had pain with intercourse. On evaluation, it emerged that intercourse often lasted about 30 minutes, until the intensity of Elena's pain made them stop. On these occasions Mark had not yet ejaculated. Sexual problems worsened shortly after marriage, when Mark told Elena about his HPV infection. Elena was angry that Mark had not shared this information with her. She insisted that they use condoms until Mark was "medically cleared." Mark felt "controlled" but consented to use condoms. During the initial evaluation, it was explained to Mark and Elena that her pain after 10 minutes of intercourse, even with lubricants, was understandable. Mark's inability to ejaculate and his obsessive worry about genital warts became the focus of clinical attention.

In individual sessions Mark described the pornography he was viewing. Pornography had given Mark unrealistic expectations of sex and intercourse. Mark had difficulty seeing that the problem was something other than the fact that Elena was overweight and sexually unappealing, whereas the women in pornography were young, sexy, and appeared to be easily orgasmic. Mark acknowledged resentment regarding Elena's insistence on condom use and her "requirement" that he stop viewing pornography. Mark also disclosed that his HPV status made him feel inferior to Elena and made his past experiences tawdry rather than successful; and he felt relegated to never being as good as Elena in all facets of their marriage.

Sex therapy began with sensate focus. The early exercises did not involve genital contact or stimulation, and Mark's HPV was not a concern. The exercises proceeded slowly, with Mark being increasingly able to attend to Elena's sensual pleasure and Elena being able to learn how to pleasure Mark. Elena learned to communicate more effectively and empathically instead of being instructional. Because the touching was more pleasurable than the sex they had had previously, both Mark and Elena were patient with the slow pace (each sensate focus exercise took 4 weeks and two sessions of therapy).

As the therapy moved toward genital stimulation, Mark began to obsess about infecting Elena, and she worried about this as well. Mark asked Elena to wear latex gloves while stimulating his condom-sheathed penis. Needless to say, whereas Elena experienced considerable pleasure from sensate focus that progressed to include genital stimulation, Mark did not. Elena in fact experienced orgasm for the first time with Mark, an event that pleased her greatly but left Mark feeling that now Elena was also "better at sex than me." This turn of events was reframed as a sign that Mark was now a good lover, in that he could bring pleasure to Elena.

At this point, the sex therapist suggested a pause in the sensate focus treatment and referred Mark and Elena to a physician with whom he comanaged cases of chronic STI.

The comanaging physician met with Mark and Elena and discussed a number of HPV issues that provided reassurance and reduced guilt. First, the physician conveyed the medical certainty that HPV is extremely prevalent, with something like 60% of sexually active individuals acquiring one or more strains of the virus, often in their first sexual encounter with a sexually experienced partner. Second, the physician discussed recent advances, including findings that condoms may be much more effective than once believed in reducing HPV transmission (Winer et al., 2006) and the possible benefit to Elena and Mark of getting HPV vaccinations, as it was unlikely that they had been infected with all of the vaccine-preventable strains of the virus. The physician also counseled Elena to continue with routine follow-up gynecological care to reduce serious consequences of any HPV infection. Mark and Elena were also informed that his genital warts might spontaneously clear at some point.

In conjoint sessions, Mark and Elena were able to talk to one another about their feelings regarding HPV, and Mark was able to educate Elena about this topic on the basis of further research he had done on the issue, which made him feel that he was taking charge. He also negotiated with her regarding pornography, and they agreed that his pornography use was only problematic when he used it to avoid having sex with Elena. Elena told Mark that she was willing to accept the risk of getting HPV as long as she knew that they were both doing all they could do to minimize the risk of transmission. Sex therapy exercises progressed to include more genital stimulation, including condom-protected oral sex and intercourse. Mark took charge of asking Elena for the kinds of stimulation he wanted: He routinely asked Elena to lubricate the tip of his penis with saliva to increase his sensation and then he put on a condom. Mark was ultimately able to ejaculate intravaginally after 7 minutes of intercourse. He continued to consult his physician regularly to "reality check" his suspicions that he might have a wart. Treatment lasted for 18 months, during which time Mark did not ever have a wart. Follow-up a year later found that Mark and Elena were having mutually satisfying sex about once a month. Although Mark continued to worry about transmitting HPV to his wife, he was able to act on this concern in a constructive manner, by using condoms and visiting his physician. Both he and Elena now viewed his worry as a sign that he was "taking charge" of their mutual sexual health.

AN STI PRIMER: CHARACTERISTICS OF COMMON INFECTIONS

This section provides an overview of the characteristics of common STIs, grouped by causative agents, and outlines their prevalence, clinical presentation, and measures to prevent, treat, or suppress the infections and their consequences. Further information about characteristics and management of specific STIs may be obtained from the Centers for Disease Control and Prevention (2012b) and Health Canada (2012).

Bacterial STIs

Chlamydia, gonorrhea, and syphilis are caused by bacteria, and a defining characteristic of bacterial STIs is that they may be cured by antibiotic treatment. Early detection and treatment of bacterial STIs may prevent their more serious medical consequences.

Chlamydia

Chlamydia trachomatis is a prevalent bacterial STI in both women and men and is most commonly transmitted via penis–vagina and penis–anus sexual contacts, although oral sexual transmission is also possible. Young heterosexual males and females have the highest rates of chlamydia (Centers for Disease Control, 2012d; Fisher & Steben, 2014). More than two-thirds of chlamydia infections are asymptomatic; some chlamydia infections will present with a mild discharge from the vagina, penis, or anus, and urinary symptoms (burning or itching) in men and women and vaginal bleeding after intercourse in women may also be present.

Chlamydia can cause pelvic inflammatory disease (PID), fallopian tube scarring, ectopic pregnancy, and infertility in women (Baraitser, Alexander, & Steringham, 2011). Chlamydia also manifests itself in urethritis (inflammation of the urethra) and epididymitis (inflammation of the epididymis), with penile discharge or scrotal pain in men; lymphogranuloma venereum, a serious invasive chlymdial infection preferentially affecting the lymph tissue, may also occur. Chlamydia has historically been diagnosed in women by doing a pelvic examination and swabbing the cervix or by swabbing the man's ure-thra. The development of urine testing for chlamydia as well as self-collected vulval swabs has made screening for infections much easier and less intrusive. Chlamydia can be prevented with consistent use of latex condoms and is cur-able with antibiotics.

Gonorrhea

Gonorrhea is the second most common bacterial STI. It is transmitted in penis–vagina and penis–anus sexual contact and may be transmitted in oral sexual contact as well (Centers for Disease Control, 2012b; Fisher & Steben, 2014). It is commonly found as a coinfection with chlamydia (Sadeghi-Nejad, Wasserman, Weidner, Richardson, & Goldmeier, 2010). Gonorrhea is most common in men who have sex with men (MSM) and individuals who have had sex while traveling abroad and is less common, though increasing, in het-erosexual individuals. Gonorrhea is more often symptomatic than chlamydia, with a more pus-like yellow–green genital discharge than in chlamydia. Medi-cal consequences are similar to chlamydia for both men and women, with acute PID symptoms in women being more severe with gonorrhea. PID can lead to deep dyspareunia for women. Gonorrhea can be prevented with con-sistent use of latex condoms and is curable with antibiotics.

Syphilis

Syphilis presents with a painless genital ulcer. When syphilis is left untreated, it becomes asymptomatic and latent for decades (Centers for Disease Control and Prevention, 2012b; Fisher & Steben, 2014). Late manifestations of syphilis cause myriad symptoms, including cardiac and neurological problems. Syphi-lis can be transmitted from mother to infant. Syphilis is uncommon in the general population, though it is more frequent in MSM, in travelers who have had sex in endemic areas, and in individuals having sex in areas with geo-graphic outbreaks. The incidence of syphilis has also been increasing among heterosexuals, with the greatest increase in the United States among black and Hispanic men ages 20–29 (Su, Beltrami, Zaidi, &Weinstock, 2011). Syphilis is considered to be infectious for up to 2 years if left untreated. It can be pre-vented with consistent use of latex condoms and is curable with antibiotics.

Viral STIs

Herpes Simplex Virus

Herpes simplex virus (HSV) is quite common and causes painful blisters on the genitals that ulcerate, crust, and gradually heal (Centers for Disease Con-trol, 2012b; Fisher & Steben, 2014). Historically, HSV type 1 (HSV-1) was localized around the mouth, causing "cold sores," while HSV-2 caused genital herpes. These divisions have blurred over the past decades. Herpes can be transmitted during oral, vaginal, and anal sex, and it can be transmitted to infants during childbirth. It is transmissible while the individual is symptomatic or during asymptomatic periods when the individual may still be shedding virus. Herpes outbreaks can recur, though subsequent outbreaks gradually become less frequent and less painful. Both primary and recurrent events lead to painful sex, as well as fears of passing on the infection. Xu et al. (2006) report that 17% of Americans ages 14–49 had evidence of HSV-2 infection, with 90% not knowing that they had contracted it. HSV may occur in women who have had sex with women (Marrazzo, 2010). Individuals with herpes should inform their partners.

HSV screening of asymptomatic individuals is not routine, and management and prevention implications of a positive HSV test for the individual and his or her partner are not clear. The adverse psychological effect of being screened positive for HSV has been rated as similar to that of a minor automobile accident (Richards et al., 2007). Reduction of the burden of genital herpes through screening and subsequent adoption of either safer sex practices or continuous suppressive antiviral therapy has not been proven. Antiviral drug treatment at the first sign of an outbreak can reduce outbreak symptoms. For those with recurrent attacks, continuous use of medications reduces morbidity, as well as decreasing viral shedding and partner infectivity (Mindel & Marks, 2005). People with recurrent genital herpes can reduce the risk of passing HSV to their partners by using latex condoms. Abstention during an outbreak still carries a 5% annual partner infection rate due to asymptomatic shedding of viral particles. This rate can be halved if the infected partner takes ongoing antiviral medications (Corey et al., 2004).

Human Papillomavirus

Human papillomavirus (HPV) is an exceedingly common sexually transmitted infection (Dunne et al., 2007; Fisher, 2012; Giuliano et al., 2011; Richardson et al., 2003; Winer et al., 2006) that may have serious medical consequences (Palefsky, 2010; Parkin & Bray, 2006). HPV prevalence among U.S. women ages 14–59 is estimated to be 26.8%, with both low-risk HPV types (15.2% prevalence), which can cause genital warts, and high-risk HPV types (17.8% prevalence), which can cause cervical, vaginal, penile, anal, and head and neck cancers, quite common (Dunne et al., 2007). A recent multinational study of men ages 18–70 showed a 50% prevalence of HPV infection in men, with 38% prevalence of low-risk types and a 30% prevalence of high-risk types (Giuliano et al., 2011). The medical consequences of HPV infection, including genital warts and precancerous changes of the cervix, which require investigation and treatment, are common as well.

The approval of two HPV vaccines in recent years offers the potential to prevent most cervical cancer and genital warts and possibly other HPV-related conditions as well. Gardasil, which prevents infection with the most common cancer-causing and wart-causing HPV types, and Cervarix, which prevents infection with the most common cancer-causing HPV types, are presently available. HPV vaccine is approved for immunization of girls and women ages 9–45 for the prevention of cervical cancer and genital warts and for boys and men ages 9–26 for the prevention of genital warts. It may also be of benefit to older individuals depending upon individual circumstances. For example, a middle-aged male or female who is leaving a 20-year-long relationship and reentering the dating scene may wish to speak with his or her health care provider about the potential benefit of HPV vaccination. Note that HPV vaccine may be of benefit to individuals who have already been sexually active, as acquisition of all vaccine-preventable HPV types has not necessarily occurred. In addition to prophylactic vaccination, latex condom use may reduce the risk of HPV infection (but not entirely, as HPV infects areas of the body not covered by condoms; see Winer et al., 2006, for findings concerning condom protection from HPV infection). Treatment of HPV-related medical conditions, but not cure of the virus per se, is possible.

Human Immunodeficiency Virus

Human immunodeficiency virus (HIV) is passed from an infected to an uninfected individual in penile–anal (highest risk), penile–vaginal (high risk), and oral sex (low risk but not risk free) contacts; through sharing paraphernalia for intravenous drug use; and from mother to infant (Centers for Disease Control and Prevention, 2012b; Fisher & Steben, 2014). Any sexual or drug-injection activity that has the potential to transfer bodily fluids, particular semen, vaginal fluid, or blood from one person to another poses risk for HIV infection. HIV infection, if untreated, leads to compromise of the immune system, opportunistic infections, and very high mortality. Highly active anti-retroviral therapy (HAART), developed in the mid-1990s, represents an effective treatment for HIV that has turned the disease into a chronic manageable condition that requires a high degree of adherence to the drug regimen over the lifespan. Individuals adhering to HAART may be much less infectious to others, though this depends upon adherence to medication and therapeutic efficacy in lowering the individual's viral load (Granich et al., 2009). The U.S. Centers for Disease Control reported that at the end of 2009 there were 784,701 people living with HIV in the 46 reporting states, meaning that about 1 million Americans are living with HIV (Centers for Disease Control and Prevention, 2012c) and that a significant proportion of people living with HIV are not aware that they are infected.

Male-to-male sexual contact, injection-drug paraphernalia sharing, and heterosexual contact are all relatively common routes of HIV infection, with male-to-male contact the most common route of infection among men. Heterosexual contact and intravenous-drug paraphernalia sharing are the most common routes of HIV infection among women (Centers for Disease Control and Prevention, 2012b). Latex condoms are effective in preventing HIV infection, and avoidance of risky sexual practices, mutual HIV testing, partner serosorting (having sex with persons of like HIV status), and viral load lowering via adherence to HAART are all harm-reduction possibilities (Fisher,

2012). The use of postexposure prophylaxis with HAART within 72 hours for individuals who have experienced sexual assault, and potentially for those who have simply had unprotected intercourse, should also be explored when indicated. Preemptive pre-exposure prophylaxis for individuals who practice risky behavior may be explored as well. HIV antibody testing can be used to screen or test for HIV infection. We again note that HIV testing detects antibodies to infection and is regarded as definitively negative only when conducted some 3 months after an individual's last potential exposure to risk.

Hepatitis

Hepatitis A, B, and C are viral infections that can cause liver disease and can be sexually transmitted (Centers for Disease Control and Prevention, 2012d; Fisher & Steben, 2014). Hepatitis A and B are relatively common among MSM, and hepatitis C is relatively common among HIV-infected MSM. Hepatitis may also be common among individuals who share injection-drug paraphernalia and among individuals who come from countries in which the infection is endemic. Chronic hepatitis B can lead to cirrhosis and is a common cause of liver cancer. The lag time between exposure to hepatitis via intimate sexual, blood, or fecal contact may make it difficult for patients to know how, or from whom, they contracted the infection. Hepatitis A and B are vaccine preventable. Most schoolchildren in North America have received hepatitis B vaccine in school-based vaccination programs, and the rate of new hepatitis B infections has declined by 82% in the United States since 1991, when the recommendation to routinely vaccinate all children was introduced (Centers for Disease Control and Prevention, 2012e).

Other Genital Concerns

Trichomonas Vaginalis

Trichomonas vaginalis (Centers for Disease Control and Prevention, 2012b) is a protozoan infection that is often transmitted sexually but can be contracted nonsexually. Trichomonas is often asymptomatic, but it can cause symptoms similar to yeast infections in women and can cause burning on urination or ejaculation in men and discomfort during sex for both men and women. It can be transmitted in both heterosexual and same-sex sexual contacts; condoms can help prevent trichomonas but not with complete effectiveness. Trichomonas can cause preterm labor and low-birth-weight infants and can be treated with oral antibiotics.

Vulvovaginal Candidiasis

Vulvovaginal candidiasis, or "yeast infection," is caused by the overgrowth of bacteria that normally live in the vagina (Centers for Disease Control and Prevention, 2012f). Up to 75% of women will experience a genital yeast infection at some point in their lives, with up to half of all women suffering more than once. Yeast vulvovaginitis is characterized by vaginal irritation and itching, a white discharge, and inflammation and redness of the vaginal mucosa. Vulvovaginal candidiasis is *not* an STI per se. A sizable increase in risk of genital yeast infections does occur when women become sexually active, but sexual intercourse itself, and the frequency of coitus, are not clearly causative agents (Sobel, 2003; Sobel et al., 1998). Antibiotics can also cause vulvovaginal candidiasis. Men can get yeast infections on the glans penis, especially if they are uncircumcised. For both sexes, vulvovaginal candidiasis can lead to painful intercourse. Genital yeast infections can be treated with both topical and oral medications. Treating both partners can prevent "ping-pong" reinfections.

IMPACT OF STIs ON SEXUAL AND RELATIONSHIP FUNCTION

Systematic evidence concerning the impact of STIs on sexual and relationship function has begun to appear in the professional literature in recent years (Fisher, 2012; Goldmeier & Leiblum, 2005; Graziottin & Serafini, 2009; Sadeghi-Nejad et al., 2010).

With respect to the impact of bacterial—and therefore curable—STIs on sexual and couple relationships, Gottlieb and colleagues (2011) recruited women testing positive for chlamydia at a U.S. midwestern family planning clinic. Approximately 90% of these women felt that it would be difficult to trust future partners, 7 out of 10 felt betrayed by their current partners, and 1 in 3 women who tested positive for chlamydia reported breaking up with their partners the following month. More than 75% of the women who tested positive for chlamydia reported that they "were not very proud" of their actions, more than 50% felt guilty that they might have infected someone else with chlamydia, and one in four of these women were very scared about telling their partners about their infections. Gottlieb et al. (2011, p. 1009) note that "tailored counseling might minimize psychosocial impact. For example, discussing the fact that most people are unaware that they have Chlamydia and that infection may last for > 1 year may help to alleviate concerns about partner fidelity and trust for some patients." The clinical wisdom of emphasizing the ambiguity of timing of a chlamydia infection, a point also raised by Duncan, Hart, Scoular, and Bigrigg (2001), may depend upon the specifics of an individual's and couple's situation. The clinician would not necessarily want to obscure an incident of infidelity that resulted in the importation of chlamydia into a relationship, nor would the clinician wish to encourage this conclusion if unwarranted by ambiguous timing of infection. The issue of possible harm resulting from false-positive results in low-prevalence populations has also been discussed by Gottlieb et al. (2011) and Sadeghi-Nejad et al. (2010).

With respect to the impact of viral—and therefore manageable but not curable—STIs on sexual and relationship health, recent research on the effects of HPV infection is informative. Sexual and relationship impact of HPV infection may stem from the infection and its clinical symptoms, from anxiety about transmission of the virus to or from a sexual partner, from extended, painful, and sometimes ineffective treatment of symptoms, or from all of these (Linnehan & Groce, 2000).

Research on men and women recently diagnosed with HPV-related anogential warts indicates that this condition has a significant negative impact on quality of life, mental health, and sexual health measures (Drolet et al., 2011a). The negative impact of anogenital warts on these factors dissipated among those whose warts cleared during a prospective arm of study but remained elevated among those whose warts had not resolved. Women with HPV-related abnormal Pap tests have been found to experience significant negative impact on quality of life and mental health, as well as negative impact on their sexuality and concerns about their partners and HPV transmission (Drolet et al., 2011b). HPV-infected women report stigma (e.g., "I feel the need to hide the fact that I have HPV"), shame (e.g., "I am ashamed of having HPV"), self-blame (e.g.,"With HPV, I feel that I am paying for past behaviors"), and feelings that "my body is disgusting to me" and of being "unclean" (Daley et al., 2010, p. 285). In related findings, McCaffery and colleagues (2004) found that HPV-infected women felt worse about their current sexual partners, worse about their past sexual partners, and worse about their future sexual relationships, compared with uninfected women. Sexual disturbances have also been reported by women who have HPV infection and cervical intraepithelial neoplasia (CIN), precancerous cervical changes. Campion and colleagues (1988) found that HPV-infected women with CIN reported significant decreases in sexual desire, sexual frequency, sexual arousal, and orgasm, as well as greater discomfort and more negative feelings about sexual intercourse, 6 months after treatment.

Findings for the negative psychosexual impact of HPV infection in women may be of considerably increased significance to sex therapists in coming years. HPV testing is currently being phased in as a routine measure to augment or replace the traditional Pap smear for detecting precursors of cervical cancer (Cuzick et al., 2006). As a consequence of routine HPV screening, we anticipate that a substantial number of women and their partners will have to deal with psychosexual sequelae of an HPV diagnosis.

Systematic research on psychosexual consequences of other viral STIs, including genital herpes (e.g., Melville et al., 2003; Mindel & Marks, 2005) and HIV (Sadeghi-Nejad et al., 2010; Shindel, Horberg, Smith, & Breyer, 2011; Jena, Goldman, Kamdar, Lakdawalla, & Lu, 2010) has also been reported in recent years. In a review of the literature concerning psychosexual consequences of genital herpes infection, Mindel and Marks (2005) conclude that the "studies suggest that, at presentation, at least some patients with genital herpes will have psychological and psychosexual problems and that these may be more clinically significant and more common than those occurring in patients routinely attending genitourinary medicine departments with other complaints. . . . Individuals with many recurrences continued to be anxious and concerned, as they had been at first visit" (Mindel & Marks, 2005, p. 306). These authors also review research on management options, including psychoeducational approaches and suppressive antiviral therapy for ameliorating the negative psychosexual impact of genital herpes, and report favorable evidence for the latter approach. This may suggest the utility of comanagement of the psychosexual sequelae of genital herpes with a medical provider experienced in this area.

The possible sexual consequences of HIV infection have been the subject of a number of studies (e.g., Shindel et al., 2011) and have been reviewed in detail by Sadeghi-Nejad and colleagues (2010). This review concludes that rates of sexual dysfunction appear to be sharply elevated among HIV-infected MSM compared with uninfected MSM and among HIV-infected women compared with uninfected women. Causes of sexual dysfunction among HIV-infected individuals may include affective disorders associated with HIV diagnosis, direct effects of HIV infection on sexual function, and effects of HIV treatment that result in distinctive body fat accumulations, body image disturbance, and visible disclosure that the individual is infected, as well as HIV-associated hormonal disturbances and HAART-associated iatrogenic HSDD. Critical issues for sex therapists treating HIV-infected individuals and HIV-discordant couples are several. First, sex therapists may need to increase awareness that their scope of practice could include welcoming HIV-infected individuals and HIV-affected couples and bringing to bear sex therapy skills in assisting such individuals and couples with issues of sexual adjustment. Second, whether for an HIV-infected individual or an HIV-discordant couple, counseling and coaching may be in order in connection with managing sexual relationships and avoiding transmission of infection. Third, addressing HIV-related and HIV-unrelated sexual disturbances will require clinical judgment about predisposing and maintaining factors without necessarily concluding that HIV infection is the primary factor at play. Fifth, active management of safer and risky sexual behavior with HIV-infected individuals may be a significant clinical objective (Fisher et al., 2006). Finally, active comanagement with HIV care medical personnel may be a desirable option. The creation of clinical liaisons that increase awareness in the HIV-affected community that there is a source of professional support for HIV-related sexual function and relationship challenges would be a welcome addition to the sex therapy and HIV care landscape.

We note in closing this section on psychosexual impact of STIs that we have observed that the effect of an STI on sexual and relationship health is heavily influenced by the meanings that the individuals involved ascribe to the infection. At some level, it is the role of a therapist working with a couple dealing with an STI to help each individual make meaning of the diagnosis. An STI arising within a relationship may appear overwhelming to many. Helping a couple find perspective and acknowledge the other dimensions and connections of their relationship may help them move forward. The diagnosis of an

STI is often a crisis for the couple. In addition to myriad negative impacts, such a crisis may provide an opportunity for the couple to start dealing with secrets, improve communication, and deal with shame and hurt. Therapists can help both members of the couple generate a new narrative as they work to move forward with their new reality.

SEX THERAPY, STIs, AND ETHICAL AND LEGAL RAMIFICATIONS

Sex therapists need to be knowledgeable and respectful of their particular discipline's and jurisdiction's rules with respect to situations in which the clinician becomes aware of STI transmission risk behavior. Such professional and legal regulations differ across differing jurisdictions and must be considered and respected.

CONCLUSIONS

We conclude our discussion with a summary of STI counseling principles in the sex therapy setting.

1. Sex therapy may unintentionally enable sexual behavior in clients who are unaware of their STI risk. The sex therapist should assess STI risk for all clients and counsel STI prevention strategies as appropriate.
2. Assessing STI risk behavior and the epidemiological setting of such risk behavior can guide evaluation of a client's level of risk and suggest appropriate prevention and testing strategies.
3. Monogamy with known and trusted partners is not necessarily an effective STI prevention strategy.
4. Latex condom use may be a reassuring method of prevention of STI. However, condom use must be consistent; it effectively prevents some STIs, but not others; and condoms do not prevent oral transmission of STI unless employed as a barrier in oral sexual contacts.
5. For optimum STI prevention, latex condom use should be maintained at least until mutual STI testing, joint agreement on monogamy, and discussion of how to handle any unintended breach of mutual monogamy have taken place in couples in which one or both partners have been sexually active in the past.
6. STI testing can be an effective and reassuring means of STI prevention if testing takes place prior to sexual contact and if posttest monogamy is adhered to. STI testing, however, can detect some but not all STIs; it is retrospective; and the HIV–hepatitis–syphilis window periods may be factors in relying on STI test results.

7. Sex therapists may employ existing counseling skills to rehearse and motivate safer sex client—partner communication concerning condom use, STI testing, posttest monogamy, and incident STI infection.
8. Specific suggestions, including HPV vaccination, hepatitis A and B vaccination, and reminding sexually active women about the importance of routine Pap tests, should be considered.
9. Sex therapists may find that management of the sexual and relationship impacts of STIs benefits from comanagement with knowledgeable and supportive medical providers who can contribute to comprehensive care for those experiencing consequences of an infection.
10. Laboratory tests for STIs can identify the infective agent but cannot always definitively state when the infection was contracted or who gave it to whom.
11. Sex therapists may deal with couples in whom an STI acquired historically surfaces within a sexual relationship. They can inform clients that the infection is historical and does not represent an importation from an unfaithful partner. Sex therapists may also deal with a situation in which an acute STI acquired in extrarelationship sexual contact provokes a primary relationship crisis exacerbated by the STI.
12. An STI arising in a relationship appears overwhelming to many. Helping a couple find perspective and acknowledge the many other dimensions and connections of their relationship may help them move forward.
13. The role of a therapist working with a couple dealing with an STI is to help each individual, as well as the dyad, make meaning of the diagnosis.

CODA

I'm dealing a lot better with my situation since my original e-mail, largely brought upon the support of the people I chose to share the news with and with the information I got through you. The realization that life will and has continued on as it did before, for the most part, helps in dealing with this. . . . Still a lot of anxiety in relation to the possibility of a future outbreak, not knowing when it may come, how bad it will be, and being aware perhaps too much of signs that another outbreak is coming. The only other source of anxiety is associated with fear surrounding the idea of even entering the dating scene again (and even though I'm in a happy relationship there's a lot of pressure to make sure this relationship works out, just to avoid finding someone else while having the STI. I see this as not so problematic for me personally but could see how some women may be influenced to stay in an abusive/bad relationship because of this). Also upon talking with some close friends about it I found out one had had a run in with a treatable STI in the past and another who had a friend who had gotten genital warts. Hearing that I'm not the only one was sort of helpful and as it turns out my story has convinced all my friends to consistently use condoms so that's a silver lining as well, as much worse STIs are out there and I would hate any of my friends to catch them. Only other thing I can think of is that there is still a minor effect on my sex life, as oral sex is still off limits (and was previously enjoyed) but other than that most things remain the same.

—ANONYMOUS (personal communication, 2011)

REFERENCES

Annon, J. (1976). The PLISSIT model: A proposed conceptual scheme for the behavioural treatment of sexual problems. *Journal of Sex Education and Therapy*, 2(1), 1–15.

Baraitser, P., Alexander, S., & Sheringham, J. (2011). Chlamydia trachomatis screening in young women. *Current Opinions Obstetrics and Gynecology, 23,* 315–320.

Black, A., Yang, Q., Wu Wen, S., Lalonde, A. B., Guilbert, E., & Fisher, W. A (2009). Contraceptive use among Canadian women of reproductive age: Results of a national survey. *Journal of Obstetrics and Gynaecology Canada, 31,* 627–640.

Campion, M. J., Brown, J. R., McCance, D. J., Atia, W., Edwards, R., Cuzick, J., et al. (1988). Psychosexual trauma of an abnormal cervical smear. *British Journal of Obstetrics and Gynaecology, 95,* 175–181.

Canadian STI Guidelines. (2012a) *Primary care and sexually transmitted infections*. Retrieved April 2, 2012, from *www.phac-aspc.gc.ca/std-mts/sti-its/pdf/secii-eng.pdf.*

Canadian STI Guidelines. (2012b) *Human immunodeficiency virus infections*. Retrieved April 2, 2012, from *www.phac-aspc.gc.ca/std-mts/sti-its/pdf/508hiv-vih-eng.pdf.*

Centers for Disease Control and Prevention. (2012a). *Male latex condoms and sexually transmitted diseases*. Retrieved April 2, 2012, from *www.cdc.gov/condomeffectiveness/latex.htm.*

Centers for Disease Control and Prevention. (2012b). *Sexually transmitted diseases*. Retrieved August 16, 2012, from *www.cdc.gov/std.*

Centers for Disease Control and Prevention. (2012c). *HIV surveillance United States 1981–2008*. Retrieved April 2, 2012, from *www.cdc.gov/mmwr/preview/mmwrhtml/mm6021a2.htm.*

Centers for Disease Control and Prevention. (2012d). *Hepatitis information for the public*. Retrieved April 2, 2012, from *www.cdc.gov/hepatitis/publicinfo.htm#whatishep.*

Centers for Disease Control and Prevention. (2012e). *Hepatitis B FAQ for health professionals*. Retrieved April 2, 2012, from *www.cdc.gov/hepatitis/hbv/hbvfaq.htm.*

Centers for Disease Control and Prevention. (2012f). *Genital/vulvovaginal candidiasis (VVC)*. Retrieved April 2, 2012, from *www.cdc.gov/fungal/candidiasis/genital.*

Cochran, S. D., & Mays, V. M. (1990). Sex, lies, and HIV. *New England Journal of Medicine, 322*(11), 774–775.

Corey, L., Wald, A., Patel, R. H., Sacks, S. L., Tyring, S. K, Warren, T., et al. (2004). Once-daily valacyclovir to reduce the risk of transmission of genital herpes. *New England Journal of Medicine, 350,* 11–20.

Cuzick, J., Clavel, C., Petry, K.-U., Meijer, C. J. L. M., Hoyer, H., Ratnam, S., et al. (2006). Overview of the European and North American studies on HPV testing in primary cervical cancer screening. *International Journal of Cancer, 119,* 1095–1101.

Daley, E. M., Perrin, K. M., McDermott, R. J., Vamos, C. A., Rayko, H. L., & Packing-Ebuen, J. L. (2010). The psychosocial burden of HPV. *Journal of Health Psychology, 15*(2), 279–290.

Drolet, M., Brisson, M., Maunsell, E., Franco, E. L., Coutlee, F., Ferenczy, A., et al. (2011a). The impact of anogenital warts on health-related quality of life: A 6-month prospective study. *Sexually Transmitted Diseases, 38*(10), 949–956.

Drolet, M., Brisson, M., Maunsell, E., Franco, E. L., Coutlée, F., Ferenczy, A., et al. (2011b). The psychosocial impact of an abnormal cervical smear result. *Psychooncology, 21*(10), 1071–1081.

Duncan, B., Hart, G., Scoular, A., & Bigrigg, A. (2001). Qualitative analysis of psychosocial impact of diagnosis of chlamydia trachomatis: Implications for screening. *British Medical Journal, 322,* 195–199.

Dunne, E. F., Unger, E. R., Sternberg, M., McQuillan, G., Swan, D. C., Patel, S. S., et al. (2007). Prevalence of HPV infection among females in the United States. *Journal of the American Medical Association, 298*(8), 813–819.

Fisher, J. D., Fisher, W. A., Cornman, D. H., Amico, K. R., Bryan, A., & Friedland, G. H. (2006). Clinician-delivered intervention during routine clinical care reduces unprotected sexual behavior among HIV-infected patients. *Journal of Acquired Immune Deficiency Syndrome, 41*(1), 44–52.

Fisher, W. A. (2012). "I think having the option available is a no-brainer": Will gay and bisexually active men at high risk of infection use over-the-counter rapid HIV tests to screen sexual partners? *Journal of Sex Research, 49*(4), 388–389.

Fisher, W. A. (2012). Understanding HPV vaccine uptake in developed countries. *Vaccine, 305,* F149–F156.

Fisher W. A., & Steben, M. (2014). Sexually transmitted infection: At the junction of biology and behavior. In C. Puckall (Ed.), *Human sexuality: Research and theory.* New York: Oxford University Press.

Giuliano, A. R., Lee, J.-H., Fulp, W., Villa, L. L., Lazcano, E., Papenfuss, M. R., et al. (2011). Incidence and clearance of genital human papillomavirus infection in men (HIM): A cohort study. *The Lancet, 377*(9769), 932–940.

Golden, M. R., Stekler, J., Hughes, J. P., & Wood, J. P. (2008). HIV serosorting in men who have sex with men: Is it safe? *Journal of Acquired Immune Deficiency Syndromes, 49,* 212–218.

Goldmeier, D., & Leiblum, S. R. (2005). STIs and sexual dysfunction. *Sexually Transmitted Diseases, 81,* 364.

Gottlieb, S. L., Stoner, B. P., Zaidi, A. A., Buckel, C., Tran, M., Leichliter, J. S., et al. (2011). A prospective study of the psychosocial impact of a positive chlamydia trachomatis laboratory test. *Sexually Transmitted Diseases, 38*(11), 1004–1011.

Granich, R. M., Gilks, C. F., Dye, C., De Cock, K. M., & Williams, B. G. (2009). Universal voluntary HIV testing with immediate antiretroviral therapy as a strategy for elimination of HIV transmission: A mathematical model. *The Lancet, 373,* 48–57.

Graziottin, A., & Serafini, A. (2009). HPV infection in women: Psychosexual impact of genital warts and intraepithelial lesions. *Journal of Sexual Medicine, 6,* 633–645.

Health Canada. (2012). *Canadian guidelines on sexually transmitted infections.* Retrieved April 2, 2012, from *www.phac-aspc.gc.ca/std-mts/sti-its.*

Jena, A. B., Goldman, D. P., Kamdar, A., Lakdawalla, D. N., & Lu, Y. (2010). Sexually transmitted diseases among users of erectile dysfunction drugs: Analysis of claims data. *Annals of Internal Medicine, 153,* 1–7.

Laumann, E.O., Gagnon, J.H., Michael, R.T., & Michaels, S. (1994). *The social organization of sexuality: Sexual practices in the United States.* Chicago: University of Chicago Press.

Linnehan, M. J., & Groce, E. (2000). Counseling and educational interventions for women with genital human papillomavirus infection. *AIDS Patient Care and STDs, 14*(8), 439–445.

MacDonald, N. E., Wells, G. A., Fisher, W. A., Warren, W. K., King, M. A., Doherty, J. A., et al. (1990). High-risk STD/HIV behavior among college students. *Journal of the American Medical Association, 263,* 3155–3159.

Marrazzo, J. M. (2010). Even NHANES evolves: Some surprising findings about women who have sex with women. *Sexually Transmitted Diseases, 37*(7), 414–415.

McCaffery, K., Waller, J., Forrest, S., Cadman, L., Szarewski, A., & Wardle, J. (2004). Testing positive for human papillomavirus in routine cervical screening: Examination of psychosocial impact. *British Journal of Obstetrics and Gynaecology, 111,* 1437–1443.

Melville, J., Sniffen, S., Crosby, R., Salazar, L., Whittington, D., Dithmer-Schreck, D., et al. (2003). Psychosocial impact of serological diagnosis of herpes simplex virus type 2: A qualitative assessment. *Sexually Transmitted Infections, 79,* 280–285.

Mindel, A., & Marks, C. (2005). Psychological symptoms associated with genital herpes virus infections: Epidemiology and approaches to management. *CNS Drugs, 19*(4), 303–312.

Misovich, S. J., Fisher, J. D., & Fisher, W. A. (1997). Close relationships and HIV risk behavior: Evidence and possible underlying psychological processes. *General Psychology Review, 1,* 72–130.

Palefsky, J. M. (2010). Human papillomavirus-related disease in men: Not just a women's issue. *Journal of Adolescent Health, 46*(4, Suppl.), S12–S19.

Parkin, D. M., & Bray, F. (2006). Chapter 2: The burden of HPV-related cancers. *Vaccine, 24*(Suppl. 3), S3/11–S3/25.

Parsons, J. T., Schrimshaw, E. W., Wolitski, R. J., Halkitis, P. N., Purcell, D. W., Hoff, C. C., et al. (2005). Sexual harm reduction practices of HIV-seropositive gay and bisexual men: Serosorting, strategic positioning, and withdrawal before ejaculation. *AIDS, 19*(Suppl. 1), S13–S25.

Richards, J., Scholes, D., Caka, S., Drolette, L., Margaret, A. M., Yarbro, P., et al. (2007). HSV-2 serologic testing in an HMO population: Uptake and psychosocial sequelae. *Sexually Transmitted Diseases, 34*(9), 718–725.

Richardson, H., Kelsall, G., Tellier, P., Voyer, H., Abrahamowicz, M., Ferenczy, A., et al. (2003). The natural history of type-specific human papillomavirus infections in female university students. *Cancer Epidemiology, Biomarkers and Prevention, 12,* 485–490.

Rollnick, S., Miller, W. R., & Butler, C. C. (2008). *Motivational interviewing in health care: Helping patients change behavior.* New York: Guilford Press.

Sadeghi-Nejad, H., Wasserman, M., Weidner, W., Richardson, D., & Goldmeier, D. (2010). Sexually transmitted diseases and sexual function. *Journal of Sexual Medicine, 7,* 389–413.

Shindel, A. W., Horberg, M. A., Smith, J. F., & Breyer, B. N. (2011). Sexual dysfunction, HIV, and AIDS in men who have sex with men. *AIDS Patient Care and STDS, 6,* 341–349.

Sobel, J. D. (2003). Management of patients with recurrent vulvovaginal candidiasis. *Drugs, 63*(11), 1059–1066.

Sobel, J. D., Faro, S., Force, R. W., Foxman, B., Ledger, W. J., Nyirjesy, J. R., et al. (1998). Vulvovaginal candidiasis: Epidemiologic, diagnostic, and therapeutic considerations. *American Journal of Obstetrics and Gynecology, 178*(2), 203–211.

Su, J. R., Beltrami, J. F., Zaidi, A. A., & Weinstock, H. S. (2011). Primary and secondary syphilis among Black and Hispanic men who have sex with men: Case report data from 27 states. *Annals of Internal Medicine, 155,* 145–151.

Winer, R. L., Hughes, J. P., Feng, Q., O'Reilly, S., Kiviat, N. B., Holmes, K. K., et al. (2006). Condom use and the risk of genital human papillomavirus infection in young women. *New England Journal of Medicine, 354.* 2645–2654.

Xu, F., Sternberg, M. R., Kottiri, B. J., McQuillan, G. M., Lee, F. K., Nahmias, A. J., et al. (2006). Trends in herpes simplex virus type 1 and type 2 seroprevalence in the United States. *Journal of the American Medical Association, 296,* 964–973.

Lifespan Changes

CHAPTER 23

Sexual Problems in Adolescents and Young Adults

Lucia F. O'Sullivan and Vickie Pasterski

"**A** sexually active adolescent female who feels no desire, has never had an orgasm, and experiences no pleasure from her sexual life is unlikely to be viewed as experiencing sexual problems," O'Sullivan and Pasterski point out. They say that what constitutes a sexual dysfunction in adulthood is often viewed as normative (or perhaps even ideal) in adolescence. Their review of the available research on adolescent sexuality finds that it is narrowly focused on high-risk behaviors and problematic outcomes (e.g., STIs, pregnancy, rape). O'Sullivan and Pasterski nevertheless do a masterful job of integrating the adult treatment literature with an understanding of the unique issues facing adolescents in order to provide sound treatment recommendations for conducting sex therapy with young adults and teens. Improving our understanding of adolescent sexuality (normal, healthy, ideal, and dysfunctional) will necessarily improve our understanding of how sexual problems develop and have a positive impact on therapeutic efficacy.

Lucia F. O'Sullivan, Ph,D, is Professor of Psychology at the University of New Brunswick in Canada. She also holds a Canada Research Chair in Adolescents' Sexual Health Behaviour. Her work centers primarily on sexual functioning, health, and risk behavior among adolescents and young adults. Dr. O'Sullivan serves on the editorial boards of eight journals, has published over 72 scientific articles and chapters, and has also won outstanding teaching awards from Columbia University and the University of New Brunswick.

Vickie Pasterski, PhD, is a recognized authority on normative and non-normative psychosexual development in children and adolescents and has published widely on these topics. She is a Research Psychologist in Paediatrics at Addenbrooke's Hospital,

University of Cambridge, where she has most recently focused on outcomes in disorders of sex development (DSD). She also holds affiliated lecturer status in the Department of Psychology, University of Cambridge.

OVERVIEW OF SEXUAL PROBLEMS
AMONG ADOLESCENTS AND YOUNG ADULTS

Despite the wealth of research on the sexual lives of adolescents and young adults, it is surprising how little is known about the sexual functioning of young people. "Adolescence" refers here to the period of development between childhood and adulthood and captures the teenage years. "Young adulthood" typically refers to the period between late adolescence through the mid-20s (Centers for Disease Control and Prevention, 2012; UN Population Information Network, 1997). The gap in this literature is also notable in light of the high rates of sexual dysfunctions among adults. Sexual experiences in adolescence and young adulthood are the foundation on which adult sexual lives are based. Positive sexual functioning is clearly an essential component of sexual health; however, there is a dearth of research on the sexual functioning of young adult populations and almost none among adolescents. Although their sexual lives have garnered considerable research attention, it has been through a very selective prism focusing on high-risk behaviors and problem outcomes, such as early onset of partnered activity, unwanted pregnancy, sexually transmitted infections (STIs), and coercion. In some respects, the same sexual problems that are considered to be indicative of dysfunction among adults, such as lack of pleasure, rapid ejaculation, anorgasmia, and pain, are viewed as normative conditions among young people.

Society fosters a deep and abiding distrust and discomfort about issues related to sexual development, privileging sexual experience to the realm of adulthood. Thus sexually active young people are viewed with some disdain, their sexual behaviors referred to as irresponsible or problems in themselves, and they are not viewed as having rights to sexual pleasure (or absence of pain). Sexual problems that arise are in some respects viewed as if they are deserved or to be expected ("the wages of sin"). This period of life is replete with many related psychosocial and relational challenges, including establishing one's sexual identity, learning to negotiate issues such as contraceptive access and use, fear of pregnancy or contraceptive/condom failure, use and exposure to sexually explicit media, and changes in dating norms. Problems in sexual functioning may compromise young people's romantic and sexual relationships and exacerbate questions relating to gender identity, body image, and fertility—all factors central to positive development, identity, and adjustment in this period of life. We use a developmental focus and a sexual-rights perspective to address issues relevant to sexual functioning among adolescents and young adults and explore the challenges and limitations to advancing treatment among this population.

EPIDEMIOLOGY

Several large-scale studies of sexual functioning have included late adolescents or young adults. However, they tend to be small in number and include rates that are obscured in the analyses of older adults (e.g., Mercer et al., 2003). For example, a U.S. national probability sample analyzed rates from men and women 18–29 years of age (Laumann, Paik, & Rosen, 1999). These rates combine those of late adolescents, young adults, and adults. Even so, the following rates were obtained for men and women, respectively, for the preceding year in several domains: lack of interest in sex (14%, 32%), inability to orgasm (7%, 26%), experience of pain during sex (30%, 21%), finding sex not pleasurable (10%, 27%), anxiety about performance (19%, 16%), trouble lubricating (19%, women only), and trouble maintaining or achieving an erection (7%, men only). Sexual difficulties were more prevalent among women (43%) than among men (31%).

In an analysis of data from the National Longitudinal Study of Adolescent Health, researchers examined the regularity of orgasm among 3,237 respondents ages 18–26 years, who reported being in heterosexual relationships of at least 3 months' duration (Galinsky & Sonenstein, 2011). Ages, again, were not separated for adolescents and young adults alone, as the range includes those up to 26 years of age. Sex was defined as including vaginal, oral, or anal sex. Fifteen percent of the young women reported having orgasms less than half the time or never compared with 2.6% of the young men. A survey of 18 to 24-year-old women found that 31% were unable to have orgasms during intercourse, 33% reported low sexual desire, and 22% reported physical pain during intercourse (Fisher, Boroditsky, & Morris, 2004). No data on men were available. Although unclear, these studies suggest moderate to high rates of problems in sexual functioning among young people and possibly rates that are comparable to those of adults.

In one of the few known studies addressing sexual problems among young people directly, 171 late-adolescent men and women (17–21 years) were surveyed regarding lifetime experiences of sexual difficulties (O'Sullivan & Majerovich, 2008). The prevalence of difficulties among men that occurred "sometimes" or "always" included: climaxing too quickly (41.9%), anxiety about performing sexually (32.6%), difficulty maintaining an erection (23.1%), engaging in unwanted sexual activity (18.7%), and inability to climax (16.3%). Chronic difficulties were uncommon in this sample of men, although occasional experiences of sexual difficulties, such as rapid ejaculation and performance anxiety, were fairly common. Problems reported "sometimes" or "always" for women were: inability to climax (53.1%) or climaxing too quickly (23.2%), insufficient lubrication (31.3%), performance anxiety

(31.2%), painful intercourse (25.8%), unwanted sexual activity (23.5%), and lack of interest (22.9%) or pleasure (11.2%). Like the young men, few young women reported "always" experiencing a given sexual problem. The most common persistent difficulty was inability to have an orgasm.

Follow-up qualitative interviews with 30 of these individuals revealed that (1) pleasure increased with sexual experience; (2) sexual difficulties frequently led to sex avoidance; (3) sexual activity may have been high even when sexual interest was low; and (4) pain was often linked to low arousal. A female participant said, "If we don't do it for a couple days it'll hurt sometimes, just starting off . . . or actually on the inside wall sometimes it hurts after I've reached orgasm. I don't know why. . . . I just work through it." A man explained, "Her sex drive is still very, um, high and mine's falling off. Which is kind of ironic, since the guy's supposed to be the sexual animal. . . . It's a point of stress, which makes it worse, so I'm beginning to hide out, avoid even touching her." A young woman explained, "Uh, one of the reasons why I believe I can't orgasm during sex is because I haven't . . . there's not much to it. I don't feel a whole lot during sex." Another young woman told us: "He has [laughs] a very large penis. And it hurt. . . . It wasn't enjoyable. I thought he hit an organ for god's sake. [Laughs] So, we only had sex twice. I . . . I . . . I just wasn't happy with the relationship in many ways and that was one of them." Additional research is needed to explore further the impact of sexual problems on the psychological and relationship functioning of young people.

An ongoing longitudinal study of 406 youth (16–21 years) is under way to help track the onset and progression of sexual problems among adolescents and young adults (O'Sullivan, Brotto, Byers, Majerovich & Wuest, in press). Analyses of baseline data for sexually active youth revealed that 50% reported a sexual problem and 50% of those reported distress associated with a sexual problem. Using a standard measure of sexual dysfunction (Rosen et al., 2000), young women's scores revealed problems in desire, arousal and satisfaction, lubrication, orgasm, and genital pain that more closely resembled those of women with sexual dysfunction than those of controls. The young men's scores more closely resembled those obtained from the adult controls (Rosen et al., 1997). Overall, 19% of the young men were classified as having symptoms of premature ejaculation (PE) or possible PE. No other studies that address a range of sexual problems among adolescents and young adults were found.

Finally, there are several studies linking specific sexual dysfunctions among young people to medical disorders; gynecological or genitourinary problems or abnormalities (e.g., pelvic inflammatory disease, testicular cancer, endometriosis); conditions requiring surgical treatments, such as congenital anomalies or ovarian cysts or tumors (Greydanus & Matytsina, 2010), complications of medications, such as selective serotonin reuptake inhibitors (SSRIs); antipsychotic medication; and long-term oral contraceptive use. Other studies provide less direct evidence of sexual dysfunctions, such as sildenafil use among late adolescent males (Peters, Johnson, Kelder, Meschack, & Jefferson, 2007).

ASSESSMENT AND DIAGNOSTIC ISSUES

A sexually active adolescent female who feels no desire, has never had an orgasm, and experiences no pleasure from her sexual life is unlikely to be viewed as experiencing sexual problems. Tolman argues, "Female adolescent sexual dysfunction is an oxymoron" (Tolman, 2001, p. 197). Sexual problems among adolescent males are frequently the object of ridicule or depicted humorously in popular books or movies, such as *American Pie* and *Fast Times at Ridgemont High*. Adolescence is viewed as a period in which young people transform from sexually inexperienced to sexually inept to sexually competent. Upon reaching adulthood, they are expected to have sexual experience, expertise, even prowess (for men at least), perhaps contributing in part to the high rates of adult sexual dysfunctions.

These assumptions are particularly clear when reviewing the diagnostic criteria of the DSM. There are no age criteria for any of the sexual dysfunctions included in DSM-5 (American Psychiatric Association, 2013) or its predecessors. As we argued earlier, many of the hallmark features of the dysfunctions appear to be typical of many young people, especially early in their sexual lives, such as "marked delay in, marked infrequency of or absence of orgasm" (female orgasmic disorder, p. 429); "persistent or recurrent pattern of ejaculation occurring during partnered sexual activity within approximately one minute following vaginal penetration and before the individual wishes it" (early ejaculation, p. 443); "absent/reduced interest in sexual activity" (sexual interest/arousal disorder in women, p. 433); "persistently or recurrently deficient (or absent) sexual/erotic thoughts or fantasies and desire for sexual activity" (male hypoactive sexual desire disorder, p. 440); and "persistent or recurrent difficulties with vaginal penetration during intercourse" (p. 437); or "marked vulvovaginal or pelvic pain during vaginal intercourse or penetration attempts" (genito-pelvic pain/penetration disorder, p. 437). Even if there were age-related specifiers (e.g., age at onset), underlying assumptions within the DSM-5 criterion-based diagnostic system present challenges to the case of adolescence and/or early adulthood.

The DSM diagnoses require that an individual experience the symptoms for at least 6 months for a diagnosis to be warranted. Thus many adolescents and young adults in their first half year following the onset of sexual activity could meet this requirement for diagnosis of a sexual dysfunction. We recommend that clinicians not be put off by the lack of specificity and review presenting symptoms in the context of an individual's broader sexual and relationship life. Particularly important in the case of young people is to take into account patterns of sexual functioning from the onset of their sexual lives—across partners, if applicable—while bearing in mind that many young people have little consistency in sexual frequency and experience long periods of abstinence at first. The 6-month criterion assumes regular sexual activity to assess frequency of symptoms, which is much less likely in younger adolescents. It may be a year or two once activity has commenced before there is a sustained period across which one may judge the course of the complaint. Thus clinicians should apply that criterion cautiously. It is likely that some problems are encountered in the process of learning how to control timing and to communicate effectively with a partner in order to maximize pleasure and while developing preferences for positions and activities in general. We recommend that clinicians always be cognizant of the potentially strong stigmatizing or inhibiting impact of applying diagnostic labels at this (early) point of life. Clinicians should communicate these labels cautiously, if at all.

Central to the diagnostic system is an assessment in each case that an individual has experienced "clinically significant distress or impairment" as a result of the problem. This feature likely ensures that many young people who are learning "how sex works," developing skills, learning how to communicate about sexual matters with a partner, and overcoming various sexual problems across partners, activities, and time are unlikely to report the high level of distress that warrants diagnosis. This is only an assumption based on our own research, however, as there is scant research to indicate whether distress is characteristic of their early sexual lives, and certainly no discourse on this matter in the field. A challenge to clinicians is to assess the nature and severity of distress related to established problems in sexual functioning among adolescents and young adults.

We recommend that clinicians employ existing measures designed for adults, with a few changes (e.g., wording to reflect the knowledge or lexicon of a teenager) as necessary. We like the comprehensiveness of the Golombok–Rust Inventory of Sexual Satisfaction (GRISS; Rust & Golombok, 1985), but it has a strong relationship focus, which may not always be appropriate. We have also used successfully the Female Sexual Functioning Inventory (Rosen et al., 2000), and the Brief Index of Sexual Functioning for Women (Taylor, Rosen, & Leiblum, 1994). For young men, we recommend the International Index of Erectile Function (IIEF; Rosen et al., 1997), the Premature Ejaculation Diagnostic Tool (Symonds et al., 2007) or the Brief Sexual Function Questionnaire (Reynolds et al., 1988). The Female Sexual Distress Scale (FSDS; Derogatis, Rosen, Leiblum, Burnett, & Heiman, 2002) can measure sexual functioning distress in both young women and men.

The potential impact of DSM-5 diagnostic criteria on adolescents and young adults is likely minimal, given that the dysfunctions have unknown applicability. However, in the case of the new diagnoses for female orgasmic disorder and sexual interest/arousal disorder in women, changes recognizing the substantial variation across women in sexual response cycles will likely benefit young women who may have response cycles that look quite different from adult women's. There is also now greater recognition of variation in the expression of interest and desire, especially in the form of fantasy and erotic thoughts. Researchers find both overlap in interest, arousal, and desire, inconsistent sequencing, and variation in spontaneity/responsiveness (Graham, Sanders, Milhausen, & McBride, 2004). The new genito-pelvic pain/penetration disorder is far more expansive and descriptive than before and now may capture young people's experiences, given the high rates of sexual pain among both male and female adolescents (O'Sullivan & Majerovich, 2008). The new "other specified sexual dysfunction" category addresses fear and anxiety related to sexual contact rather than loss of sexual feelings despite "otherwise normal" arousal and orgasm. Once again, there is no comparative model to capture "normal" response cycles in young people, but fear and anxiety are known components of early sexual expression and avoidance for adolescents, if not young adults.

ETIOLOGY/THEORIES/MODELS OF THE SEXUAL PROBLEM

Young people face a host of age-related factors that appear to be linked to the experience of sexual problems. These include inadequate sex education and family communication concerning issues pertaining to sexual functioning, lack of experience across time and partners, less sophisticated communication and intimacy/relationship skills, and high rates of compromising health factors, such as STIs, and anxiety and depression. Compared with adults, sexual problems among young people might be less attributable to organic breakdown associated with long-term medical conditions, although we simply do not yet know.

Important to understanding etiology is the host of psychosocial factors central to the experience of youth, including the sexual objectification of girls to represent targets of male desire; socialization with heavy emphasis on a range of romantic myths surrounding sex, such as that sex should always be perfect, spontaneous, and fulfilling; and the myriad messages that young people receive through the media equating sex with personal value. There continues to be strong endorsement of what Simon and Gagnon (1986) have termed the traditional sexual script, which positions men as adversarial sexual agents in heterosexual encounters with girls and positions girls as sexual ascetics, targets of male sexual attention, or negotiators of sex for love and security. Endorsing such scripts has negative consequences for both young women and men, such as agreeing to unwanted or painful sex, silencing oneself concerning sexual interests and needs, abuse and coercion, poor body image, guilt, resignation, resentment, and anxiety (Dworkin & O'Sullivan, 2005; Elmerstig, Mijma, & Berterö, 2008).

Dysfunctions may also be the result of biomedical factors, such as inherent pathophysiological abnormalities. These would include mild congenital defects, such as hypospadias in males or the more complex case of abnormalities of the urogenital tract due to a disorder of sex development (DSD; Pasterski, Prentice, & Hughes, 2010). Genetic impairments may also result in the inability to reduce inflammatory responses or in variations in pain-regulatory mechanisms or thresholds (Landry & Bergeron, 2011).

APPROACHES TO TREATMENT

Young people are not expected to have sexual lives, so it is expected, if not subtly reinforced, that they may experience pain or lack of desire. Standard approaches to the treatment of sexual problems among young people are often medical ones, and health care providers are the first (and often only) to know of sexual problems (Brown & Brown, 2006). Although desire and arousal are important components of a healthy sexual life, the focus with youth tends to be on issues of contraception and reproductive health. Young people require assurances that the care they receive is confidential, yet it is only when the provider suspects that the individual has a sexual problem to discuss that clinicians typically request that a parent leave the room, offer time alone, or assure an adolescent or young person that the information that they provide is kept private (McKee, Rubin, Campos, & O'Sullivan, 2011).

Because youth may not present with sexual problems, clinicians need to ask the essential questions that can uncover problems in sexual functioning. An excellent approach is to incorporate this line of questioning into inquiries for related presenting issues, backed by more random and comprehensive inquiries into all areas of medical or psychosocial functioning that include sexuality. Neither parental nor partner consent is required to talk to or counsel an individual below the age of majority about sexual problems or to discuss a young person's relationship. Clinicians need to be aware of age-of-consent laws relevant to sexual activity, as they vary regionally (e.g., 16 in Canada and the United Kingdom; 16–18 in the United States) and need to clarify the limitations of their privacy assurances with the youth whom they counsel. Similarly, the issue of parental involvement for adolescents can be a difficult one. We recommend encouraging open communication with a parent or other trusted family member or offering to facilitate communication about sexual problems that require more serious intervention or treatment.

Without a body of literature upon which to draw, it is exceedingly difficult to outline treatment approaches. Tailoring standard psychological therapies that are used with adults with dysfunctions to address the unique issues faced by adolescents and young adults (as described earlier) is a sound starting point. Therapy might best be combined with pharmacological management of cases, but we know of no medications that are approved for treatment of sexual dysfunctions among young people and recommend again that clinicians take a longer term perspective to truly understand the sexual problem in the context of a young person's developing sexual life. In the absence of a literature to which to refer, treatment protocols may be developed drawing on other related bodies of literature or by developing theoretical models. In the case of structural anomalies in sexual functioning, there is a growing consensus about psychological treatment relating to psychosexual health in young patients (Hughes, Houk, Ahmed, & Lee, 2006). The approach is one of full disclosure (with the permission of parents where necessary) and openness regarding sexual functioning. Talk-based therapy is often used to address psychological sequelae of these dysfunctions (e.g., Hughes et al., 2012). Interestingly, in this context, sexual activity is generally seen as a healthy and natural part of early adult life. The goal of the health care provider is to promote healthy sexual functioning. In the absence of structural abnormality, frank discussion regarding sexual functioning, treatment options, and general sexual health apply.

Although there are as yet no reports of outcomes specific to psychological therapeutic approaches in counseling adolescents and young adults with possible sexual dysfunction secondary to DSD, one successful approach has incorporated cognitive theory. According to cognitive theory, general positive beliefs about the self are central to healthy psychological functioning and should be considered in parallel with treatments aimed at specific sexual problems. Open communication with one's partner(s) may be difficult or impossible for a young person experiencing dysfunction. Improving the self- and body image by restructuring beliefs and underlying assumptions may be valuable here. In many cases, sex therapy requires that both partners participate and work together toward solving sexual functioning problems. Although such an approach requires trust and a degree of stability in the relationship, we recommend incorporating partners wherever possible.

Some useful resources include books such as *Sex, Therapy, and Kids: Addressing Their Concerns through Talk and Play,* by Sharon Lamb (Norton, 2006); *It's Perfectly Normal: Changing Bodies, Growing Up, Sex, and Sexual Health,* by Robie H. Harris and Michael Emberley (Candlewick, 2009); and *Nurturing Queer Youth: Family Therapy Transformed,* by Linda Stone Fish and Rebecca G. Harvey (Norton, 2005). Excellent Web resources include those of the College of Sexual and Relationship Therapists, the Sex Information and Education Council of Canada, the Sex Information and Education Council of the United States, American Association of Sexuality Educators, Counselors and Therapists, *sexualityandU.ca*, and Advocates for Youth.

CASE DISCUSSIONS

We reiterate here that there is no systematic report of sexual dysfunction or its treatment in adults younger than 17 years old. We present two cases and outcomes here, but these are only examples and not evidence of treatment success. Larger samples and systematic implementation of treatment protocols are needed to establish guidelines beyond our recommendations.

Case 1

Here we present a case of a 17-year-old female, JL, who presented upon referral from her general practitioner and at her mother's insistence. The primary complaint was that, for about 8 weeks, JL had been exhibiting symptoms of what her mother feared might be depression. JL had withdrawn from most activities with her family, spent much of her free time by herself in her bedroom, had fallen behind in her homework, and showed no outward signs of distress at her failing grades. Most notably, however, was that she had cut off contact with her boyfriend, who also expressed concern to her family. In JL's first meeting with the psychologist, she calmly and quietly confirmed what her mother had reported. In this case, a standard psychological assessment was administered, confirming clinical depression. However, upon hearing the results of the assessment, JL broke down in tears and revealed that, contrary to her presentation heretofore, she was keenly aware of the factors contributing to her withdrawal and low mood.

In the prior 4–5 months, JL had become sexually active with the boyfriend who she had been dating for 2 years. She made it clear that she had consented and that the two loved each other. The problem was that JL was left with severe abrasions after each episode. The psychologist quickly assessed that the abrasions were likely due to lack of lubrication and began a line of questioning about JL's sexual response from the desire to arousal to orgasm. Not surprisingly, JL reported that most encounters began quickly and passionately, but without sufficient arousal (or time for arousal) to allow for lubrication. JL was unaware of the relationship between arousal and lubrication, nor did she report experiencing orgasm during intercourse. In any case, the abrasions became infected, and intercourse became incredibly painful for JL. Not wanting to disappoint her boyfriend, she gave excuses for withdrawal from him that led to feelings of sadness and despair. JL's mood lifted very quickly upon realization that there was nothing mysteriously wrong with her, as she had tested negative for STIs.

This case illustrates several points critical to the conceptualization of sexual dysfunction in adolescents and young adults. First, JL would not meet the standard criterion that suggests that the "dysfunction" should be noted in comparison with previous satisfactory functioning. JL had only been sexually active for a very short time. Second, JL, as with many young women, may not have been exposed to features of healthy sexual functioning. In fact, she was unaware of the necessity for lubrication to facilitate coitus. She was also seemingly unaware that her own sexual response was critical to her sexual satisfaction. She seemed to be under the impression that women should "have sex" with their partners because that is what the partner desires. Finally, this case illustrates the fragility of the sexual response in the context of depressed mood, or, in this case, apparent clinical depression. In many cases, the clinician has trouble discerning which factors lead to the other, that is, whether low arousal contributes to relationship difficulties and/or depression or whether depression completely unrelated to relationships can decrease desire and arousal. In this case, confusion, pain, and fear of disappointing her partner clearly led to the depressed mood. Once this cascade of events was set in motion, it likely turned into a cycle difficult to break.

JL was a bright and insightful young woman. She was visibly affected by the short course of sexual education that she received in the therapist's office. She took advice with respect to taking some control of the sexual encounters.

She, surprisingly, was also open to having a discussion with her boyfriend explaining what she had kept secret for several months. At follow-up, JL reported that she had taken some time for the abrasions to heal, although she very quickly became romantically engaged with her boyfriend again. The reunion had a very positive effect on her mood and self-esteem. Once she and her partner resumed sexual relations, she felt more in control and better understood her own sexuality. Her report suggested that she now had what appeared to be a healthy sexual relationship. One final point should be noted: Without the education JL received from the psychologist, she may well have gone on to have further difficulty in other areas of her life in addition to romantic/sexual relationships. This, again, illustrates the importance of education for a healthy beginning to sexual life.

Case 2

Our second case is that of a 16-year-old male, TM, who presented to a community mental health clinic with complaints of erectile dysfunction. This young man presented of his own accord without hesitation regarding his inability to maintain an erection during heterosexual encounters. He reported that he had never suffered from a psychological disorder, nor was there any such history in his family. TM reported that he came from an intact family including three children, two boys and one girl. TM was the oldest. There was no history of sexual abuse, and his parents appeared to him to have a loving relationship. TM's family was of middle income, which afforded him the ability to focus on his studies and social affairs. He planned at the time to go to a university to study art history. TM presented with no obvious personality or psychological dysfunction. He was engaged and measured with regard to the frank discussion about his sexual problem.

When asked to describe the problem specifically, TM said that on several occasions he had been unable to maintain an erection to the point of climax and had had to end the encounters with attractive young women prematurely. He found this embarrassing, although he had been able to attribute the dysfunction to alcohol consumption, allowing him to save face. It became clear that he had a tight circle of friends and that these episodes occurred with girls in his social network. He had asked for help, as he felt he could no longer engage sexually in his network without solving this problem first. Although he recognized, from popular culture, that young males need to find their way about sexual relations, he believed that the problems he was experiencing reflected something more than inexperience. At the completion of the general assessment, TM was offered a referral to a sex therapy center. TM expressed that the couple-oriented nature of sex therapy did not appeal to him, as he had no regular partner and no one with whom he might comfortably implement treatment strategies. It was at this point that TM offered his impression that there was a psychological conflict at the root of his problem and suggested that he would like to further explore his sense of self as a sexual person.

It later came to light that TM had concerns regarding his sexual orientation but had yet to explore them for fear of a homosexual orientation. He was not bigoted toward homosexuality, nor did he maintain beliefs about the superiority of heterosexuals. He said that the thought of letting his parents down when it came to having a family of his own someday had caused him some concern. It also came to light that TM perceived that his male friends were engaging completely successfully in sexual relations. This apparently had become a topic of discussion among the young men on a regular basis. It was also the case that the sought-after girls were in the same network and that gossip traveled quickly. TM had put immense pressure on himself to perform before he had even begun his sexual life in full.

Although there was no clear evidence of anxiety disorder, this preoccupation had become a type of obsession for TM. The therapist proposed a combination of schema therapy and cognitive-behavioral therapy. The aim was for TM to first explore his relationship with his parents and his sense of self in that context. Next steps involved assessing TM's beliefs about himself in his cohort as a successful male. Both therapist and patient agreed that to relieve the pressure might alleviate the problem. Twelve sessions were proposed.

Given TM's general intelligence and insight, the case took clear form and resolved. He reevaluated his parents' expectations, which were clearly that he grow into a happy, healthy adult. He also had the insight that his male companions were likely presenting as socially desirable in competing for females. The greatest relief came with the insight that he could explore his sexual orientation if he wanted to, albeit in a context outside his social set. TM's dysfunction abated in the sense that he no longer felt pressured to perform nor distressed about the prospects of maintaining an erection during intercourse with women. He carried on with his goals toward becoming an art historian. In this case, we were able to watch this young man's sexuality as it first developed. This likely provided a strong foundation for a healthy sex life, although no follow-up has been completed. Although in this case the therapist was confronted with the inability to apply traditional couple or sex therapy, we can see that the application of schema and cognitive theories was successful, at least in the short term. TM was never diagnosed with ED, which, in our view, was to his benefit.

CONCLUSIONS

Our current understanding of sexual problems in adolescents and young adults is based on a small, but growing, body of research and to some extent extrapolation from the adult literature on dysfunctions. Many sexual problems among young people likely reflect a steep learning curve emanating from a dearth of information about how sex works; however, rates of sexual problems appear high and no gender differences in rates are noted. Our strongest recommendation is to provide extensive, comprehensive, and explicit information about healthy, pleasurable sexual functioning, with an emphasis on effective and clear partner communication and negotiation, as well as strategies for seeking treatment. Connecting with health care providers, who are likely to learn first of any problems that emerge, and encouraging frank discussions about sexual matters among youth in one's practice are also recommended. Until intervention research has advanced, clinicians must adapt standard approaches for adults to the unique contexts of young people's lives. We also strongly suggest that clinicians treating young people connect to organizations aimed at improving the sexual lives of youth for resources, support, and continued education.

REFERENCES

American Psychiatric Association. (2013). *Diagnostic and statistical manual of mental disorders* (5th ed.). Arlington, VA: Author.

Brown, R. T., & Brown, J. D. (2006). Adolescent sexuality. *Primary Care: Clinics in Office Practice, 33,* 373–390.

Centers for Disease Control and Prevention. (2013). *Vaccines for college students and young adults (19 to 26 years old).* Available at *www.cdc.gov/vaccines/adults/rec-vac/college.html.*

Derogatis, L. R., Rosen, R., Leiblum, S., Burnett, A., & Heiman, J. (2002). The Female Sexual Distress Scale (FSDS): Initial validation of a standardized scale for assessment of sexually related personal distress in women. *Journal of Sex and Marital Therapy, 28,* 317–330.

Dworkin, S. L., & O'Sullivan, L. (2005). Actual versus desired initiation patterns among a sample of college men: Tapping disjunctures within traditional male sexual scripts. *Journal of Sex Research, 42,* 150–158.

Elmerstig, E., Mijma, B., & Berterö, C. (2008). Why do young women continue to have sexual intercourse despite pain? *Journal of Adolescent Health, 43,* 357–363.

Fisher, W.A., Boroditsky, R., & Morris, B. (2004). The 2002 Canadian Contraception Study: Part B. *Journal of Obstetrics and Gynaecology of Canada, 26*(6), 580–590.

Galinsky, A. M., & Sonenstein, F. L. (2011). The association between developmental assets and sexual enjoyment among emerging adults. *Journal of Adolescent Health, 48,* 610–615.

Graham, C. A., Sanders, S. A., Milhausen, R. R., & McBride, K. R. (2004). Turning on and turning off: A focus group study of the factors that affect women's sexual arousal. *Archives of Sexual Behavior, 33,* 527–538.

Greydanus, D. E., & Matytsina, L. (2010). Female sexual dysfunction and adolescents. *Current Opinion in Obstetrics and Gynecology, 22,* 375–380.

Hughes, I. A., Davies, J. D., Bunch, T. I., Pasterski, V., Mastroyannopoulou, K., & MacDougall, J. (2012). Androgen insensitivity syndrome. *Lancet, 380,* 1419–1428.

Hughes, I. A., Houk, C., Ahmed, S. F., & Lee, P. A. (2006). Consensus statement on the management of intersex disorders. *Journal of Pediatric Urology, 2,* 148–162.

Landry, T., & Bergeron, S. (2011). Biopsychosocial factors associated with dyspareunia in a community sample of adolescent girls. *Archives of Sexual Behavior, 40,* 877–889.

Laumann, E. O., Paik, A., & Rosen, R. C. (1999). Sexual dysfunction in the United States: Prevalence and predictors. *Journal of the American Medical Association, 281*, 537–544.

McKee, M. D., Rubin, S., Campos, G., & O'Sullivan, L. F. (2011). Challenges of providing confidential care to adolescents in urban primary care: Clinicians' perspectives. *Annals of Family Medicine, 9*, 37–43.

Mercer, C. H., Fenton, K. A., Johnson, A. M., Wellings, K., Macdowall, W., McManus, S., et al. (2003). Sexual function problems and help seeking behavior in Britain: National Probability Sample Survey. *British Medical Journal, 327*, 426–427.

O'Sullivan, L. F., Brotto, L., Byers, E. S., Majerovich, J. A., & Wuest, J. (in press). Problems in sexual functioning among adolescents and young adults. *Journal of Sexual Medicine*.

O'Sullivan, L. F., & Majerovich, J. (2008). Difficulties with sexual functioning in a sample of male and female late adolescent and young adult university students. *Canadian Journal of Human Sexuality, 17*, 109–121.

Pasterski, V., Prentice, P., & Hughes, I. A. (2010). Impact of the consensus statement and the new DSD classification system. *Best Practices and Research Clinical Endocrinology and Metabolism, 24*, 187–195.

Peters, R. J., Johnson, R. J., Kelder, S., Meschack, A. F., & Jefferson, T. (2007). Beliefs and social norms about sildenafil citrate (Viagra) misuse and perceived consequences among Houstonian teenage males. *American Journal of Men's Health, 1*, 208–212.

Reynolds, C. F., Frank, E., Thase, M. E., Houck, P. R., Jennings, J. R., & Howell, J. R. (1988). Assessment of sexual function in depressed, impotent, and healthy men: Factor analysis of a Brief Sexual Function Questionnaire for men. *Psychiatry Research, 24*, 231–250.

Rosen, R., Brown, C., Heiman, J., Leiblum, S., Meston, C., Shabsigh, R., et al. (2000). The Female Sexual Function Index (FSFI): A multidimensional self-report instrument for the assessment of female sexual function. *Journal of Sex and Marital Therapy, 26*, 191–208.

Rosen, R., Riley, A., Wagner, G., Osterloh, I. H., Kirkpatrick, J., & Mishra, A. (1997). The International Index of Erectile Function (IIEF): A multidimensional scale for assessment of erectile dysfunction. *Urology, 49*, 822–830.

Rust, J., & Golombok, S. (1985). The Golombok–Rust Inventory of Sexual Satisfaction (GRISS). *British Journal of Clinical Psychology, 24*, 63–64.

Simon, W., & Gagnon, J. (1986). Sexual scripts. *Archives of Sexual Behavior, 15*, 97–120.

Symonds, T., Perelman, M. A., Althof, S., Giuliano, F., Martin, M., May, K., et al. (2007). Development and validation of a premature ejaculation diagnostic tool. *European Urology, 52*, 565–573.

Taylor, J. R., Rosen, R. C., & Leiblum, S. R. (1994). Self-report assessment of female sexual dysfunction: Psychometric properties of the brief index of sexual functioning for women. *Archives of Sexual Behavior, 23*, 627–643.

Tolman, D. L. (2001). Female adolescent sexuality: An argument for developmental perspective on the New View of women's sexual problems. *Women and Therapy, 24*, 195–209.

United Nations Population Information Network. (2007). *HIV prevalence (females 15–24)*. Available at *http://data.un.org/data.aspx?q=15-24&d=unaids&f=inid %3a346*.

CHAPTER 24

Sexuality and Aging

Marc E. Agronin

"**S**exuality continues to play a vital role in the lives of aging individuals," writes Agronin. He details the physiological, psychological, and relational changes that affect the sexuality of older adults. Throughout the chapter the message is clear. Although aging is associated with declines in frequency and function, sexual satisfaction often remains high. Agronin suggests multiple roles for the sex therapist, including reassurance, education, counseling and therapy. It is important for the sex therapist to be able to function in a multidisciplinary setting and adapt interventions to the physical and social realities associated with aging. In addition, Agronin discusses special issues related to aging, including how to deal with sexuality in long-term-care settings and how to cope with the complex interpersonal and ethical issues related to sexuality and dementia. He also points out that aging individuals may be less aware of the dangers of sexually transmitted infection but are still at risk. Agronin is optimistic about the possibility that sexuality can continue to contribute to quality of life throughout the lifespan, noting that it is the ability to adapt to physical, social, and interpersonal changes that is the key to sexual longevity.

Marc E. Agronin, MD, is a board-certified adult and geriatric psychiatrist who has served since 1999 as Medical Director for Mental Health and Clinical Research at the Miami Jewish Health Systems. He is also Affiliate Associate Professor of Psychiatry and Neurology at the University of Miami Miller School of Medicine. In 2008, Dr. Agronin was named the "Clinician of the Year" by the American Association for Geriatric Psychiatry, and in 2011, he was elected as a Distinguished Fellow of the American Psychiatric Association. Dr. Agronin is a nationally recognized expert in psychiatric illnesses in the elderly and has authored several books, including *How We Age: A Doctor's Journey into the Heart of Growing Old* (2011), *Alzheimer's Disease and Other Dementias: A Practical Guide*, 3rd edition (2014), and *Therapy with Older Clients: Key Strategies for Success*

(2010) and is the coeditor of the textbook *Principles and Practice of Geriatric Psychiatry, 2nd edition* (2011). He has published widely on sexuality and aging, including a chapter coauthored with the noted TV and radio personality Dr. Ruth Westheimer.

The impact of aging on sexual function has historically been regarded as an inevitable process of decline that robbed individuals of any possible or enjoyable sexuality in late life. Both the science and the attitudes toward sex and sexual disorders in late life have evolved considerably, however, pushed along by the sexual and feminist revolutions in the 1960s and 1970s, the fact of longer and healthier lifespans for most elders, and the development and popularization of medications to treat erectile dysfunction (ED), the most common age-related sexual dysfunction. With the advent of 77 million members of the baby-boom generation beginning to turn 65, we can expect to see sexuality playing an increasingly active and vital role in the lives of most elders.

AGE-RELATED CHANGES IN SEXUAL RESPONSE

Normal aging is associated with a general decline in physiological sexual response and more variable declines in sexual activity. For women, the experience of sexuality in late life is fundamentally shaped by the physiological and psychological changes that occur with menopause. For men, no comparable midlife change in physiological function occurs. With aging, however, many men can experience important changes in bodily function that are linked to declines in testosterone production.

Menopause leads to important changes in female genital anatomy and function, including atrophy of urogenital tissue; decreased uterine and vaginal size; and decreases in vaginal lubrication, vasocongestion, and the erotic sensitivity of nipple, clitoral, and vulvar tissue during sexual activity (Wilson, 2003a). Accompanying changes in sexual function include declines in libido, sexual responsiveness, and the frequency of sexual activity (Hayes & Dennerstein, 2005; Dennerstein, Guthrie, Hayes, DeRogatis, & Lehert, 2008). During menopause up to 85% of women also experience symptoms such as hot flashes, head and neck aches, transient disruptions in mood (e.g., anxiety, irritability, and depression), sleep disturbances, and excess fatigue. Although these changes are primarily attributed to the loss of estrogen production, the role of age-related disruption in hypothalamic function has also been investigated for many menopausal symptoms, particularly hot flashes. Declines in testosterone production in premenopausal women may also lead to changes that affect sexual function, including loss of libido; decreased clitoral, vulvar, and nipple sensitivity; and fatigue (Morley, 2003).

As men age, there are gradual declines in sexual function that have variable impacts on sexual activity. There are no predictable changes in sexual desire, although it remains relatively stable in most men. Erections are less reliable and durable and require more stimulation to achieve and sustain. Ejaculation during orgasm involves decreased amounts of seminal fluid, and the refractory period between orgasms can increase by hours to days. By middle age, testosterone levels begin to decrease by 1–2% per year, meaning that anywhere from 35 to 70% of men over the age of 70 suffer from hypogonadism, defined by a testosterone level less than 200 ng/dL (Morley, 2003; Harman, Metter, Tobin, Pearson, & Blackman, 2001). Terms such as *andropause, male climacteric, partial androgen deficiency of the aging male,* and *late-onset hypogonadism* have all been coined to refer to a symptom complex that results from age-related declines in testosterone levels (Pines, 2011). Clinical symptoms include decreased libido and sexual function; depression; decreased lean body mass, body hair, muscle power, and bone density; and increased visceral fat distribution. Some researchers also believe that andropause brings an increased risk for osteoporosis, bone fractures, obesity, insulin resistance, and cardiovascular disease (Shabsigh, 2003; Sternbach, 2003). Some individuals will react negatively to these age-related changes, viewing them as harbingers of physical decline or sexual dysfunction. For men, declines in erectile function can symbolize a threat to their sense of masculinity and lead to excessive worry, anger, or even depression. Some women grieve the loss of potential motherhood at menopause, particularly if they never had children. Negative reactions may reinforce stereotypes about late-life sexuality being inappropriate or dangerous and may lead to less frequent and less enjoyable sexual relations (Agronin, 2005). On the other hand, aging can bring increased emotional maturity and a heightened capacity for intimacy that can enhance sexual relationships. Older couples may also have greater privacy and more time for intimacy. Individuals who understand that certain changes in sexual function are normal are less fearful and better able to adapt. For example, instead of dreading the effects of menopause, a woman may welcome the freedom from worry about contraception and unwanted pregnancy. Instead of focusing solely on sexual intercourse as the end-all and be-all of sexuality, a man may be able to shift his focus to the pleasurable sensual intimacy of sexual foreplay. Couples who communicate well can adjust sexual practices in order to maintain or even improve on previous levels of enjoyment (Agronin, 2005).

PREVALENCE OF SEXUALITY IN LATER LIFE

For both men and women, the impact of age-related changes in sexual function has a variable effect on sexual attitudes and behaviors. In general, there is a decline in the frequency of sexual activity after the age of 65, but not as much as might be imagined (National Council on Aging, 1998; Jacoby, 1999; American Association for Retired Persons [AARP], 2005; Fisher, 2010; Lindau et al., 2007). For example, a study of late-life sexuality by Lindau and colleagues (2007) involved a representative probability sample of 3,005 individuals ages 57–85 (1,550 men and 1,455 women) who agreed to comprehensive interviews by trained individuals. The definition of being sexually active was not limited to intercourse or orgasm but included any mutual sexual activity. The percentages of individuals who had been sexually active within the previous 12 months were quite high but declined with age, from 83.7% of men and 61.6% of women ages 57–64 to 67% of men and 39.5% of women ages 65–74 to 38.5% of men and 16.7% of women ages 75–85. Of those individuals in the oldest age group who were sexually active with partners, 54% of them were sexually active at least 2–3 times per month, while 23% were sexually active at least once a week.

In the Lindau (2007) and other studies, older men were found to be more sexually active than older women, although sexual satisfaction was relatively high in both sexes. The major predictors of sexual activity have included previous level of sexual activity, an individual's physical and psychological health, and the availability, interest level, and health of a partner (Lindau et al., 2007; Schick et al., 2010). Physical health appears to be the most influential factor for older men, while the quality of the relationship is most important for older women (Lindau et al., 2007; Schick et al., 2010).

HOMOSEXUALITY

There are an estimated 1–3 million gay and lesbian individuals over the age of 60 in the United States, and this number is expected to double in the next 30 years. In a 2009 survey conducted by the AARP, 5% of the roughly 2,000 respondents described themselves as having same-sex partners (8% of men, 2% of women), with 3% identifying as gay, less than 0.5% as lesbian, and 1% as bisexual (Fisher, 2010). Gay and lesbian individuals and couples face similar issues as heterosexuals in terms of age-associated changes in sexual function and sexual relationships. Several studies indicate that older gay and lesbian individuals feel high levels of satisfaction with both their identities and lifestyles, and high levels of sexual satisfaction. For example, in one study of over 100 older gay men, 86% of respondents 60 years and older were sexually active, with two-thirds of them reporting sexual activity at least once a month (Adelman, 1991).

SEXUALITY IN LONG-TERM-CARE SETTINGS

Compared with elderly individuals living in the community, nursing home residents are significantly less likely to be sexually active (Hajjar & Kamel, 2003a; Spector & Fremeth, 1996). In one study of 250 nursing home residents, less than 10% reported being sexually active in the preceding month, although nearly 20% reported a desire for sexual activity but were limited by the lack of a partner or privacy (White, 1982). Barriers to sexuality in long-term care include loss of interest, poor health, sexual dysfunction, lack of partners, lack of privacy, and the negative attitudes of staff (Hajjar & Kamel, 2003a; Richardson & Lazur, 1995). Older gay and lesbian individuals in long-term care face additional challenges, as they fear being rejected and neglected (Stein, Beckerman, & Sherman, 2010). In addition, one small study suggested that staff members tend to have more negative views of same-sex intimacy (Hinrich & Vacha-Haase, 2010). Long-term-care facilities have the responsibility, however, to educate both staff and residents about the residents' rights to privacy and to engage in intimate relationships. There are many accommodations that can be provided in a facility to appropriate individuals, such as beauty services, private rooms for conjugal visits, and medical and mental health consultation for sexual dysfunction (Schick et al., 2010).

SEXUALLY TRANSMITTED DISEASES

Sexually transmitted diseases (STDs) are at epidemic levels in the United States, affecting over 65 million people, many with incurable viral infections (Wilson, 2003b). The Centers for Disease Control and Prevention (CDC) and other research groups indicate that individuals 65 and older account for less than 2% of reported STDs, including chlamydia, gonorrhea, syphilis, and HIV (Centers for Disease Control and Prevention, 2009; Xu, Schillinger, Aubin, St. Louis, & Markowitz, 2001). The differences in STD rates between young and old might be largely attributed to the fact that older individuals have fewer sexual encounters with fewer partners.

Despite low prevalence rates, older people remain at risk for acquiring STDs, especially as they are increasingly sexually active. There are numerous reasons for this, including the fact that many older people never received the sex education provided to today's younger population. In addition, the knowledge that STDs are most prevalent in younger people may lead to a false sense of safety among older couples, causing them to neglect safe-sex practices. Older couples may also be less apt to use barrier contraceptives that protect against some STDs because they do not have to worry about unwanted pregnancy. In fact, a large study that looked at nearly 6,000 individuals ages 14–94 found that 91% of older men and a majority of older women did not use a condom when having sex with a date or acquaintance, and some didn't even use one when they knew their partner had an STD (AARP, 2005). Given these lapses in safe-sex measures, education about sexuality, STDs, and safe-sex practices remains critical throughout the entire adult life cycle.

SEXUAL DYSFUNCTION

ED is the most common form of sexual dysfunction in older men, affecting 20–40% of men in their 60s and 50–70% of men in their 70s and 80s

(Lewis et al., 2004; Feldman, Goldstein, Hatzichristou, Krane, & McKinlay, 1994; Laumann & Waite, 2008). In older women, the most common forms of sexual dysfunction include hypoactive sexual desire, inhibited orgasm, and dyspareunia (Bitzer, Platano, Tschudin, & Alder, 2008; Lindau et al., 2007). The percentage of women with low sexual desire jumps from 10% of women under 50 to nearly 50% of women in their late 60s and 70s (Lewis et al., 2004). One study found that 43% of women ages 57–85 years reported low desire, 39% had difficulty with lubrication, and 34% had anorgasmia (Lindau et al., 2007).

The causes of sexual dysfunction in late life are typically multifactorial, involving the physical effects of medical illness and/or medications, comorbid psychiatric illness, and underlying maladaptive attitudes and/or dysfunctional relationships. Any medical illness that impairs the blood supply or nervous innervation of genital tissue can potentially serve as a primary cause of sexual dysfunction. Secondary sexual dysfunction may result from fatigue, pain, physical disability, or some other effect of a medical illness. For example, a man with chronic obstructive pulmonary disease may become short of breath during sexual activity, causing him to become less aroused, with resultant ED. Another example would be a woman with a history of cervical cancer who has pain during sex and subsequent loss of libido due to scarring and contractures of her vaginal tissue from surgery and radiation.

There are numerous medical conditions commonly associated with sexual dysfunction in late life, including cardiac and pulmonary disease, vascular damage due to atherosclerosis or diabetes mellitus, endocrine disorders that affect estrogen or testosterone levels, urological or gynecological conditions that require surgical or chemotherapeutic intervention that alters or damages urogenital tissues, and neurological disorders such as peripheral neuropathy, multiple sclerosis, and Parkinson's disease that can diminish nervous innervation of genital tissue and lead to diminished physical mobility that in turn impairs sexual activity. Orthopedic problems and joint disease can also cause pain and physical disability that can similarly affect sexual activity.

Medications often play a role in precipitating sexual dysfunction, and they can affect both sexes at any point in the sexual response cycle (Crenshaw & Goldberg, 1996; Goodwin & Agronin, 1997; Thomas, 2003). Some of the most common culprits include antihypertensives (e.g., ß-blockers, diuretics), antiandrogens, and many psychotropic medications, particularly antidepressants (Thomas, 2003; Montejo, Llorca, & Izquierdo, 2001; Ferguson, 2001). One prospective study found that nearly 60% of individuals on selective serotonin reuptake inhibitors (SSRIs) or venlafaxine suffered from various forms of sexual dysfunction, such as low desire, ED, and delayed orgasm, with higher rates in men (Montejo et al., 2001). By contrast, up to 25% of those on mirtazapine and only 8% on nefazodone reported such forms of sexual dysfunction. Bupropion has also been associated with lower rates of sexual dysfunction, in the 5–15% range (Kavoussi, Segraves, Hughes, Ascher, & Johnston, 1997).

Initial episodes of sexual dysfunction in the elderly are often precipitated by a major psychosocial stress, such as the loss of a job or loved one, a medical crisis or prolonged illness, or a hospitalization. Such major stresses may break sexual patterns and lead to uncertainty as to how to resume sexual activity. The loss of a partner is particularly devastating, making the idea of sexuality moot in the short term and often suppressing sexual desire and the willingness to seek out a new partner in the long run if grief or survivor guilt persists. In the face of an acute illness, such as a recent heart attack or respiratory compromise, older individuals can suffer from performance anxiety if they anticipate pain, self-injury (or injury to a debilitated partner), or even death during sex. Some people may feel less sexual because they are embarrassed by changes in their personal appearance (e.g., due to a surgical scar or colostomy bag) or are fearful of body odors or incontinence during sex. Chronic illness can also sap one's energy and enthusiasm for sex.

Sexual dysfunction in late life is often comorbid with psychiatric illness, particularly mood and anxiety disorders, in which loss of libido is a frequent symptom (Clayton, 2001). At baseline, 40–50% of individuals suffering from depression experience loss of sexual desire as a cardinal symptom, but up to 90% may experience any form of sexual dysfunction prior to being started on antidepressants (Montejo et al., 2001). Individuals with schizophrenia and other psychotic disorders may have fewer problems with sexual function per se but more difficulty with managing sexual relationships.

SEXUAL DYSFUNCTION AND DEMENTIA

The effect of dementia on sexual function poses a number of complex issues. On the one hand, sexual function and sexual needs continue throughout the course of most dementias and can play an important role as a nonverbal form of communication and intimacy for couples. As dementia progresses, however, individuals become more prone to sexual dysfunction and to sexually disinhibited behaviors. Caregivers bear the brunt of these changes, as they struggle to maintain a relationship in the face of uncertainty about the appropriateness of sex with someone who is slowly losing the capacity to understand and consent to mutual sexual relations (Davies et al., 2010). In addition, caregivers may lose the desire for sex with a cognitively impaired partner, perhaps due to being "turned off" by the effects of the disease or frustrated by a partner who acts inappropriately, has lost all desire for sex, or repeatedly or perhaps uncharacteristically requests sexual gratification. Some partners may be torn by conflicting feelings of love and fidelity for the partner with dementia and desires for both emotional and physical intimacy from an individual without dementia.

In the early and middle stages of Alzheimer's disease (AD) and other dementias, there is no predictable change in sexual desire, with it declining in some individuals and increasing in others, perhaps due to changes in the degree of cognitive disinhibition. Sexual activity does decline, however; one study found that 46% of couples with a partner suffering from dementia were sexually active 3 years after diagnosis, dropping to 41% after 5 years and 28% after 7 years (Eloniemi-Sulkava et al., 2002). ED and female orgasmic disorder are the two most commonly reported forms of sexual dysfunction in men and women with dementia, respectively (Zeiss, Davies, Wood, & Tinklenberg, 1990). Sexual dysfunction may result in part from the cognitively impaired individual's declining ability to maintain a coherent focus on physical or mental stimulation during sex or to initiate and sequence components of lovemaking (Duffy, 1995; Rosen, Lachs, & Pillemer, 2010).

The ability to consent to sexual activity is a particularly sensitive issue for many partners, who fear that they may be coercing their loved one into something they can no longer fully understand (Rosen et al., 2010). This is also an important issue in long-term-care facilities, where an individual with dementia may be engaging in or attempting to engage in sexual activity with another individual with cognitive impairment. This behavior raises sensitive ethical dilemmas when neither individual can truly consent to sexual activity and when there is a spouse or partner without dementia living outside of the facility who might not approve. Both legally and ethically, the rights of an individual in a long-term-care facility to engage in sexual activity depend on his or her ability to understand the nature of the relationship and provide reasonable consent. When there is concern about an individual's capacity to provide such consent, clinicians should attempt to determine how well the individual is able to understand the nature of the relationship, including its risks, and to what degree the individual with cognitive impairment can avoid coercion or exploitation (Lichtenberg & Strzepek, 1990).

Sexually disinhibited behaviors include inappropriate sexual comments or requests, public exposure or masturbation, and aggressive fondling, groping, or forced sexual activity. Not surprisingly, such behaviors generate a considerable amount of anxiety on the part of caregivers. They have been reported in 2–7% of individuals with dementia and in 25% of residents in dementia units, and they tend to be more common in men (Guay, 2008; Kumar, Koss, Metzler, Moore, & Friedland, 1988; Hajjar & Kamel, 2003b). Risk factors include frontal and temporal lobe impairment, mania, psychosis, substance abuse, stroke, head trauma, premorbid sexual aggression, and certain medications, such as dopaminergic agents used to treat Parkinson's disease (Guay, 2008; Hashmi, Krady, Qayum, & Grossberg, 2000; Bowers, Woert, & Davis, 1971; Uitti et al., 1989).

ASSESSMENT

The assessment of sexual problems in late life will generally follow guidelines for younger individuals, varying by the type of disorder being addressed. These are discussed in detail in other chapters, but several age-specific issues are reviewed here. The assessment of sexual dysfunction in an older individual depends, first and foremost, on an educated clinician who is comfortable and knowledgeable about late-life sexuality. If the clinician is embarrassed or uncomfortable asking questions about sexual function to aged individuals, it is unlikely that an adequate history will be gathered. The clinician must be able to ask direct questions using common language and to listen carefully and patiently, keeping in mind that older people will have many of the same sexual concerns as younger people (Swabo, 2003). An indispensable source of information about a sexual problem is the partner. The partner's presence during an interview will help facilitate open communication with the affected partner that will prove critical during the treatment phase.

The role of the clinician in the treatment of sexual dysfunction is to provide reassurance, education, and counseling or formal sex therapy as necessary. Sometimes this approach is sufficient; in other cases, a specialist is needed to treat physical causes related to other comorbid disorders. For example, an endocrinologist may be needed to address low testosterone, which is more common in late life, or a urologist might be consulted for a prostate problem. Reassurance of the patient depends on an enlightened clinician who understands that sexuality in general and sexual intercourse in particular remain important to many older patients. The clinician should listen empathically and then emphasize, in clear and nontechnical language, the normality of sexuality in late life and the possibility of effective treatment for sexual problems. In addition, the clinician should emphasize the wide range of potential expressions of sexuality, in addition to sexual intercourse. Keep in mind that many older patients have internalized negative perspectives on late-life sexuality. The act of providing reassurance builds trust between patient and clinician, and this relationship will lay the basis for the patient's feeling comfortable with being open about emotional reactions to the problem and seeking follow-up treatment.

The current cohort of individuals in their 80s and 90s grew up in an era when any mental health issue carried tremendous stigma and psychotherapy was not the norm. Thus the very act of going to see a clinician may seem foreign and threatening. This reluctance is amplified by a fear of ageism, the fear that the younger clinician will not take the older patient seriously or will see his or her problem as only a normal consequence of old age. Such stereotypes often become internalized, prompting further pessimism on the part of patients.

Educating patients about both normal and pathological changes in sexual function in late life can reduce excessive fear and increase acceptance of these changes (Bitzer et al., 2008; Swabo, 2003). For example, a man who does not understand the normal changes in erectile function may misinterpret them and believe he is suffering from a sexual problem. Similarly, a woman may misinterpret the experience of vaginal dryness to mean that she does not want to have sex. The clinician should review with the patient the normal changes in sexual function throughout each stage of the sexual response cycle and discuss ways in which the patient's physical or mental state may be influencing these changes. For example, an older man with diabetes or atherosclerotic disease may have a more pronounced decline in erectile function or even ED, given possible compromise of penile blood flow. An older woman with a history of an arthritic hip might experience more limited pelvic movement or even pain during sex, in addition to potential discomfort due to decreased vaginal lubrication. A depressed patient may report significant reductions in libido. In each case, the patient can be reassured that his or her sexual changes have clearly identified causative factors and that treatment can improve or even alleviate these concerns.

Education should also focus on improving the quality of an individual's sexual relationship with his or her partner. Sometimes the clinician can provide a forum for the couple to discuss basic difficulties during sexual activity and strategize about ways to improve them. When there is significant discord, couple therapy should be the initial therapeutic modality. The clinician should emphasize to the couple that sex can be more than just intercourse and that physically pleasing each other can occur through massage and masturbation and does not always have to be mutual. Couples often have to adapt sexual techniques and refocus more time on foreplay in order to preserve previous levels of sexual function and enjoyment.

When one or both partners suffer from chronic medical illness or disability, sexual practices may need to be adapted to account for physical limitations, fatigue, loss of muscle strength, and pain (Schover & Jensen, 1988). A physician who treats the condition in question should be consulted on ways to minimize pain or discomfort and maximize function, perhaps by taking analgesics or other treatments (e.g., specific muscle stretches, nasal oxygen, inhalers) prior to sex. The couple can be instructed to find sexual positions that minimize physical exertion or stress on certain parts of the body.

Case Discussion

Mr. J, a 78-year-old widower, was seen in a geriatric psychiatry clinic for symptoms of depression. He was started on an antidepressant but thought it was not helping. During the initial assessment, the psychiatrist asked Mr. J about his sexual functioning, which prompted an outpouring of grief. Mr. J confided that he had suffered from ED ever since undergoing a prostatectomy 6 months prior to the appointment. Mr. J had asked the surgeon about changes in his sexual function, and he paraphrased the surgeon's response as, "Impotence is quite common after this surgery, but why would you worry about that anyway at your age?" Feeling humiliated and hopeless about regaining his sexual function, Mr. J broke up with his girlfriend and lapsed into a depression. The subsequent use of an antidepressant reduced his libido further and felt like a double blow.

The sex therapist spent a session reassuring Mr. J that treatment was available and encouraged him to see a urologist who specialized in ED in order to consider an oral erectogenic agent. He also educated Mr. J about erectile physiology and discussed with him other potential causes of his ED, such as medication effects and unresolved grief over the death of his wife that manifested in anger directed toward his girlfriend. Even before treatment for his ED began, Mr. J reported feeling less depressed and more hopeful. Eventually, Mr. J got involved in another relationship and felt more confident and positive about being intimate. However, he was not as focused on sexual intercourse as the only means of intimacy and was able to enjoy kissing and caressing without thinking that he needed to have an erection to feel like a man. His depression lifted, and he was able to stop the antidepressant. As the relationship progressed, he was able to have satisfying sexual relations that sometimes involved sexual intercourse. He used an oral erectogenic agent to strengthen his erection but did not feel dependent upon it.

SEX THERAPY

Sex therapy is described in detail elsewhere in this book, but several age-associated issues are worthy of mention. The use of sex therapy has been eclipsed by the introduction of oral erectogenic agents, because many older couples believed incorrectly that the simple correction of ED with a pill would resolve long-standing sexual and other relationship problems. In those situations and many others, enduring issues such as low desire, relationship discord, physical deconditioning, and medical problems must be dealt with at the outset of sex therapy. In order to accomplish this, a multidisciplinary approach is particularly critical with older individuals in order to identify and address these various conditions.

For the older individual or couple, an initial supportive and educational approach can help in building a crucial alliance with the therapist and in promoting understanding of the problem and optimism about improvement. Sometimes practical suggestions on sexual technique can bring immediate improvement; in other situations, the therapist needs to impose a moratorium on sex to reduce tension and eventually reintroduce a more relaxed and sensuous approach. In some cases, intensive couple therapy is necessary; in others, pharmacological treatment of debilitating psychiatric symptoms (e.g., depression, panic attacks, psychosis) is needed, or the patient may need to be referred back to a specialist for further treatment of an enduring medical issue (e.g., joint or chest pain or shortness of breath during exertion). In general, these approaches to sexual dysfunction will not differ substantially across the age span.

Case Discussion

Mr. and Mrs. B, a couple in their late 70s, had been married for 45 years. They had previously experienced an enjoyable sexual relationship into their early 70s but had stopped having sexual intercourse several years ago after Mrs. B was treated for breast cancer with a mastectomy and radiation therapy. Mrs. B began seeing a geriatric psychiatrist for treatment of depression and became quite tearful when describing the impact of her experience with breast cancer, feeling that it had ruined her as a sexual being. A hip fracture had only made things worse for her, she believed, as any sexual activity was associated with pain. The psychiatrist referred the couple to a colleague trained in sex therapy.

After taking a careful sex history, the therapist felt that although Mrs. B's medical problems had disrupted the couple's sex life, they were not insurmountable obstacles. Mrs. B's poor sexual desire was attributed to the loss of her breast being a blow to her body image and self-confidence. The therapist also learned that although Mrs. B experienced limited hip movement and pain after her surgery, this had largely resolved, whereas her fear of recurrent pain had not.

After discussing these issues with the couple, a series of sensate focus exercises were prescribed. The couple was amazed to find that just by gently massaging each other in bed without any expectation of sex, their sexual desire improved. The therapist encouraged Mrs. B to wear loose-fitting lingerie that made her feel sexy and minimized the contour of her chest, helping her to lessen the focus on her surgical scars. After consulting with Mrs. B's orthopedist, the therapist recommended that the couple engage in mutual massage and genital fondling in a sexual position that put minimal stress on Mrs. B's hip joint. Within several sessions Mr. and Mrs. B had progressed to sexual intercourse, which they both described as being comfortable and satisfying.

CONCLUSIONS

Sexuality continues to play a vital role in the lives of aging individuals, and most surveys show that although the frequency of sexual activity declines with age, satisfaction continues to be quite strong. Despite the predictable changes in physiology that may slow sexual response and the increase in medical disorders and medication use associated with sexual dysfunction, there are many ways in which individuals can adapt sexual activity or seek treatment to mitigate sexual problems. Dementia presents unique limitations on sexual activity and the potential for inappropriate sexual behaviors that require attention by specialists.

REFERENCES

Adelman, M. (1991). Stigma, gay lifestyles, and adjustment to aging: A study of late-life gay men and lesbians. *Journal of Homosexuality, 20,* 7–32.

Agronin, M. E. (2005). Geriatric psychiatry: Sexuality and aging. In B. J. Sadock &

V. A. Sadock (Eds.), *Kaplan and Sadock's comprehensive textbook of psychiatry* (8th ed., pp. 3834–3838). Philadelphia: Lippincott Williams & Wilkins.

American Association for Retired Persons. (2005). *Sexuality at midlife and beyond: 2004 update of attitudes and behaviors.* Retrieved August 1, 2012, from *www.aarp.org/relationships/love-sex/info-05–2005/2004_sexuality.html.*

Bitzer, J., Platano, G., Tschudin, S., & Alder, J. (2008). Sexual counselling in elderly couples. *Journal of Sexual Medicine, 5*(9), 2027–2043.

Bowers, M. B., Woert, M. V., & Davis, L. (1971). Sexual behavior during L-dopa treatment for Parkinsonism. *American Journal of Psychiatry, 127,* 1691–1693.

Centers for Disease Control and Prevention. (2009). *Sexually transmitted disease surveillance 2009.* Retrieved February 1, 2011, from *www.cdc.gov/std/stats09/surv2009-complete.pdf.*

Clayton, A. H. (2001). Recognition and assessment of sexual dysfunction associated with depression. *Journal of Clinical Psychiatry, 62*(Suppl. 3), 5–9.

Crenshaw, T. L., & Goldberg, J. P. (1996). *Sexual pharmacology: Drugs that affect sexual function.* New York: Norton.

Davies, H. D., Newkirk, L. A., Pitts, C. B., Coughlin, C. A., Sridhar, S. B., Zeiss, L. M., et al. (2010). The impact of dementia and mild memory impairment (MMI) on intimacy and sexuality in spousal relationships. *International Psychogeriatrics, 4,* 618–628.

Dennerstein, L., Guthrie, J. R., Hayes, R. D., DeRogatis, L. R., & Lehert, P. (2008). Sexual function, dysfunction, and sexual distress in a prospective, population-based sample of middle-aged, Australian-born women. *Journal of Sexual Medicine, 5*(10), 2291–2299.

Duffy, L. M. (1995). Sexual behavior and marital intimacy in Alzheimer's couples: A family theory perspective. *Sexuality Disability, 13,* 239–254.

Eloniemi-Sulkava, U., Notkola, I. L., Hämäläinen, K., Rahkonen, T., Viramo, P., Hentinen, M., et al. (2002). Spouse caregivers' perceptions of influence of dementia on marriage. *Psychogeriatrics, 14*(1), 47–58.

Feldman, H. A., Goldstein, I., Hatzichristou, D. G., Krane, R. J., & McKinlay, J. B. (1994). Impotence and its medical and psychosocial correlates: Results of the Massachusetts Male Aging Study. *Journal of Urology, 151,* 54–61.

Ferguson, J. M. (2001). The effects of antidepressants on sexual functioning in depressed patients: A review. *Journal of Clinical Psychiatry, 62*(Suppl. 3), 22–34.

Fisher, L. L. (2010). *Sex, romance, and relationships: 2009 AARP survey of midlife and older adults* (Publication No, 19234). Retrieved February 1, 2011, from *http://assets.aarp.org/rgcenter/general/srr_09.pdf.*

Goodwin, A. J., & Agronin, M. E. (1997). *A women's guide to overcoming sexual fear and pain.* Oakland, CA: New Harbinger Press.

Guay, D. R. (2008). Inappropriate sexual behaviors in cognitively impaired older individuals. *American Journal of Geriatric Pharmacotherapy, 6*(5), 269–1288.

Hajjar, R. R., & Kamel, H. K. (2003a). Sexuality in the nursing home: Part 1. Attitudes and barriers to sexual expression. *Journal of the American Medical Directors Association, 5*(Suppl. 2), 152–156.

Hajjar, R. R., & Kamel, H. K. (2003b). Sexuality in the nursing home: Part 2. Managing abnormal behaviour—legal and ethical issues. *Journal of the American Medical Directors Association, 5*(Suppl. 2), 203–206.

Harman, S. M., Metter, E. J., Tobin, J. D., Pearson, J., & Blackman, M. R. (2001). Longitudinal effects of aging on serum total and free testosterone levels in healthy men: Baltimore Longitudinal Study of Aging. *Journal of Clinical Endocrinology and Metabolism, 86,* 724–731.

Hashmi, F. H., Krady, A. I., Qayum, F., & Grossberg, G. T. (2000). Sexually disinhibited behavior in the cognitively impaired elderly. *Clinical Geriatrics, 8*(11), 61–68.

Hayes, R., & Dennerstein, L. (2005). The impact of aging on sexual function and sexual dysfunction in women: A review of population-based studies. *Journal of Sexual Medicine, 2*(3), 317–330.

Hinrich, K. L., & Vacha-Haase, T. (2010). Staff perceptions of same-gender sexual contacts in long-term care facilities. *Journal of Homosexuality, 57*(6), 776–789.

Jacoby, S. (1999, September–October). Great sex. What's age got to do with it? *Modern Maturity,* pp. 43–48.

Kavoussi, R. J., Segraves, R. T., Hughes, A. R., Ascher, J. A., & Johnston, J. A. (1997). Double-blind comparison of bupropion sustained release and sertraline in depressed outpatients. *Journal of Clinical Psychiatry, 58,* 532–537.

Kumar, A., Koss, E., Metzler, D., Moore, A., & Friedland, R. P. (1988). Behavioral symptomatology in dementia of the Alzheimer type. *Alzheimer's Disease and Associated Disorders, 2,* 363–365.

Laumann, E. O., & Waite, L. J. (2008). Sexual dysfunction among older adults: Prevalence and risk factors from a nationally representative United States probability sample of men and women 57–85 years of age. *Journal of Sexual Medicine, 5*(10), 2300–2311.

Lewis, R. W., Fugl-Meyer, K. S., Bosch, R., Fugl-Meyer, A. R., Laumann, E. O., Lizza, E., et al. (2004). Epidemiology/risk factors of sexual dysfunction. *Journal of Sexual Medicine, 1*(1), 35–39.

Lichtenberg, P. A., & Strzepek, D. M. (1990). Assessments of institutionalized dementia patient's competencies to participate in intimate relationships. *Gerontologist, 30,* 117–120.

Lindau, S.T., Schumm, L.P., Laumann, E.O., Levinson, W., O'Muircheartaigh, C. A., & Waite, L. J. (2007). A study of sexuality and health among older adults in the United States. *New England Journal of Medicine, 357,* 762–774.

Montejo, A. L., Llorca, G., & Izquierdo, J. A. (2001). Incidence of sexual dysfunction associated with antidepressant agents: A prospective multicenter study of 1022 outpatients. *Journal of Clinical Psychiatry, 62*(Suppl. 3), 10–21.

Morley, J. E. (2003).Testosterone and behavior. *Clinics in Geriatric Medicine, 19*(3), 605–661.

National Council on Aging. (1998). *Healthy sexuality and vital aging: Executive summary.* Washington, DC: Author.

Pines, A. (2011). Male menopause: Is it a real clinical syndrome? *Climacteric, 13*(6), 15–17.

Richardson, J. P., & Lazur, A. (1995). Sexuality in the nursing home patient. *American Family Physician, 51*(1), 121–124.

Rosen, T., Lachs, M. S., & Pillemer, K. (2010). Sexual aggression between residents in nursing homes: Literature synthesis of an underrecognized problem. *Journal of the American Geriatric Society, 58*(10), 1970–1979.

Schick, V., Herbenick, D., Reece, M., Sanders, S. A., Dodge, B., Middlestadt, S. E., et al. (2010). Sexual behaviors, condom use, and sexual health of Americans over 50: Implications for sexual health promotion for older adults. *Journal of Sexual Medicine, 7*(Suppl. 5), 315–329.

Schover, L.R., & Jensen, S.B. (1988). *Sexuality and chronic illness*. New York: Guilford Press.

Shabsigh, R. (2003). Urological perspectives on andropause. *Psychiatric Annals, 33*(8), 501–509.

Spector, I. P., & Fremeth, S. M. (1996). Sexual behavior and attitudes of geriatric residents in long-term care facilities. *Journal of Sex and Marital Therapy, 22,* 235–246.

Stein, G. L., Beckerman, N. L., & Sherman, P. A. (2010). Lesbian and gay elders and long-term care: Identifying the unique psychosocial perspectives and challenges. *Journal of Gerontological Social Work, 53*(5), 421–435.

Sternbach, H. (2003). Psychiatric manifestations of low testosterone in men. *Psychiatric Annals, 33*(8), 517–524.

Swabo, P. A. (2003). Counseling about sexuality in the older person. *Clinics in Geriatric Medicine, 19*(3), 595–604.

Thomas, D. R. (2003). Medications and sexual function. *Clinics in Geriatric Medicine, 19,* 553–562.

Uitti, R. J., Tanner, C. M., Rajput, A. H., Goetz, C. G., Klawans, H. L., & Thiessen, B. (1989). Hypersexuality with antiparkinsonian therapy. *Clinical Neuropharmacology, 12,* 375–383.

White, C. B. (1982). Sexual interests, attitudes, knowledge, and sexual history in relation to sexual behavior in the institutionalized aged. *Archives of Sexual Behavior, 11,* 11–21.

Wilson, M. G. (2003a). Menopause. *Clinics in Geriatric Medicine, 19*(3), 483–506.

Wilson, M. G. (2003b). Sexually transmitted diseases. *Clinics in Geriatric Medicine, 19*(3), 637–655.

Xu, F., Schillinger, J. A., Aubin, M. R., St. Louis, M. E., & Markowitz, L. E. (2001). Sexually transmitted diseases of older persons in Washington state. *Sexually Transmissable Diseases, 28,* 287–291.

Zeiss, A. M., Davies, H. D., Wood, M., & Tinklenberg, J. R. (1990). The incidence and correlates of erectile problems in patients with Alzheimer's disease. *Archives of Sexual Behavior, 19,* 325–332.

CONCLUSION

Sex Therapy in Transition
Are We There Yet?

Marta Meana, Kathryn S. K. Hall,
and Yitzchak (Irv) M. Binik

From its first edition in 1980, *Principles and Practice of Sex Therapy* (Leiblum & Pervin, 1980) has observed a tradition of stepping back from individual treatment-focused chapters to gauge the overall temperature of sex therapy as a discipline. How is it doing? How has it changed? Where is it going? A sense of momentum has always been recorded, arguably accelerated over the past two editions in concert with advances in sexual medicine. This state of perpetual transition may be the hallmark of a healthy discipline adjusting to and incorporating new knowledge. It can also indicate a failure to effectively chart a unified direction—a stalling of sorts. In the past decade, the latter concern has informed some commentaries that have sounded alarms about the state of sex therapy and its possibly threatened future (e.g., Binik & Meana, 2009; Kleinplatz, 2003; Rowland, 2007). The discipline is clearly undergoing a period of existential self-reflection that stands in stark contrast to its self-assured origins.

The heady early days of sex therapy held the promise of targeted interventions for clearly defined sexual problems with easily assessed outcomes. Masters and Johnson had taken sexual function and dysfunction out of the morass of psychodynamic constructions and into the supposed clarity of behaviorism and stimulus control. The journey from dysfunction to function was sequentially mapped, with the estimated arrival time much earlier than that indicated by previous treatment approaches.

Over the ensuing 50 years, research and practice in a number of disciplines effected numerous modifications to the traditional models proposed by Masters and Johnson (1966) and later Kaplan (1977) and Lief (1977). The accumulation of empirical data invariably resulted in downward revisions of inflated original outcome predictions. Sexuality and the treatment of its problems appeared to be not so simple, after all. The complexity that traditional sex therapy had eschewed would not be denied (if not psychoanalyzed), and its sources would be far more numerous than imagined. This multifactorial complexity is evidenced in the literature, from the very questioning of an archetypal sexual response and associated constructs to deliberations about what constitutes successful treatment outcome. The acknowledgement of complexity may result in a reconfiguration of sex therapy that elevates its relevance, or it may result in its disintegration. A review of factors that are driving or complicating the current transition is here offered in the hope that we can collectively rise to the very real challenges facing our still young, though somewhat weathered, discipline.

QUESTIONS ABOUT CONSTRUCT UTILITY

The past couple of decades have witnessed the emergence of questions about the nature of basic constructs that had long been taken for granted in sexology. The very notions of function and dysfunction have been reevaluated as potentially problematic imports from a medical model that cannot capture the nuances of human sexuality. The concept of sexual function has been criticized as reductive in its emphasis on the mechanics and hydraulics of sex. The concept of dysfunction has been called into question for failing to encompass gender differences in sexual function and for altogether missing the possibility that both sexual difficulties and associated distress may be culturally defined and influenced (Tiefer, 2001).

Constructs within the traditional sexual response model are also teetering under scrutiny. Research indicates that sexual desire, once considered a biological drive that sprung spontaneously and had sexual activity and/or orgasm as its goal, is much more unwieldy. With few reliable physiological, cognitive, and behavioral referents in women, sexual desire is now a construct undergoing reconsideration as a simple motivational state with clear goals (Meana, 2010). Furthermore, the difficulty reported by both men and women in differentiating desire from subjective or even physiological arousal has raised concerns about the utility of distinguishing between the two (Brotto, Heiman, & Tolman, 2009; Graham, Sanders, Milhausen, & McBride, 2004; Janssen, McBride, Yarber, Hill, & Butler, 2008). Even when a clear demarcation can be made between desire and arousal, their temporal sequence in the triphasic model of the sexual response is now in doubt. Clinical case reports and empirical data emanating from research on the incentive model of the sexual response suggest that arousal may often precede desire (Basson, 2007; Both, Everaerd, & Laan, 2007). Whether this rearrangement of the sequence is warranted or simply further evidence that desire and arousal are hard to tease apart remains a question.

The third phase of the triphasic sexual response, orgasm, appears to be a little sturdier, although attempts to define this construct have failed to reach consensus (Mah & Binik, 2001; Levin, 2004). When this failure is coupled with the minimal empirical research on orgasm, the perception of sturdiness may be illusory. The sexual pain disorders have also posed some conceptual problems. They have underlined the difficulty in establishing how we define a sexual dysfunction in the first place. The research of the past 15 years has effectively demonstrated that, in most cases, dyspareunia constitutes a pain disorder whose connection with sexuality is mostly incidental (Binik, Meana, Berkley, & Khalife, 1999). The hyperalgesic genital area happens to interfere with sexual intercourse. This interference can undoubtedly result in myriad sexual and relational difficulties, but there are few data to suggest that its origins are psychosexual. The question then becomes: Why is dyspareunia considered a sexual dysfunction instead of a pain disorder that happens to interfere with sexual function, as undoubtedly many other pain disorders do (Binik et al, 1999)? This raises an even broader question as to what the nine sexual dysfunctions share, other than their nonunique interference with sexual activity and the experience of pleasure therein. After all, what does premature ejaculation (PE) really share with dyspareunia, other than an interference with sexual activity and pleasure? Couldn't this interference with sex also be claimed by headaches and lower back pain, which are not categorized as sexual dysfunctions? Anxiety (about sex, sexual performance and/or intimacy), once thought to be the common denominator of sexual dysfunction, has given way to a biopsychosocial model that postulates multiple contributing factors, many of them unique to each dysfunction.

The DSM-5 (American Psychiatric Association, 2013) sub-work group on sexual dysfunction did not really address the question of construct validity in the concept of sexual dysfunction. Their response has essentially consisted of tinkering with existing diagnostic categories. This has included creating a greater differentiation between men and women (each now have their own desire-related dysfunction category) and collapsing across dysfunctions for which differentiation has been problematic (hypoactive sexual desire disorder and female sexual arousal disorder into sexual interest/arousal disorder in women; dyspareunia and vaginismus into genito-pelvic pain/penetration disorder). Whether the gender differentiation or dysfunction collapsing is an effective clinical response to the complexity of the sexual experience only research and field trials will tell. Some have argued that complexity calls for more rather than fewer distinctions (Derogatis, Clayton, Rosen, Sand, & Pyke, 2011).

The debunking of these once sacrosanct constructs challenges clinicians to modify, amend, or devise (new) treatments. Women worried about the loss of spontaneous sexual desire are now counseled to focus on responsive desire that may coincide with or even follow sexual arousal. Understanding that dyspareunia is primarily a pain disorder rather than an anxious, avoidant sexual response rooted in intrapsychic or relational difficulty has also had important treatment ramifications. Informed by the literature on chronic pain, psychological therapies and medical treatment now dovetail to improve clinical outcomes. The clinical isolationism that once defined sex therapy appears to be over, as mindfulness meditation, eye movement desensitization and reprocessing (EMDR), and various cognitive-behavioral therapy (CBT) strategies continue to be incorporated in sex therapy.

ENCOMPASSING MULTIDIMENSIONALITY AND DIVERSITY

The idea of an archetypal sexual response that crosses individual, gender, age, sexual orientation, relationship longevity, health/ability status, or cultural boundaries has definitely been challenged in the past few years. The aforementioned recognition that men and women may have differing sexual responses has been a catalyst for the consideration of diversity beyond gender. Even within gender, individuals speak of significantly different experiences and endorse different models of the sexual response as reflective of their experience (e.g., Sand & Fisher, 2007). The ages of individuals and of their relationships may be central to the "morphology" of their sexual response. Although this type of diversity is probably endemic to many psychophysiological phenomena, the simplicity that had been attributed to the sexual response probably delayed what should have been relatively obvious considerations of its diversity across individuals and groups.

Cultural diversity has been difficult to address, as there are precious few cross-cultural data or even data from different ethnic groups within North America. The few we do have are plagued by a Western-centric focus. This is certainly true of surveys asking and finding that Western-defined sexual dysfunctions exist elsewhere in the world. However, the importance placed on these dysfunctions varies. In many parts of the world sexual dysfunctions that interfere with reproduction are deemed worthy of treatment, whereas dysfunctions that interfere with pleasure, especially for women, are not universally considered problematic. Culture-specific sexual dysfunctions, relegated to an appendix of DSM-IV-TR (American Psychiatric Association, 2000) under the rubric "culture-bound syndromes," are as yet little known or understood in the West. Regardless, there does appear to be a growing consciousness in sex therapy of the potential diversity of sexual response and expression. The search for one model that captures the experience of all individuals seems less of a concern and maybe even a dubious endeavor.

In direct response to this complexity, the DSM-5 Work Group on Sexual Dysfunctions has removed the overly simplistic and often categorical etiological specifiers in the DSM-IV (American Psychiatric Association, 1994; i.e., due to psychological or combined factors). Instead, the descriptive text emphasizes contextual factors (e.g., culture, relationships, stressors) for all dysfunctions. The consideration of individual vulnerability, relationship, medical, and sociocultural and religious mediators is a testament to the growing, though dispersed, body of research indicating that sexuality is heavily influenced by multiple contextual factors (e.g., Bancroft, 2009). It also acknowledges the difficulty (and possible futility) in distinguishing between psychological and physical etiological factors in a literature that has found single-cause pathways elusive.

The new view of women's sexual problems had been espousing this type of multidimensional coverage for years, in reaction to mechanistic and medicalized models of human sexuality and its problems (Tiefer, 2001). The impact, however, on actual DSM-5 (American Psychiatric Association, 2013) diagnoses was not that significant. The descriptive text that mentions contextual factors appears to be little more than a reminder to clinicians to consider the multiple forces potentially acting on or affected by the sexual difficulty. Because these contextual factors are not included as specifiers in the actual diagnosis, we wonder if many clinicians will continue to ignore these factors.

THE RISE OF SEXUAL MEDICINE AND INTERDISCIPLINARITY

The multidimensionality of sexuality necessarily calls for assessment and treatment strategies that can account for all the potential dimensions at play when an individual encounters sexual difficulties. Evident though this may seem, there has been much hand-wringing over the meteoric rise of medical approaches to sexual problems. Some have argued that the latter risks making sex therapy obsolete, unless sex therapy is able to empirically demonstrate added value (Rowland, 2007). One could alternately argue that sexual medicine has increased sex therapy's relevance in light of high rates of medical treatment failures (Althof & Rosen, 2010). There are no empirical data evaluating the impact of medical approaches on sex therapy or how it is playing out. It is, however, undeniable that the PDE5 inhibitors and the use of androgens for desire and erection problems in men and desire difficulties in women have changed the treatment landscape.

On the surface, there does not appear to be a crisis, with sexuality journals flourishing and professional sexology conferences bursting at the seams. Clients who want medical solutions and for whom these solutions are deemed sufficiently effective will simply not seek out sex therapy. Some clients for whom these solutions do not work will consider sex therapy as alternative or adjuvant treatment. Others will not. It is hard to know how the numbers compare with those of the pre-sexual-medicine era. It is quite possible that the popularization of treatment for sexual dysfunction effected by the sexual-medicine juggernaut has mitigated what otherwise may have been a reduction in the number of clients who sought sex therapy for lack of any other choice.

If nothing else, the rise of sexual medicine has accelerated the movement of sex therapy toward interdisciplinarity, and that is a roundly positive development from a patient care perspective. The expansion of treatment options puts appropriate pressure on the sex therapy enterprise to demonstrate effectiveness and on sex therapists to expand their knowledge base so that they can collaborate with other health professionals.

As the preceding chapters have shown, combination treatments for erectile dysfunction (ED) and PE are state of the art. The treatment for the sexual pain disorders now calls for the involvement of physical therapists, as well as gynecologists and, possibly, dermatologists. Curiously, these interdisciplinary approaches are relatively new to the treatment of sexual problems. Sex therapy has lagged well behind the treatment of other psychological difficulties (e.g., depression, anxiety), which have involved combination therapy for decades (Althof & Rosen, 2010). The delay may be in part explained by the faux simplicity of early models of the sexual response or, alternately, by the historic reticence of nonpsychological fields to consider sexual function as an integral part of health. Regardless, all relevant disciplines are relatively new to the interdisciplinary treatment of sexual problems, and there is much to learn about how to do it well. The most important guideline may be that the multiple disciplines coming to bear on a problem do so concurrently. The theory behind combination therapy posits that the best outcome is likely to occur when treatments are concurrently rather than sequentially administered, allowing for a positive interaction of the different strategies. For example, the PDE5 may provide the physical trigger that encourages the client to entertain and address, through sex therapy, the psychological and relationship factors that in turn facilitate or even make possible the erectile function. Without the PDE5 facilitated erection, the client might have had little patience for what felt like indirect psychological and couple interventions. Without the psychological and couple work, the erection may have been beside the point, even if attained. Such an approach is best described as "interdisciplinary," rather than "multidisciplinary" as it concurrently capitalizes on the contributions of multiple disciplines. One of the burdens of interdisciplinarity is the expansion of our knowledge base to include a working, if not in-depth, familiarity with the expertise of our health care coproviders and vice versa. Another is the investment of time needed to coordinate and integrate client care. These are not insignificant concerns, and they require a commitment to the interdisciplinary model and a willingness to share in both the success and the failure of our outcomes. Theory and research, however, increasingly point to interdisciplinary treatment of sexual problems as the appropriate and expected standard of care.

RECONCEPTUALIZING TREATMENT OUTCOME

A research and theoretical literature questioning definitions of sexual function and dysfunction and its constructs, their generalizability, and the extent to which they are sociopolitically determined is inevitably going to raise questions about appropriate treatment outcome variables. If we are not sure what the sexual problem is or whether there is even a sexual problem, it can be questionable to speak categorically about solutions. Some cases are clear: A woman presents with dyspareunia or a man presents with PE and both are incapable of having desired intercourse. A reduction in her pain or its resolution and the extension of his ejaculation latency would be evidently reasonable goals. Other instances are trickier. Is the goal of sex therapy to increase a woman's supposed low desire? Why not decrease her husband's higher desire?

The point here is that either in cases of clear dysfunction (e.g., pain) or in cases of questionable dysfunction (e.g., desire discrepancy), sometimes we do succeed in improving "function," and sometimes we do not because improvement is outside the reach of available treatments (e.g., some cases of provoked vestibulodynia; normal differences in sexual drive). What we can always target, however, is the individual's and couple's level of adjustment to circumstances and the ways in which they process their problem and their relationship dynamics.

On some level, the ultimate goal of sex therapy is increasing sexual satisfaction. Although sexual satisfaction and sexual function are positively correlated, some studies with women have found the association to be less than hardy (Ferenidou et al, 2008). Dundon and Rellini (2010) found that psychological well-being and relationship adjustment were strong predictors of sexual satisfaction over and above sexual function. Rosen and Bachmann (2008) have gone as far as to deemphasize function in a conceptual paradigm that focuses on the relationship of sexual satisfaction to overall health and happiness.

The current focus on sexual satisfaction is also emerging in discussions about eroticism and the meanings attached to sexuality on the part of both researchers and clinicians. The work of Kleinplatz and colleagues (2009) on "optimal sexuality" is decidedly free of references to "function," and her respondents describing great sex are more likely to speak of "transcendence" than lubrication. Sexual function may even be a problem, as she proclaims that "Nothing kills desire more than doing what works—relentlessly" (Kleinplatz, 2006, p. 345). Leonore Tiefer (2009) bemoans our abandonment of the art of sex for its mechanics. Esther Perel (2006) privileges eroticism over function when discussing the sexual problems of long-term relationships with floundering sex lives. It is noteworthy that the eroticism that these authors allude to was actually present in early sex therapy interventions, such as sensate focus, that sought to deemphasize function and focus on sensuality. Perhaps we have come full circle, or perhaps those early interventions inadvertently stifled eroticism with their directives and homework exercises.

LACK OF SEX THERAPY OUTCOME RESEARCH

As most of the chapters in this volume attest, there is a troubling lack of sex therapy outcome research. A review of the randomized controlled trials of the past 15 years reveals an impressive number of studies investigating the impact of pharmacological agents on sexual function, a much smaller number comparing pharmacological or other nonpsychological interventions with sex therapy, and a handful focusing exclusively on some version of sex therapy or combination therapies. The current reasons for this are relatively clear. Pharmacological interventions are far easier to administer and likely to be funded by an industry interested in promoting the use of its products. In contrast, there is no organized profit motive for sex therapy research. Nonindustry funding for sexuality research continues to be minimal. It is simply not a priority area for governmental funding (at least in the United States). This, however, does not explain why, in the heyday of sex therapy and ample U.S. federal funding, such research was not carried out. Perhaps sex therapists believed their own rhetoric about simple and easy cures. On the other hand, there does appear to be significant and recent therapy outcome research mostly outside the United States, at least with respect to the sexual pain disorders (e.g., van Lankveld et al., 2006; Masheb, Kerns, Lozano, Minkin, & Richman, 2009; Bergeron et al., 2001; ter Kuile et al., 2009).

The complexity of psychological interventions for sexual problems may, however, also pose a significant challenge to the identification of effective interventions. Generally, sex therapy includes cognitive reframing, emotional regulation, stimulus control techniques, and relationship skill building. Researchers interested in isolating active ingredients are hard-pressed to parse these treatments, and replication invariably requires manualization. However, these challenges are no different from those encountered by treatment outcome researchers for any number of psychological disturbances.

Importantly, the proliferation of pharmacological studies has had some benefits outside of the testing of its agents. It has spawned the development and standardization of numerous self-administered measures that are now widely used both in research and clinical practice. Outcomes in these studies have also been expanded from mere function to satisfaction and well-being. All of this speaks well of the impact of sex therapists on the development and investigation of pharmacological agents, but is it enough? Sex therapy is likely to remain on the sidelines if it does not reenter the randomized clinical outcome study arena.

It is possible that, even without outcome data, sex therapy will survive as long as people continue to seek help in figuring out their sexual problems and dilemmas; as long as people find it gratifying and useful to consult with smart, caring people about issues they cannot share with anyone else. In terms of psychotherapy, surveys show that client satisfaction with general psychotherapy often outstrips its demonstrated efficacy in symptom reduction (Lunnen, Ogles, & Pappas, 2008). If this is also true of sex therapy, it may reflect a failure of outcome research to effectively measure psychotherapeutic change or to adequately measure sexual satisfaction over and above sexual performance. This is potentially easily remediable, given the development of several psychometrically promising inventories to measure sexual satisfaction (Byers, 2005; Meston & Trapnell, 2005).

INABILITY OF SEX THERAPY TO ARTICULATE
ITS UNIQUE CONTRIBUTION

In 2009, two of us (Binik & Meana, 2009) wrote a target article in the *Archives of Sexual Behavior* about the future of sex therapy. Within that article, we argued that sex therapy might have overstated its claim to specialization, with the attendant consequences of (1) inhibiting general psychologists from engaging in the treatment of sexual problems, which happen to be more prevalent than depression or anxiety, and (2) marginalizing sex therapy to the extent that it is not included in anthologies of types of psychological treatments. We also questioned its claim to uniqueness given its use of interventions (e.g., CBT, stimulus control, communication skills) common to the treatment of myriad other difficulties, not to mention their undifferentiated use across all dysfunctions.

If, in fact, sex therapy has a unique contribution to make, it has to date failed to articulate it as well as it could. The commentaries on our target article and our consequent self-reflection have led us to conclude that the unique contribution of sex therapy may be the willingness to talk about sex with clients. On the surface, this may sound simplistic, but the general societal discomfort with sexuality appears to pervade the health professions, including psychology. It has been consistently documented that medical doctors fail to ask questions about sexual health during history taking and routine check ups and that patients are reticent to raise the issue if doctors do not (Moreira, Glasser, & Gingell, 2005; Moreira, Glasser, Nicolosi, Duarte, & Gingell, 2008). Although no such data are available on general psychologists, the lack of sexuality training in clinical psychology programs would indicate that the discomfort in all likelihood extends to them as well (Miller & Byers, 2010). It is common for even couple therapists to refer clients out to sex therapists when sexual issues come to the fore.

Perhaps the unique contribution of sex therapy extends beyond comfort with discussing sexual concerns. Perhaps sex therapy stands out as the ultimate integrative and interdisciplinary psychological intervention with tendrils into more disciplines than other mental health areas. With physical therapy, urology, gynecology, dermatology, and endocrinology as common collaborators, sex therapy could position itself at the vanguard of interdisciplinary treatment. It has yet to do so. The ongoing failure to properly articulate what sex therapy does and how it does it could result in a true marginalization of a practice with much to offer for very mainstream problems.

DEFENSIVENESS AND FRAGMENTATION

Although sex therapists understandably rail against reductive and overmedicalized approaches to the treatment of sexual problems, we need to ensure that such criticisms emanate from evidence-based clinical concerns rather than from a defensive stance against the encroachment of other disciplines. Sexual medicine has as much to offer as does sex therapy. The benefits of interdisciplinarity notwithstanding, some cases will not require sex therapy at all. In some men with uncomplicated erectile difficulties, a PDE5 inhibitor will be all that is needed. In some women whose desire has tanked with menopause, low-dose androgen therapy may restore desire levels to their satisfaction as well as that of their partners. There may be nothing to talk about or to process. The principle of interdisciplinarity does not imply that all potentially relevant disciplines will in fact be needed in any given case. It is their consideration that is imperative, just in case.

Undoubtedly, sexual medicine and sex therapy have different orientations, which may sometimes complement each other but at other times clash. Sexual medicine is based upon a disease model and aims to "cure" or ameliorate the effects of said disease. Sex therapy has always considered the enhancement of sexual pleasure as a worthwhile treatment goal. When these two different approaches zero in on the same sexual problem, there may be contention. Nowhere has this been more evident than in the treatment of low sexual desire in women. The standard applied by the Food and Drug Administration (FDA) envisions sexual function, but not sexual pleasure, as a health issue. In fact, the virulent debate that occurred during the FDA hearings regarding Flibanserin (a drug proposed for the treatment of low desire in women) was characterized by one side insisting that low desire in women is a disease worthy of treatment and the other side decrying the "disease mongering" attitude of "big pharma." In an eloquent post on a sex therapy listserv, Margaret Nichols (2010) suggested: "perhaps we could reconcile these positions by taking a different stance about drug use, and admit that people, more and more, will want medications for 'enhancement' purposes, much like surgery for cosmetic purposes. . . . If we could even discuss the merits of medications/'good drugs' used for enhancement, we might be able to give up the pretense that, for example, the desire to increase sexual desire has to be a 'disease.'"

In other words, if we do not chastise sex therapy for dealing in the enhancement of people's sex lives (disordered or not), why should we chastise sexual medicine for its version of the same endeavor? The problem remains that, although sexual medicine physicians indeed prescribe "off label" medications for improved sexual pleasure, the discipline has remained mum on the subject of pleasure. Perhaps this will not always be the case, and sex therapy and sexual medicine will be able to join forces to improve the sexual lives of men and women without first diagnosing them with a disease. For the moment, the "better loving through chemistry" niche is occupied by herbal and holistic remedies that have yet to undergo the scrutiny of randomized controlled clinical trials.

Another potential threat to the progress of those of us interested in the interdisciplinary treatment of sexual problems is the fragmentation of sexology and sexual medicine into professional factions that inevitably compete with each other. Despite the fact that health professionals interested in the treatment of sexual problems remain few in number, comparatively speaking, our efforts are divided into numerous professional societies, each vying for members and conference attendees and each appealing to different types of sex researchers and therapists. Within North America there is the Society for Sex Therapy and Research (SSTAR), the Society for the Scientific Study of Sex (SSSS), the Canadian Sex Research Forum (CSRF), the American Society of Sexuality Educators, Counselors and Therapists (ASSECT), the International Academy of Sex Research (IASR), the International Society for the Study of Women's Sexual Health (ISSWSH), and the Society for Sexual Medicine (SSM). It is questionable whether this type of fragmentation serves our discipline or splinters and disempowers it. Although some of these groups strive for multidisciplinarity in their membership, the extent to which they promote one vision (sexual health, medicine, therapy) over another does not speak to the interdisciplinary unification that the literature seems to be calling for.

As a group, sex therapists have not systematically attempted to set standards for interdisciplinary treatment. Even when definitive treatments are lacking, other groups have organized consensus conferences in an attempt to instruct and guide the field. It is time for sex therapists to do the same through existing journals, professional groups, and conferences. Imagine the effect if representatives from all the professional groups just listed sat down and developed a set of standards for the assessment and treatment of DSM-5 (American Psychiatric Association, 2013) defined sexual dysfunctions.

The certification of sex therapists may also be working against the principles of interdisciplinarity. Most licensing for the health professions is general in nature and occurs at the state and provincial levels. Individual practitioners can then decide to claim areas of particular competence based on their training and experience. We do not *certify* individuals as being depression or anxiety specialists, as the treatment of these disorders is expected of the general mental health practitioner. Considering that most sexual dysfunctions are more prevalent than depression or anxiety disorders, it is hard to rationalize special certification for the treatment of sexual difficulties. More important, the insistence on certification is likely to dissuade many other health care providers from assisting their clients with sexual problems, when in fact the treatment of sexual problems draws liberally from the arsenal of general psychotherapy interventions (Binik & Meana, 2009). These attempts at formalizing specialization, although possibly driven by concerns over quality control, may in the end only serve to marginalize sex therapy and restrict the help available to clients.

POLEMIC/POLITICAL/DISCIPLINARY DEBATES

Discussions of sexual dysfunction, especially in regard to women, have become highly politicized and emotionally charged. This was most evident in the debates during the DSM-5 (American Psychiatric Association, 2013) development process concerning the proposal to collapse desire and arousal problems in women into one diagnostic category. The reason that the arguments became heated is clear. The construct of desire is sociopolitically loaded, as we have yet to tease apart gendered social constructions about its experience and expression and its more essential characteristics. Perhaps we never will. Perhaps these debates about distinguishing what clients want from what we think they might want, given different social and power structures, are ultimately of little immediate clinical relevance. How likely is it that an individual requesting treatment for what he or she considers a problem, regardless of its sociopolitical framing, will be interested in or helped by these debates? It is hard to know.

The situation can be further complicated by different disciplines being exposed to and "seeing" the same supposed disorder in markedly different ways. For example, the sex therapist who sees a heterosexual couple presenting with distress over the woman's comparatively low desire level may hear a set of circumstances quite divergent from that of the gynecologist who sees a woman reporting low desire in the context of a routine checkup. Furthermore, each discipline will be biased toward the consideration of etiologies in which they have the greater expertise and for which their specific help is sought. The loss of the female sexual arousal disorder in DSM-5 (American Psychiatric Association, 2013) as a stand-alone dysfunction may seem of little consequence to sex therapists who rarely see arousal problems decoupled from desire ones. On the other hand, this change may seem incomprehensible to gynecologists who are consulted more often by women who suffer exclusively from physical arousal problems.

Once entrenched, interdisciplinarity in the treatment of sexual dysfunctions should moderate these disagreements, with outcome research focusing on the effectiveness of interactions. The natural tension among disciplines is precisely why interdisciplinary treatment is likely to be more effective than a unidisciplinary approach. The key, however, will be the extent to which the relevant disciplines can come together as a team, with the optimization of client care as the primary goal.

PUBLIC DEMAND FOR EASY SOLUTIONS

If the exaggerated claims of early sex therapy primed the public for easy solutions, the advent and widespread promotion of pharmacotherapies may have come perilously close to cementing that expectation. It is an expectation that can only frustrate both clients and their health care providers, as the empirical literature and clinician reports consistently indicate that easy solutions are few and far between. Sex therapy outcome research remains scarce and boasts moderate success. The outcome research on pharmacotherapies is actually quite impressive in comparison, but it also suggests that drugs fail to be a panacea for many patients. In the case of the PDE5 inhibitors, research has shown that they are not efficacious in 30% of men with ED and that many others discontinue treatment even when the drug significantly improves erectile function (Althof & Rosen, 2010).

As disciplines reach the realization that the treatment of sexual difficulties is a complex endeavor and that we need each other to succeed, we must communicate effectively with clients so as to dispel damaging myths. Aligning the expectations of our clients with reality, while maintaining hope, will be crucial to client care. It is essential to distinguish actual treatment failure from negative outcomes that arise out of client impatience and/or misunderstanding about the full nature of the problem. It is undeniable that in our consumer culture, this effort will be up against the formidable foe of industry advertising efforts that promise quick solutions. Our interdisciplinary story is harder to tell and to sell.

ACCESS TO AND COST
OF INTERDISCIPLINARY TREATMENT

Perhaps the biggest threats to the transition that sex therapy is attempting to make into interdisciplinarity are cost and access to services. Teams of health care providers specializing in the treatment of sexual problems are likely to be mostly confined to large urban centers. Even within these, sex therapists are not very numerous. This makes it likely that the interdisciplinary approach will remain an ideal outside of the reach of many clients. Furthermore, in countries in which both medical care and sex therapy are costly, the majority of individuals may not be able to afford the kind of interdisciplinary care we believe to be optimal.

Although at first hand it may seem as if this problem is outside the power of sex therapy to address, the Internet may provide partial solutions to the problems of access and cost. It was clear 20 years ago that technology (Binik, Meana, & Sand, 1994) could provide help where services were not available. Research into interactive Internet-delivered sex therapy is growing and showing promising results (Jones & McCabe, 2011). There are likely other types of applications yet to be investigated that may be able to fill some of the holes in the interdisciplinary net. This will require that sex therapists and their collaborators collectively think about ways to deliver services that at first may appear unusual or even counterintuitive. Innovation in health care delivery is a concern across health areas (Hwang & Christensen, 2008). It may be a speeding train that sex therapy cannot afford to miss.

CONCLUSIONS

The tongue-in-cheek title of this chapter implied a number of possibilities: that sex therapy may be stuck; that there is impatience with our progress; that we appear to be in a constant state of transition. We think that there is some truth to all of these.

At times, sex therapy has appeared to be stuck. With hardly any outcome data to support our claims to relevance, some have wondered whether we could end up becoming obsolete (Rowland, 2007). There is little doubt that sex therapy is being outresearched by pharmacology. The reasons for that are not hard to invoke (e.g., industry funding and ease of delivery), but the reasons do not change the fact. Two of us (Binik & Meana, 2009) have bemoaned sex therapy's claim to specialization and wondered whether this turf entrenchment has resulted in less rather than more progress. Sexuality is barely covered in general psychology graduate programs and has all but disappeared from medical training. These are not heartening developments.

On the other hand, documented concerns about sexual dysfunction and its treatment date back to the earliest written records in history. Currently, sexuality and its problems are covered by the media at unprecedented levels, and the public's thirst for knowledge about sex seems insatiable. There are numerous publications about the adaptation of sex therapy to non-Western cultures and groups (Hall & Graham, 2012; So & Cheung, 2005). North American-based sexuality journals are receiving a large number of foreign submissions, even from countries in which issues of sexuality have been traditionally suppressed. All of this bodes well for our discipline, at least in terms of demand.

Sex therapists and researchers, however, need to remain impatient with their progress, as this impatience may be central to momentum. A perpetual state of agitated, outward-reaching transition may be exactly where we need to be to ensure that we do not recede into the shadows of insularity and marginalization. The relatively dramatic changes in DSM-5 (American Psychiatric Association, 2013) speak to a lively research effort in the past 20 years, although one woefully short on treatment outcome. With a lack of field trials to test the new, proposed categories, we are assured of continuing controversy and more changes in the sixth edition.

We are definitely not *there* yet, but there is likely no *there*, no bacteria or virus to target. The treatment of sexual dysfunctions is no different from the treatment of any disorder with a diagnostic category in the DSM. It involves whole individuals with complex lives and histories, and it targets perhaps the most socioculturally loaded of human experiences; sexuality. May the state of transition never ease up. May we never think we have arrived.

REFERENCES

Althof, S. E., & Rosen, R. C. (2010). Combining medical and psychological interventions for the treatment of erectile dysfunction. In S. B. Levine (Ed.), *Handbook of clinical sexuality for mental health professionals* (2nd ed., pp. 251–266). New York: Routledge/Taylor & Francis.

American Psychiatric Association. (1994). *Diagnostic and statistical manual of mental disorders* (4th ed.). Washington, DC: Author.

American Psychiatric Association. (2000). *Diagnostic and statistical manual of mental disorders* (4th ed., text rev.). Washington, DC: Author.

American Psychiatric Association. (2013). *Diagnostic and statistical manual of mental disorders* (5th ed.). Arlington, VA: Author.

Bancroft, J. (2009). *Human sexuality and its problems* (3rd ed.). London: Elsevier.

Basson, R. (2007). Sexual desire/arousal disorders in women. In S. R. Leiblum (Ed.), *Principles and practice of sex therapy* (4th ed., pp. 25–53). New York: Guilford Press.

Bergeron, S., Binik, Y. M., Khalife, S., Pagidas, K., Glazer, H. I., Meana, M., et al. (2001). A randomized comparison of group cognitive-behavioral therapy, surface electromyographic biofeedback, and vestibulectomy in the treatment of dyspareunia resulting from vulvar vestibulitis. *Pain, 91*(3), 297–306.

Binik, Y. M., & Meana, M. (2009). The future of sex therapy: Specialization or marginalization? *Archives of Sexual Behavior, 38*(6), 1016–1027.

Binik, Y. M., Meana, M., Berkley, K., & Khalifé, S. (1999). The sexual pain disorders: Is the pain sexual or the sex painful? *Annual Review of Sex Research, 10*, 210–235.

Binik, Y. M., Meana, M., & Sand, N. (1994) Interaction with a sex-expert system changes attitudes and may modify sexual behavior. *Computers in Human Behavior, 10*, 1–16.

Both, S., Everaerd, W., & Laan, E. (2007). Desire emerges from excitement: A psychophysiological perspective on sexual motivation. In E. Janssen (Ed.), *The psychophysiology of sex* (pp. 327–339). Bloomington: Indiana University Press.

Brotto, L. A., Heiman, J. R., & Tolman, D. (2009). Narratives of desire in mid-age women with and without arousal difficulties. *Journal of Sex Research, 46*, 387–398.

Byers, E. S. (2005). Relationship satisfaction and sexual satisfaction: A longitudinal study of individuals in long-term relationships. *Journal of Sex Research, 42*(2), 113–118.

Derogatis, L. R., Clayton, A. H., Rosen, R. C., Sand, M., & Pyke, R. E. (2011). Should sexual desire and arousal disorders in women be merged? [Comment/Reply]. *Archives of Sexual Behavior, 40*, 217–219.

Dundon, C. M., & Rellini, A. H. (2010). More than sexual function: Predictors of sexual satisfaction in a sample of women age 40–70. *Journal of Sexual Medicine, 7*, 896–904.

Ferenidou, F., Kapoteli, V., Moisidis, K., Koutsogiannis, I., Giakoumelos, A., & Hatzichristou, D. (2008). Presence of a sexual problem may not affect women's satisfaction from their sexual function. *Journal of Sexual Medicine, 5*, 631–639.

Graham, C. A., Sanders, S. A., Milhausen, R. R., & McBride, K. R. (2004). Turning on and turning off: A focus group study of the factors that affect women's sexual arousal. *Archives of Sexual Behavior, 33*, 527–538.

Hall, K. S., & Graham, C. A. (Eds.). (2012). *The cultural context of sexual pleasure and problems: Psychotherapy with diverse clients*. New York: Routledge.

Hwang, J., & Christensen, C. M. (2008). Disruptive innovation in health care delivery: A framework for business-model innovation. *Health Affairs, 27*(5), 1329–1335.

Janssen, E., McBride, K. R., Yarber, W., Hill, B. J., & Butler, S. M. (2008). Factors that influence sexual arousal in men: A focus group study. *Archives of Sexual Behavior, 37*(2), 252–265.

Jones, L. M., & McCabe, M. P. (2011). The effectiveness of an Internet-based psychological treatment program for female sexual dysfunction. *Journal of Sexual Medicine, 8,* 2781–2792.

Kaplan, H. S. (1977). Hypoactive sexual desire. *Journal of Sex and Marital Therapy, 3,* 3–9.

Kleinplatz, P. J. (2003). What's new in sex therapy?: From stagnation to fragmentation. *Sexual and Relationship Therapy, 18,* 95–106.

Kleinplatz, P. J. (2006). Learning from extraordinary lovers: Lessons from the edge. *Journal of Homosexuality, 50*(2–3), 325–348.

Kleinplatz, P. J., Menard, A. D., Paquet, M.-P., Paradis, N. C., Zuccarino, D., & Mehak, L. (2009). The components of optimal sexuality: A portrait of great sex. *Canadian Journal of Human Sexuality, 18,* 1–13.

Leiblum, S. R., & Pervin, L. A. (Eds.). (1980). *Principles and practice of sex therapy.* New York: Guilford Press.

Levin, R. J. (2004) An orgasm is . . . who defines what orgasm is? *Sexual and Relationship Therapy, 19,* 101–107.

Lief, H. I. (1977). Inhibited sexual desire. *Medical Aspects of Human Sexuality, 7,* 94–95.

Lunnen, K. M., Ogles, B. M., & Pappas, L. N. (2008). A multiperspective comparison of satisfaction, symptomatic change, perceived change, and end-point functioning. *Professional Psychology: Research and Practice, 39,* 145–152.

Mah, K., & Binik, Y. M. (2001). The nature of human orgasm: A critical review of major trends. *Clinical Psychology Review, 21*(6), 823–856.

Masheb, R. M., Kerns, R. D., Lozano, C., Minkin, M. J., & Richman, S. (2009). A randomized clinical trial for women with vulvodynia: Cognitive-behavioral therapy vs. supportive psychotherapy. *Pain, 141,* 31–40.

Masters, J., & Johnson, V. (1966). *Human sexual response.* Boston: Little, Brown.

Meana, M. (2010). Elucidating women's (hetero)sexual desire: Definitional challenges and content expansion. *Journal of Sex Research, 47,* 104–122.

Meston, C., & Trapnell, P. (2005). Development and validation of a five-factor sexual satisfaction and distress scale for women: The Sexual Satisfaction Scale for Women (SSS-W). *Journal of Sexual Medicine, 2*(1), 66.

Miller, S. A., & Byers, E. S. (2010). Psychologists' sexual education and training in graduate school. *Canadian Journal of Behavioural Science, 42*(2), 93–100.

Moreira, E. D., Glasser, D. B., & Gingell, C. (2005). Sexual activity, sexual dysfunction and associated help-seeking behaviours in middle-aged and older adults in Spain: A population survey. *World Journal of Urology, 23,* 422–429.

Moreira, E. D., Glasser, D. B., Nicolosi, A., Duarte, F. G., & Gingell, C. (2008). Sexual problems and help-seeking behaviour in adults in the United Kingdom and continental Europe. *British Journal of Urology International, 101,* 1005–1011.

Nichols, M. (2010, June 17). Push to market pill stirs debate on sexual desire. Message posted to *sstargaze-maurice@interchange.ubc.ca.*

Perel, E. (2006). *Mating in captivity: Reconciling the erotic + the domestic.* New York: HarperCollins.

Rosen, R. C., & Bachmann, G. A. (2008). Sexual well-being, happiness, and satisfaction in women: The case for a new conceptual paradigm. *Journal of Sex and Marital Therapy, 34,* 291–297.

Rowland, D. L. (2007). Will medical solutions to sexual problems make sexological care and science obsolete? *Journal of Sex and Marital Therapy, 33,* 385–397.

Sand, M., & Fisher, W. A. (2007). Women's endorsement of models of female sexual response: The nurses' sexuality study. *Journal of Sexual Medicine, 4*(3), 708–719.

So, H. W., & Cheung, F. M. (2005). Review of Chinese sex attitudes and applicability of sex therapy for Chinese couples with sexual dysfunction. *Journal of Sex Research, 42*, 93–101.

ter Kuile, M. M., Bulte, I., Weijenborg, P. T. M., Beekman, A., Melles, R., & Onghena, P. (2009). Therapist-aided exposure for women with lifelong vaginismus: A replicated single-case design. *Journal of Consulting and Clinical Psychology, 77*(1), 149–159.

Tiefer, L. (2001). Arriving at a "new view" of women's sexual problems: Background, theory and activism. *Women and Therapy, 24*, 63–98.

Tiefer, L. (2009). *The marketing of female sexual dysfunction: Illuminating current issues in sex and public health.* Retrieved April 15, 2009, from *www.fsd-alert.org.*

van Lankveld, J. J., ter Kuile, M. M., de Groot, H. E., Melles, R., Nefs, J., & Zandbergen, M. (2006). Cognitive-behavioral therapy for women with lifelong vaginismus: A randomized waiting-list controlled trial of efficacy. *Journal of Consulting and Clinical Psychology, 74*(1), 168–178.

Index

The letter *f* following a page number indicates figure; the letter *t* indicates table.